Gottfried O.H. Naumann, Leonard M. Holbach, Friedrich E. Kruse (Eds.)
Applied Pathology for Ophthalmic Microsurgeons

G.O.H. Naumann, L.M. Holbach, F.E. Kruse (Eds.)

Additional main authors: Claus Cursiefen, Ludwig M. Heindl,
Antonia M. Joussen, Anselm Jünemann, Christian Y. Mardin,
and Ursula Schlötzer-Schrehardt

Applied Pathology for Ophthalmic Microsurgeons

With 317 figures in 1063 parts mostly in color and 108 tables

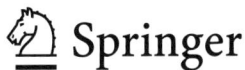

GOTTFRIED O.H. NAUMANN, PROF. (EMER.) DR. MED. DR. HC. (MULT.)
Department of Ophthalmology, University of Erlangen-Nürnberg
Schwabachanlage 6, D-91054 Erlangen, Germany

LEONARD M. HOLBACH, PROF. DR. MED.
Department of Ophthalmology, University of Erlangen-Nürnberg
Schwabachanlage 6, D-91054 Erlangen, Germany

FRIEDRICH E. KRUSE, PROF. DR. MED.
Department of Ophthalmology, University of Erlangen-Nürnberg
Schwabachanlage 6, D-91054 Erlangen, Germany

ISBN 978-3-540-24189-8   Springer-Verlag Berlin Heidelberg New York

Library of Congress Control Number: 2007941808

This work is subject to copyright. All rights are reserved, whether the whole or part of the material is concerned, specifically the rights of translation, reprinting, reuse of illustrations, recitation, broadcasting, reproduction on microfilm or in any other way, and storage in data banks. Duplication of this publication or parts thereof is permitted only under the provisions of the German Copyright Law of September 9, 1965, in its current version, and permission for use must always be obtained from Springer-Verlag. Violations are liable for prosecution under the German Copyright Law.

Springer is a part of Springer Science+Business Media
springer.com

© Springer-Verlag Berlin Heidelberg 2008

Printed in Germany

The use of general descriptive names, registered names, trademarks, etc. in this publication does not imply, even in the absence of a specific statement, that such names are exempt from the relevant protective laws and regulations and therefore free for general use.

Product liability: The publishers cannot guarantee the accuracy of any information about the application of operative techniques and medications contained in this book. In every individual case the user must check such information by consulting the relevant literature.

Editor: Marion Philipp, Heidelberg
Desk Editor: Martina Himberger, Heidelberg
Copy-editing: WS Editorial Ltd, Shrewsbury, UK
Illustrations: Jörg Kühn, Heidelberg
Production Editor: Joachim W. Schmidt, Munich

Cover design: eStudio Calamar, Spain

Typesetting: FotoSatz Pfeifer GmbH, Gräfelfing
Printed on acid-free paper – 24/3150 – 5 4 3 2 1 0

To competent and compassionate ophthalmic microsurgeons committed to the preservation and restoration of sight – everywhere

Preface

Interaction of Pathology and Ophthalmic Microsurgery

Ophthalmic pathology means the study of the symptoms and morphologic signs of diseases of the eye and ocular adnexae both biomicroscopically and in the laboratory. Precise definition of the phenotype is a prerequisite for correlation to the genotype, helping to design clinical studies. Spectacular progress is considered a hallmark of both conservative medicine and surgery today. This is driven by the application of both the methods of molecular biology and the new approaches in biotechnology.

Microsurgical magnification and miniaturization of instruments and non-mechanical tools, e.g., lasers, have made possible procedures beyond our imagination a few years ago. They are characterized by small-access wounds into the eye and only minimal threshold trauma beyond the targeted intraocular tissue. In view of all the glittering advances of biotechnology, the details of critical anatomy morphology are too often neglected or forgotten although they are essential for the success of our microsurgical manipulations.

This book is intended for ophthalmologists in training and also for mature eye physicians. Hopefully, this should help them to avoid pre-, intra- and postoperative complications and make them more alert to explaining the risks to their patients before surgery. It attempts to remind the ophthalmic microsurgeon that knowledge of the minutiae of structures is a prerequisite to achieving the intended outcome. Microsurgical landmarks need to be defined more precisely than in conventional ophthalmic surgery without microscopic magnification. Awareness of the specific pathology is crucial for the appropriate indications and suitability of instrumentation to overcome the specific tissue resistance.

Finally, while biotechnology is always changing, the morphologic elements of the eye and ocular adnexae in health and disease remain essentially the same. However, wound healing, scars and complications are also modified by new microsurgical approaches.

Our intention is not to compile a complete list of references but instead to give the reader a selection of textbooks and review articles that may be helpful for further study.

We have not concentrated on the details of instrumentation and surgical techniques. Both are developing continuously. As an exception the reader is referred to sections on non-mechanical trephination penetrating keratoplasty with the excimer laser along metal masks and direct surgery of the ciliary body (see Chapters 5.1 and 5.4).

Clinical findings including imaging by biomicroscopy, "biocytology", ultrasound, OCT, CT, MRI etc. of the phenotype – supported by knowledge of the "third dimension" supplied by ophthalmic pathology – therefore are essential for patient care. They present in vivo *and* in the laboratory the foundation for solving diagnostic and therapeutic challenges for the clinician and microsurgeon: *Ophthalmic pathology is also a clinical subspecialty*.

We want to emphasize that demanding and complex "*ophthalmic microsurgery is applied ophthalmic pathology.*" This is particularly true if intra- or postoperative complications need to be corrected or minimized.

Therefore we have tried to do the following:

1. Alert the ophthalmic microsurgeon to the *critical surgical anatomy and pathology, landmarks* and *potential complications before* he or she plans and starts to discuss the indications with the patient and then the procedure itself.
2. Emphasize *respect for the structure of the eye and ocular adnexae* and point out the *most vulnerable cell populations* in the various microsurgical interventions.
3. Point out the peculiar and *unique features of intraocular microsurgery* in the "*closed* system" and "*open* eye," focusing on acute ocular hypotony-paracentesis effects and the influence on *blood-ocular barriers*.
4. Illustrate the consequences of the *movement of the iris-lens diaphragm* ("vis a tergo") in relation to the systemic arterial pressure in the open eye; also the significance of maintaining or *restoring the anterior chamber at the end of all intraocular procedures involving the anterior segment*.
5. Show how knowledge of the *specific pathology modifies* microsurgical interventions. We mention here only a few examples and refer the reader to the relevant chapters.
   - *Loss of Bowman's layer – focal or diffuse* – recognized before corneal incisions or grafting makes a surplus of interrupted sutures advisable: because suture loosening is more likely. Running sutures can then be particularly annoying, because if one loop becomes loose the entire suture and wound will be unstable. Single loose interrupted sutures can be easily removed at the slit lamp – the architecture of the wound beyond one loose suture is usually not endangered.
   - Calcifications within Bowman's layer in band degeneration of the cornea can usually be chemically dissolved and do not justify sacrifice of this structure, e.g., by excimer laser.
   - *Limbal stem cell insufficiency* alerts one to serious ocular surface problems.
   - Avascular corneal lesions after herpes corneae may more likely harbor *herpes simplex-virus in the stroma, which may lead to recurrence* after keratoplasty. In contrast vascularized herpetic scars indicate an increased risk for postoperative immune reactions following corneal transplantation.
   - *Granulomatous reaction against Descemet's membrane* in herpes corneae leads to defects and signals imminent corneal perforation. This may be an argument for urgent curative perforating keratoplasty.
   - Tumors of the "iris root" de facto involve the anterior face of the ciliary body and need to be treated by block excision of iris *and* ciliary body.
   - Cystic and diffuse *epithelial ingrowth* into the anterior chamber usually reach the angle and cover the anterior surface of the ciliary body. Therefore "block excisions" are necessary including removal of the adjacent pars plicata of the ciliary body, iris, cornea and sclera – acting as a "shell." Only small epithelial implantations in the central iris region can be cured by iridectomy if the angle is not involved.
   - Fibrous pseudo-metaplasia of the anterior subcapsular lens epithelium results in mechanical properties such as sclera; it may divert the standard capsulorrhexis around the anterior subcapsular cataract.
   - *Pseudoexfoliation syndrome* (PEX) is a generalized disease of the extracellular matrix. It affects *all tissues of the anterior segment of the eye*. Although common, it may very often be overlooked and may manifest asymmetrically but in fact is always present bilaterally. It is not a harmless anomaly but a disease leading in its advanced stages to potentially catastrophic complications.
   We need to consider not only the risk of *secondary open angle* and *angle closure glaucomas*, but also the *zonular instability, blood-aqueous barrier breakdown*, anterior segment *hypoxia, poor mydriasis*, and *reduced mobility of the iris*. The vulnerability of the directly involved corneal endothelium contributes to the increased risk of corneal decompensation. To miss the diagnosis of PEX or disregard it may imply many unpleasant surprises or "recklessly running into a trap."

- *Intraocular neovascularization* commonly develops in the end stages of many ocular and systemic diseases. Until recently medical and laser therapy attempted to eliminate angiogenic factors originating from hypoxic retina. The new capillaries did not disappear but were less recognizable because of decreased blood flow in the persisting vascular scaffold. A spectacular advance currently is evolving by new local application of specific inhibitors of vascular endothelial growth factors (VEGFs) in the therapy of these entities. The endothelial capillary sprouts can actually regress as long as a capillary basement membrane has not yet been formed.
- Defining structures ("*Leitstrukturen*") of the retina help to better interpret optical coherence tomography (OCT), retinal thickness analysis (RTA) and fluorescence angiography to outline indications for microsurgery.
- *Uveal malignant melanomas* almost always invade the sclera, although their degree often is not detectable clinically – particularly if they are unpigmented.

6. Not to forget: All cataract surgeons exert some tension on the lens capsule and thus exert *traction on the vitreous base via Wieger's ligaments* – but many are not really aware of this in their daily routine. The peripheral retina also should be inspected before and after cataract surgery.
7. Features of normal and pathologic *wound healing* ("*scar wars*") deserve attention in the various tissues following mechanical or non-mechanical (laser, cryo-, diathermia coagulation) interventions in the closed and open eye constellations.

Beyond the practical implications these pages might also encourage our colleagues to study the living eye and ocular adnexae – with a conscious knowledge of the third dimension – and with enlightened curiosity and magnified attention.

We sincerely hope that our book might be helpful in the clinical care of patients.

Erlangen, Summer 2007

Gottfried O.H. Naumann
Leonard Holbach
Friedrich E. Kruse

Acknowledgements

We would like to thank our numerous coworkers at the Departments of Ophthalmology of the Universities of Hamburg (1961–74), Tübingen (1975–80) and Erlangen (since 1980), who have made such a large contribution to this book. It is impossible to mention them all.

Our colleagues from the European Ophthalmic Pathology Society (EOPS), the Verhoeff-Zimmerman Society and the German Speaking Ophthalmic Pathologists (DOP) and many ophthalmologists from around the world were a great source of inspiration in the preparation of the book.

Frau Carmen Rummelt of the Ophthalmic Pathology Laboratory in Erlangen made expert technical contributions to the cutting and staining of specimens for the figures and helped with the digital microphotographs and SEM. The excellent work of our photographers, particularly H. Strahwald and M. Vogler in Erlangen, is evident from their clinical pictures, and Jörg Kühn, Heidelberg, created some fine graphical work by modifying sketches mainly from previous publications by the authors, unless mentioned otherwise.

Most of the schematic drawings and tables are based on drafts by the First Editor/Author, who also supplied numerous microphotographs.

We are very grateful to Frau Marion Philipp and Frau Martina Himberger, Springer-Verlag, Heidelberg, for their encouragement and tolerance with unforeseeable delays; Mr. W. Shufflebotham, who with great patience transferred our teutonic version of the manuscript into correct English; and Herr Joachim W. Schmidt, Munich, who combined the text, figures, tables and references very efficiently into the book in its present form.

Frau Iris Schmitt not only typed many of the chapters but was essential in maintaining orderly communications during the long process of preparing the text and arranging tables, figures and literature of the manuscript. Her experience in preparing books and publications since 1975 proved invaluable. Without her untiring support this book would not yet be finished.

Finally, we are very grateful for the support of our partners and families for their understanding and patience during the completion of this project.

Condensed Table of Contents

1 Introduction
G.O.H. Naumann, Friedrich E. Kruse 1

2 General Ophthalmic Pathology: Principal Indications and Complications, Comparing Intra- and Extraocular Surgery
G.O.H. Naumann, F.E. Kruse 7

3 Special Anatomy and Pathology in Surgery of the Eyelids, Lacrimal System, Orbit and Conjunctiva
L.M. Holbach 29

3.1 Eyelids
L.M. Heindl, L.M. Holbach 30

3.2 Lacrimal Drainage System
L.M. Heindl, A. Jünemann, L.M. Holbach 45

3.3 Orbit
L.M. Holbach, L.M. Heindl, R.F. Guthoff 49

3.4 Conjunctiva and Limbus Corneae
C. Cursiefen, F.E. Kruse, G.O.H. Naumann 67

4 General Pathology for Intraocular Microsurgery: Direct Wounds and Indirect Distant Effects
G.O.H. Naumann, F.E. Kruse 76

5 Special Anatomy and Pathology in Intraocular Microsurgery

5.1 Cornea and Limbus
C. Cursiefen, F.E. Kruse, G.O.H. Naumann 97

5.2 Glaucoma Surgery
A. Jünemann, G.O.H. Naumann 131

5.3 Iris
G.O.H. Naumann 152

5.4 Ciliary Body
G.O.H. Naumann 176

5.5 Lens and Zonular Fibers
U. Schlötzer-Schrehardt, G.O.H. Naumann 217

5.6 Retina and Vitreous
A.M. Joussen and G.O.H. Naumman
with Contributions by S.E. Coupland, E.R. Tamm, B. Kirchhof, N. Bornfeld ... 255

5.7 Optic Nerve and Elschnig's Scleral Ring
C.Y. Mardin, G.O.H. Naumann 335

6 Influence of Common Generalized Diseases on Intraocular Microsurgery
G.O.H. Naumann, U. Schlötzer-Schrehardt 350

6.1 Diabetes Mellitus
G.O.H. Naumann 351

6.2 Arterial Hypertension and "Vis A Tergo"
G.O.H. Naumann 353

6.3 Pseudoexfoliation Syndrome: Pathological Manifestations of Relevance to Intraocular Surgery
U. Schlötzer-Schrehardt, G.O.H. Naumann 354

6.4 Other Generalized Diseases
G.O.H. Naumann 378

6.4.1 Infectious Disorders (AIDS, Sepsis) 378

6.4.2 Hematologic Disorders 378

6.5.3 Neurologic and Muscular Diseases 378

General References 379

List of Figures 381

List of Tables 387

Subject Index 391

Contents

1 Introduction
G.O.H. Naumann, F.E. Kruse 1
1.1   Ophthalmic Pathology in Clinical Practice, Teaching and Research 1
1.1.1 Confirmation and Quality Control of Clinical Diagnoses 1
1.1.2 Modern Ophthalmomicrosurgery is Applied Ophthalmopathology 1
1.1.3 Ophthalmic Pathology is the Science of the Phenotype 1
1.1.4 Ophthalmic Pathology also Connects Experimental and Clinical
      Ophthalmology 2
1.2   Historical Sketch of Ophthalmic Surgery from Antiquity to Modern
      Times 2
1.3   Overview of Advances in Ophthalmic Pathology in the Nineteenth
      and Twentieth Centuries 4
References 6

2 General Ophthalmic Pathology: Principal Indications and Complications, Comparing Intra- and Extraocular Surgery
G.O.H. Naumann, F.E. Kruse 7
2.1   Principal Indications: Clinico-pathologic Correlation 7
2.1.1 Defects 7
2.1.2 Excess of Tissue 8
2.1.3 Altered Tissue In Situ 8
2.1.4 Displaced Tissue 8
2.1.5 Neovascularization and Scars 9

2.2   Intraocular Compared with Extraocular Surgery: Distinguishing
      Features and Potential Complications 11
2.2.1 Anterior Movement of the Iris-Lens Diaphragm ("Vis a Tergo") 13
2.2.2 Paracentesis Effect 14
2.2.3 Expulsive Choroidal Hemorrhage and Uveal Effusion 17
2.2.4 Pupillary and Ciliary Block 17
2.2.5 Purulent Endophthalmitis 18
2.2.6 Sympathetic Uveitis 19
2.2.7 Diffuse and Cystic Epithelial Ingrowth 19
2.2.8 Hemorrhage from Vasoproliferative Processes 21
2.2.9 "Toxic Anterior Segment Syndrome" (TASS) 22
2.2.10 "Intraoperative Floppy Iris Syndrome" (IFIS) 22

2.3   Choice of Anesthesia and Knowledge of Ophthalmic Pathology 24

2.4   Instrumentation and Physical Principles 26
References 27

3 Special Anatomy and Pathology in Surgery of the Eyelids, Lacrimal System, Orbit and Conjunctiva
L.M. Holbach 29

3.1 Eyelids
L.M. Heindl, L.M. Holbach 30
- 3.1.1 Surgical Anatomy 30
- 3.1.1.1 Arterial Supply 32
- 3.1.1.2 Venous Drainage 32
- 3.1.1.3 Lymphatic Drainage 32
- 3.1.1.4 Motor Nerve Supply 32
- 3.1.1.5 Sensory Nerve Supply 32

- 3.1.2 Surgical Pathology 33
- 3.1.2.1 Disorders of Eyelid: Position and Movement 33
- 3.1.2.1.1 Surgical Pathology and Anatomic Principles of Ectropion Repair 34
- 3.1.2.1.2 Surgical Pathology and Anatomic Principles of Entropion and Distichiasis Repair 37
- 3.1.2.1.3 Surgical Pathology and Anatomic Principles of Blepharoptosis Repair   39
- 3.1.2.2 Eyelid Tumors 40
- References 44

3.2 Lacrimal Drainage System
L.M. Heindl, A. Jünemann, L.M. Holbach 45
- 3.2.1 Surgical Anatomy 45
- 3.2.2 Surgical Pathology 46
- 3.2.3 Principles of Lacrimal Surgery 47
- 3.2.3.1 External Dacryocystorhinostomy (with or without Silicone Tube Intubation) 47
- 3.2.3.2 External Canaliculo-Dacryocystorhinostomy 47
- 3.2.3.3 External Dacryocystorhinostomy with Bypass Tube Insertion 48
- References 48

3.3 Orbit
L.M. Holbach, L.M. Heindl, R.F. Guthoff 49
- 3.3.1 Surgical Anatomy 49
- 3.3.2 Surgical Pathology 50
- 3.3.2.1 Orbital Tumors 50
- 3.3.2.2 Thyroid-Associated Orbitopathy – Endocrine Orbitopathy/ Ophthalmopathy – Graves' Ophthalmopathy 62

- 3.3.3 Principles of Orbital Surgery 64
- 3.3.3.1 Surgical Approaches to the Orbit in Orbital Tumor Surgery 64
- 3.3.3.1.1 Anterior Orbitotomy 64
- 3.3.3.1.2 Lateral Orbitotomy 65
- 3.3.3.2 Surgical Management in Thyroid Eye Disease 65
- 3.3.3.2.1 Orbital Decompression 65
- 3.3.3.2.2 Extraocular Muscle Surgery 65
- 3.3.3.2.3 Eyelid Surgery to Prevent Lagophthalmus 65
- 3.3.3.3 Surgical Approaches in Anophthalmic Socket Surgery 65
- 3.3.3.3.1 Enucleation with Orbital Implants 65
- 3.3.3.3.2 Evisceration 66
- 3.3.3.3.3 Exenteration 66
- References 66

3.4 Conjunctiva and Limbus Corneae
C. Cursiefen, F.E. Kruse, G.O.H. Naumann 67
- 3.4.1 Introduction 67
- 3.4.2 Surgical Anatomy, Landmarks, Nerve Supply, and Vascular Supply with Blood Vessels and Lymphatics, Including Regional Lymph Nodes and Aqueous Episcleral Veins 67
- 3.4.2.1 Limbal Stem Cells, Vogt's Palisades, Cornea Verticillata, Tear Film 69
- 3.4.2.2 Langerhans Cells in the Limbal and Corneal Epithelium 69
- 3.4.2.3 Bowman's Layer as Mechanical Barrier 69
- 3.4.2.4 Keratocyte Distribution, Reaction to Trauma 69
- 3.4.2.5 Nerve Supply of Superficial Cornea 69
- 3.4.2.6 Anatomic Landmarks for Surgical Limbus: Edge of Bowman's Layer, Schlemm's Canal, Scleral Spur 69
- 3.4.3 Surgical Pathology 69
- 3.4.3.1 Hereditary Anomalies of the Conjunctiva: Conjunctival Lymphangioma 70
- 3.4.3.2 Conjunctival Inflammations 70
- 3.4.3.3 Sarcoidosis and Conjunctival Involvement in Systemic Disease 71
- 3.4.3.4 Pterygium 72
- 3.4.3.5 Conjunctival Cysts 72
- 3.4.3.6 Conjunctival Tumors 72
- 3.4.3.6.1 Melanocytic Lesions 72
- 3.4.3.6.2 Acquired Epithelial Melanosis 72
- 3.4.3.7 Amniotic Membrane Transplantation 73
- 3.4.3.8 Limbal Stem Cell Transplantation 73
- 3.4.3.9 Dry Eye 73
- 3.4.3.10 Superior Limbal Keratitis (Theodore) 74
- 3.4.3.11 Ligneous Conjunctivitis (Conjunctivitis Lignosa) 74
- 3.4.4 Indications for Smear Cytology, Incisional or Excisional Biopsies, Autologous or Homologous Transplantation, Radiation, and Local and Systemic Chemotherapy 74
- 3.4.4.1 Conjunctival Oncology: Melanocytic Processes 75
- 3.4.4.2 Limbus Stem Cell Insufficiency 75
- 3.4.4.3 Amnion Transplantation 75
- 3.4.5 Wound Healing: Influence of Basic Disease and Adjunct Therapy (Radiation, Chemotherapy) 75

References 75

4 General Pathology for Intraocular Microsurgery: Direct Wounds and Indirect Distant Effects
G.O.H. Naumann, F.E. Kruse 76
- 4.1. **Access** into the Eye: Principal Options and Anterior Segment Trauma 76
- 4.1.1 Direct Incisions and Wounds 76
- 4.1.1.1 Transcorneal Access 76
- 4.1.1.2 Access via Corneal "Limbus," Fornix and Limbus Based Conjunctival Flaps 86
- 4.1.1.3 Pars Plana Transscleral Approaches 90
- 4.1.2 Indirect Distant Effects 90

- 4.2 Obvious and Potential **Compartments** of the Intraocular Space 90

- 4.3 **Variants** of Intraocular Microsurgery 90
- 4.3.1 Wide Open Sky Approach 90
- 4.3.2 Minimally Invasive Intraocular Microsurgery 91
- 4.3.3 Intraocular Surgery Without Opening of the Eye Wall 91

4.4	Microsurgical Manipulations in the **Anterior Chamber**: Critical Structures and Vulnerable Cell Populations	92
4.4.1	Free Access to Trabecular Meshwork in Open Angle and Free Flow in the Pupillary Zone and Between the Pars Plicata and Lens Equator	92
4.4.2	Corneal Endothelium	92
4.4.3	Iris Microanatomy	93
4.4.4	Lens Capsule and Anterior Zonular Insertion	93
4.5	Surgical Manipulation in the **Vitreous Cavity**: Critical Structures and Vulnerable Cell Populations	93
4.5.1	Vitreous Attachments	93
4.5.2	Sensory Retina, Retinal Pigment Epithelium and Optic Nerve Head	93
4.5.3	Posterior Lens Capsule and Posterior Zonula Insertion	94
4.5.4	Choroidal Hemorrhage	94
4.6	Role of the **Size of the Eye**	94
4.7	**Wound Healing** After Intraocular Microsurgery and Trauma	94
4.7.1	"Surgically Induced Necrotizing Scleritis" (SINS)	96
4.7.2	Concept of a "Minimal Eye"	96
References		96

5 Special Anatomy and Pathology in Intraocular Microsurgery

5.1 Cornea and Limbus
C. CURSIEFEN, F.E. KRUSE, G.O.H. NAUMANN 97

5.1.1	**Surgical Anatomy** of the Cornea and Limbus	97
5.1.1.1	Corneal Epithelium	97
5.1.1.2	Bowman's Layer	98
5.1.1.3	Corneal Stroma	100
5.1.1.4	Descemet's Membrane	100
5.1.1.5	Endothelial Cells	101
5.1.1.6	Limbal Vascular Arcade	101
5.1.1.7	Tear Film	102
5.1.1.8	Anterior Chamber Associated Immune Deviation (ACAID), Corneal Immune Privilege, Corneal Antiangiogenic Privilege	105
5.1.1.9	Limbal Epithelial and Corneal Stromal Stem Cells U. SCHLÖTZER-SCHREHARDT	107
5.1.1.10	Corneal Innervation	108
5.1.1.11	Antigen Presenting Cells in the Cornea (Dendritic Cells and Macrophages)	108
5.1.1.12	Corneal Landmarks (Definition of Limbus)	109
5.1.1.13	Corneal Dimensions	110
5.1.2	**Surgical Pathology** of the Cornea	110
5.1.2.1	Hereditary Diseases of the Cornea	110
5.1.2.1.1	Corneal Dystrophies	110
5.1.2.1.2	Ectatic Disorders (Keratoconus, Keratoglobus, Keratotorus)	113
5.1.2.2	Acquired Corneal Pathologies	114
5.1.2.2.1	Degenerations	114
5.1.2.2.2	Corneal Neovascularization (Angiogenesis and Lymphangiogenesis)	114
5.1.2.2.3	Neurotrophic Keratopathy	116
5.1.2.2.4	Keratitis/Infections	116
5.1.2.2.5	Trauma	118
5.1.2.2.6	Immune Reactions	119
5.1.3	**Surgical Procedures**	121
5.1.3.1	Penetrating Keratoplasty	121
5.1.3.1.1	Surgical Technique	121

5.1.3.1.2	Suturing Technique	123
5.1.3.1.3	Complications	123
5.1.3.2	Lamellar Keratoplasty	123
5.1.3.3	Refractive Surgery and Phototherapeutic Keratectomy	125
5.1.3.4	Corneal Abrasion	125
5.1.3.5	Amniotic Membrane Transplantation	125
5.1.3.6	Stem Cell Transplantation and Donor Limbal Stem Cell Procurement	126
5.1.4	**Wound Healing**	126
5.1.4.1	Epithelial-Stromal Interactions	126
5.1.4.2	Epithelial Invasion (LASIK, Keratoplasty)	127
5.1.4.3	Reinnervation After Penetrating Keratoplasty and Refractive Surgical Procedures	127
5.1.4.4	Hem- and Lymphangiogenesis After Keratoplasty	127
5.1.4.5	Recurrence of Corneal Dystrophy	128
5.1.4.6	Replacement of Donor by Host Tissue After Keratoplasty	128
References		128

5.2 Glaucoma Surgery
A. Jünemann, G.O.H. Naumann 131

5.2.1	**Principal Aspects** of Glaucomas and Their Terminology	131
5.2.2	**Surgical Anatomy**	131
5.2.2.1	Landmarks for Gonioscopy	131
5.2.2.2	Landmarks for Surgical Corneal Limbus	135
5.2.3	**Surgical Pathology**	136
5.2.3.1	Angle Closure Glaucomas (ACG)	136
5.2.3.2	Open Angle Glaucomas (OAG)	138
5.2.3.3	Secondary Open Angle Glaucomas (SOAG)	138
5.2.3.4	Congenital Open Angle Glaucomas	140
5.2.4	**Indications and Contraindications** for Microsurgery of Glaucomas	143
5.2.4.1	YAG-Laser Iridotomy	143
5.2.4.2	Mechanical Peripheral Iridotomy/Iridectomy	143
5.2.4.3	Laser Trabeculoplasty	144
5.2.4.4	Transscleral Thermic Diode Laser	144
5.2.4.5	Mechanical Goniotomy and Trabeculotomy	144
5.2.4.6	Procedures for Acute Secondary Open Angle Glaucomas	145
5.2.4.7	Filtrating Glaucoma Surgery	146
5.2.4.8	Concept of a Transtrabecular Shunt Between the Anterior Chamber and Schlemm's Canal	148
5.2.4.9	Transscleral Coagulation of the Ciliary Body	148
5.2.4.10	Contraindication to Filtering Procedures	149
5.2.5	**Complications** with Excessive and Deficient Wound Healing	149
5.2.5.1	Acute Postoperative Decompensation of Intraocular Pressure	149
5.2.5.2	Late Conjunctival Bleb Wound Dehiscence	150
5.2.5.3	Failure of Goniotomy	150
5.2.5.4	Failure of Filtering Surgery for Chronic Open Angle Glaucoma	150
5.2.5.5	Postoperative Peripheral Anterior Synechiae	150
5.2.5.5.1	Thermic Laser Trabeculoplasty	150
5.2.5.5.2	Subsequent Filtering Procedures	150
5.2.5.6	Consequences of Acute and Persistent Ocular Hypotony Following Filtrating Glaucoma Surgery	151
5.2.5.7	Corneal Endothelial Proliferation and Migration After Filtrating Surgery	151
References		151

5.3 Iris
G.O.H. Naumann 152
- 5.3.1 **Surgical Anatomy** 153
- 5.3.1.1 Blood-Aqueous Barrier 154
- 5.3.1.2 "Biocytology" of Normal Pigmented Cells of the Iris 155

- 5.3.2 **Surgical Pathology** 156
- 5.3.2.1 "Biocytology" of Minimal Microsurgical Trauma 156
- 5.3.2.2 Melanin Dispersion from the Iris Pigment Epithelium 156
- 5.3.2.3 Rubeosis Iridis Followed by Secondary Open and Angle Closure Glaucomas ... 156
- 5.3.2.4 Angle Closure Glaucomas Via Pupillary and Ciliary Block 158
- 5.3.2.5 Iridodialysis 159
- 5.3.2.6 Tumors of the Iris 161
- 5.3.2.7 Epithelial Ingrowth, Diffuse and Cystic 164
- 5.3.2.8 Non-invasive In Vivo Diagnostic Procedures for Processes of the Iris .. 166

- 5.3.3 **Indications** for Surgical Procedures Involving the Iris 169
- 5.3.3.1 YAG-Laser Iridotomy and Iridoplasty 169
- 5.3.3.2 Mechanical Iridotomy and Iridectomy 170
- 5.3.3.3 Mechanical Mydriasis 171
- 5.3.3.4 Sector Iridectomy 171
- 5.3.3.5 Closure of Iridodialysis 171
- 5.3.3.6 Localized Excision and Block Excisions of Iris Tumors and Epithelial Implantation Cysts ... 171

- 5.3.4 Wound Healing and Complications of Procedures Involving the Iris .. 172
- 5.3.4.1 Iris Sutures 172
- 5.3.4.2 Laser-Idirotomy and Hemorrhage from Iris 173
- References 175

5.4 Ciliary Body
G.O.H. Naumann 176
- 5.4.1 **Surgical Anatomy** 178

- 5.4.2 **Surgical Pathology** 182
- 5.4.2.1 Presbyopia 182
- 5.4.2.2 Cataract Surgery 182
- 5.4.2.3 Contusion Deformity 183
- 5.4.2.4 Traumatic Cyclodialysis 183
- 5.4.2.5 Pseudoadenomatous Hyperplasia ("Fuchs' Adenoma") 186
- 5.4.2.6 Tumors of the Ciliary Body 186
- 5.4.2.7 Epithelial Ingrowth Involving the Anterior Chamber 193
- 5.4.2.8 Zonular Apparatus in Pseudoexfoliation Syndrome and Homocystinuria ... 193
- 5.4.2.9 Non-invasive In Vivo Diagnostic Procedures 193

- 5.4.3 **Indications** for Procedures Involving the Ciliary Body 193
- 5.4.3.1 Posterior Sclerotomy 193
- 5.4.3.2 Pars Plana Vitrectomy 193
- 5.4.3.3 Direct Cyclopexy for Treating Persisting Ocular Hypotony Resulting from Traumatic or Iatrogenic Cyclodialysis ... 193
- 5.4.3.4 "Block Excision" of Tumors and Epithelial Ingrowth of Anterior Uvea .. 195
- 5.4.3.4.1 Block Excision of Localized Tumors 204
- 5.4.3.4.2 Block Excision of Epithelial Ingrowth 204
- 5.4.3.5 Cyclodestruction 213

- 5.4.4 **Wound Healing** and Complications After Procedures Involving the Ciliary Body ... 215

5.4.4.1	Intraoperative Hemorrhage	215
5.4.4.2	Local Recurrence and Metastasis of Tumors	215
5.4.4.3	Prevention of Retinal Detachment	215
5.4.4.4	Corneal Endothelium Proliferation and Migration in Traumatic Postcontusional Cyclodialysis	215
5.4.4.5	Ocular Hypotony After Block Excision for Tumors or Epithelial Ingrowth	215
5.4.4.6	Relative Ocular Hypertension After Block Excision	215
5.4.4.7	Lens Decentration/Subluxation and Cataract Formation After Block Excision	216
References		216

5.5 Lens and Zonular Fibers
U. Schlötzer-Schrehardt, G.O.H. Naumann 217

5.5.1	**Key Features** of the Lens	217
5.5.2	**Basic Aspects of Intraocular Anatomy** for Microsurgery of the Lens	219
5.5.2.1	Position of the Lens and the Lens-Iris Diaphragm	219
5.5.2.2	Characteristics of the Lens Capsule	219
5.5.2.3	Hyalocapsular Ligament (Wieger's Ligament)	219
5.5.2.4	Features of Lens Epithelial and Fiber Cells	220
5.5.2.5	Iatrogenic Mydriasis	220
5.5.2.6	Pseudophakic Lens Implants	220
5.5.3	**Surgical Anatomy** of the Lens	220
5.5.3.1	Gross Anatomy	220
5.5.3.2	Lens Capsule	221
5.5.3.3	Lens Epithelium	222
5.5.3.4	Lens Fibers	224
5.5.3.5	Suspensory Apparatus	225
5.5.3.5.1	Zonular Fibers	225
5.5.3.5.2	Wieger's Ligament	226
5.5.4	**Aging Changes**	226
5.5.4.1	Gross Anatomy	226
5.5.4.2	Lens Capsule, Epithelium, Fibers, and Zonules	227
5.5.4.3	Biochemical Changes	228
5.5.5	**Surgical Pathology of the Lens**	229
5.5.5.1	Anomalies of Size and Shape	229
5.5.5.1.1	Aphakia	229
5.5.5.1.2	Duplication of the Lens (Biphakia)	229
5.5.5.1.3	Microspherophakia	229
5.5.5.1.4	Lens Coloboma	229
5.5.5.1.5	Lenticonus and Lentiglobus	230
5.5.5.1.6	Persistent Hyperplastic Primary Vitreous	230
5.5.5.2	Lens Dislocations (Ectopia Lentis)	232
5.5.5.2.1	Isolated Dislocation	232
5.5.5.2.2	Systemic Diseases and Lens Dislocation	232
5.5.5.2.3	Traumatic Luxation	234
5.5.5.3	Cataracts	234
5.5.5.3.1	Basic Mechanisms of Cataract Formation	236
5.5.6	**Basic Aspects of Cataract Surgery**	244
5.5.6.1	Preoperative Examinations	244
5.5.6.2	Indications for Removal of the Lens and Artificial Lens Implantation	244
5.5.6.2.1	Extracapsular Cataract Extraction	245
5.5.6.2.2	Intracapsular Cataract Extraction	246

5.5.7	**Complications After Cataract Surgery** and Wound Healing	246
5.5.7.1	Complications	247
5.5.7.1.1	Corneal Endothelial Cell Loss	247
5.5.7.1.2	Iris Damage	247
5.5.7.1.3	Retinal Damage	247
5.5.7.1.4	Endophthalmitis	247
5.5.7.2	Secondary Cataract After Extracapsular Cataract Surgery	247
5.5.7.2.1	Fibrosis-Type of Posterior Capsular Opacification (PCO)	248
5.5.7.2.2	Pearl-Type PCO	249
5.5.7.2.3	Soemmerring's Ring	249
5.5.7.2.4	Other Causes of PCO	251
5.5.7.2.5	Prevention and Treatment of PCO	251
5.5.7.3	Pseudophakia and Complications	251
5.5.7.3.1	True Pseudophakic Accommodation and Pseudoaccommodation	252
5.5.7.4	Complications After Intracapsular Cataract Extraction	252
References		252

5.6 Retina and Vitreous

A.M. JOUSSEN and G.O.H. NAUMANN
with Contributions by S.E. COUPLAND, E.R. TAMM, B. KIRCHHOF, N. BORNFELD 255

5.6.1	**Surgical Anatomy**	255
5.6.1.1	Vitreous Attachments at the Base of the Ora Serrata and Martegiani's Ring	255
5.6.1.2	Bursa Macularis	256
5.6.1.3	Bergmeister Disc	256
5.6.1.4	Potential Subretinal Spaces: Foveolar and Ora Clefts	256
5.6.1.4.1	Potential "Ora Cleft"	256
5.6.1.4.2	Potential "Foveola Cleft"	256
5.6.1.5	Horizontal Barriers ("*Leitstrukturen*")	257
5.6.1.6	Vertical Barriers ("*Leitstrukturen*")	257
5.6.1.7	Subretinal Immune Privilege	258
5.6.2	**Surgical Pathology**	260
5.6.2.1	Peripheral Retinal Degenerations and Vitreous Traction	260
5.6.2.1.1	Lattice Degeneration	260
5.6.2.1.2	Cystic Retinal Tuft	261
5.6.2.1.3	Peripheral Microcystoid Degeneration	262
5.6.2.2	Peripheral Retinal Holes and Tears	263
5.6.2.3	Retinal Detachment	266
5.6.2.3.1	Effects of Detachment of the Ocular Tissues	267
5.6.2.3.2	Histopathology of Rhegmatogenous Detachment	267
5.6.2.3.3	Exudative Detachment	268
5.6.2.3.4	Central Serous Retinopathy	268
5.6.2.3.5	Traction Detachment	269
5.6.2.3.6	Special Forms of Retinal Detachment	269
5.6.2.4	Retinoschisis	270
5.6.2.4.1	X-Linked Retinoschisis	272
5.6.2.5	Macular Hole	273
5.6.2.6	Vitreoschisis and Both Macular and Peripheral Pucker	279
5.6.2.7	Retinal Vascular Abnormalities and Neovascularization	281
5.6.2.7.1	Central Retinal Vein Occlusion	287
5.6.2.7.2	Retinopathy of Prematurity (ROP)	287
5.6.2.7.3	Hemoglobinopathies	287
5.6.2.7.4	Diabetic Retinopathy	287
5.6.2.7.5	Radiation Retinopathy	289
5.6.2.7.6	Eales' Disease	289
5.6.2.7.7	Norrie's Disease	289

5.6.2.7.8	Coats' Disease	290
5.6.2.7.9	Familial Exudative Vitreoretinopathy	290
5.6.2.8	Choroidal Neovascularization	291
5.6.2.9	Tumors of Choroid and Retina	294
5.6.2.10	Dyes, Vitreous Substitutes and Infusion Fluids	299
5.6.2.10.1	Dyes for Intravitreal Use	299
5.6.2.10.2	Vitreous Substitutes and Tamponades	300
5.6.2.10.3	Infusion Fluids	302
5.6.3	**Principal Indications**	302
5.6.3.1	Closure of Defects	302
5.6.3.1.1	Buckling or Scleral Indentation	303
5.6.3.1.2	Vitrectomy Procedure	303
5.6.3.2	Release of Vitreous Traction	305
5.6.3.3	Removal of Internal Limiting Membrane	306
5.6.3.4	Removal of Vitreous Opacities	307
5.6.3.5	Retinal Hypoxia	310
5.6.3.6	Choroidal Neovascularization and Atrophy	311
5.6.3.7	Chorioretinal Biopsy	311
5.6.3.8	General Concepts in the Treatment of Tumors of Choroid and Retina	312
5.6.3.8.1	Controversies in the Management of Malignant Melanomas of the Posterior Uvea	312
5.6.4	**Wound Healing** and Complications of Therapy	314
5.6.4.1	Retinal Pigment Epithelium Scars	314
5.6.4.2	Proliferative Vitreoretinopathy	314
5.6.4.3	Active Cell Populations	316
5.6.4.3.1	Retinal Pigment Epithelial Cells	316
5.6.4.3.2	Hyalocytes	317
5.6.4.3.3	Müller Cells and Their Functions	317
5.6.4.3.4	Endothelial Cells, Astrocytes and Vascular Development	318
5.6.4.4	Distant Defects	318
5.6.4.4.1	Nuclear Cataracts After Vitrectomy	318
5.6.4.4.2	Angle Closure Glaucoma After Vitreoretinal Surgery	319
References		320

5.7 Optic Nerve and Elschnig's Scleral Ring
C.Y. Mardin, G.O.H. Naumann 335

5.7.1	**Anatomy,** Landmarks, Harmless and Other Anomalies, Age Related Changes, Juxtapapillary Coni	335
5.7.1.1	Anomalies of the Optic Disc Are Associated with the Disc's Size	337
5.7.2	**Surgical Pathology** and **Indications for Microsurgery**	339
5.7.2.1	The Glaucomatous Optic Disc	339
5.7.2.1.1	Glaucomatous Disc Damage	340
5.7.2.1.2	Juxtapapillary Glaucoma Damage	340
5.7.2.2	Giant Cell Arteritis and Biopsy of the Temporal Artery	342
5.7.2.2.1	Biopsy and Histology of the Temporal Artery	342
5.7.2.3	Optic Disc in Non-/Ischemic Central Retinal Vein Occlusion and Opticotomy	343
5.7.2.3.1	Non-ischemic Central Vein Occlusion	343
5.7.2.3.2	Ischemic Central Vein Occlusion	343
5.7.2.4	Congenital Pits of the Optic Nerve	344
5.7.2.4.1	Vitreoretinal Microsurgery	345
5.7.2.5	Tumors of the Optic Nerve	345
5.7.2.6	Intracranial Hypertension: Acute and Chronic Variants Must Be Distinguished	346

5.7.2.6.1	Acute Intracranial Pressure Rise and Terson's Syndrome	346
5.7.2.6.2	Benign Chronic Intracranial Hypertension and Optic Disc Swelling (Pseudotumor Cerebri)	346
5.7.3	**Wound Healing** and Complications	347
5.7.3.1	Pseudocavernous Optic Neuropathy	347
5.7.3.2	Radiation Opticoneuropathy	347
References		348

6 Influence of Common Generalized Diseases on Intraocular Microsurgery
G.O.H. Naumann, U. Schlötzer-Schrehardt 350

6.1 Diabetes Mellitus
G.O.H. Naumann 351

6.1.1	Diabetic Retinopathy	351
6.1.2	Diabetic Iridopathy	351
6.1.3	Recurrent Corneal Erosions	351
6.1.4	Cataracts	351
6.1.5	Risk of Infection	352

6.2 Arterial Hypertension and "Vis A Tergo"
Gottfried O.H. Naumann 353

6.3 Pseudoexfoliation Syndrome: Pathological Manifestations of Relevance to Intraocular Surgery
U. Schlötzer-Schrehardt, G.O.H. Naumann 354

6.3.1	Introduction	354
6.3.2	Pathobiology of PEX Syndrome	355
6.3.3	Clinical Diagnosis and Early Recognition	357
6.3.3.1	Manifest PEX Syndrome	357
6.3.3.2	Masked PEX Syndrome	359
6.3.3.3	Early Stages of PEX Syndrome	359
6.3.3.4	Asymmetry of Involvement	359
6.3.4	Surgical Pathology	360
6.3.4.1	Lens, Ciliary Body, and Zonular Apparatus	360
6.3.4.2	Iris	364
6.3.4.3	Trabecular Meshwork	368
6.3.4.4	Cornea	371
6.3.5	Microsurgical Considerations	374
6.3.5.1	Intraoperative Complications	374
6.3.5.2	Postoperative Complications	375
6.3.6	Conclusions	375
References		375

6.4 Other Generalized Diseases
G.O.H. Naumann 378

6.4.1	Infectious Disorders (AIDS, Sepsis)	378
6.4.2	Hematologic Disorders	378
6.4.3	Neurologic and Muscular Diseases	378

General References 379

List of Figures 381

List of Tables 387

Subject Index 391

List of Contributors

Norbert Bornfeld, Prof. Dr. med.
Department of Ophthalmology, University of Essen
Hufelandstrasse 55, D-45122, Essen, Germany

Sarah E. Coupland, MBBS, PhD
School of Cancer Studies, University of Liverpool
5 049, Duncan Building, Daulby Street, Liverpool
L69 3GA, UK

Claus Cursiefen, Priv.-Doz. Dr. med.
Department of Ophthalmology, University of
Erlangen-Nürnberg, Schwabachanlage 6
D-91054 Erlangen, Germany

Rudolf F. Guthoff, Prof. Dr. med.
Department of Ophthalmology, Rostock University
Doberaner Strasse 140, D-18057 Rostock, Germany

Ludwig M. Heindl, Dr. med.
Department of Ophthalmology, University of
Erlangen-Nürnberg, Schwabachanlage 6
D-91054 Erlangen, Germany

Leonard M. Holbach, Prof. Dr. med.
Department of Ophthalmology, University of
Erlangen-Nürnberg, Schwabachanlage 6
D-91054 Erlangen, Germany

Antonia M. Joussen, Prof. Dr. med.
Department of Ophthalmology, Heinrich-Heine
University, Moorenstrasse 5, 40225 Düsseldorf
Germany

Anselm Jünemann, Prof. Dr. med.
Department of Ophthalmology, University of
Erlangen-Nürnberg, Schwabachanlage 6
D-91054 Erlangen, Germany

Bernd Kirchhof, Prof. Dr. med.
Department of Vitreoretinal Surgery, Center for
Ophthalmology, University of Cologne, Joseph-
Stelzmann-Strasse 9, D-50931 Cologne, Germany

Friedrich E. Kruse, Prof. Dr. med.
Department of Ophthalmology, University of
Erlangen-Nürnberg, Schwabachanlage 6
D-91054 Erlangen, Germany

Christian Y. Mardin, Prof. Dr. med.
Department of Ophthalmology, University of
Erlangen-Nürnberg, Schwabachanlage 6
D-91054 Erlangen, Germany

Gottfried O.H. Naumann, Prof. (emer.) Dr. med. Dr. h.c. (mult.)
Department of Ophthalmology, University of
Erlangen-Nürnberg, Schwabachanlage 6
D-91054 Erlangen, Germany

Ursula Schlötzer-Schrehardt, Prof. Dr. rer. nat.
Department of Ophthalmology, University of
Erlangen-Nürnberg, Schwabachanlage 6
D-91054 Erlangen, Germany

Ernst R. Tamm, Prof. Dr. med.
Department of Anatomy, University of Regensburg
Universitätsstrasse 31, D-93053 Regensburg, Germany

List of Abbreviations

AMD	Age related macula degeneration	PAS	Periodic Acid Schiff Stain
ARMD	Age related macula degeneration	PCO	Posterior Capsular Opacification
BAB	Blood-aqueous barrier	PDGF	Platelet-derived growth factor
BM	Bruch's membrane	PEDF	Pigment epithelium-derived factor
BRB	Blood-retina barrier	PKP	Perforating keratoplasty
CM	Ciliary muscle	POAG	Primary open angle glaucoma
CNTF	Ciliary neurotrophic factor	PVR	Proliferative vitreoretinopathy
CNV	Choroidal neovascularization	RAM	Relative anterior microphthalmus
CPC	Clinicopathologic correlation	ROP	Retinopathy of prematurity
CRVO	Central retinal vein occlusion	ROP	Retinopathia of prematurity
EMZL	Extranodal marginal zone B-cell lymphoma	RPE	Retinal pigment epithelium
FEVR	Familial exudative vitreoretinopathy	RTA	Retinal thickness analysis
FR	Fuchs' roll	SC	Schlemm's canal
GFAP	Glial fibrillary acid protein	SEM	Scanning Electromikroscopy
HE	Haematoxylin and Eosin	SINS	Surgically induced necrotizing scleritis
ICG	Indocyanine green	SL	Schwalbe line
ILM	Inner limiting membrane	SOAG	Secondary open angle glaucoma
IFIS	Intraoperative floppy iris syndrome	SS	Sclera spur
LASIK	Laser in situ keratomileusis	TASS	Toxic anterior segment syndrome
MLM	Intermediate (middle) limiting membrane	TM	Trabecular meshwork
NHL	Non-Hodgkin lymphoma	TTT	Transpupillary thermotherapy
NVD	Neovascularization of the disk	USB	Ultrasound biomicroscopy
NVE	Neovascularization elsewhere	VEGF	Vascular endothelial growth factor
OCT	Optical coherence tomography	VIP	Vasoactive intestinal polypeptide
OLM	Outer limiting membrane		

Chapter 1

Introduction

G.O.H. NAUMANN, F.E. KRUSE

1.1
Ophthalmic Pathology in Clinical Practice, Teaching and Research

As ophthalmologists we are fascinated by the structures of the normal and diseased eye. The clear optical media allow almost all tissues within the eye to be *observed directly* in vivo. The interpretation of *clinical* observations obtained by echographic techniques, fluorescein angiography (FA), optical coherence-laser tomography (OCT), confocal laser scanning in vivo microscopy, polarimetry, etc., requires a precise knowledge and *direct correlation* with the ophthalmopathologic basis. This is true for quantitative pathology and in vivo "*biomorphometry*" as well as for quantitative *in vivo cytology* – "biocytology" – such as corneal endothelial microscopy. Ophthalmic pathology comprises the *entire spectrum* of structural changes, ranging from slit lamp microscopy and "biocytology" to the available laboratory methods of general pathology including macroscopy, light and electron microscopy, immune histochemistry as well as modern molecular and cell biology. Ophthalmopathology thus offers a *three-dimensional framework* for morphologic differential diagnosis, and also for the training of medical students and ophthalmologists.

The necessity for clinicopathologic correlations (CPCs) with excised tissues and enucleated eyes is particularly obvious for the following reasons:

1.1.1
Confirmation and Quality Control of Clinical Diagnoses

Confirmation and quality control of clinical diagnoses are indispensable in infectious diseases and oncology for the appropriate therapy. The correction of misdiagnoses is also one of the most effective tools in teaching.

1.1.2
Modern Ophthalmomicrosurgery is Applied Ophthalmopathology

This is no exaggeration, as ophthalmic microsurgery today is done with the same magnifications as for low light microscopy in the laboratory. In fact, the main purpose of this book is to illustrate this everyday experience. As a prerequisite for the recognition and prevention of potential complications, we can modify the surgical approaches – keeping in mind the vulnerability of the most critical cell populations involved.

We shall not discuss and illustrate the whole spectrum of morphologic elements but confine ourselves mainly to the magnifications of both light microscopy and the operating microscope. We shall illustrate simple stains such as the standard hematoxylin and eosin (HE), and periodic acid–Schiff (PAS), to outline the resistant structures of outstanding basement membranes like Descemet's and Bruch's membrane, the inner limiting membrane of the retina, and the lens capsule. The Masson stain facilitates the distinction between epithelial (red) and connective mesenchymal tissue (blue).

Studies of *wound healing* after ophthalmic microsurgery and its complications in and around the eye are of particular interest – "scar wars" – by being excessive or insufficient.

1.1.3
Ophthalmic Pathology is the Science of the Phenotype

Defining the phenotype in a reproducible fashion therefore has become more important than ever if a meaningful correlation to a genotype is sought. Criteria for the phenotype in ophthalmology rely mainly on morphologic features: Today refined methods for quantification are available, e.g. for measuring corneal endothelial density, size of the optic disc and its intra- and peripapillary alterations. And one might add: *ophthalmic examination and microsurgery are concerned with the morphologic phenotype*. Microsurgical manipulations of the genotype are a topic for the future and might potentially require the appropriate nanotechniques.

1.1.4
Ophthalmic Pathology also Connects Experimental and Clinical Ophthalmology

In view of the very close interrelation between clinical practice and ophthalmic pathology, it is highly desirable that the ophthalmic pathology laboratory should be closely integrated, also geographically, into departments of ophthalmology "in situ."

Obviously a close cooperation with the general pathologist is necessary and fruitful, especially in the differential diagnosis of orbital processes and peculiar lid alterations.

On the other hand, we know from many consultations with general pathologists that they experience difficulties in the differential diagnoses of conjunctival and even common intraocular diseases. The specific pathology of the "eye" mandates this interdisciplinary exchange and makes it a rewarding experience.

As in all paths of life we need to know the history to better understand the present and also to judge the opportunities and risks of the future.

A very brief sketch of the history of ophthalmic (micro-)surgery may be of interest (Tables 1.1, 1.2).

Table 1.1. Historical overview of ophthalmic surgery from antiquity to 1800

1700 B.C.	Codex Hammurabi, Mesopotamia
500 B.C.	Susrata, India: cataract couching
25 B.C.–50 A.D.	Aulus Cornelius Celsus (25–35 A.D.): first description of cataract couching via the "pars plana approach"
1163	Council of Tours: "*Ecclesia abhorret a sanguine*"
1583	George Bartisch, oculist to the Court of Saxony in Dresden: *Ophthalmodouleia* textbook: enucleation, exenteration, cataract couching, triachiasis, ptosis, blepharochalasis surgery
1750	Jacques Daviel: extracapsular cataract surgery
1793	Ecole Santé, Paris: surgery in addition to medicine included in the university curriculum of the Medical Faculty

1.2
Historical Sketch of Ophthalmic Surgery from Antiquity to Modern Times

During the last century (from 1900 to 2000), advances in ocular surgery were more rapid and spectacular than in the entire previous history. The following pioneers and their procedures represent milestones for this period:

- 1905 Zirm was the first to perform corneal transplantation as the first transplantation in humans. He used the clock-driven trephine developed by Arthur von Hippel 1877.

Table 1.2. Selected overview of ophthalmic surgery after 1800

1839	Johann Friedrich Dieffenbach, Berlin: extraocular muscles/squint surgery
1856	Albrecht von Graefe, Berlin: iridectomy for angle closure glaucoma
1858	George Critchett, London: principle of filtrating surgery
1860	William Bowman, London: optical sector iridectomy for keratoconus inferiorly. Superior location for antiglaucomatous iridectomy
1866	Alexander Pagenstecher, Wiesbaden: intracapsular cataract surgery
1884	Carl Koller, Vienna: local anesthesia with cocaine
1905	Eduard Zirm, Olmütz: successful corneal grafting (5.0 mm) as the very first successful human tissue transplantation
1916	Jules Gonin, Lausanne: first successful procedure for retinal detachment
1927	Wladimir P. Filatow, Odessa: donor cornea from cadaver
1949	Gerd Meyer-Schwickerath, Essen: light coagulation and light surgery for retinal disease without opening the eye
1949	Harold Ridley, London: pioneer of intraocular lens implant after extracapsular cataract removal with PMMA
1952	Ernst Custodis, Düsseldorf: external implant for retinal detachment
1958	Joaquin Barraquer, Barcelona: erysophake and α-chymotrypsin for zonulolysis facilitating intracapsular cataract extraction
1956	Tadeusz Krwawicz: intracapsular cryoextraction of cataract
1950/60	Heinrich Harms and Gunter Mackensen, Tübingen; Joaquim Barraquer, Barcelona; Jörg Draeger, Hans Sautter, Hamburg; et al.: operating microscope for ophthalmic microsurgery
1965	Charles Kelmann, New York: phakoemulsification revolutionizing extracapsular cataract extraction
1965	José Barraquer, Bogota: mechanical keratomileusis
1969	Robert Machemer, Göttingen, Miami, Durham: pars plana vitrectomy for vitreal and retinal disease
1970	Hugo Hager, Tübingen: laser trabeculoplasty
1975	Trokel and Srinivasan: excimer laser 193 nm – experimental ablation of cornea
1975	Franz Fankhauser, Bern, and Aron-Rosa, Paris: YAG-laser iridotomy and capsulotomy for secondary cataract
1985	Theo Seiler and Josef Wollensak, Berlin: excimer-laser corneal refractive ablation (PRK) in patients
1988	Ioannis Pallikaris, Crete: LASIK

- 1916 Gonin developed the first cure for retinal detachment.
- 1949 Ridley started the era of lens implantation.
- 1949 Meyer-Schwickerath pioneered light coagulation as the precursor of laser medicine.

1952 Custodis proposed episcleral implants for the closure of retinal defects causing retinal detachment.
1956 Kwrawicz initiated cryotherapy in cataract extraction.
1960 José Barraquer started mechanical refractive surgery of the cornea, and 25 years later, Seiler and Wollensak used photorefractive keratectomy (PRK) to treat myopia.
1969 Robert Machemer opened up a new era in intraocular surgery by devising the "pars plana vitrectomy."
1975 Fankhauser developed the YAG-laser, opening up a new era in antiglaucomatous iridotomy and in the treatment of secondary cataracts of extracapsular surgery.

Surgery in and around the eye started in antiquity; only a few names can be mentioned (Table 1.1).

The Codex Hammurabi lists the drastic punishments for surgical failures and complications.

Susratra first documented cataract surgery in India in 500 B.C.

During the Council of Tours (1163 A.D.), a Medical Faculty was accepted for the first time in the medieval university, but surgery was excluded because it was considered an ordinary craft: "*Ecclesia abhorret a sanguine!*".

Long-term effects are evident to this day: British tradition in medicine still distinguishes between "Mr." and "Ms." for surgeons and "Doctor" for conservative physicians. Georg Bartisch, an oculist at the Saxonian Court in Dresden, in 1583 wrote *Ophthalmoduleia* – the first textbook of ophthalmic surgery – but was not considered a physician. He described procedures for lid processes, extraocular muscles and enucleations. A somewhat condescending arrogant attitude of non-surgical medical colleagues towards surgeons can be observed occasionally even in our time. The editors of the *New England Journal of Medicine* in January, 2000, in their article "Looking back at the Millennium in Medicine" omit surgery and anesthesia completely – and this is probably not only a different linguistic tradition.

Only after 600 years in 1793 did the Ecole Santé, Paris, finally welcome surgery in the Medical Faculty as an academic entity at the European university.

A tabulated overview of the advances in ophthalmic (micro-) surgery in the nineteenth and twentieth centuries outlines some of the spectacular advances made in ophthalmic surgery in the last 200 years. They are highlighted by some of the outstanding pioneers (Table 1.2).

Hermann von Helmholtz, Königsberg (1850), developed the ophthalmoscope (*Augenspiegel*), allowing the fundus of the eye to be observed for the first time – making visible diseases of the retina. This made diseases of the eye, such as retinal detachments, a goal of therapy.

Albrecht von Graefe in Berlin, Bowman in London, Donders in Utrecht, et al. pioneered modern ophthalmology. In 1856 von Graefe cured acute angle closure glaucomas by iridectomy. George Critchett, London (1858), proposed the principle of filtrating surgery which was later modified by Heine, Holt, Lagrange, Elliot and others.

William Bowman, London, published in 1849 "Lectures on the parts concerned in the operation on the eye." He performed optical sector iridectomy inferiorly for keratoconus; he also suggested performing iridectomy for acute glaucomas superiorly to be partially covered by the lids (1860).

Eduard Zirm, Olmütz (1905), demonstrated successful *corneal grafting* 5 mm in diameter as the very first successful human tissue transplantation.

Jules Gonin, Lausanne (1916), proposed the first successful procedure for retinal detachment.

Tsutomu Sato, Tokyo (1930), attempted refractive surgery of the cornea by incisions in Descemet's membrane.

Gerd Meyer-Schwickerath, Hamburg, Bonn and Essen (1949), pioneered light coagulation and non-mechanical "light surgery" for retinal diseases without opening the eye. This principle was later enhanced in 1960 by various lasers applied to the anterior and posterior segment of the eye and in all medical specialties (Fig. 1.1).

Harold Ridley, London (1949), first inserted an intraocular lens implant consisting of polymethylmethacrylate (PMMA) into extracapsular aphakic eyes.

Ernst Custodis, Düsseldorf (1952), introduced an external implant for retinal detachment. Arruga and Schepens modified this approach.

Heinrich Harms (1955/1960), Günter Mackensen (Tübingen), Joaquim Barraquer (Barcelona), José Barraquer (Bogota), Jörg Draeger and Hans Sautter (Hamburg) and other Europeans together with E. Malbran and R. Troutman introduced and perfected the use of the operating microscope and microinstruments within ophthalmic surgery (Fig. 1.2).

Charles Kelman, New York (1965), revolutionized cataract extraction with phakoemulsification.

Hugo Hager, Tübingen (1970), introduced laser trabeculoplasty (which was further developed by Krasnow and Wise in 1976).

Robert Machemer, Göttingen, Miami and Durham (1969ff), developed pars plana vitrectomy a pioneering new treatment of vitreal and retinal diseases, that were considered hopeless. He gave a chance to help patients with massive vitreal hemorrhage from diabetic retinopathy and trauma etc.

Trokel and Srinivasan used a 193-nm excimer laser in the experimental ablation of cornea in rabbits.

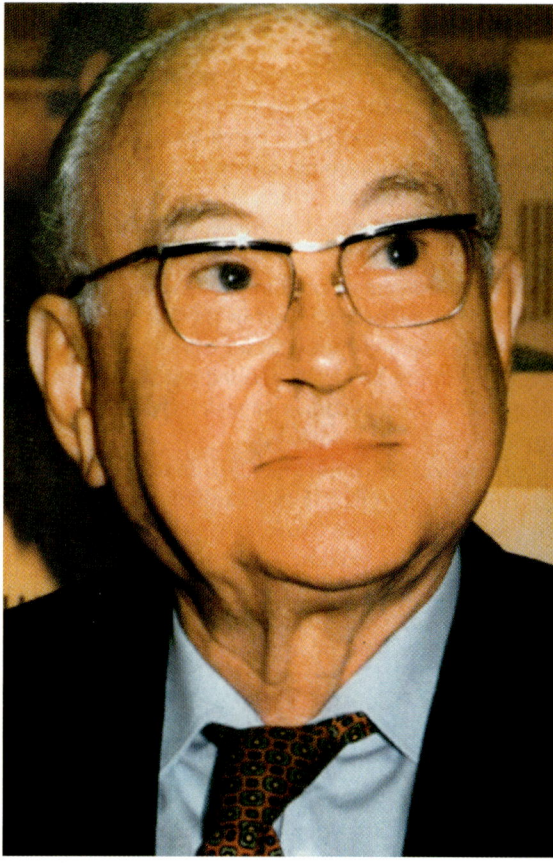

Fig. 1.1. Gerd Meyer-Schwickerath, 1920–1992, Hamburg, Bonn, Essen, Germany. Pioneer of "light surgery" initially with the "heliostat" using the light of the sun (1949), later with the xenon high pressure lamp. Afterwards modified by laser technology

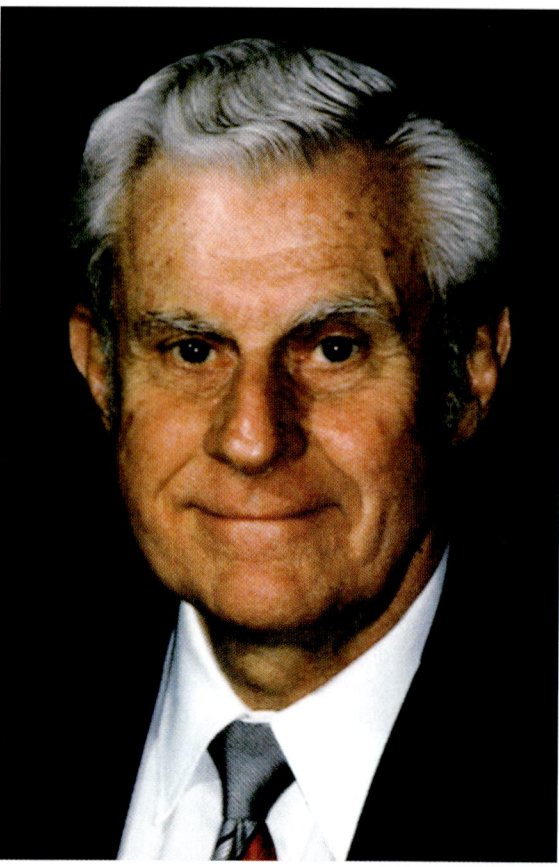

Fig. 1.3. Lorenz E. Zimmerman (1920–): Chairman, Department of Ophthalmic Pathology, Armed Forces Institute of Pathology, Washington, DC/USA, mentor of a generation of ophthalmic pathologists from around the world

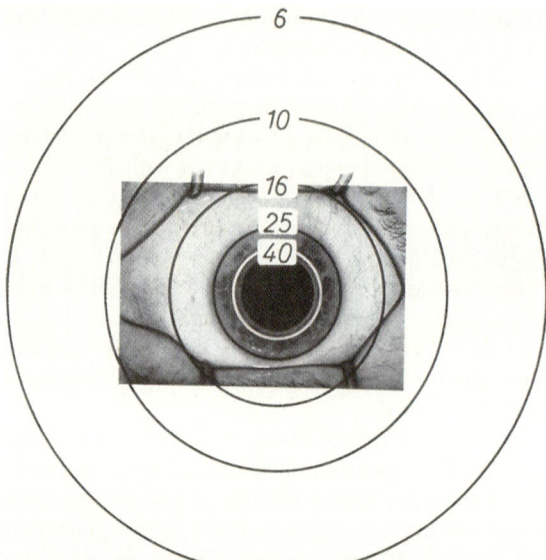

Fig. 1.2. Operating microscope: range of magnification from 6- to 40-fold projected on the eye (modified after Harms and Mackensen 1966)

Franz Fankhauser, Bern, and Aron-Rosa, Paris (1975), performed YAG-laser iridotomy and capsulotomy for secondary cataracts, and carried out non-mechanical and non-thermal intraocular surgery without opening the eye.

1.3
Overview of Advances in Ophthalmic Pathology in the Nineteenth and Twentieth Centuries

Some milestones and personalities in ophthalmic pathology/anatomy are listed to give an indication of how much interest this subject has received despite its small size (Table 1.3).

Rudolph Virchow, Berlin: recognized retinoblastoma, which he termed "glioma" – and uveal melanoma as a malignant tumor.

Theodor Leber, Heidelberg: defined inflammatory processes and angiogenesis in the cornea and coined the term "chemotaxis" (1879).

Ernst Fuchs, Vienna: father of modern ophthalmic

1.3 Overview of Advances in Ophthalmic Pathology in the Nineteenth and Twentieth Centuries

Table 1.3. Milestones and personalities in ophthalmic pathology and anatomy from antiquity to the present

Date	Person and contribution
131–201 A.D.	Claudius Galen: Pergamum, Rome: anatomy
1620–1689	Theophile Bonet, Geneva: pathologic anatomy of the eye (published before 1700, Lyon)
1720	Albrecht von Haller, Bern, Switzerland: ophthalmic artery
1727–1759	Johann Gottfried Zinn, Schwabach, Göttingen: anatomy book (1755)
1755–1830	Samuel Thomas Soemmerring, Frankfurt: atlas (1881)
1761	Giambattista Morgagni, Padua: 13th letter: pathology eye and orbit
1832	Julius Arnold, Leipzig: microscopy
1811–1982	Samuel Moritz Pappenheim, Breslau: histology of the eye (1842)
1847	Ernst von Brücke, Berlin, Vienna: anatomy of the eye
1849	William Bowman, London: "Lectures on the Parts Concerned in the Operations on the Eye"
1782–1869	James Wardrop: Edinburgh 1808/1818: pathology of eye: retinoblastoma
1799–1828	Friedrich August von Ammon, Göttingen, Dresden: pathology of eye
1820–1864	Heinrich Müller, Würzburg: modern histopathology of the eye
1851–1930	Ernst Fuchs, Vienna: father of ophthalmic pathology, many editions of textbooks
1849–1852	John Dalrympe and Edward Nettleship, J. Herbert Parson, E. Treacher Collins: textbooks in English Alan William Sichel: textbook in French
1854	Georg Theodor Ruette, Adolf Alt, Wedl and Block, Otto Haab, Leipzig: textbooks in German
1860	Rudolf Virchow, Berlin: "glioma retinae"
1861	Carl Wedl and Stellwag von Carion, Vienna: atlas
1879	Theodor Leber, Heidelberg: "chemotaxis," textbook on inflammation
1884–1971	Georgiana Dvorak-Theobold; Edward Nettleship; J. Herbert Parsons; E. Treacher Collins, London; H. Stephan Mayou, Paris: textbooks
1897–1955	Jonas Stein Friedenwald, Baltimore: experimental eye pathology
1874–1968	Frederick Verhoeff, Boston: father of ophthalmic pathology in the USA
1907–1975	Michael Hogan
1913–2001	Norman Ashton: diagnostic and experimental pathology
1917–1994	Frederick C. Blodi, Austrian emigrated to USA: Clin.-Path. Correlations
1930–1938	Karl von Wessely: three volume textbook on pathology of the eye (part of the Henke-Lubarsch series in German)
1960ff	Hogan and Zimmerman, Washington; Spencer, San Francisco; Yanoff and Fine, Philadelphia, Washington: textbooks
1920–	Lorenz E. Zimmerman, Washington: "put the house of ocular structure in order." Mentor of many ophthalmic pathologists around the world
1990	Thaddeus P. Dryja: identified the "retinoblastoma suppressor gene"

pathology (together with Parsons, London, and Frederic Verhoeff, Boston). He described sympathetic uveitis, and many entities bear his name.

Eugen v. Hippel, Göttingen: phakomatoses (1895).

Frederick Verhoeff, Boston: defined "*retinoblastoma*" as originating from photoreceptors. Established criteria for so-called "endophthalmitis phacoanaphylactica."

Karl von Wessely, Munich: immune ring of the cornea. Edited a three-volume textbook on ophthalmic pathology, 1930–1938.

Norman Ashton, London (1950ff–2001): established an experimental model of retinopathia praematurorum based on reactive retinal hypoxia following excess oxygen exposure. Pioneer of experimental ophthalmic pathology.

Helen Wilder, Washington (1953): identified toxoplasmosis retinochoroiditis and *Toxocara canis* endophthalmitis in enucleated eyes.

Lorenz E. Zimmerman (Fig. 1.3), Washington (1953ff): "put the house of ophthalmopathology in systematic order" based on morphologic criteria of the phenotype. Created a school of ophthalmic pathology around the world, emphasizing clinicopathologic correlations (CPCs)!

Thaddeus P. Dryja (1990): identified the retinoblastoma suppressor gene.

References (see also page 379)

Albert DM and Edwards DD. The History of Ophthalmology. Blackwell, London, 1996

Apple David J. Sir Harold Ridley and His Fight For Sight: He changed the world so that we may better see it, Slack Incorp., USA, 2006

Apple DJ, Kincaid MC, Mamalis N, Olson RJ. Intraocular lenses. Evolution designs, complications, and pathology, Williams & Wilkins, Baltimore, 1989

Birkmeyer NJO and Birkmeyer JD. Strategies for Improving Surgical Quality – Should Payers Reward Excellence or Effort? NEJ Med 2006; 354: 864–868

Forrester JV, Dick AD, McMenamin PG, Lee WR. The Eye, 2nd edition. Saunders, London, 2002

Gieler J, Heuser D. Verschiebungen des Iris-Linsen-Diaphragmas unter Einfluss vasoaktiver Pharmaka. Vorläufige Mitteilung tierexperimenteller Befunde. In Naumann GOH and Gloor B loc. cit.

Grossniklaus A.E. (Editor): Ophthalmic Pathology and intraocular tumors, Section 4, Basic and Clinical Science Course, American Academy Ophthalmology, 2004–5

Guthoff RF, Baudouin C, Stave J. Atlas of Confocal Laser Scanning In-vivo Microscopy in Ophthalmology. Springer Heidelberg, 2006

Heuser D, Gieler J, Jehnichen R. Ein Verfahren zur kontinuierlichen Registrierung sagittaler Verschiebungen des Iris-Linsen-Diaphragmas im tierexperimentellen Modell. In Naumann GOH and Gloor B loc. cit.

Hirschberg J (translated by FC Blodi). History of Ophthalmology, Wayenborg Pub, Belgium 1986

Hirschberg J: Geschichte der Augenheilkunde, Georg Olms, Hildesheim-New York, 1977 Bd. I–VII (Nachdruck der Ausgabe Berlin 1918)

Johnson GJ, Miniassian DC, Weale R, et al.: The Epidemiology of Eye Disease. Chapman & Hall Medical, London, 1998; and Arnold, London, 2003

Kelman CD. Phacoemulsification and aspiration: A new technique of cataract removal. Am J Ophthalmol 1967; 64: 23–25

Kelman CD. The history and development of phacoemulsification. Int Ophthalmol Clinics 1994; 34: 1–12

Küchle HJ.: Ophthalmology Departments of German Universities, 19th and 20th century (in German), 450 pages, Bierman Pub., Köln, 2005

Lebensohn JF. An anthology of Ophthalmic Classics. William & Wilkins, Baltimore, 1969

Lee, P. Into the Looking Glass: Factors and Opportunities to Reshape Eye Care in the next 25 Years. Ophthalmology 2007; 114:1–2

Lervin LA, Ritch R, Richards JE, Borrás T. Stem Cell Therapy for Ocular Disorders. Arch Ophthalmol 2004; 122:621–627

Lim, KH and Lim A. Ophthalmology awakens in Asia. Singapore National Eye Center, 1999

Machemer R (1972) Vitrectomy. A pars plana approach. Grune & Stratton, New York, pp 1–136

Münchow W. History of Ophthalmology (in German), 755 pages, Enke, Stuttgart, 1984

Naumann GOH and Gloor B (eds) Wound Healing of the Eye and its Complications, pp. 71–72; 73–75, Bergmann Verlag, München, 1980

Naumann GOH et al. Pathology of the Eye, Springer-Verlag Heidelberg: German 1980 and 1997; English 1986, Japanese 1987 and 2003

Ridley NHL. Intraocular acrylic lenses – 10 years development. Br J Ophthalmol 1960; 44: 705-712

Ridley NHL. Intraocular acrylic lenses. Trans Ophthalmol Soc UK LXXI-617-621, 1951

Sing KD, Logan NS, Gilmartin B. Three-Dimensional Modelling of the Human Eye Based on Magnet Resonance Modelling. Invest Ophthalmol Vis Sci 2006; 47:2272–79

Spencer WA, Albert DM. The Armed Forces Institute of Pathology. An Appreciation. Arch Ophthalmol 2006; 124: 1332–1334

Zerhoumi EA: Translational and Clinical Science – Time for a New Vision. N Engl J Med 2005; 335:1621–23

General Ophthalmic Pathology: Principal Indications and Complications, Comparing Intra- and Extraocular Surgery

G.O.H. NAUMANN, F.E. KRUSE

The principal indications for extra- and intraocular surgery are similar to those of surgery for other purposes. However, surgical procedures inside the eye are associated with a unique pattern of complications. They not only affect the site of entry but tissue distant to this location.

Obviously, clinical ophthalmology, ophthalmic pathology and ophthalmic microsurgery share principal approaches in the spectrum of conservative medicine and macrosurgery. The eye requires a different approach from other organs in the body because of: (1) its *small dimensions*, (2) the *delicate structure* of the intraocular tissues and, importantly, (3) the fact that the *intraocular pressure is significantly higher* than the tissue pressure of other organs (Tab. 2.1).

Use of the operating microscope was pioneered by ophthalmologists and has contributed to the spectacular progress not only in microsurgery of the eye but also in other specialties in the last 50 years (see Chapter 1, Sect. 2). The magnification used covers part of the range used in light-microscopic histopathologic study. Approaches for the eye range from morphologic in vivo diagnosis with the slit lamp, A- and B-echography, optical coherence tomography (OCT), ultrasound biomicroscopy, laser in vivo confocal microscopy, ultrasound biomicroscopy (USB) and fluorescence angiography, etc., to observation and action under the operating microscope. Thus either excised tissue or the entire eye can be studied in the ophthalmic pathology laboratory. The surgical anatomy with lines, planes and spaces as landmarks has particular importance for the ophthalmic microsurgeon for orientation; the anatomy for each tissue is discussed under the relevant section.

Discussions in this book are confined to light microscopic dimensions enhanced by electron microscopy if necessary, e.g., in the pseudoexfoliation syndrome (see Chapter 6.3). "*Biocytology*" means the non-invasive study of *single* cells in vivo, e.g., specular microscopy of the corneal endothelium or of individual benign or malignant melanocytes on the surface of the gray-blue iris or the anterior lens capsule.

We shall *not* discuss *proteomics* with the imaging of molecules. Nanomedicine on a scale of less than 100 nm may have exciting potential for diagnosis and therapy and will probably demand further sophistication of ophthalmic microsurgery beyond our current imagination. These channels of current interdisciplinary "high risk research" will lead to investigations which will also include and fascinate the ophthalmic microsurgeon and the pathologist. Our current state of knowledge does not allow us to speculate on how these paths will develop in the future.

"*Robotic surgery* – squeezing into tight places" – making microsurgery "go digital," may also have great potential for the future. Currently it is good for extirpation but not for reconstruction (Berlinger 2006).

2.1
Principal Indications: Clinico-pathologic Correlation

The principal indications in ophthalmic microsurgery are similar to those in macrosurgery concerning other organs of the body. We shall briefly outline these obvious principal indications.

2.1.1
Defects

Defects in the scleral wall of the globe or in the cornea due to trauma or surgery cause more or less pronounced ocular hypotony. Hemorrhage into the anterior chamber and vitreous from damaged vascularized tissue may be profuse due to the suddenly decreased tissue pressure. Prolonged ocular hypotony always causes uveal effusion followed by progressive choroidal

Table 2.1. Special features of the eye's normal function

1. Blood-ocular barrier (Fig. 2.6)
2. Avascularity of cornea, anterior chamber, lens and vitreous
3. All vascularized tissues spare the optical axis
4. Increased tissue pressure maintains a smooth refractive surface of the cornea and properly aligned photoreceptors
5. Sensory retina is transparent

hemorrhage. Drastic pressure release in eyes with acute glaucomas increases the risk of expulsive choroidal hemorrhage (see below). To prevent infection and indirect distant complications, e.g., traumatic tears, perforations of necrotizing keratitis or insufficiently closed surgical wounds, water-tight closure is required as soon as possible (see Chapters 2.2, 4).

Defects in the sensory retina, such as horseshoe tears or foramina, are one reason for retinal detachments. The other is anteriorly displaced vitreous tissue, causing traction on the sensory retina separating it from the retinal pigment epithelium (RPE). "Locations of minor resistance" are the potential "*ora slit*" and "*foveola slit*" (see below and Chapter 5.6). Various methods of extrascleral indentations by implants and intravitreal cutting and aspiration release the traction to the margins of the retinal defects (see Chapter 5.6). Other methods, like cryocoagulation (diathermy) or laser therapy, induce necroses of RPE, sensory retina and choroid followed by scar formation between the reattached sensory retina and the viable margin of underlying RPE and choroid.

2.1.2
Excess of Tissue

Congenital anomalies – hamartomas and choristomas – inflammatory or oncologic processes, abnormal wound healing and neovascularization may lead to an excess of tissue. Malignant neoplasias may impair the function of the eye or even pose a risk for life. Depending on the dimension, removal of such processes requires "*excisional biopsy*," which means *complete* removal of larger lesions, or *limited* biopsy to establish the histologic diagnosis. If a wide defect results, wound closure with mobilization of the adjacent tissue or transplantation may be necessary (for details see Chapters 3 and 5 for the individual tissue).

2.1.3
Altered Tissue In Situ

Opacities of the lens may present at birth or are acquired following trauma, other ocular or generalized diseases, or – most commonly – are associated with aging. *Cataract extraction* is the most frequently performed surgical procedure of all medical disciplines. Today the cloudy lens tissue is removed and a lens implant of plastic is inserted into the empty lens capsular bag. With current methods the lens epithelium cannot be removed completely. Reactive proliferation of the remaining lens epithelium *always* occurs. The resulting *secondary cataract* can be considered the product of a wound healing process of the lens epithelium and often requires a non-mechanical YAG-laser capsulotomy to reestablish a clear axis of the optic media (see Chapter 5.5). All attempts to avoid secondary cataract would require removal of *all* lens epithelial cells. This, however, may interfere with a reliable fixation of the lens implant and/or its haptic.

Other examples of altered tissue are those in the *trabecular meshwork* for chronic open angle glaucomas (see Chapter 5.2), *opacities of the cornea* from hereditary dystrophies or acquired as a consequence of infectious or non-infectious inflammation causing scar formation (see Chapter 5.1). In 1905 Zirm demonstrated that the corneal obstacle to vision can be removed and replaced by a clear corneal graft – achieving the first successful and today by far the most often performed human tissue transplantation.

2.1.4
Displaced Tissue

Most commonly the retina or the lens is involved.

Detachment of the sensory retina used to be a cause of irreversible blindness until 1916, when Gonin showed that closure of the *retinal defect* can achieve a cure.

Anatomical variations explain the *locations of "minor resistance"* for detachment of the sensory retina:

"*Ora slit*": In the pre-equatorial area the photoreceptors are only rudimentary and cannot achieve the usual interdigitation between the processes of the pigment epithelium and the outer segments of rods. As a result the adhesion is relatively weak predisposing to separation. This explains why rhegmatogenous retinal detachments usually start in the equatorial region following traction from the anteriorly displaced vitreous body, creating a retinal defect at its base.

"*Foveola slit*": The outer segments of foveolar cones – unlike rods, do not develop the relatively tight interdigitation with the processes of the foveolar pigment epithelium. This predisposes the macular region to the common "disciform" separation of the sensory retina from the RPE.

The sensory retina can also be displaced by *traction* from preretinal granulation tissue – retinopathy proliferans – particularly with diabetes mellitus or after traumatic vitreal hemorrhage (see Chapters 5.6, 6.1).

Dislocation of the clear lens may occur after blunt trauma, or with metabolic defects like homocystinuria or Marfan syndrome. As this may seriously disturb the optical axis, it may require removal of a clear lens (see Chapter 5.5).

More subtle displacements of the lens develop with the frequently overlooked *pseudoexfoliation syndrome,* which is a generalized disorder of the extracellular matrix. The zonular instability caused by this process leads to *phacodonesis* and an increased incidence of vitreous loss during extracapsular cataract surgery and its consequences (see Chapters 5.5, 5.6, 6.3).

2.1.5
Neovascularization and Scars

Intraocular neovascularization most often originates (1) either from the retinal vessels – always toward the vitreous, never to the outer layer of the sensory retina, or (2) from the choriocapillaris beyond Bruch's membrane under the RPE, never to the outer choroidal layer (Fig. 2.1).

The process of *preretinal* vascularization into the vitreous, originating from the retinal vessels, is the cause of *retinopathia proliferans* particularly in diabetes mellitus, Eales and sickle-cell disease. Angiogenic factors originating from the hypoxic retina initiate also neovascularization of the ciliary body – *cyclitic membranes* – or on the surface of the iris – *rubeosis iridis*. As long as the basic metabolic and angiogenic pathology in diabetes mellitus is not sufficiently understood, prevention of proliferative retinopathy remains unsatisfactory. The disturbing excessive scar tissue can be removed by pars plana vitrectomy (see Chapter 5.6).

Subretinal neovascularization originating from the choriocapillaries is the irreversible feature of so-called *age related disciform macular degeneration*.

Scars do not only follow mechanical or non-mechanical trauma, but also inflammatory processes in the cornea, iris, anterior chamber, vitreous and in the border zone between the sensory retina and vitreous or RPE and choroid.

After trauma and intraocular surgery, restoration of the anterior chamber must achieve access to the surface of the trabecular meshwork in an open angle. This is essential to prevent scar formation between Fuchs' roll of the iris and the trabecular meshwork, causing irreversible anterior synechiae and angle closure glaucoma. With current microsurgical methods adhesions

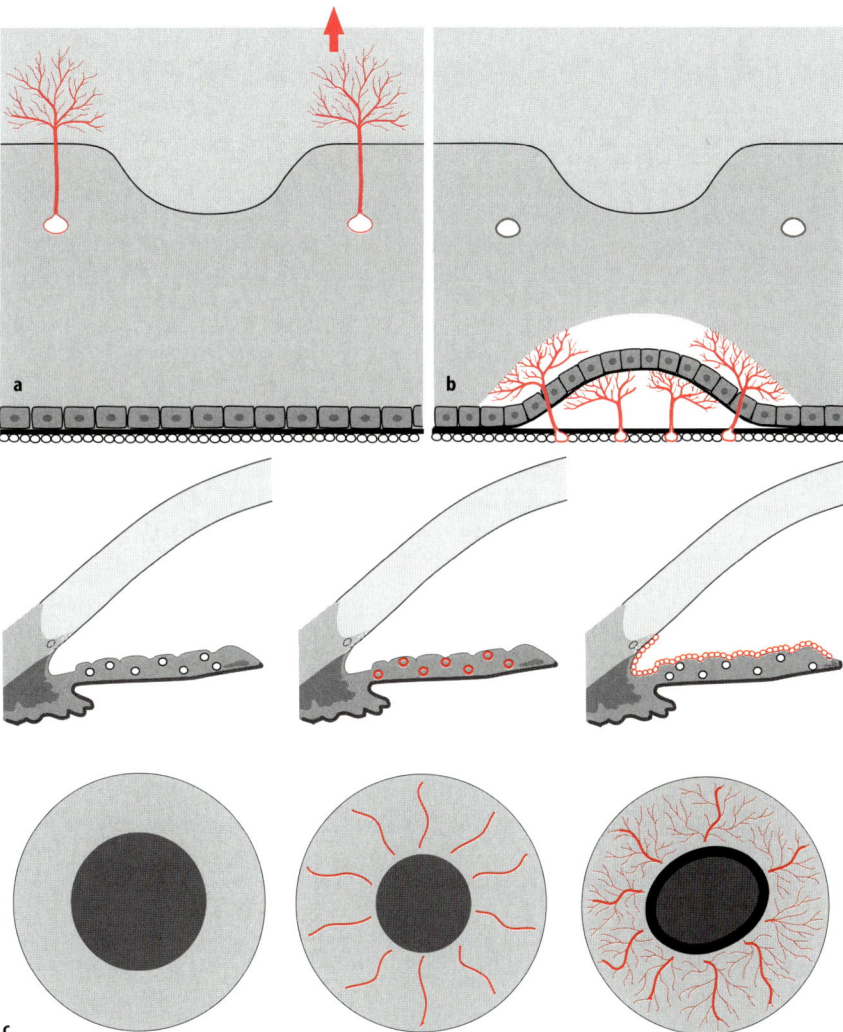

Fig. 2.1. Intraocular neovascularization. **a** Retinopathia proliferans originating from the retinal vessels reaching into the vitreous. **b** Choroidal neovascularization originating from the choriocapillary reaching below the retinal pigment epithelium and sensory retina. **c** Rubeosis iridis (*right*) in comparison to hyperemia (*middle*) and normal iris vascularization

following loss of the anterior chamber can only be separated within the first hours and days. In later stages vascular fibrotic scars within the trabecular meshwork become irreversible even after the angle is opened mechanically.

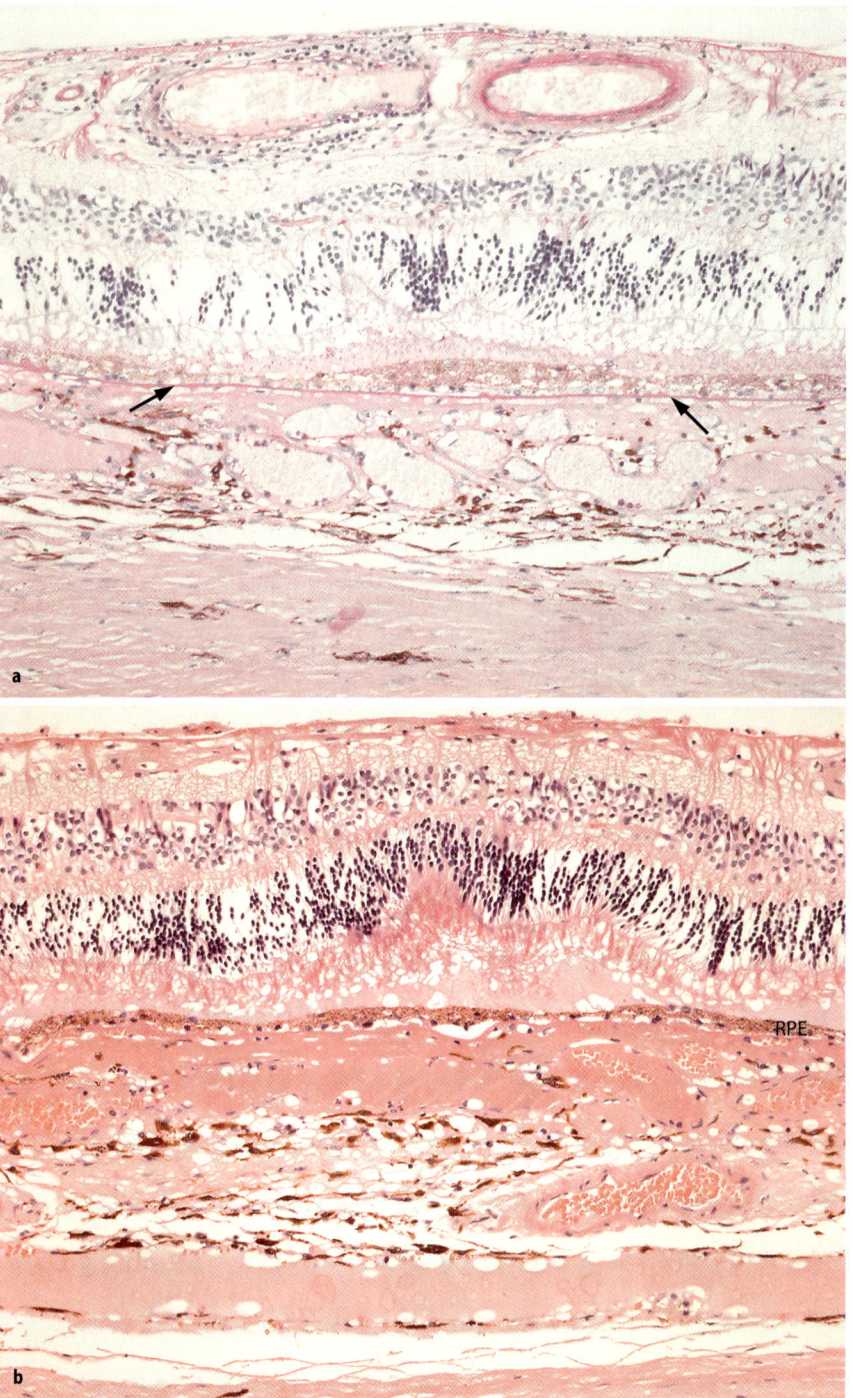

Fig. 2.2. Choroidal and retinal changes with ocular hypotony due to anterior segment trauma with wound leakage. **a** Early uveal effusion: hyperemia of choroidal vessels and exudation with retinal periphlebitis Bruch membrane (*arrow*) (PAS). **b** Pronounced exudation and thickening, retinal folds. Retinal pigment epithelium (RPE)

2.2 Intraocular Compared with Extraocular Surgery: Distinguishing Features and Potential Complications

Extraocular surgery of lid, orbit and the epibulbar procedures not opening the intraocular space take into consideration the special surgical anatomy and pathology, but otherwise follow the same pattern as in general surgery in the various organs of the body (see Chapter 3).

Intraocular microsurgery with an opening in the eye wall alters the peculiar equilibrium of the tissues and spaces within the eye (Fig. 2.2, 2.3, 2.4). The normal function of the eye depends on some special features (Table 2.1): (1) blood-ocular barriers in analogy to the *blood-brain barrier*; (2) *avascularity* of the cornea, anterior chamber, lens and vitreous in order to maintain

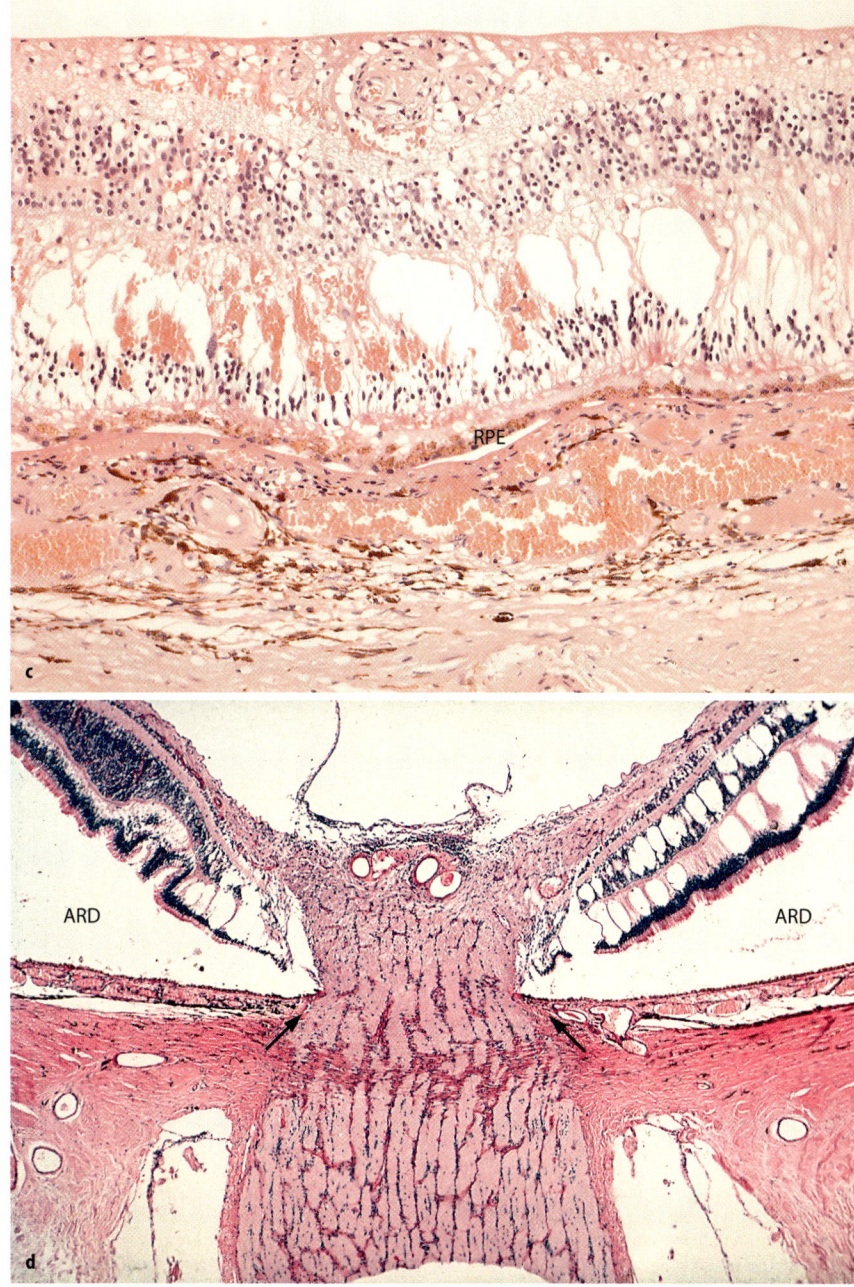

Fig. 2.2. c Beginnings of choroidal hemorrhage, cystoid changes and hemorrhage into the outer retinal layers.
d Papilledema, retinal folds, and cystoid alteration of the outer and inner plexiform layers of the sensory retina 10 weeks after perforating injury with wound leakage. Notice thin sclera behind Elschnig's spur (*arrow*). Retina arteficially detached (ARD) (PAS)

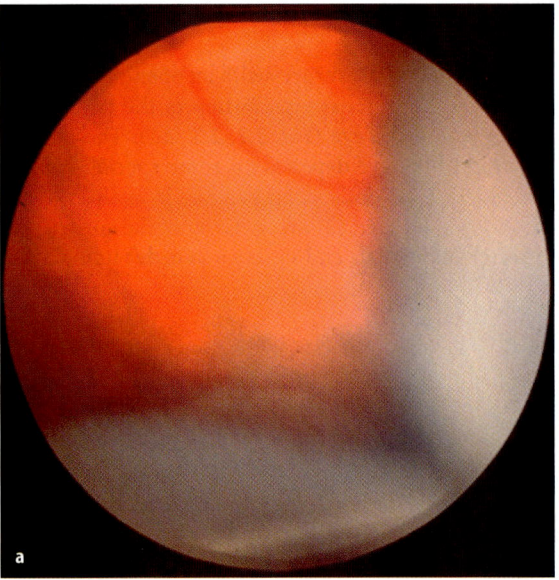

optical transparency; (3) localization of all vascularized tissues in a thin layer inside the wall of the eyeball, clearing a broad transparent zone around the optical axis; and (4) *increased tissue* pressure in comparison to other organs, keeping the optical surfaces of the cornea smooth and the alignment of the photoreceptors in the proper direction – modified by the foveal stretch steered by the ciliary muscle (historic term "musculus tensor chorioideae").

The following is a brief discussion of the special risks of any open eye microsurgery (Table 2.2).

Ocular hypotony and its immediate consequences are also outlined in the following points.

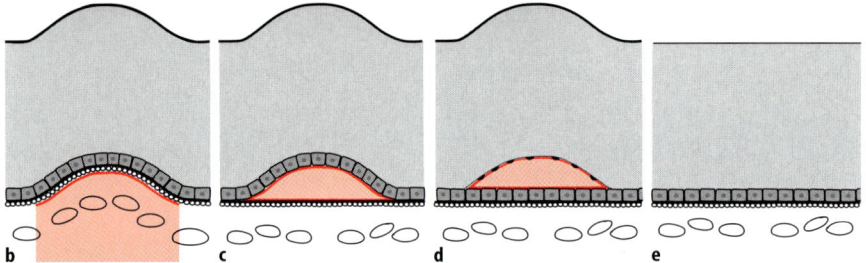

Fig. 2.3. a Choroidal detachment following filtering procedure with hypotony. **b–e** Differential diagnosis of choroidal edema: **b** True choroidal edema. **c** Detachment of retinal pigment epithelium. **d** Detachment of sensory retina with retinal "precipitates." **e** Normal state

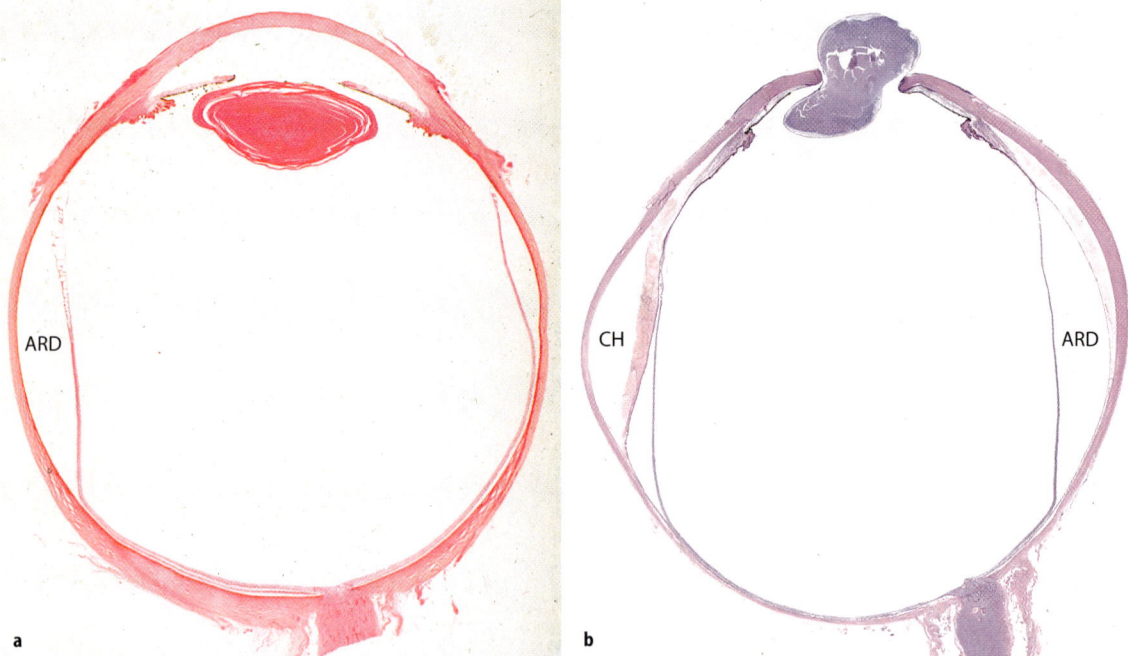

Fig. 2.4. Progression of choroidal detachment and hemorrhage in prolonged ocular hypotony syndrome following anterior segment trauma and aqueous leakage. **a** Horizontal section through normal eye (autopsy), artificial detachment of the retina. **b** Choroidal detachment and beginnings of hemorrhage between scleral spur and region behind the equator (*CH*) after perforating necrotizing keratitis with subluxation of the lens into the defect of the cornea (PAS), arteficial retinal detachment (*ARD*)

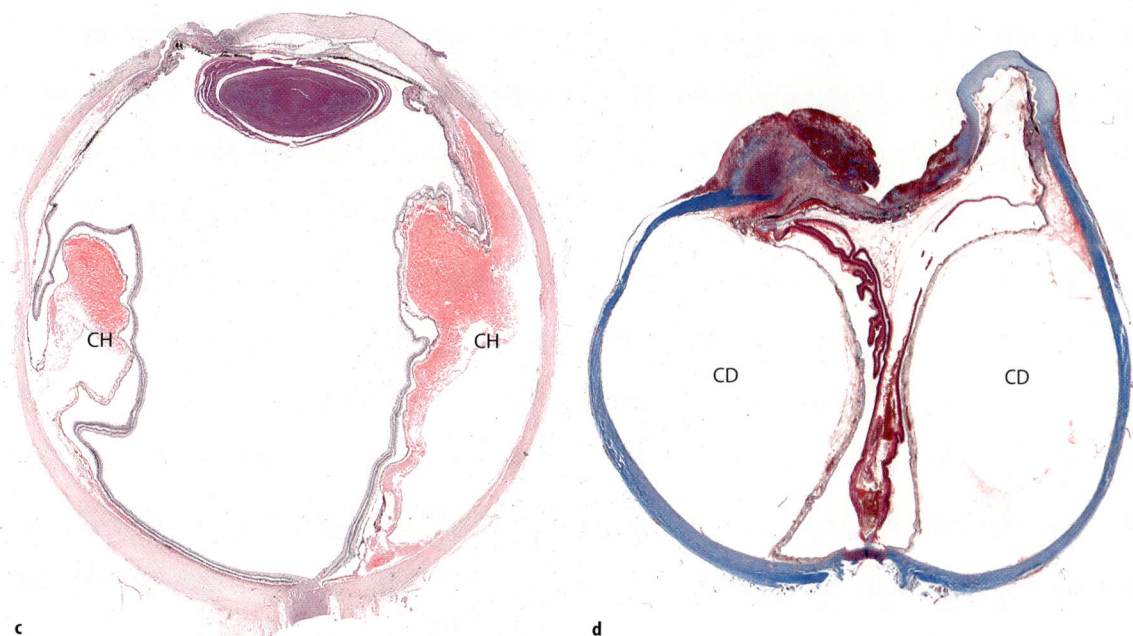

Fig. 2.4 (*cont.*) **c** Choroidal hemorrhage between scleral spur and optic nerve and collateral retinal detachment after necrotizing keratitis with perforation. **d** Almost total choroidal detachment (*CD*). Choroid with retinal detachment touching each other in the center of the eye (MASSON)

Table 2.2. Special risks of "open eye" microsurgery

1. Forward motion of iris-lens diaphragm: "vis a tergo" (Fig. 2.5)
2. Paracentesis effect: blood-aqueous barrier breakdown (Fig. 2.6)
3. Expulsive choroidal hemorrhage (Fig. 2.7)
4. Pupillary and ciliary block angle closure (Fig. 2.8)
5. Infectious endophthalmitis, acute with bacteria, subacute with fungi (Fig. 2.9)
6. Sympathetic uveitis
7. Diffuse and cystic epithelial ingrowth (Fig. 2.11–2.13)
8. Hemorrhage from vasoproliferative processes (Fig. 2.1)
9. "Toxic anterior segment syndrome" (TASS)
10. "Intraoperative floppy iris syndrome" (IFIS)

2.2.1
Anterior Movement of the Iris-Lens Diaphragm ("Vis a Tergo")

Any opening of the anterior chamber with loss of aqueous moves the iris-lens diaphragm forward. It is also mobile during intravitreal manipulation. Opening of the anterior chamber with leakage of aqueous always induces an *acute ocular hypotony*. Increased filling of the blood vessels of the posterior uvea, combined with uveal effusion, acts as an engine to push the retina, vitreous and the iris-lens diaphragm forward (Fig. 2.5).

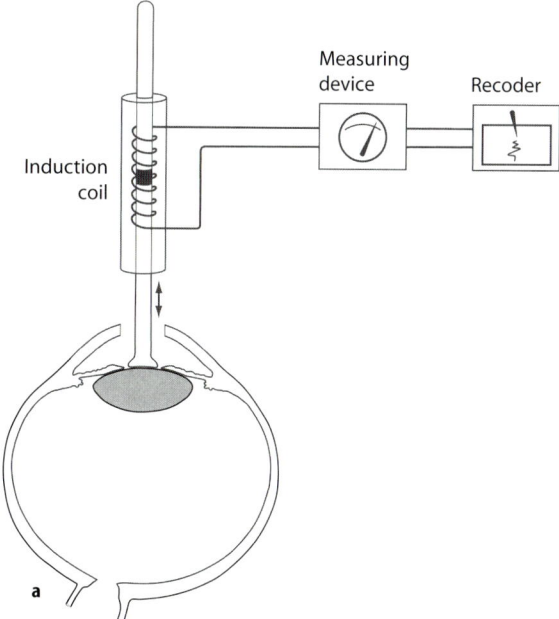

Fig. 2.5. Lens-iris diaphragm moving forward by uveal hyperemia and effusion ("vis a tergo"): During open eye surgery the mean arterial blood pressure is an important factor determining the location of the iris-lens diaphragm within the eye. Microincisions of the cornea and "positive pressure" in the anterior chamber reduce the risk of protrusion. **a** Device for measuring the movement of the iris-lens diaphragm in the cat after wide open corneal trephination (Heuser and Gieler, 1979)

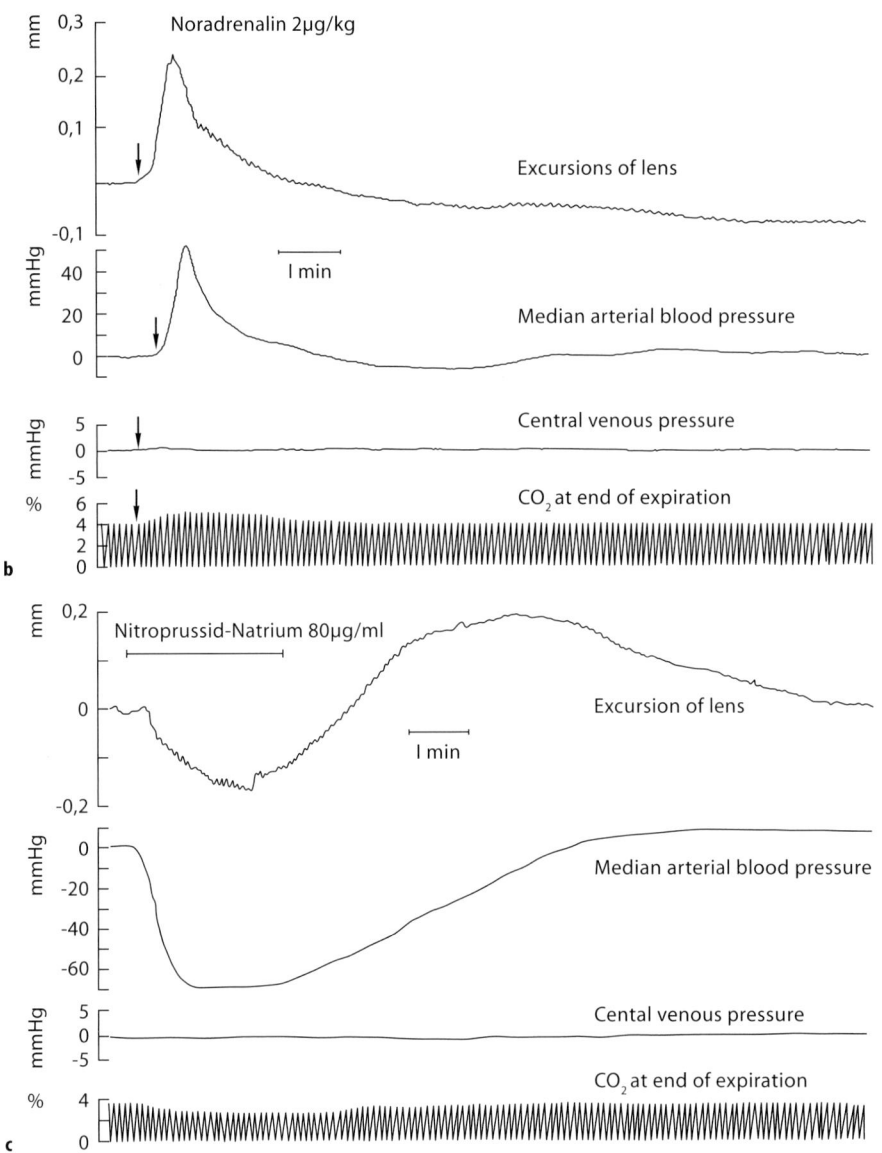

Fig. 2.5. b Movement of iris lens from forward with artificial increase of arterial blood pressure by adrenaline. **c** Lowering of the arterial blood pressure by sodium nitroprusside makes the iris-lens diaphragm move backward into the eye. The motor for anterior or posterior movement of the iris-lens diaphragm is the filling of the choroidal vessels and "uveal effusion" (Gieler and Heuser 1979)

The degree of blood filling of the choroidal vessels in the "open eye" depends on the mean arterial blood pressure. This process can be reduced by lowering the arterial and venous blood pressure and/or exerting "positive pressure" (Blumenthal) in the anterior chamber, e.g., by infusion and working in an almost "closed system."

Self-sealing cornea wound architecture achieves quick tamponade of tiny incisions in the cornea and minimizes the effects of acute ocular hypotony and paracentesis – but in principle both always occur temporarily. However, squeezing of the anterior chamber, e.g., by lid specula, may be followed by aspiration of fluid from the ocular surface ("gulp phenomenon"), particularly if located in the lidfissure increasing the risk of postoperative endophthalmitis (see 2.2.5 and Chapter 5.5).

2.2.2
Paracentesis Effect

Breakdown of the blood-ocular barriers (Fig. 2.6): A hyperemia of all intraocular vessels and a breakdown at the *blood-aqueous barrier* is associated with any *acute ocular hypotony*: the non-fenestrated endothelial layer of the iris capillaries and the zonulae occludentes of the ciliary body open up and permit a leakage of serum proteins into the tissue and posterior and anterior chamber: This can be measured in vivo by laser tyndallometry. The plasmoid aqueous reduces the transparency and increases the risk of iris-synechia. A lowering of intraocular pressure also affects the zonulae occludentes of the blood-retinal barrier in the RPE (Verhoeff's membrane) and those of the retinal capillaries:

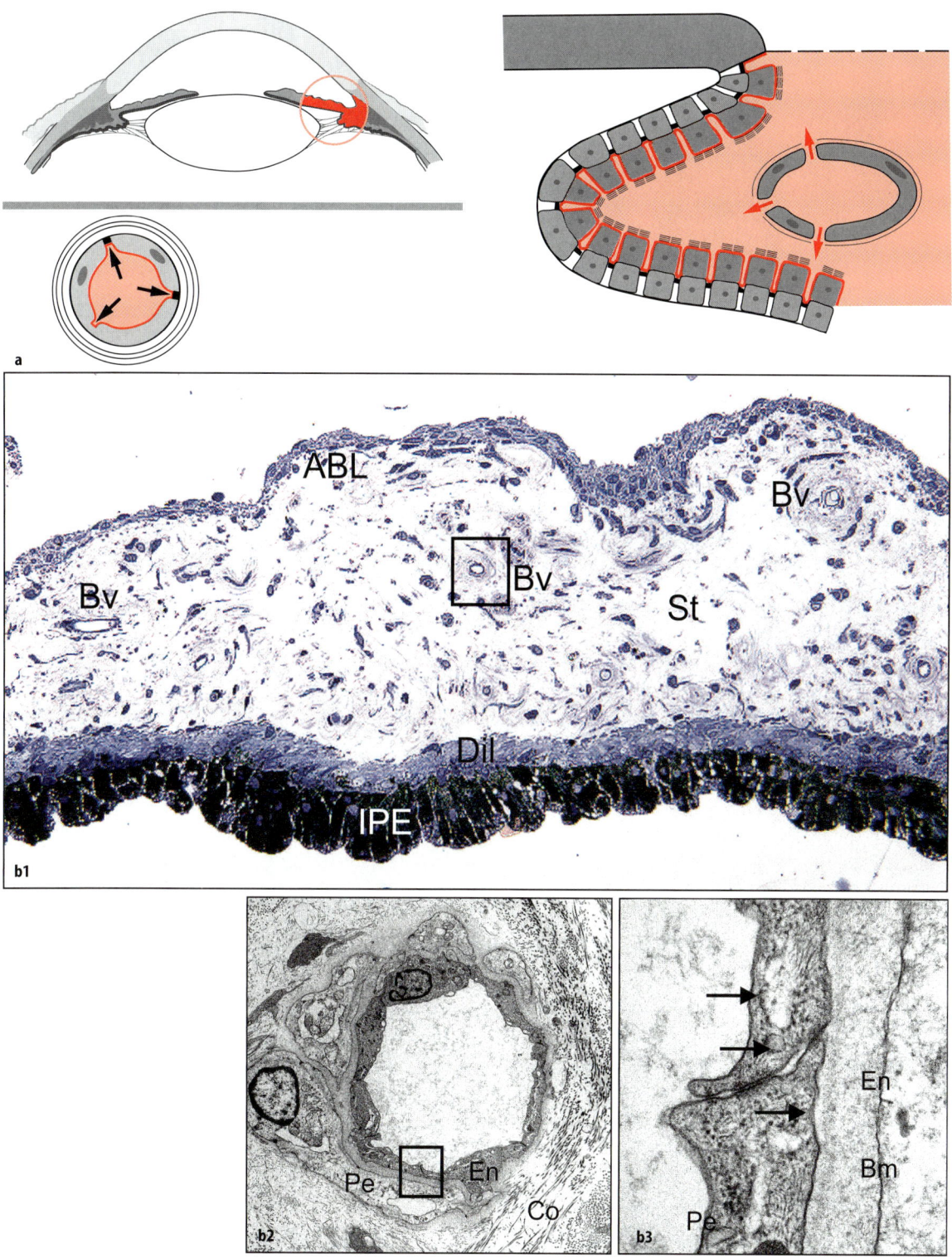

Fig. 2.6. Blood-ocular barrier breakdown ("paracentesis effect"): leakage of serum proteins into the aqueous and vitreous through the defect barrier. **a Blood-aqueous barrier:** unfenestrated endothelium lines the iris vessels and zonula occludentes close to the non-pigmented ciliary epithelium. **b Blood-aqueous barrier of the iris. b1** Semithin section of iris (*ABL* anterior border layer, *Bv* blood vessel, *Dil* dilator muscle, *IPE* iridal pigment epithelium, *St* stroma). **b2** Electron micrograph of iridal blood vessel (*Co* perivascular collagen fibers, *En* endothelium, *Pe* pericytes). (Courtesy of U. Schlötzer-Schrehardt, 2007), **b3** Detail of **b1** showing tight junctions between endothelial cells (*arrows*) (*Bm* basement membrane, *En* endothelium, *Pe* pericyte)

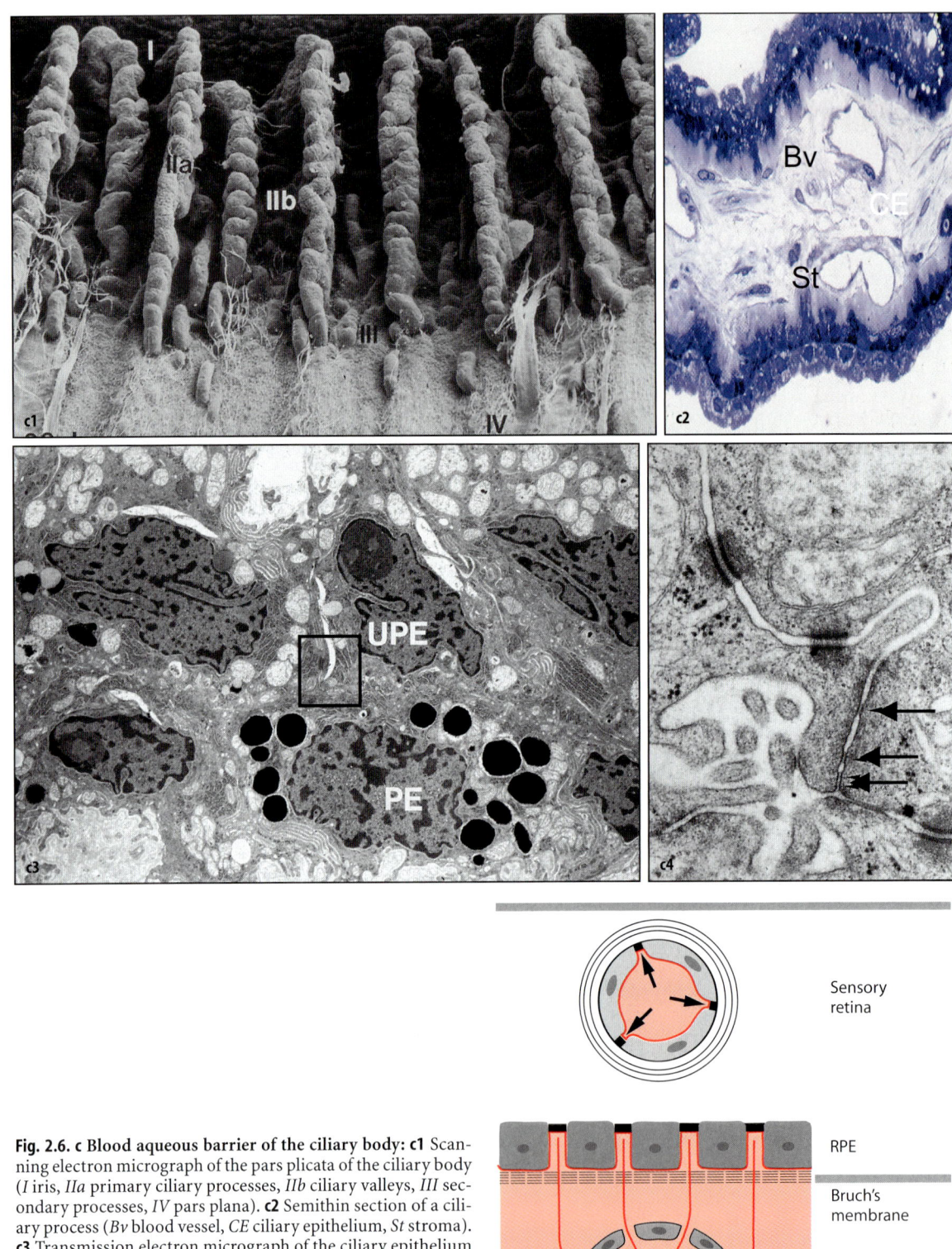

Fig. 2.6. c Blood aqueous barrier of the ciliary body: c1 Scanning electron micrograph of the pars plicata of the ciliary body (*I* iris, *IIa* primary ciliary processes, *IIb* ciliary valleys, *III* secondary processes, *IV* pars plana). **c2** Semithin section of a ciliary process (*Bv* blood vessel, *CE* ciliary epithelium, *St* stroma). **c3** Transmission electron micrograph of the ciliary epithelium with pigmented (*PE*) and unpigmented (*UPE*) layers. **c4** Detail of **c3** showing tight junctions (*arrows*) between unpigmented epithelial cells. **d Blood-retinal barrier:** non-fenestrated endothelium lining of the retinal capillaries and zonula occludentes of the retinal pigment epithelium (Verhoeff's membrane)

breakdown of the *blood-retinal barrier*: "*Physiologic defects*" of the blood-ocular barriers are recognizable in the transition of iris root to ciliary body and at the optic disc margin (see Chapter 5.7).

After reliable closure of the wound in the eye wall, blood-ocular barrier breakdown is reversible in hours, days or weeks. Cystoid maculopathy (see 4.7, and 5.6).

2.2.3
Expulsive Choroidal Hemorrhage and Uveal Effusion

Acute or chronic persisting ocular hypotony occurs if defective wound healing of the entrance results in an external fistula or cyclodialysis causes excessive uveal scleral outflow. Both acute and chronic *ocular hypotony* initiate an *uveal effusion* and can lead to an *expulsive hemorrhage* originating from a tear in the posterior ciliary artery entering into the choroidal vessels (Fig. 2.2, 2.3, 2.4, 2.7). The risk of this catastrophe is increased with high arterial blood pressure and in high myopes, where the ciliochoroidal vasculature is attenuated (Fig. 2.7). In nanophthalmus the scleral wall is thickened; this may block the outflow via the vortex veins and accelerate an uveal effusion (see above, Chapter 4.6).

2.2.4
Pupillary and Ciliary Block

Pupillary and ciliary block with acute and delayed secondary angle closure glaucoma can be the consequence of defective wound healing (see Chapter 5.2) (Fig. 2.8).

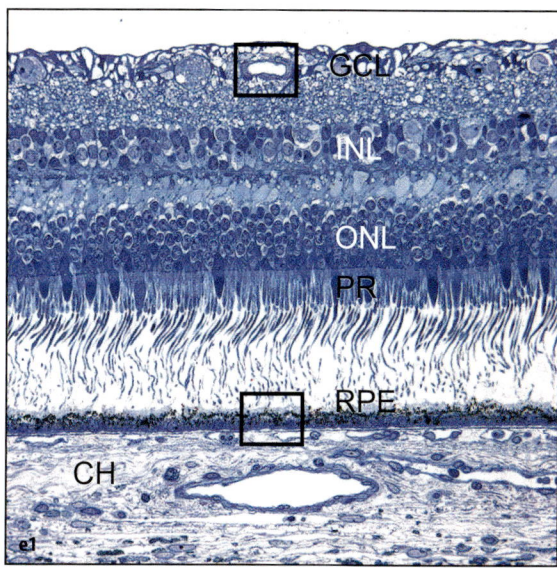

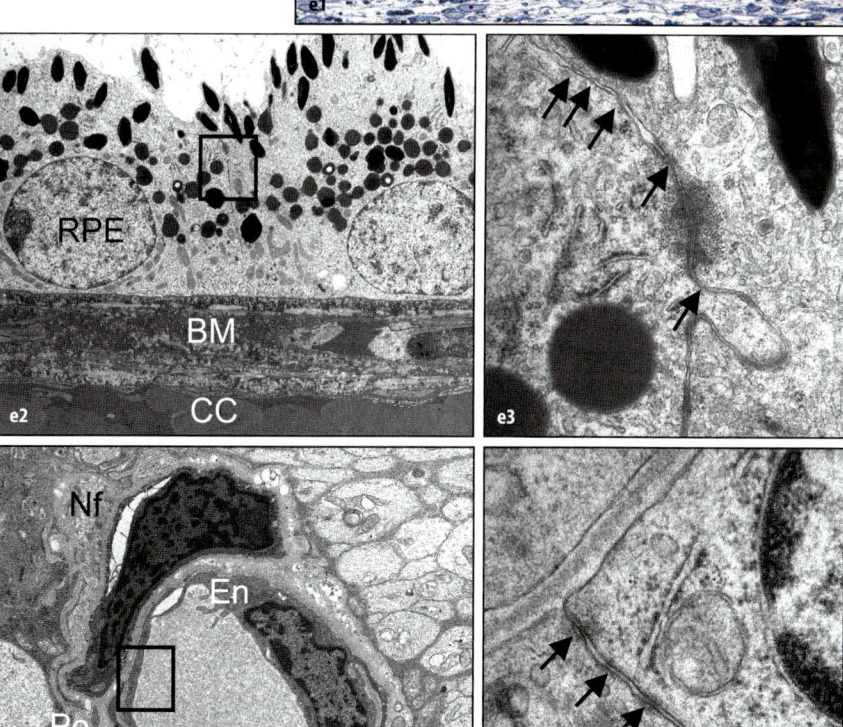

Fig. 2.6. e Blood-retinal barrier: **e1** Semithin section of the retina (*CH* choroid, *GCL* ganglion cell layer, *INL* inner nuclear layer, *ONL* outer nuclear layer, *PR* photoreceptor layer, *RPE* retinal pigment epithelium). **e2** Electron micrograph of the retinal pigment epithelium (*RPE*) (*BM* Bruch's membrane, *CC* choriocapillaris). **e3** Detail of **e2** showing tight junctions (*arrows*) between retinal pigment epithelial cells. **e4** Retinal capillary (*En* endothelium, *Nf* nerve fibers, *Pe* pericyte). **e5** Detail of **e4** showing tight junctions (*arrows*) between endothelial cells (**b–d** Courtesy of U. Schlötzer-Schrehardt 2007)

2 General Ophthalmic Pathology

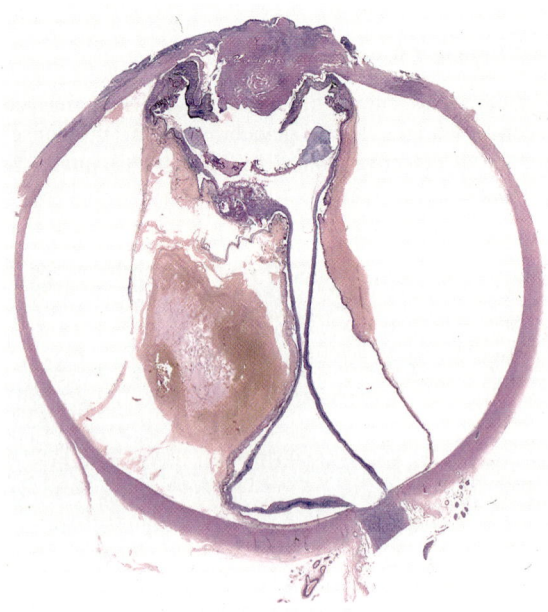

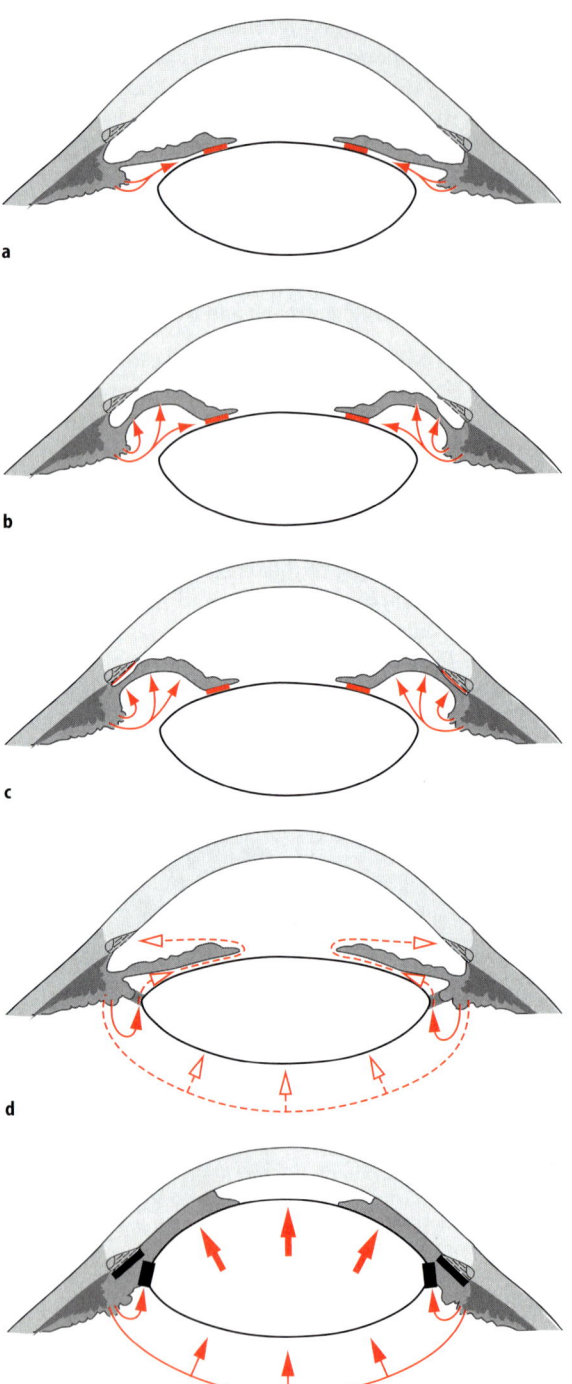

Fig. 2.7. Expulsive choroidal hemorrhage: The uveal effusion is associated with every phenomenon of vis a tergo particularly in young patients with arterial hypertension, and may induce a tear in the posterior ciliary vessels at the inner sclera entering the choroid. The resulting choroidal hemorrhage leads to a ballooning of the choroid filling the entire intraocular space and pushing the tissues of retina, lens, and iris into the wound opening anteriorly (PAS)

▷
Fig. 2.8. Pupillary and ciliary block leading to angle closure glaucoma: **a** Normal anterior chamber. **b, c** Pupillary *block* obstructs flow from the posterior into the anterior chamber by increased contact between the pupillary iris with the anterior lens capsule or, rarely, from luxation of the lens in the anterior chamber. This obstruction is increased by viscosity of the aqueous fluid, by paracentesis effect and hemorrhage. In pupillary block the position of the lens is unchanged; only the peripheral anterior chamber is occluded by the iris. **d, e** Ciliary block means obstruction of aqueous flow from the retrolental space into the posterior and anterior chamber. The contact between the ciliary body and muscle with the equator of the lens misdirects aqueous toward the vitreous, pushing the lens forward. With the forward position of the lens there is shallowing also of the central anterior chamber

2.2.5
Purulent Endophthalmitis

Theoretically every opening of the eye wall is at risk of an acute (bacterial) or chronic (mycotic) infection or inflammation. Acute infections are potentially devastating because of the small dimensions and irreversible damage (Fig. 2.9) particularly after foreign body entrance (Fig. 2.10).

In a recent interventional case series from the Wilmer Institute, it was shown that an inflow of extraocular fluid into the anterior chamber occurs *frequently* after phacoemulsification via a sutureless 2.8-mm corneal incision even after hydrosealing if located temporally. This aspiration may happen spontaneously and was observed after pressure release on the anterior chamber in *all* eyes! With minimal bleeding from the limbal capillaries this could easily be illustrated (Taban et al., 2005). In spite of all attempts at anti-infectious prophylaxis, the ciliae and glands located at the lid margins cannot be made completely free of bacterial coloniza-

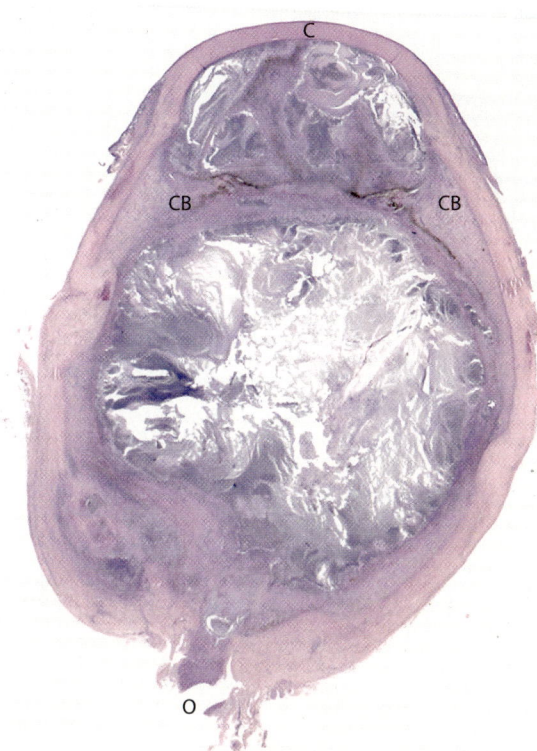

Fig. 2.9. Purulent panophthalmitis may result from exogenous inflow of bacteria or fungi or endogenously from hematogenic sepsis. All intraocular tissues are involved. *Bacterial* endophthalmitis usually follows an acute course and is characterized by diffuse leukocytic infiltration of the vitreous. *Mycotic* endophthalmitis usually develops endogenously subacutely or chronically from a retinitis septica Roth or infected infusion fluid with multiple microabscesses. Optic nerve (*O*), Cornea (*C*), Ciliary body (*CB*) (PAS)

tion. Therefore it is not surprising that at the end of the procedure bacteria can be detected in the anterior chamber aqueous in about 30% of all patients after extracapsular cataract extraction (Linda Ficker). We must assume that mechanisms exist to eliminate these minimal but common usually subclinical bacterial infections.

The rate of postoperative endophthalmitis following intraocular microsurgery apparently can be reduced by prophylactic intracameral antibiotics (see also chapter 5.5 and Lundström et al., 2007).

2.2.6
Sympathetic Uveitis

Even with meticulous microsurgical techniques the catastrophe of a bilateral sympathetic uveitis cannot be excluded with certainty in intraocular microsurgery – although the incidence today is extremely low. It has even been observed following a surgical iridectomy with a small corneoscleral incision. One hundred years ago sympathetic uveitis after perforating ocular injury occurred so frequently that early enucleation of the traumatized eye was recommended as a prevention.

2.2.7
Diffuse and Cystic Epithelial Ingrowth

Diffuse and cystic epithelial ingrowth cannot be totally excluded following punctures or extensive wounds in the cornea, or the corneoscleral or conjunctivoscleral region (Fig. 2.11–13). Rarely a non-penetrating wound in the corneal limbus may induce an extensive deep conjunctival epithelial lined cyst containing mucus-producing goblet cells, procing a sedimented horizontal level.

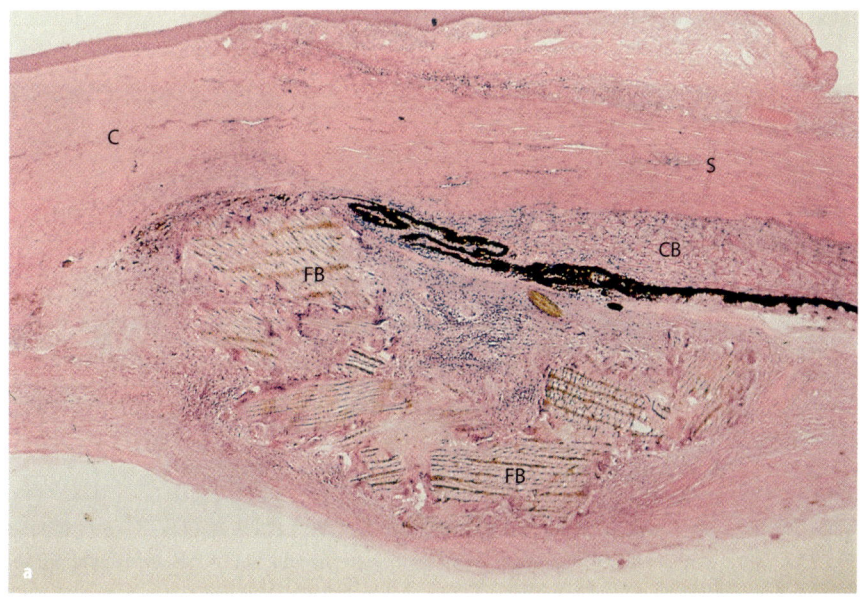

Fig. 2.10. a Intraocular foreign body granuloma due to intraocular wooden foreign body (*FB*). Cornea (*C*), Sclera (*S*), Ciliary body (*CB*)

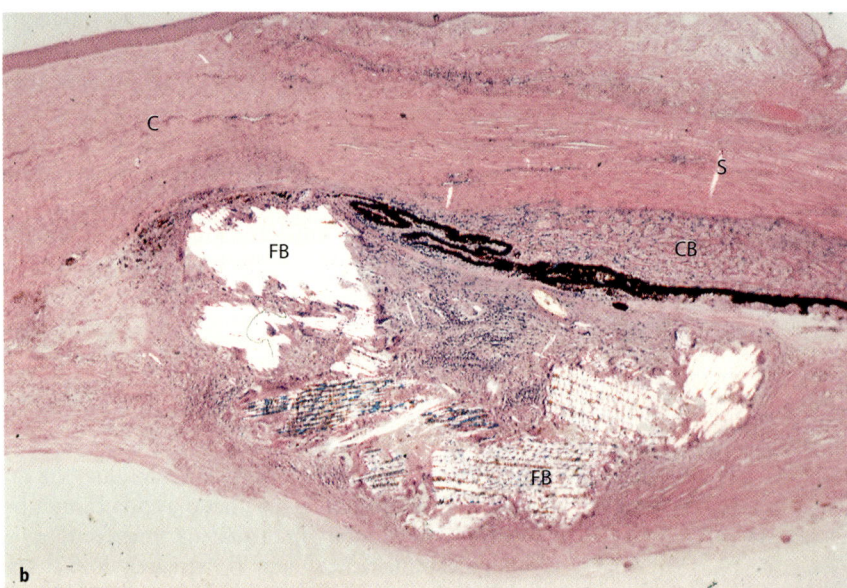

Fig. 2.10. b Polarized light

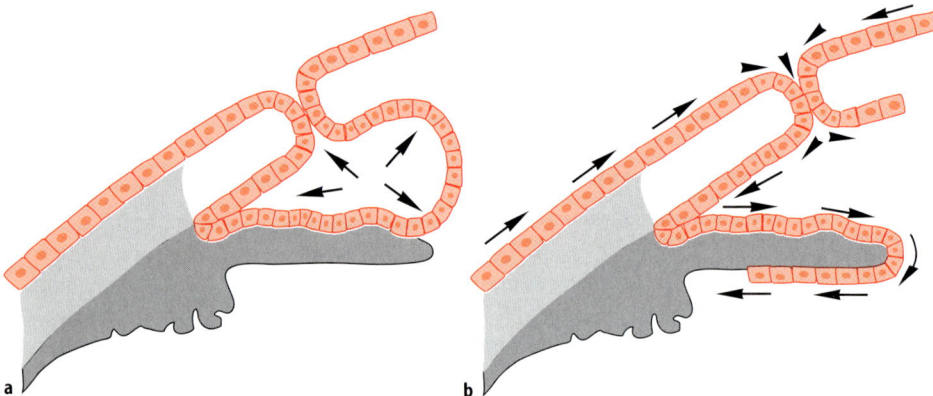

Fig. 2.11. Epithelial downgrowth or ingrowth. **a** Cystic type: Epithelial strands between surface epithelium and intraocular cyst usually not visible in histologic section. **b** Diffuse type usually outlining the anterior chamber but also extending around the pupil into the vitreous base

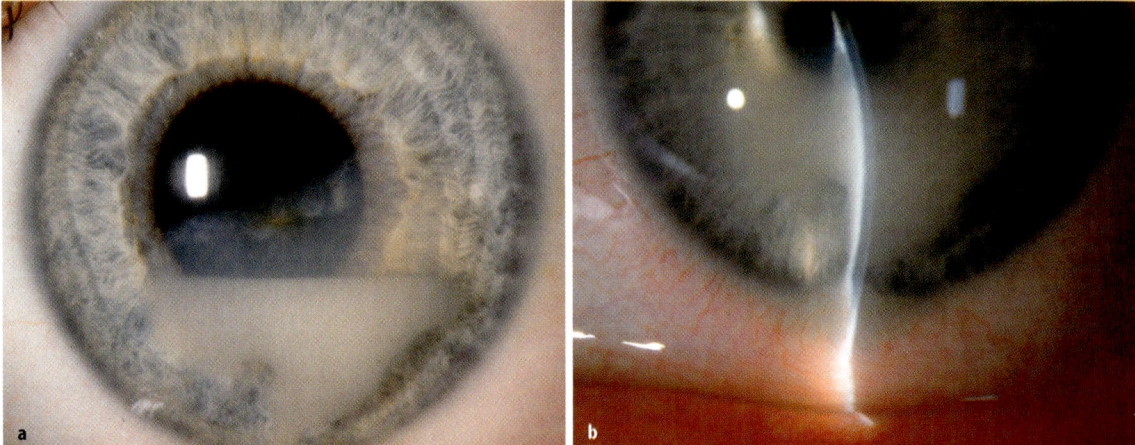

Fig. 2.12. Cystic epithelial ingrowth in the deep corneal stroma anterior to Descemet's membrane. **a** Slit lamp showing sedimented mucus with horizontal level. **b** Extension into the superficial sclera layers

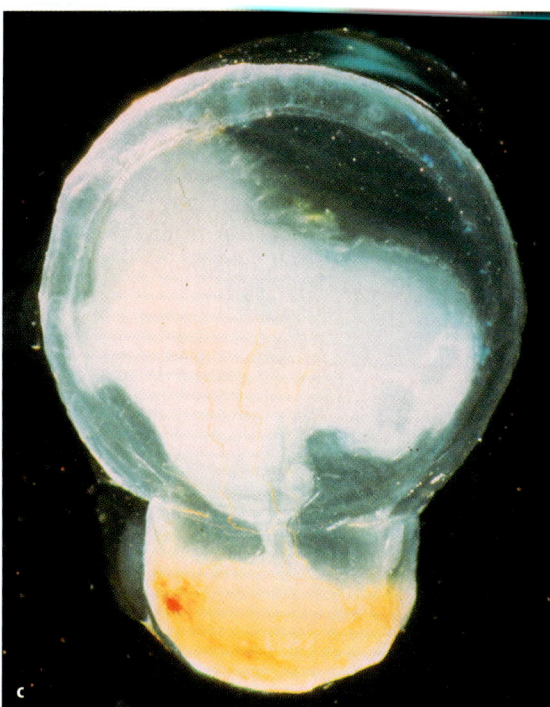
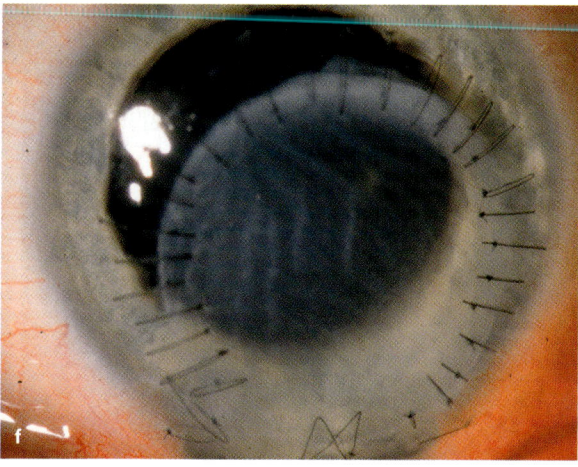

Fig. 2.12. c Excised cyst together with adjacent cornea and sclera. **d, e** Cyst lined by surface epithelium (Masson stain). **f** Corneoscleral defect closed by corresponding corneal graft (see also Chapters 5.3, 5.4)

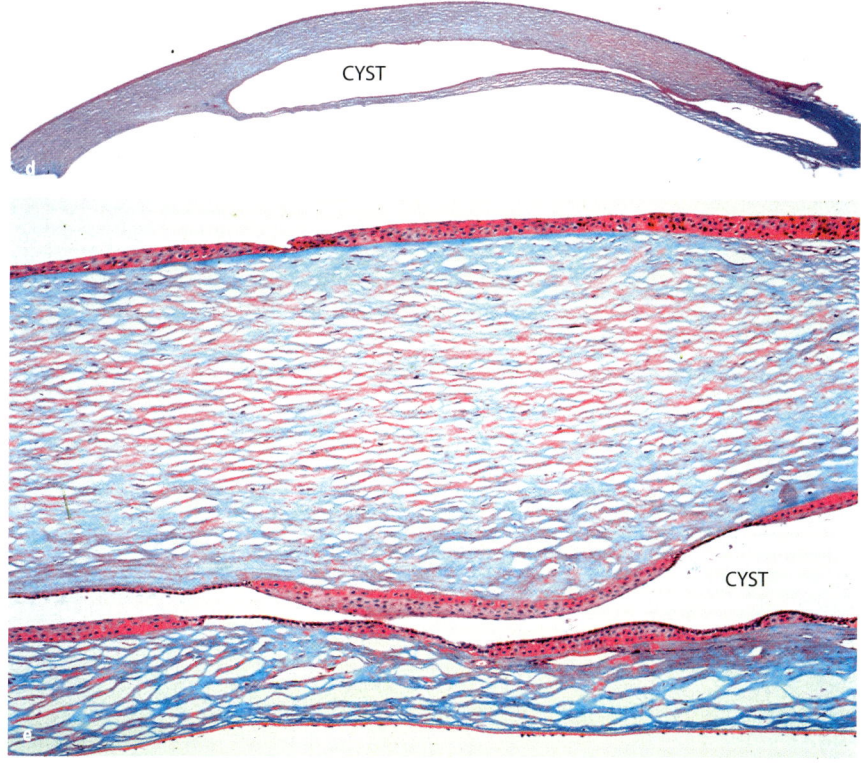

2.2.8
Hemorrhage from Vasoproliferative Processes

Hemorrhage from vasoproliferative processes (Table 2.2) into the anterior chamber and/or vitreous cavity is seen in retinopathia proliferans, cyclitic membranes and rubeosis iridis, which are all induced by a chronic focal or diffuse hypoxia of the retina or a localized trauma to the iris, ciliary body or retina (see Chap-

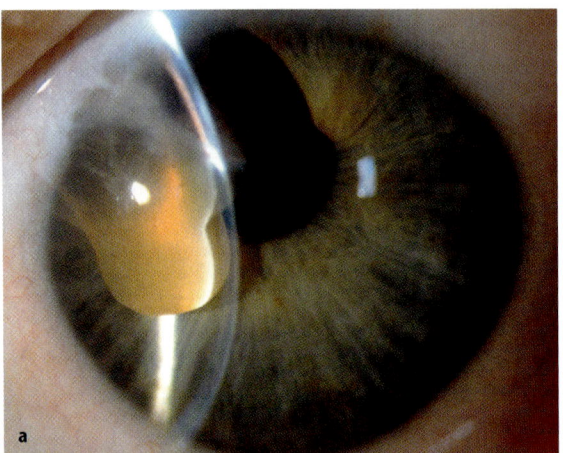

2.2.10
"Intraoperative Floppy Iris Syndrome" (IFIS)

Patients receiving systemic alpha-blocking medication develop dysfunction of the dilator muscle of the iris. This causes risks for the iris during anterior segment surgery. In extracapsular cataract surgery this can be compensated for by mechanical mydriasis, e.g., iris hooks (Chang and Campbell, 2005; Schwinn and Afshari, 2005) (see chapter 5.5).

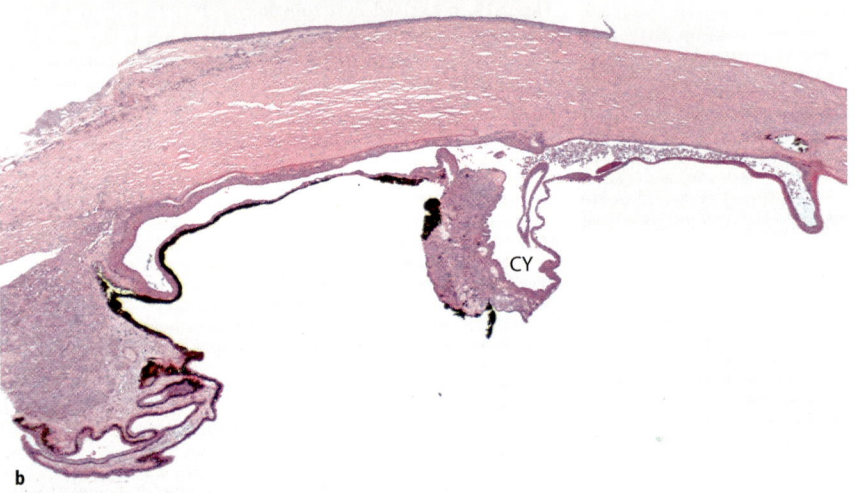

Fig. 2.13. a–b Cystic epithelial ingrowth at iris root and ciliary body following perforating trauma in a 40-year-old female patient. **a** Cyst contains mucoid and cellular debris forming a level (*CY*). **b** Complete removal of cyst with adjacent ciliary body, iris, scleral, and cornea in one piece as block excision (PAS-stain), followed by tectonic graft

ter 5.6). It is not reversible by medical therapy. As the newly formed intraocular capillary neovascularization is *fenestrated*, the leakage of serum proteins into the "plasmoid aqueous" may be very pronounced – particularly after opening the eye (Fig. 2.14–2.16).

2.2.9
"Toxic Anterior Segment Syndrome" (TASS)

Unsuitable intraocular irrigation fluid, e.g., toxic substances, pathologic osmotic concentrations, may cause catastrophic damage to tissue bordering the anterior chamber – or vitreous – resembling ischemic anterior segment necrosis! This is not an infectious process, but endotoxins from bacteria after sterilization may play a role (see also Mamalis et al., 2006).

▷
Fig. 2.14. Retinopathia proliferans – vitreoretinopathy. **a** Advanced retinopathia proliferans extending into the vitreous causing hemorrhage and a traction – detachment of the retina (RD), exudate subretinally, angle closure from rubeosis iridis. Lens arteficially subluxated

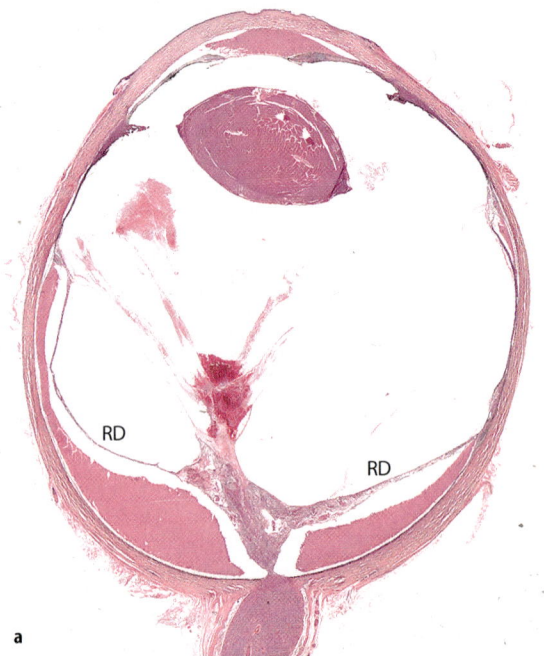

Fig. 2.14. b End stage retinopathia proliferans with total retinal detachment (*RD*), choroidal detachment (*CD*), choroidal hemorrhage (*CH*), cyclitic membrane (*CM*), massive rubeosis iridis with angle closure. Encircling episcleral implant (*EI*)

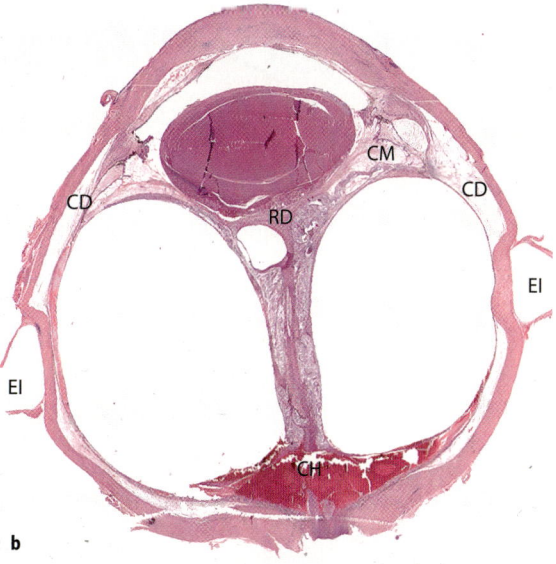

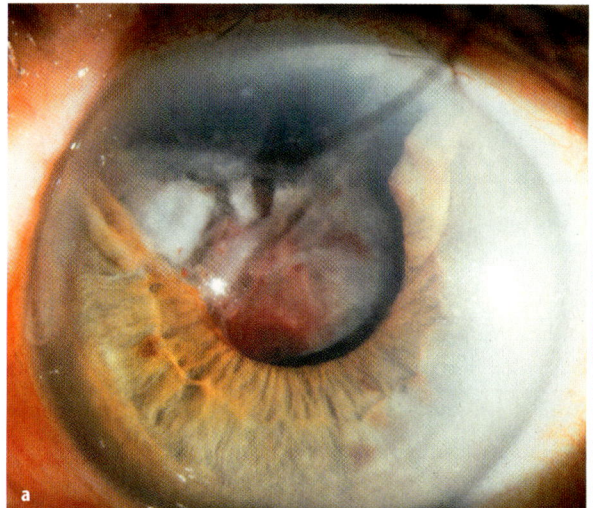

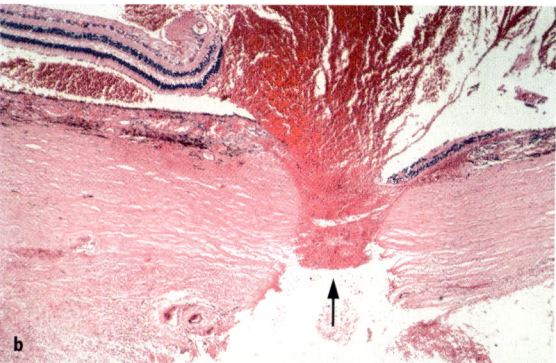

Fig. 2.15. Hemorrhage into the vitreous. **a** After attempted cataract extraction with surgical sector coloboma in a 96-year-old female patient with pseudoexfoliation syndrome. **b** Originating from perforating wounds of anterior segment and posterior sclera (*arrow*).

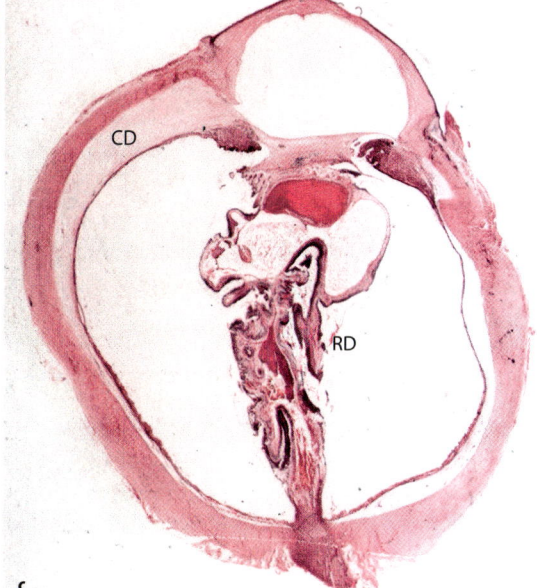

c Atrophy of the globe after traumatic aphakia, vitreal hemorrhage and total detachment

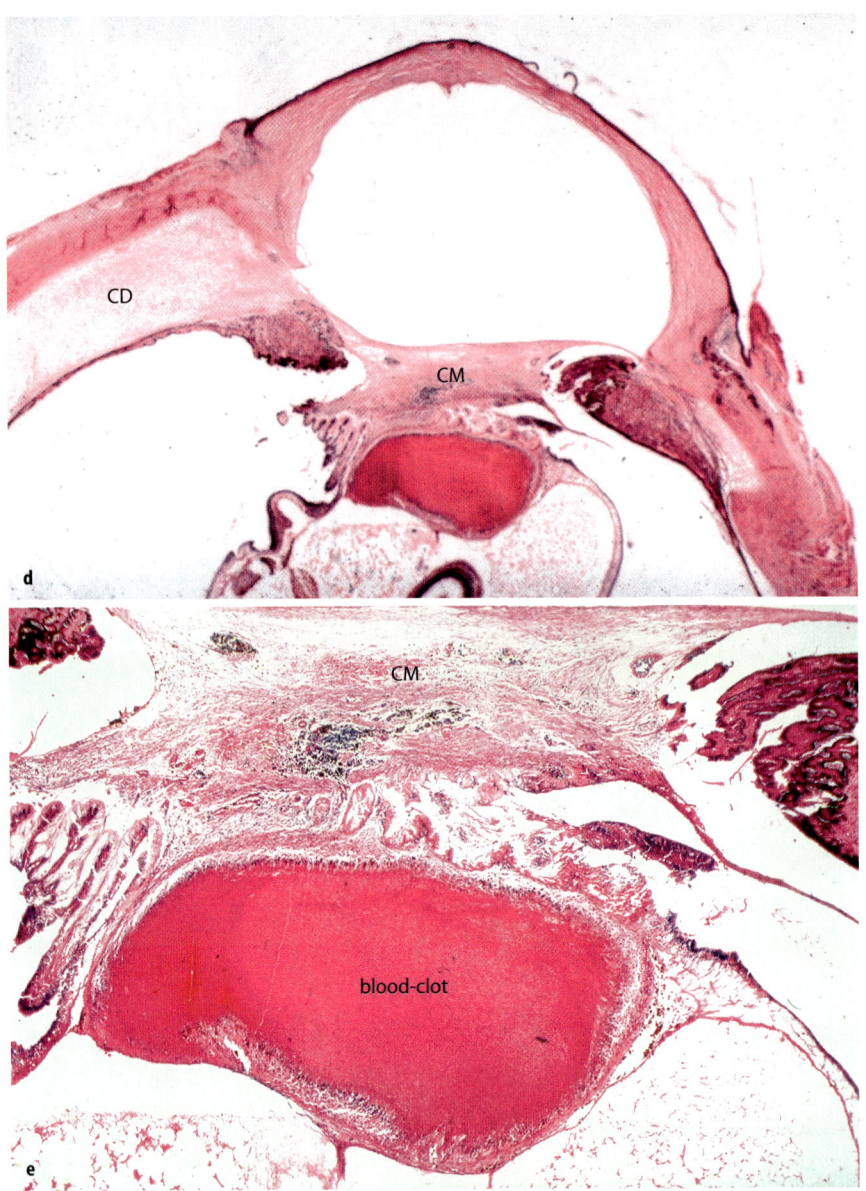

Fig. 2.15c–d "Endophthalmitis hemogranulomatosa." Choroidal detachment (*CD*), cyclitic membrane (*CM*) (PAS). **e** Higher power revealing traction on the ciliary processes. Granulomatous inflammation around blood clot. Haemosiderin in CM

2.3
Choice of Anesthesia and Knowledge of Ophthalmic Pathology

Most intraocular microsurgery today is done using local anesthesia. However, there are indications for general anesthesia – aside from the necessity in children – in the following situations. (1) preoperative *open eye*: perforating corneal trauma, or ulcers; (2) *very thin sclera*, e.g., scleral staphyloma: large globe in buphthalmus and high myopes; and (3) patients with an *only eye*. Local anesthesia today frequently is done with epibulbar drops and gels. However, if local anesthesia with parabulbar or retrobulbar injection is considered, the theoretical risk of scleral perforation by periocular needle injection cannot be totally neglected.

In analogy to severe contusion, scleral perforation occurs most easily at the three "*loci minores resistentiae*" of the sclera (Fig. 2.16, 2.17): (1) between the scleral spur and Schwalbe's line at the limbus cornea, (2) at the equator of the eye, where the sclera is thinnest underneath the insertion of the straight rectus muscles, (3) at the exit of the optic nerve through the lamina cribrosa, and (4) immediately adjacent to the optic disc margin in front of the insertion of the meninges of the optic nerve and Elschnig's scleral rim. A thin sclera is often associated with large globes such as in buphthalmus or high myopia (> 26 mm optical axis). Scleral thinning is also evident as staphyloma following scleritis, blunt

2.3 Choice of Anesthesia and Knowledge of Ophthalmic Pathology

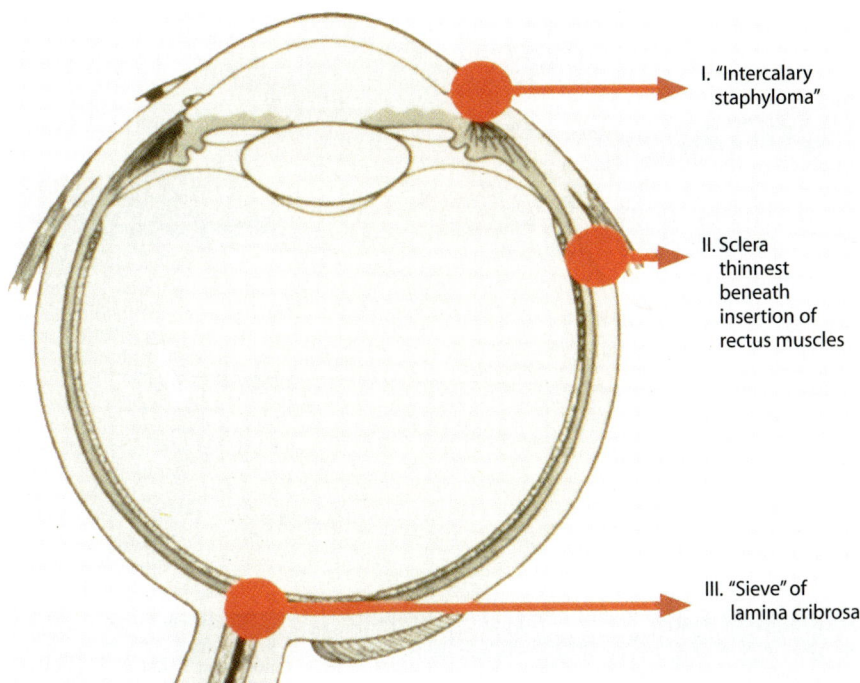

I. "Intercalary staphyloma"

II. Sclera thinnest beneath insertion of rectus muscles

III. "Sieve" of lamina cribrosa

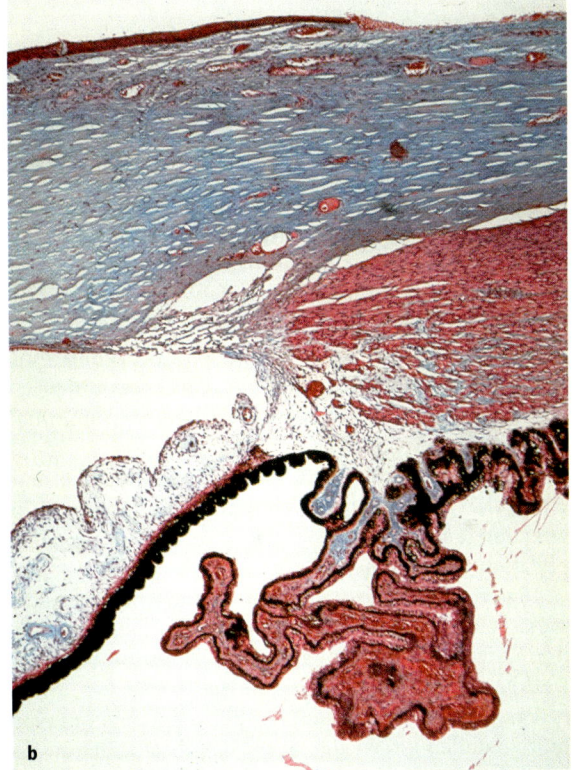

Fig. 2.16. Region of minor persistence in the biomechanics of the eye wall at limbus, insertion of straight muscles and in the optic disc region. **a** Overview. **b** Region of the limbus between peripheral edge of Bowman's layer, Schwalbe's line, scleral spur, Schlemm's canal and collector channel weakening the resistance of the scleral tissue (MASSON).

trauma and incomplete rupture of the globe, cryocoagulation or diathermy of the ciliary processes to reduce aqueous inflow or as part of retinal detachment surgery. Small caliber needles with sharp tips more easily engage with and perforate the sclera. Pronounced obesity makes orientation around the globe more demanding. Uncooperative patients present special difficulties for microsurgery with local anesthesia.

Complications of local anesthesia in ocular microsurgery may be more common than is evident from the literature. If peribulbar needle injections are done at the 12 and 6 o'clock positions adjacent to the globe, the risk of injuring the sclera is increased, because the distance from the orbital wall to the eye wall is smallest here (Fig. 2.18).

Comparing the advantages and disadvantages of local and general anesthesia (Table 2.3), we conclude that the type of local or general anesthesia we recommend to our patients must be carefully and individually considered. The advantages of local anesthesia are obvious; however, in certain selected situations general anesthesia may present an option to benefit our patients (Table 2.4). The responsibility for advice as regards choice of anesthesia lies with the ophthalmologists in close cooperation with the anesthesiologists, who always monitors the intraoperative systemic situation.

Table 2.4. Potential indications for general anesthesia

1. Children
2. "Wide open eye": perforated trauma, perforated corneal ulcers, penetrating keratoplasty, block excisions, direct surgery of ciliary body
3. Thin sclera – large globe: buphthalmus, high myopia (>26 mm), scleral staphyloma
4. Clotting defects and arterial hypertension
5. "Oculus ultimus"
6. Choice of patient (cost)

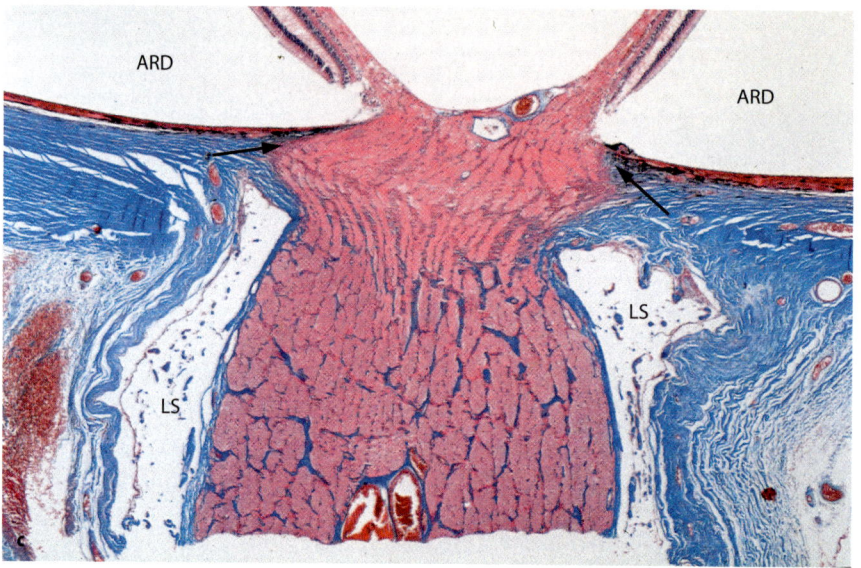

Fig. 2.16. c Weakness at the margin of the optic disc, Elschnig's spur (*arrow*): (1) lamina cribrosa with exit of axons and (2) juxtapapillary sclera between scleral spur and liquor space (*LS*). The sclera here is only half as thick as the rest of the sclera. Arteficial retinal detachment (*ARD*). MASSON-stain

Table 2.3. Advantages and disadvantages of local and general anesthesia

	Local anesthesia injection	Anesthesia with drops	General anesthesia
Advantages	Costs low Outpatient surgery	Costs low Speed	"Open eye"; thin sclera – large globe
Disadvantages	Residual risks: Perforation by needle Arterial emboli Hemorrhage	Mobile eye Residual pain	Costs high Oculocardial reflex Old age?

Although regional anesthesia appears at first glance convenient, the patient population often suffers severe comorbidity, making the perioperative management challenging. Whether regional or general anesthesia is preferable should be discussed in advance, with both the patient and the anesthesiologist. General anesthesia provided by a dedicated anesthesiologist can provide a good framework in which to perform faultless surgery without undue haste. If regional anesthesia is chosen, the anesthesiologist must be available to stabilize cardiopulmonary function immediately if necessary (Ulrich Beese, MD, personal communication, 31.12.06).

Finally: all microsurgical interventions in and around the eye can theoretically result in complications. Patient counselling following the "4R rule" – Recognition, Regret, Responsibility and Remedy – requires knowledge of the ophthalmic pathology pre-, intra- and postoperatively!

2.4
Instrumentation and Physical Principles Are *not* the Subject of Our Book

Although microsurgical instrumentation and techniques are not the subject of this book, we shall present two exceptions to this rule: "non-mechanical trephination techniques for penetrating keratoplasty with the excimer laser along a metal mask" (Chapter 5.1) and "direct surgery of the ciliary body" (Chapter 5.4) because the ciliary body until recently was considered a taboo zone. Our own experience with procedures involving the ciliary body is encouraging if certain principles and limits are respected (see Chapter 4, "minimal eye" and Chapter 5.4).

The morphologic elements of ocular disease and particularly those that are relevant for microsurgery do not change significantly over time – except for the complication of newer procedures.

In contrast, the instrumentation and technology for most ocular microsurgical procedures are undergoing dramatic and revolutionary innovations almost on a weekly basis.

Particularly the miniaturization demands an ever more detailed knowledge of the details of structural – and functional – alterations that are the target "attacked" by new microsurgical tools using both mechanical and non-mechanical principles.

2.3 Choice of Anesthesia and Knowledge of Ophthalmic Pathology

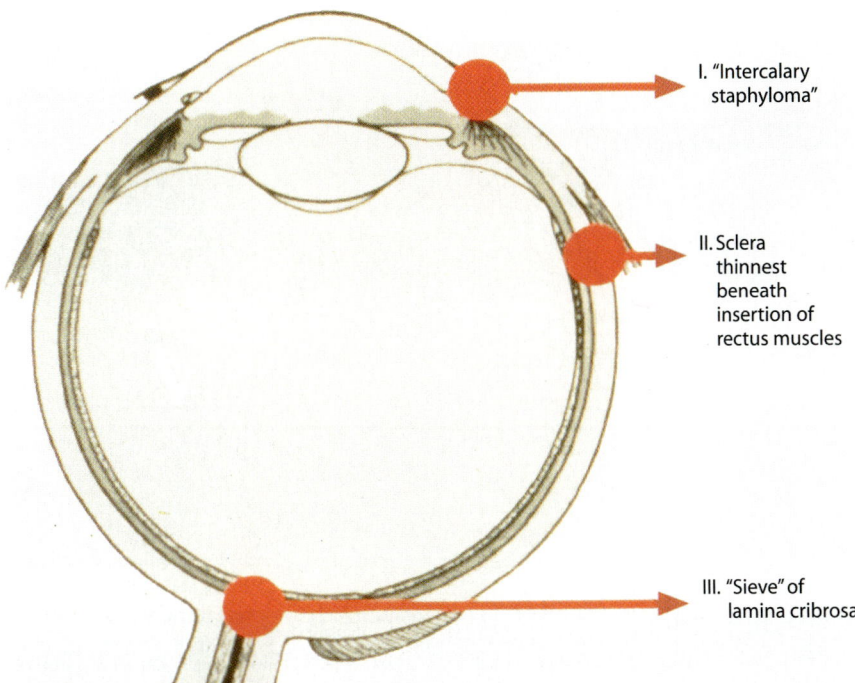

Fig. 2.16. Region of minor persistence in the biomechanics of the eye wall at limbus, insertion of straight muscles and in the optic disc region. **a** Overview. **b** Region of the limbus between peripheral edge of Bowman's layer, Schwalbe's line, scleral spur, Schlemm's canal and collector channel weakening the resistance of the scleral tissue (MASSON).

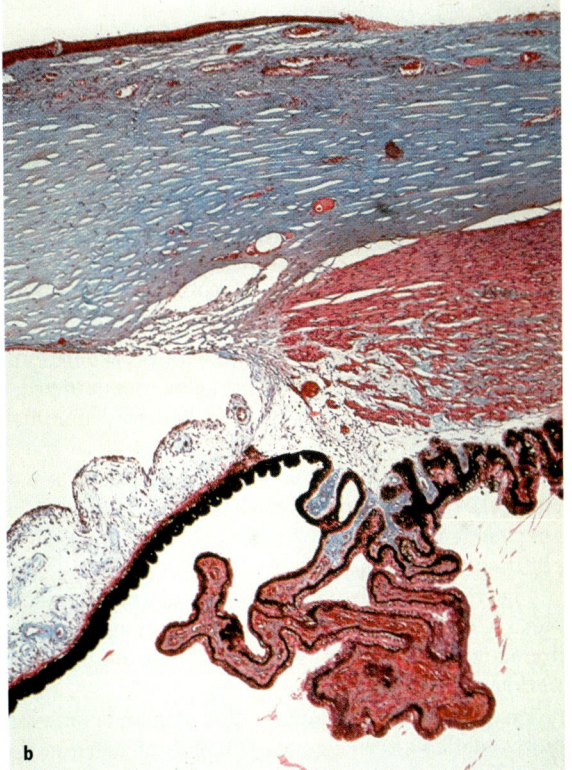

trauma and incomplete rupture of the globe, cryocoagulation or diathermy of the ciliary processes to reduce aqueous inflow or as part of retinal detachment surgery. Small caliber needles with sharp tips more easily engage with and perforate the sclera. Pronounced obesity makes orientation around the globe more demanding. Uncooperative patients present special difficulties for microsurgery with local anesthesia.

Complications of local anesthesia in ocular microsurgery may be more common than is evident from the literature. If peribulbar needle injections are done at the 12 and 6 o'clock positions adjacent to the globe, the risk of injuring the sclera is increased, because the distance from the orbital wall to the eye wall is smallest here (Fig. 2.18).

Comparing the advantages and disadvantages of local and general anesthesia (Table 2.3), we conclude that the type of local or general anesthesia we recommend to our patients must be carefully and individually considered. The advantages of local anesthesia are obvious; however, in certain selected situations general anesthesia may present an option to benefit our patients (Table 2.4). The responsibility for advice as regards choice of anesthesia lies with the ophthalmologists in close cooperation with the anesthesiologists, who always monitors the intraoperative systemic situation.

Table 2.4. Potential indications for general anesthesia

1. Children
2. "Wide open eye": perforated trauma, perforated corneal ulcers, penetrating keratoplasty, block excisions, direct surgery of ciliary body
3. Thin sclera – large globe: buphthalmus, high myopia (>26 mm), scleral staphyloma
4. Clotting defects and arterial hypertension
5. "Oculus ultimus"
6. Choice of patient (cost)

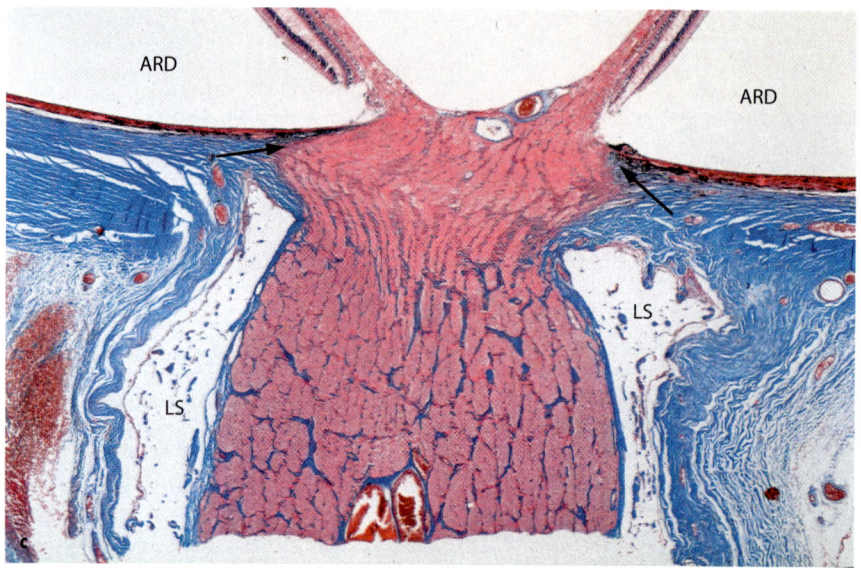

Fig. 2.16. c Weakness at the margin of the optic disc, Elschnig's spur (*arrow*): (1) lamina cribrosa with exit of axons and (2) juxtapapillary sclera between scleral spur and liquor space (*LS*). The sclera here is only half as thick as the rest of the sclera. Arteficial retinal detachment (*ARD*). MASSON-stain

Table 2.3. Advantages and disadvantages of local and general anesthesia

	Local anesthesia injection	Anesthesia with drops	General anesthesia
Advantages	Costs low Outpatient surgery	Costs low Speed	"Open eye"; thin sclera – large globe
Disadvantages	Residual risks: Perforation by needle Arterial emboli Hemorrhage	Mobile eye Residual pain	Costs high Oculocardiac reflex Old age?

Although regional anesthesia appears at first glance convenient, the patient population often suffers severe co-morbidity, making the perioperative management challenging. Whether regional or general anesthesia is preferable should be discussed in advance, with both the patient and the anesthesiologist. General anesthesia provided by a dedicated anesthesiologist can provide a good framework in which to perform faultless surgery without undue haste. If regional anesthesia is chosen, the anesthesiologist must be available to stabilize cardiopulmonary function immediately if necessary (Ulrich Beese, MD, personal communication, 31.12.06).

Finally: all microsurgical interventions in and around the eye can theoretically result in complications. Patient counselling following the "4R rule" – Recognition, Regret, Responsibility and Remedy – requires knowledge of the ophthalmic pathology pre-, intra- and postoperatively!

2.4
Instrumentation and Physical Principles Are *not* the Subject of Our Book

Although microsurgical instrumentation and techniques are not the subject of this book, we shall present two exceptions to this rule: "non-mechanical trephination techniques for penetrating keratoplasty with the excimer laser along a metal mask" (Chapter 5.1) and "direct surgery of the ciliary body" (Chapter 5.4) because the ciliary body until recently was considered a taboo zone. Our own experience with procedures involving the ciliary body is encouraging if certain principles and limits are respected (see Chapter 4, "minimal eye" and Chapter 5.4).

The morphologic elements of ocular disease and particularly those that are relevant for microsurgery do not change significantly over time – except for the complication of newer procedures.

In contrast, the instrumentation and technology for most ocular microsurgical procedures are undergoing dramatic and revolutionary innovations almost on a weekly basis.

Particularly the miniaturization demands an ever more detailed knowledge of the details of structural – and functional – alterations that are the target "attacked" by new microsurgical tools using both mechanical and non-mechanical principles.

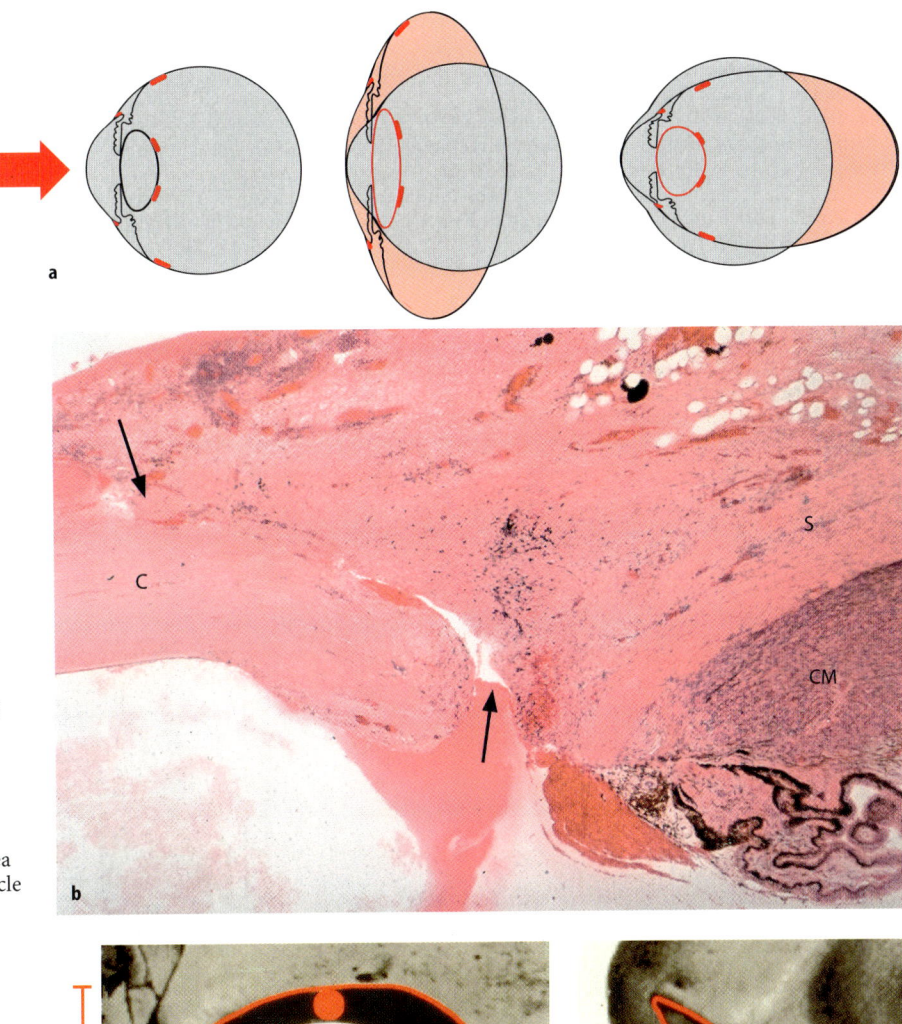

Fig. 2.17. a Deformation of globe with blunt trauma leading to defects in the weak areas shown in Fig. 2.16. **b** Rupture of the globe at the limbus from contusion (*arrows*). Cornea (*C*), sclera (*S*), ciliary muscle (*CM*)

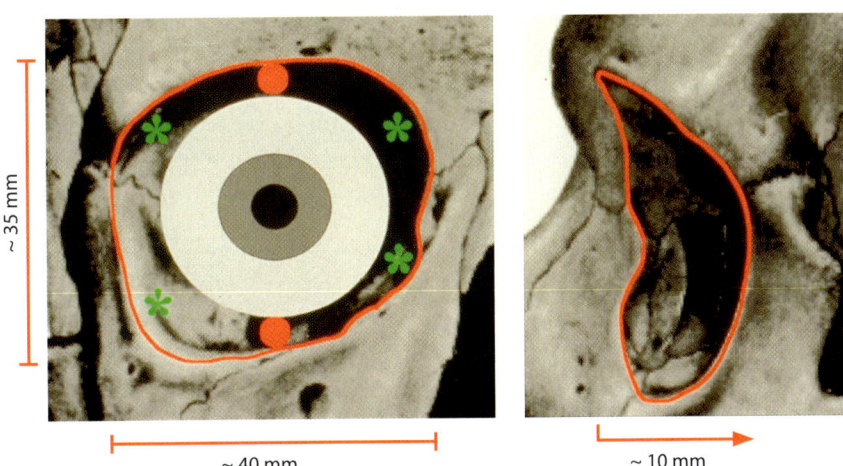

Fig. 2.18. Proximity of osseous orbital wall and globe: narrowest distance at 12 and 6 o'clock

References (see also page 379)

Berlinger NT. Robotic surgery – squeezing into tight places. N Engl J Med 2006; 354:2099

Bialasiewicz AA, Ruprecht KW, Naumann GOH. Staphylokokken-Endophthalmitis nach Schieloperation. Klin Monatsbl Augenheilkd 1990; 196: 86–88

Chang D, Campbell JR. Intraoperative Floppy Iris Syndrome (IFIS). J Cataract Refract Surgery 2005; 31:664–673

Gieler J, Heuser D. Verschiebungen des Iris-Linsen-Diaphragmas unter Einfluss vasoaktiver Pharmaka. Vorläufige Mitteilung tierexperimenteller Befunde. In Naumann GOH and Gloor B loc. cit.

Hellmund K, Frühauf A, Seiler T, Naumann GOH. Sympathische Ophthalmie 50 Jahre nach perforierender Verletzung. Eine Kasuistik Klin Monatsbl Augenheilkd 1998; 213: 182–185

Henke V, Naumann GOH, Gierth K. Intraokulare Operationen an "letzten" Augen (Bericht über 145 Eingriffe). Fortschr Ophthalmol 1988; 85: 385–389

Heuser D, Gieler J, Jehnichen R. Ein Verfahren zur kontinuierlichen Registrierung sagittaler Verschiebungen des Iris-Linsen-Diaphragmas im tierexperimentellen Modell. 1979. In Naumann GOH and Gloor B loc. cit.

Jonas JB, Holbach LM, Schönherr U, Naumann GOH. Sympathetic ophthalmia after three pars plana vitrectomies without prior ocular injury. Retina 2000; 20: 405–406

Meythaler FH, Naumann GOH. Direkte Optikus- und Retinaverletzung durch retrobulbäre Injektionen. Klin Monatsbl Augenheilkd 1987; 190: 201–204

Meythaler FH, Naumann GOH. Intraokulare ischämische Infarkte bei Injektionen in das Lid und parabulbär (ohne Bulbusperforation). Klin Monatsbl Augenheilkd 1987; 190: 474–477

Michelson G, Naujoks B, Ruprecht KW, Naumann GOH. Risikofaktoren für die vis a Tergo am "offenen Auge" bei Katarakt-Extraktionen in Lokalanästhesie. Fortschr Ophthalmol 1989; 86: 298–300

Naumann GOH and Gloor B (eds) Wound Healing of the Eye and its Complications, pp. 71–72; 73–75, Bergmann Verlag, München, 1980

Naumann GOH, Eisert S, Gieler J, Baur KF. Kontrollierte Hypotension durch Natrium-Nitroprussid bei der Allgemeinnarkose für schwierige intraokulare Eingriffe. Klin Monatsbl Augenheilkd 1977; 170: 922–925

Schwinn DA, Afshari NA. α1-Adrenergic Antagonists and Floppy Iris Syndrome: Tip of the Iceberg? Ophthalmology 2005; 112:2059–2060

Taban M, Behrens A, Newcomb RL, Nobe MY, Saedi G, Sweet PM, McDonnell PJ. Acute endophthalmitis following cataract surgery. Arch Ophthalmol 2005; 123:613–620

Völcker HE, Naumann GOH. Morphology of uveal and retinal edemas in acute and persisting hypotony. Mod Probl Ophthalmol 1979; 20: 34–41

Surgical Anatomy and Pathology in Surgery of the Eyelids, Lacrimal System, Orbit and Conjunctiva

L.M. Holbach

The eyelids, lacrimal system, orbit and conjunctiva play an important role in the protection and function of the eyes. Many diseases altering the structure or function of the eyelids, conjunctiva, lacrimal system and/or orbit threaten vision.

3.1 Eyelids

L.M. Heindl, L.M. Holbach

3.1.1 Surgical Anatomy

The anterior eyelid lamella includes the skin and orbicularis muscle (Fig. 3.1.1).

The eyelid skin is the thinnest in the body measuring less than 1 mm in thickness. The *upper eyelid skin crease* is located 6–10 mm from the lash line in an adult. It is due to the insertion of the levator aponeurosis into the orbicularis muscle at the superior border of

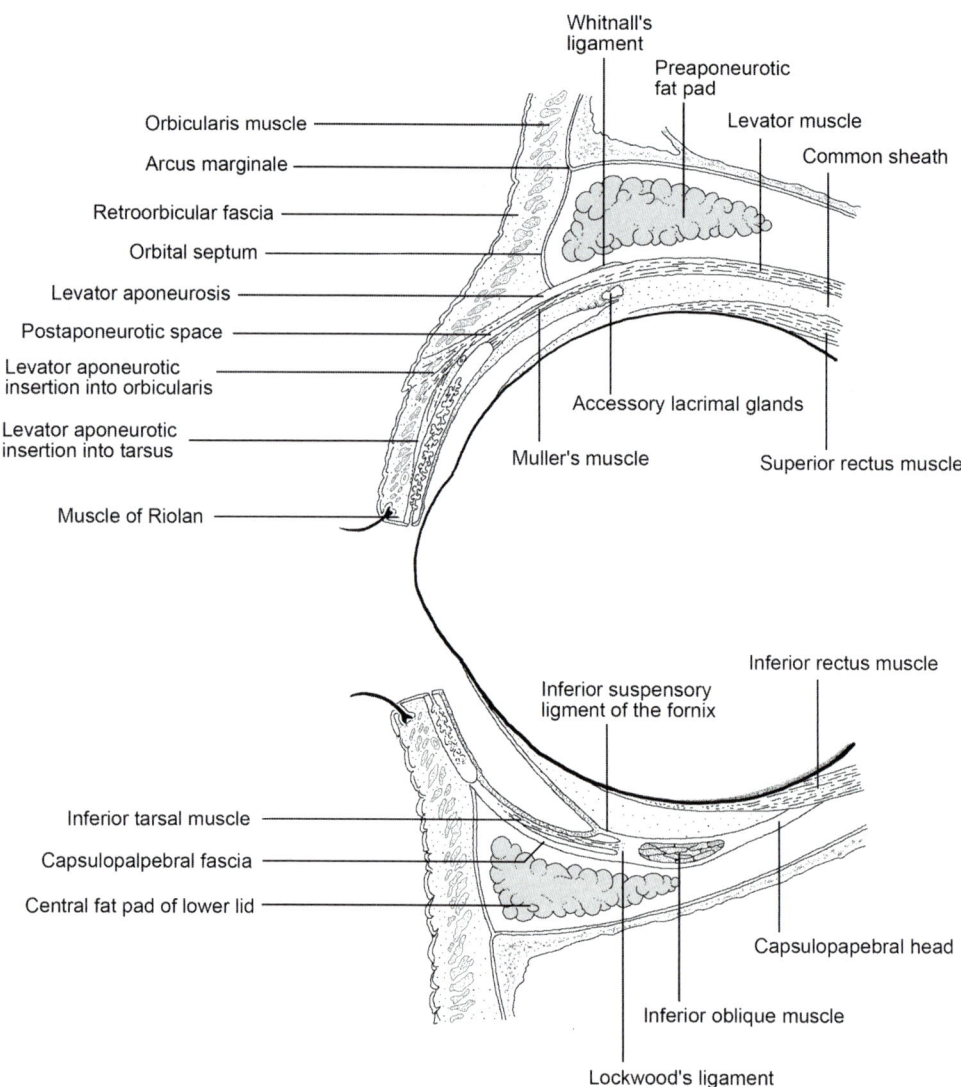

Fig. 3.1.1. Cross section of the upper and lower eyelid. (Modified from Tyers and Collin 2001)

the upper tarsus. The main difference in the oriental eyelid is the low skin crease due to the low insertion of the levator aponeurosis close to the lashes in the upper eyelid. The *lower eyelid crease* is usually located 4–5 mm from the lash line along the lower border of the inferior tarsal plate.

The *anterior eyelid margin* holds the eyelashes. Trichiasis is a common and acquired misdirection of eyelashes arising from their normal site of origin. Sweat glands of Moll secrete between the lashes or into the ducts of the glands of Zeiss. The sebaceous glands of Zeiss secrete into the lash follicles. A gray line is visible within the eyelid margin between the anterior and posterior eyelid lamella along the mucocutaneous junction. The openings of the meibomian glands are posterior to the gray line within the *posterior eyelid margin*. Distichiasis is a rare, congenital growth of an additional row of eyelashes arising from the orifices of the meibomian glands.

The fibers of the *orbicularis muscle* lie beneath the thin eyelid skin and run circumferentially around the palpebral aperture. The palpebral part of the orbicularis muscle includes the pretarsal and preseptal areas. The orbital part lies over and beyond the orbital rim. Laterally, the pretarsal muscles insert by a common tendon into Whitnall's tubercle. Medially, the superficial pretarsal muscle fibers contribute to form the anterior or superficial part of the medial canthal tendon which inserts medially on the frontal process of the maxilla immediately adjacent to the anterior lacrimal crest. Deep pretarsal muscle fibers insert into the posterior lacrimal crest immediately behind the lacrimal sac. During eyelid closure (blinking), contraction of the deep pretarsal muscle fibers (*Horner's muscle*) pulls the eyelid medially and posteriorly. This leads to shortening of the canaliculi. The puncta close and tears in the ampullae of the canaliculi are forced medially into the sac.

The *tarsal plates* represent the skeleton of the eyelids. They lie deep to the orbicularis muscle and consist of dense collagenous connective tissue with elastic fibers and contain many sebaceous glands (meibomian glands). Laterally, they form the fibrous component of the *lateral canthal tendon* which is in connection with *Whitnall's tubercle* inside the lateral orbital rim. Medially, they continue into the *medial canthal tendon*, which is attached to the *anterior and posterior lacrimal crest* (Fig. 3.1.2).

The *septum* fuses with the periosteum and periorbita at the orbital rim superiorly. It passes inferiorly into the eyelids to separate them from the orbit (preseptal and postseptal space) and fuses with the upper or lower eyelid retractors 2–4 mm from the tarsus.

The *upper eyelid retractors* include the striated levator muscle and Müller's smooth muscle. The levator arises from the orbital roof next to the optic foramen and superiorly to the rectus muscle. It measures about 40 mm in length and ends anteriorly just behind the septum as an aponeurosis. Close to the origin of the aponeurosis the muscle sheath is thickened above the muscle to form the whitish *Whitnall's ligament*, which acts as a fulcrum for the action of the levator, inserts into the trochlea of the superior oblique muscle medially and the fibrous capsule of the lacrimal gland and the orbital wall laterally.

The *levator aponeurosis* inserts anteriorly into the orbicularis muscle at the level of the skin crease and into the anterior surface of the lower tarsal plate. The medial and lateral horns of the levator aponeurosis insert near the canthal tendons (Fig. 3.1.2).

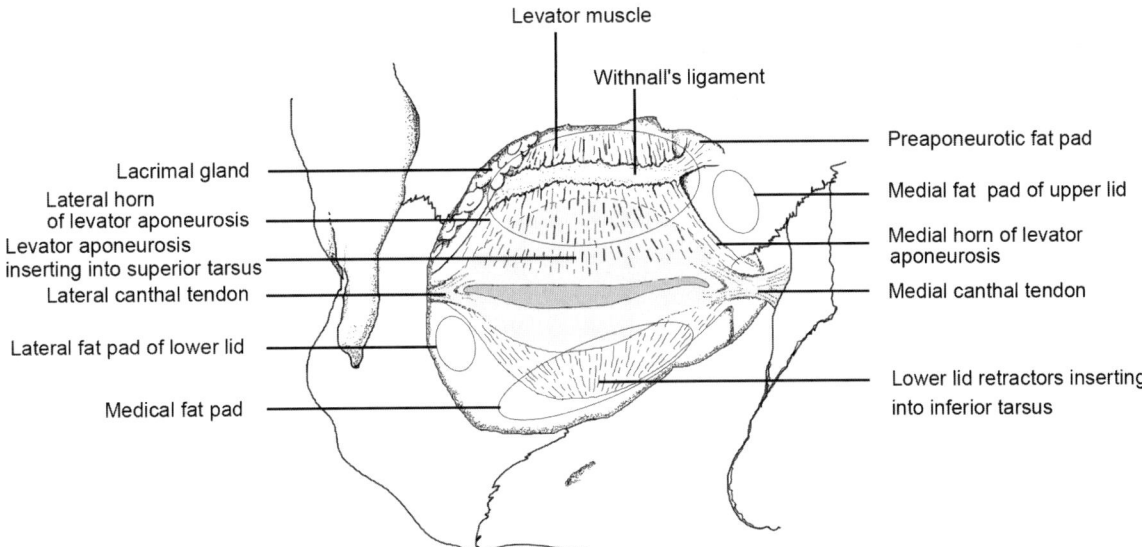

Fig. 3.1.2. Schematic illustration of the posterior eyelid lamellae. (Modified from Tyers and Collin 2001)

Müller's smooth muscle arises from the undersurface of the levator near the transition of the striated muscle fibers into the aponeurosis about 15–20 mm superior to the upper border of the tarsal plate. It descends between the levator aponeurosis and the conjunctiva to insert into the upper border of the tarsal plate.

The *fat pads of the upper eyelid* include a medial fat pad that is whitish in color and a central fat pad. The medial palpebral artery is often visible coursing through the whitish medial fat pads of the upper and lower eyelids and should be anticipated in blepharoplasty and anterior orbital operations. The lateral preaponeurotic space is filled by the pinkish gray orbital lobe of the lacrimal gland, which can prolapse into the lateral eyelid due to involutional laxity of the supporting septa.

The *lower eyelid retractors* arise from the sheath of the inferior rectus muscle and include the capsulopalpebral fascia (equivalent of the levator) and the *inferior tarsal muscle* (Müller's muscle). The latter consists mainly of fibrous tissue and a small amount of smooth muscle. The *capsulopalpebral fascia* arises from the sheath of the inferior rectus muscle, and runs forward to split and enclose the inferior oblique muscle. Thereafter it reunites to form *Lockwood's suspensory ligament*, which inserts into the orbital walls near the canthal tendons. The orbital septum fuses with the lower lid retractors below their insertion into the lower tarsal border.

In the lower eyelid the anterior orbital (postseptal) *fat* is divided into three pockets (medial, central and lateral). The medial fat is whitish in color and lies medial to the inferior oblique muscle. The lateral fat pad extends up to the inferior border of the lacrimal gland. It can prolapse into the preseptal skin and the lateral conjunctival fornix due to tissue laxity.

3.1.1.1
Arterial Supply

The *ophthalmic artery* gives origin to the *lacrimal artery* lateral to the optic nerve, to the supraorbital artery and medially to the dorsal nasal and supratrochlear arteries.

In the eyelids the *medial and lateral palpebral arteries* anastomose to form *tarsal arcades* on the surface of the upper and lower tarsal plates 2–4 mm from the lid margins. In the upper eyelid a second arcade is present at the upper border of the tarsal plate.

Blood from the *external carotid system* reaches the eyelids through anastomoses with the infraorbital and facial arteries, mainly via the *angular artery* nasally and the *superficial temporal artery*. The dense vascular supply of the face includes a network of anastomosing arterial vessels connecting the area of the internal and external carotid artery. The risk of intraarterial injections containing crystalline corticosteroid material can be associated with embolization of the ciliary and central retinal artery leading to ischemic infarctions of the retina via central artery occlusion or choroidal infarcts (Kröner, 1981).

3.1.1.2
Venous Drainage

The veins of the eyelids are located within the fornices and drain mainly to the venous network of the middle third of the face. The *angular vein* lies about 8 mm medial to the inner canthus and can often be seen through the skin. It is formed by the anastomoses of the supraorbital, supratrochlear and frontal veins at the upper nasal angle. It drains posteriorly into the superior orbital vein and inferiorly into the facial vein. In addition, venous blood drains to the inferior ophthalmic vein.

3.1.1.3
Lymphatic Drainage

The lateral two-thirds of the eyelids drain to the *preauricular and parotid lymph nodes*. The medial thirds drain to the *submandibular nodes* (Fig. 3.1.3).

3.1.1.4
Motor Nerve Supply

The orbicularis and frontal muscles are supplied by the zygomatic branches from the *facial nerve*. The levator muscle and the superior rectus muscle are supplied by the superior portion of the *third cranial nerve*. Müller's muscle is supplied by the *sympathetic nerves* travelling along the arteries.

3.1.1.5
Sensory Nerve Supply

The eyelids and orbital contents are supplied by the ophthalmic and maxillary divisions of the fifth cranial nerve. The ophthalmic division of the trigeminal nerve

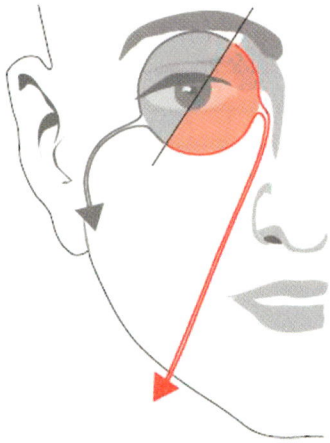

Fig. 3.1.3. Lymphatic drainage of the eyelids into the preauricular and submandibular nodes. (Modified from Völcker et al. 1980)

divides in the lateral wall of the cavernous sinus into the lacrimal, frontal and nasociliary nerves. These pass through the superior orbital fissure into the orbit. The *lacrimal nerve* runs forward along the superior border of the lateral rectus muscle to supply the lacrimal gland. It pierces the septum and supplies sensation to the *lateral part of the upper lid and conjunctiva.*

The frontal nerve runs forward between the periosteum of the orbital roof and the levator muscle. Anteriorly, it divides into the supratrochlear and supraorbital nerves. The supratrochlear nerve supplies the medial part of the eyelid, conjunctiva and skin of the forehead. The supraorbital nerve supplies the upper lid, conjunctiva, forehead and scalp.

The *nasociliary nerve* crosses medially above the optic nerve. It gives origin to several branches and then divides into the ethmoidal nerve and the supratrochlear nerve. The anterior ethmoidal nerve passes via the anterior cranial fossa to terminate as nasal nerves which supply the tip of the nose including the anterior part of the septum. The infratrochlear nerve passes below the trochlea to supply the medial ends of the lids, conjunctiva, the lacrimal sac and the root of the nose.

The infraorbital nerve is a main branch of the maxillary division of the trigeminal nerve. The maxillary nerve passes forward from the trigeminal ganglion to the foramen rotundum through which it enters the pterygopalatine fossa. The infraorbital nerve branches forward and travels in the floor of the orbita to reach the infraorbital foramen. It branches to supply the skin and conjunctiva of the lower lid, the lower part of the side of the nose and the upper lip.

3.1.2 Surgical Pathology

3.1.2.1 Disorders of Eyelid: Position and Movement

History and clinical examination are essential in the preoperative assessment of disorders in eyelid position and movement (Table 3.1.1). They are also essential for

Table 3.1.1. Differential diagnosis of disorders in eyelid position and movement

Ectropion
Involutional ectropion
Mechanical ectropion
Cicatricial ectropion
Paralytic ectropion (facial palsy)
Congenital ectropion

Entropion
Involutional entropion
Cicatricial entropion
Congenital entropion and epiblepharon

Trichiasis
Aberrant lashes
Distichiasis
Metaplastic lashes

Blepharoptosis
Aponeurotic blepharoptosis
Mechanical blepharoptosis (dermatochalasis, tumor, scar)
Myogenic blepharoptosis (progressive external ophthalmoplegia, myasthenia gravis, ocular myopathies)
Neurogenic blepharoptosis (third nerve palsy, Horner's syndrome, Marcus Gunn jaw-winking)
Dysgenetic blepharoptosis (congenital levator dystrophy with/without superior rectus weakness, blepharophimosis)

Eyelid retraction (commonly in thyroid eye disease)

the correct interpretation of histopathologic results obtained from surgical specimens.

History is essential in determining the duration and quality of symptoms. The position and movement of the eyelids are assessed using margin reflex distance and levator function. Further examination including Bell's phenomenon, jaw winking phenomenon, exclusion of myasthenia gravis, exophthalmometry, eye displacement, and determining site of skin crease or eyelid laxity (horizontal or vertical) (Fig. 3.1.4) will be helpful. Examination of the outer eye, fundus and orbit may be necessary for final diagnosis.

Histopathologic studies of surgical specimens may confirm or elucidate certain diagnoses such as in blepharoptosis caused by localized amyloid deposits of immunoglobulin lambda-light chains or in myogenic ptosis characterized histopathologically by "ragged red

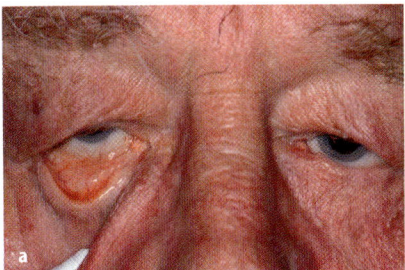
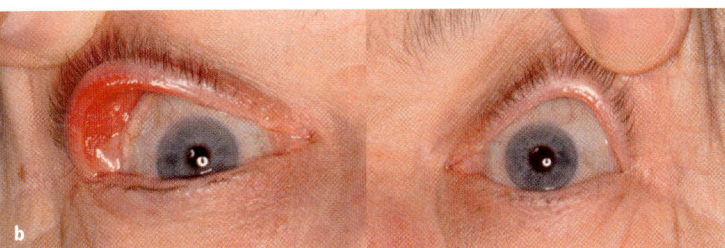

Fig. 3.1.4. Degree of horizontal eyelid laxity estimated clinically by gently pulling the lid away from the eye: **a** Abnormal laxity in the lower lid with a distance from the cornea to the posterior lid margin exceeding about 10 mm. **b** Abnormal laxity with secondary papillary conjunctivitis in the right upper lid as compared to normal findings in the left upper lid (compatible with floppy eyelid syndrome)

fibers." They may also further elucidate the pathogenesis of disorders such as lax eyelids or floppy eyelid syndrome.

If there is entropion, look for cicatricial conjunctival changes to establish the cause (e.g., ocular pemphigoid) before considering surgery. Immunofluorescent studies of conjunctival biopsies may confirm the diagnosis of ocular pemphigoid in up to 50% of cases. Horizontal laxity may include the medial and/or lateral canthus in both entropion and ectropion.

All symptoms and signs (e.g., levator function) are essential in the assessment of brow ptosis and blepharoptosis.

Surgical management of blepharoptosis may include aponeurotic repair, levator resection, frontalis suspension, and shortening of Müller's muscle.

Complete preoperative assessment of symptoms and signs with the patient sitting is essential in choosing the type of operation (repair of brow ptosis, blepharoplasty, blepharoptosis and/or ectropion). Blepharoplasty includes the removal of skin, muscle and orbital fat in varying proportions.

3.1.2.1.1
Surgical Pathology and Anatomic Principles of Ectropion Repair

Different subtypes of eyelid laxity have been reported as underlying causes of chronic ocular irritation including papillary conjunctivitis, superficial punctate keratopathy and dry eye.

Ectropion is any form of everted lid margin and may affect both the lower and/or upper lid (e.g., floppy eyelid, lax eyelid syndrome). Involutional ectropion is most commonly due to ageing changes affecting the canthal tendons, the tarsus, the lid retractors and the orbicularis muscle. A reduced tension in the lid is most probably due to a loss of elastin fibers in certain forms of ectropion such as floppy eyelid syndrome (Figs. 3.1.5 – 3.1.8). The most common principles of surgical repair include tightening or shortening procedures centrally, laterally or medially. Successful surgical management depends on the appropriate correction of the underlying anatomical defect.

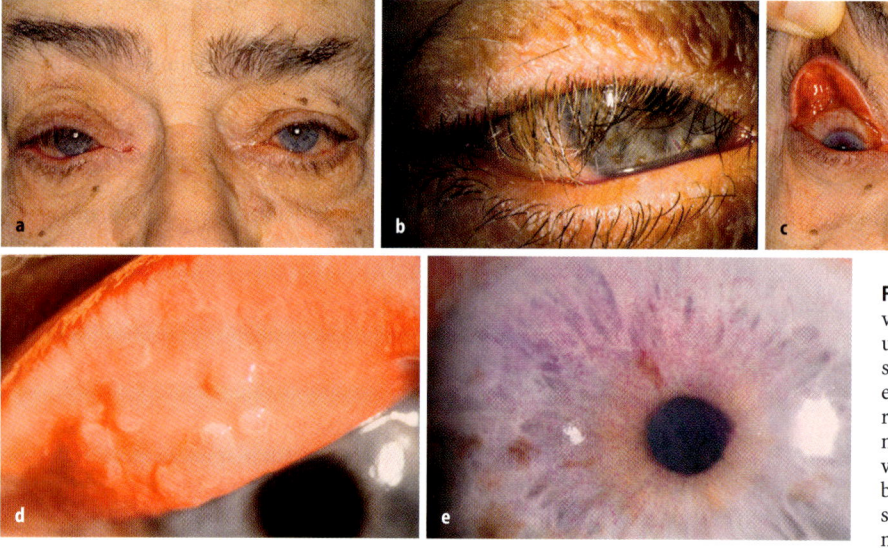

Fig. 3.1.5. Clinical signs of involutional ectropion of the upper eyelid in floppy eyelid syndrome: **a** Bilateral floppy eyelid syndrome with the right eye showing more pronounced involvement: elevated eyebrow, aponeurotic blepharoptosis, eyelash ptosis, eyelid imbrication and marked tarsal eversion. **b** Eyelash ptosis of the right eye. **c** Loss of lid margin apposition to the globe and segmental palpebral conjunctivitis confirmed by pulling the upper lid (*right→left*). **d** Papillary conjunctivitis of the upper tarsal conjunctiva. **e** Marked corneal erosions (rose bengal). (From Schlötzer-Schrehardt et al. 2005)

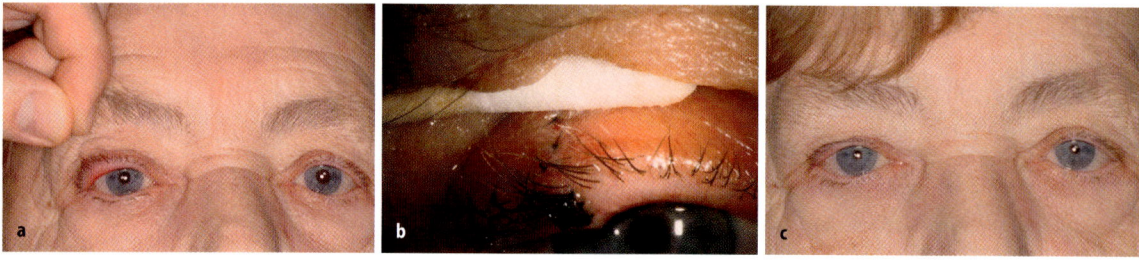

Fig. 3.1.6. Involutional ectropion of the upper eyelid in floppy eyelid syndrome – horizontal lid shortening procedure: **a** Preoperative appearance with red and thickened right upper lid margin. **b** Results 1 day postoperatively following horizontal lid shortening of the right upper lid. **c** Marked improvement of symptoms and signs 6 weeks postoperatively

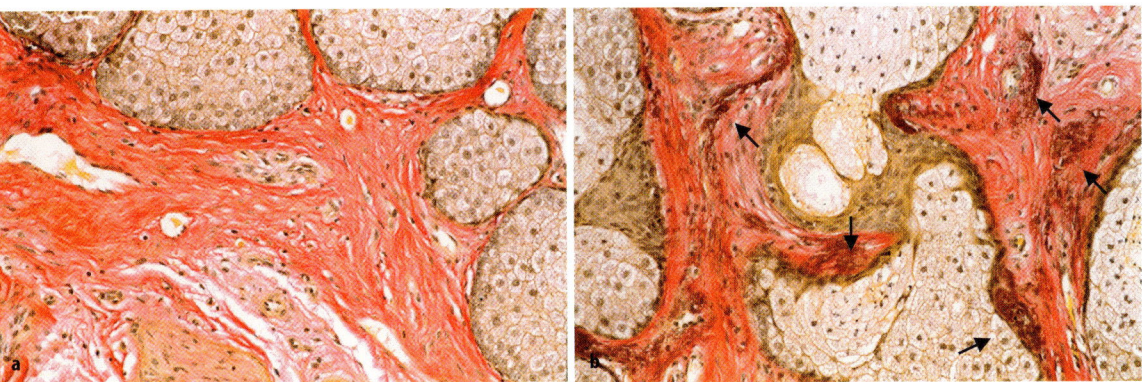

Fig. 3.1.7. Light microscopy of lid sections stained by van Gieson's method for elastic fibers in floppy eyelid syndrome (**a**) and control specimens (**b**); elastic fibers appear *dark-brown,* collagen fibers appear *red* (original magnification × 100). **a** Nearly complete absence of elastic fibers in the collagenous tarsal stroma in floppy eyelid syndrome. **b** Marked elastic fibers (*arrows*) in the collagenous tarsal stroma of control specimens. (From Schlötzer-Schrehardt et al. 2005)

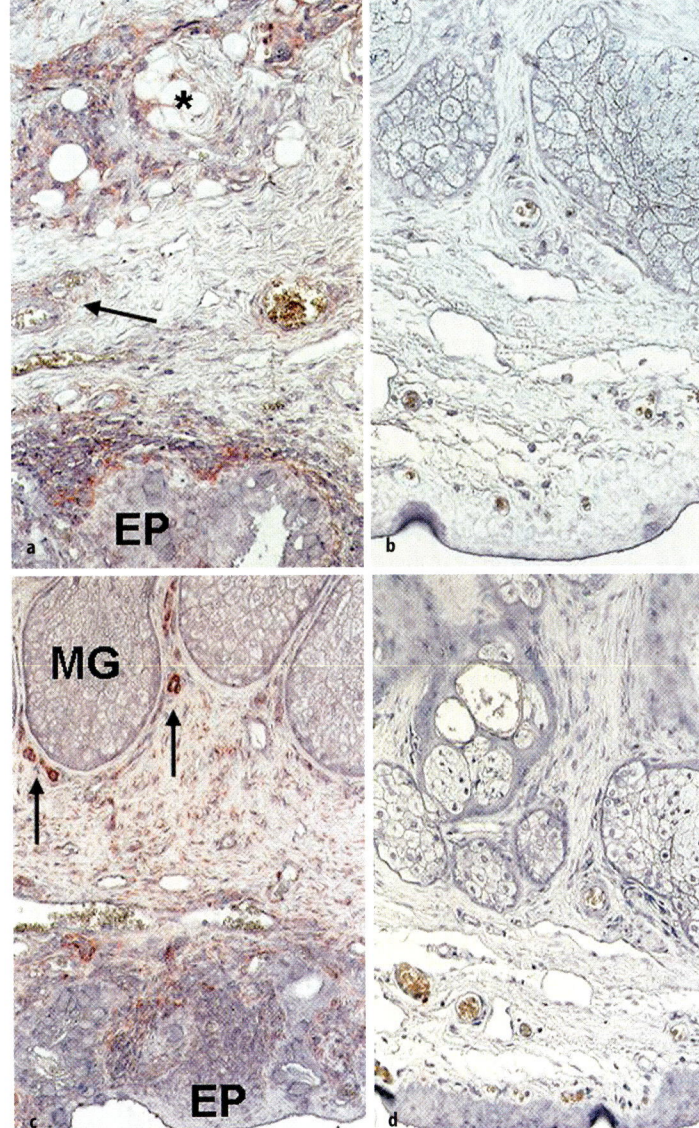

Fig. 3.1.8. Immunohistochemical localization of matrix metalloproteinases (MMPs) in the tarsal conjunctiva and tarsal plate of floppy eyelid syndrome (**a, c**) and control specimens (**b, d**) (original magnification × 50): **a** MMP-2 is expressed in the conjunctival epithelium (*EP*), in subepithelial areas of inflammatory infiltrations, in the periphery of blood vessels (*arrow*), and in stromal areas of lipogranulomatous inflammation (*star*) in floppy eyelid syndrome specimens. **b** Loss of MMP-2 expression in control specimens. **c** MMP-9 can be localized to the conjunctival epithelium (*EP*), to subepithelial inflammatory infiltrates, some blood vessel walls (*arrows*), and the stromal connective tissue adjacent to meibomian gland acini (*MG*) in a floppy eyelid syndrome specimen. **d** No MMP-9 expression in control specimens. (From Schlötzer-Schrehardt et al. 2005)

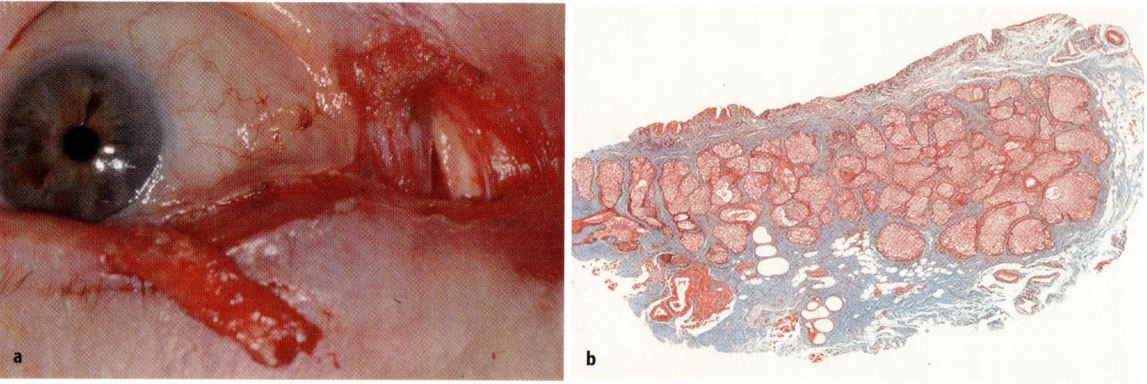

Fig. 3.1.9. Lateral tarsal strip procedure: **a** A new tendon is created from the lateral part of the tarsal plate by excising skin, orbicularis, lashes and conjunctiva from the tarsus. The periosteum over the lateral orbital rim is exposed. The lateral tarsal strip is sutured directly to the periosteum of the lateral orbital rim to tighten the lid and to obtain posterior fixation. **b** Histopathologic cross-section of the lateral tarsal strip showing collagenous tissue and meibomian glands (Masson trichrome, original magnification × 12.5)

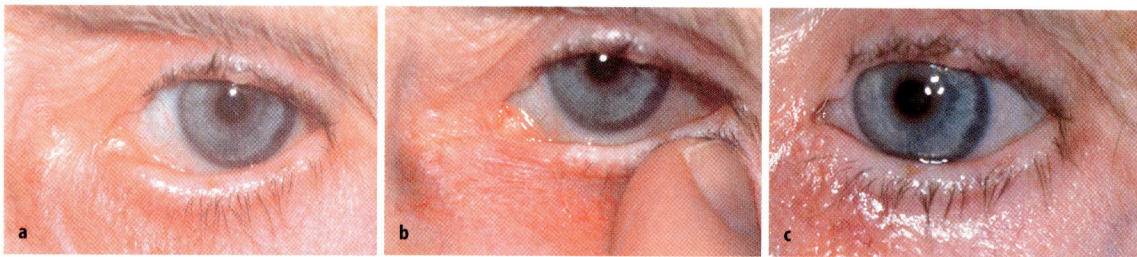

Fig. 3.1.10. Involutional ectropion of the left lower eyelid medially: **a** Everted medial lid margin. Syringe the nasolacrimal outflow system in order to exclude simultaneous obstruction prior to surgical correction of the ectropion. **b** Abnormal medial canthal tendon laxity with a punctum movable laterally to the limbus estimated clinically by gently pulling the lid laterally suggesting laxity of the anterior limb. **c** Appearance 2 weeks postoperatively following plication of the anterior limb of the medial canthal tendon

Involutional Ectropion

1. Involutional ectropion centrally: modified Bick procedure (full thickness pentagon excision and direct closure 6 mm in from the lateral canthus)
2. Involutional ectropion laterally: lateral tarsal strip procedure (Fig. 3.1.9)
3. Involutional ectropion medially: syringe the nasolacrimal outflow system to exclude any obstruction prior to surgical correction of the ectropion.
   a) Punctal ectropion without horizontal laxity: tarsoconjunctival diamond excision with a closing suture including the lower lid retractors
   b) Punctal ectropion with tarsal laxity and an intact medial canthus: full-thickness pentagon excision lateral to the punctum combined with the tarsoconjunctival diamond excision (lazy T procedure)
   c) Medial canthal tendon laxity with a punctum movable to the medial limbus: lazy T procedure
   d) Medial canthal tendon laxity with a punctum movable lateral to the limbus: plication of the anterior limb of the medial canthal tendon (Fig. 3.1.10)
   e) Medial canthal tendon laxity with a punctum movable laterally to the pupil: plication of the posterior limb of the medial canthal tendon
   f) Medial canthal tendon laxity with a punctum movable laterally beyond the pupil: medial canthal resection

Cicatricial Ectropion

Localized skin shortage: Z-plasty; if there is also horizontal laxity, combine with horizontal shortening procedure.

Diffuse Skin Shortage. Skin graft or myocutaneous flap; if there is also horizontal laxity, combine with horizontal shortening procedure (Fig. 3.1.11).

Paralytic Ectropion

Lid tightening procedure either laterally (lateral tarsal strip) (Fig. 3.1.12) or medially (medial canthal resection)

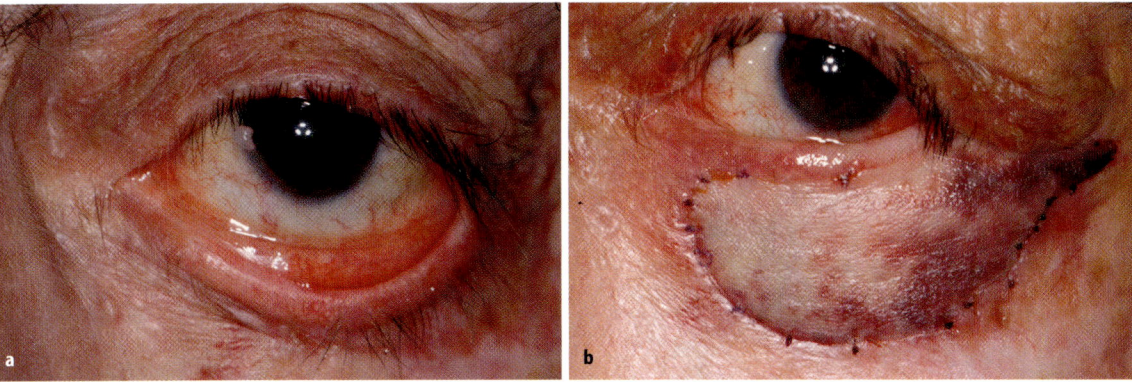

Fig. 3.1.11. Cicatricial ectropion of the left lower eyelid: **a** Generalized contraction of lower lid skin with disinsertion of the lateral canthal tendon. **b** Appearance 1 week postoperatively following skin graft combined with lateral tarsal strip procedure

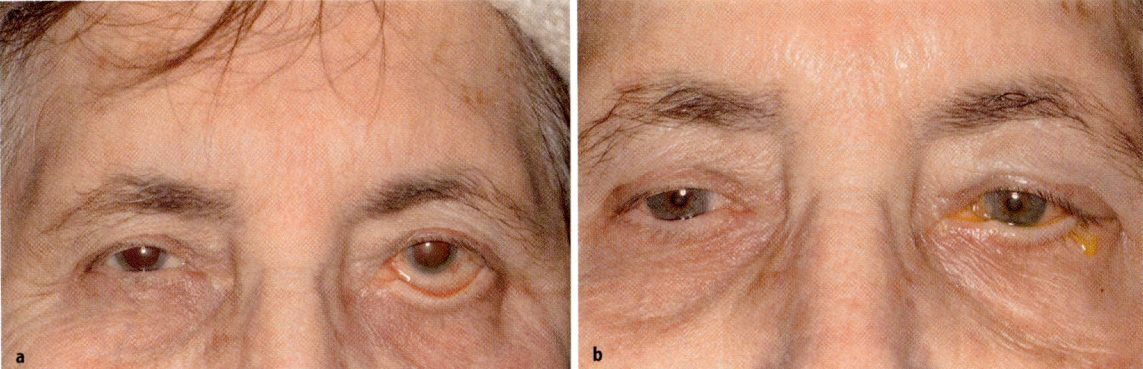

Fig. 3.1.12. Paralytic ectropion of the left lower eyelid: **a** Everted lid margin due to facial palsy. **b** Appearance 2 weeks postoperatively following lateral tarsal strip procedure

3.1.2.1.2
Surgical Pathology and Anatomic Principles of Entropion and Distichiasis Repair

Entropion of the lower or upper eyelids is any form of inverted lid margin (trichiasis). Determine if there is cicatricial entropion with conjunctival scarring and shortening of the posterior lid lamella. Try to determine its cause such as ocular pemphigoid. Involutional lower lid entropion is thought to be caused by horizontal laxity, disinsertion of the canthal tendons, vertical laxity with weakness of the lower lid retractors and overriding preseptal orbicularis muscle. Successful surgical management depends on the appropriate correction of the underlying anatomical defects. The most common principles of surgical repair include everting sutures, transverse lid split, retractor plication and horizontal shortening. Horizontal shortening is probably the most important factor in the surgical management of involutional lower lid entropion to prevent late recurrences.

Involutional Lower Lid Entropion

1. Involutional lower lid entropion without horizontal laxity:
   a) Everting sutures (temporary cure!)
   b) Transverse full thickness lid split and everting sutures (Wies procedure)
2. Involutional lower lid entropion with horizontal laxity and disinsertion of the canthal tendons (Fig. 3.1.13): determine if there is disinsertion or laxity of the canthal tendons. If yes, correct these using a tarsal strip procedure which can be combined with everting sutures.
3. Involutional lower lid entropion with horizontal laxity:
   a) Transverse full-thickness lid split, everting sutures and horizontal shortening (Quickert procedure)
   b) Retractor plication (Jones) and horizontal shortening (Fig. 3.1.14)

Cicatricial Lower Lid Entropion

1. Cicatricial lower lid entropion (minor shortening of posterior lamella): tarsal fracture and everting sutures.
2. Cicatricial lower lid entropion (major or recurrent shortening of posterior lamella) (Fig. 3.1.15): spac-

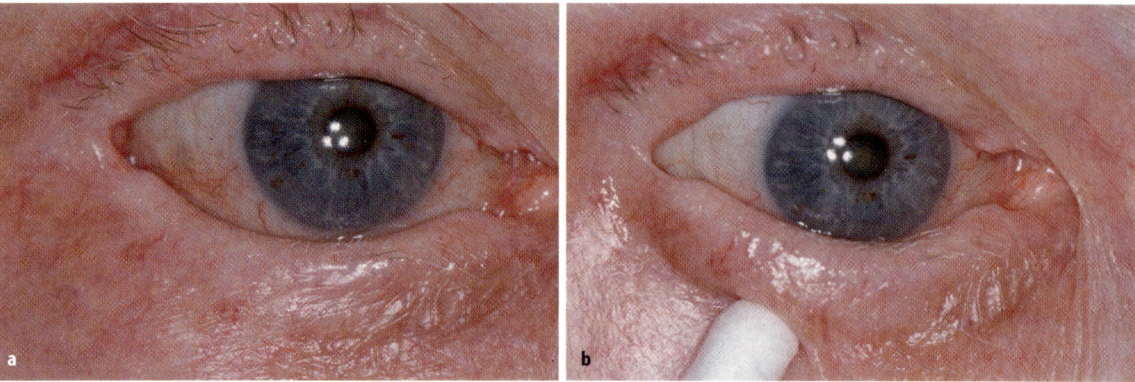

Fig. 3.1.13. Involutional entropion of the right lower eyelid: **a** Inverted lid margin with horizontal laxity and marked disinsertion of the lateral canthal tendon. **B** Disinsertion of the lateral canthal tendon is more obvious after gently pulling the eyelid medially

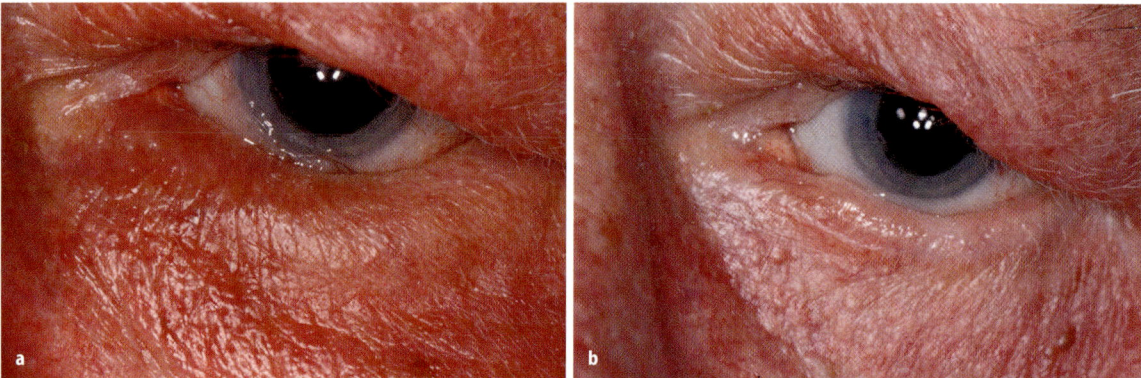

Fig. 3.1.14. Recurrent involutional entropion of the left lower eyelid with horizontal laxity – plication of lower lid retractors (Jones) with horizontal shortening: **a** Preoperative appearance. **b** Appearance 3 months postoperatively

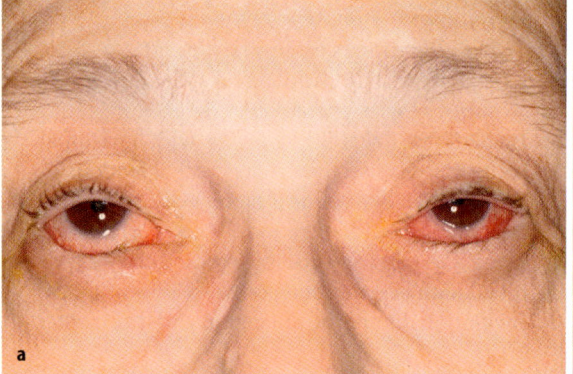 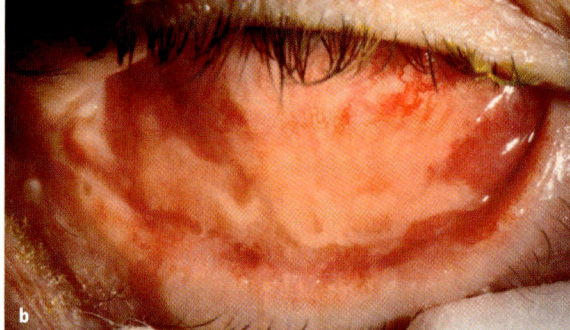

Fig. 3.1.15. Cicatricial entropion of the left lower eyelid (**a, b**)

er such as mucous membrane graft (e.g., hard palate) and everting sutures.

Upper Lid Entropion

1. Upper lid entropion (mild): anterior lamella repositioning with everting sutures
2. Upper lid entropion (moderate): anterior lamella repositioning with everting sutures and lid split in the gray line
3. Upper lid entropion with thickened tarsus: anterior lamella repositioning with tarsal wedge resection and everting sutures (Fig. 3.1.16)
4. Upper lid entropion with thinned tarsus and mild retraction: lamellar division and posterior lamella advance
5. Upper lid entropion with marked retraction and insufficient lid closure prior to keratoplasty: mucous membrane graft (e.g., hard palate or thinned nasal septal cartilage) to lengthen the posterior lamella

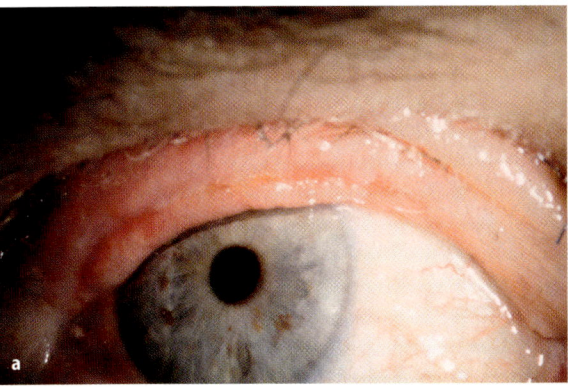 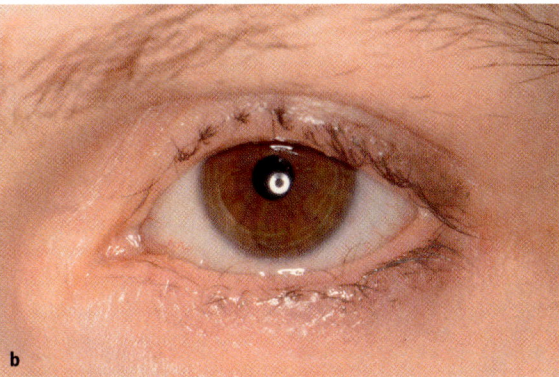

Fig. 3.1.16. Cicatricial upper lid entropion – anterior lamellar reposition, lamellar division and tarsal wedge resection: **a** Appearance 1 week postoperatively. **B** Result 6 months postoperatively

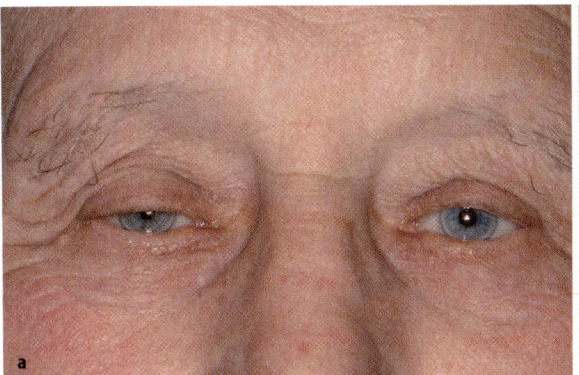 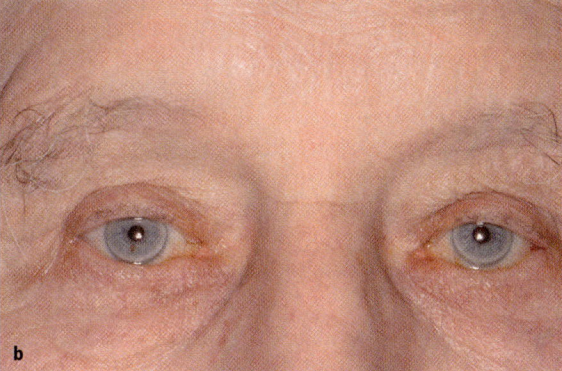

Fig. 3.1.17. Acquired aponeurotic blepharoptosis of the right eye – levator aponeurosis advancement: **a** Preoperative appearance. **b** Appearance 6 months postoperatively

Distichiasis

Lamellar division and cryotherapy to the posterior lamella.

3.1.2.1.3
Surgical Pathology and Anatomic Principles of Blepharoptosis Repair

Clinically relevant blepharoptosis with a distance from the upper lid margin to the central corneal light reflex not exceeding 2.5 mm may result in defect of peripheral visual field and in severe cases in loss of central vision. Aponeurotic, mechanical, myogenic, neurogenic and dysgenetic etiologies are responsible for acquired ptosis (Table 3.1.1). Aponeurotic ptosis as the most common type of acquired ptosis in the elderly is due to age-related disinsertion or dehiscence of the aponeurosis. In mechanical ptosis the eyelid tissues will be stretched by the increased weight due to dermatochalasis, orbital fat prolapse, eyelid tumors or scar formations. Myogenic ptosis is attributed to abnormalities of the levator muscle reducing the potential of eyelid elevation into proper position, such as chronic progressive external ophthalmoplegia (CPEO), myasthenia gravis or ocular myopathies. Neurogenic causes of blepharoptosis include dysfunction of the oculomotor nerve (third nerve palsy, Marcus Gunn jaw-winking), of the sympathetic nerves (Horner's syndrome) or of the central nervous system. Dysgenesis, such as congenital levator dystrophy with/without superior rectus weakness or blepharophimosis syndrome, may also result in blepharoptosis.

In addition to taking the history with a special look at family history, diurnal changes, diplopia and dysphagia, the levator function defined as the excursion of the upper lid from extreme downgaze to extreme upgaze is the most important factor in determining the cause of blepharoptosis and in the choice of therapy.

1. Aponeurotic blepharoptosis with good levator function (8 mm): levator aponeurosis advancement (Fig. 3.1.17)
2. Mechanical blepharoptosis with moderate (5–7 mm)/good (8 mm) levator function: removal of excess eyelid skin (blepharoplasty, Fig. 3.1.18), orbital fat prolapse, tumor or scar formation with/without adjunctive levator resection
3. Myogenic blepharoptosis with poor levator function (4 mm): frontalis sling procedure, levator resection, brow suspension (Fig. 3.1.19)
4. Neurogenic blepharoptosis with poor, moderate or good levator function: observing, causal therapy, frontalis suspension, shortening of Müller's muscle

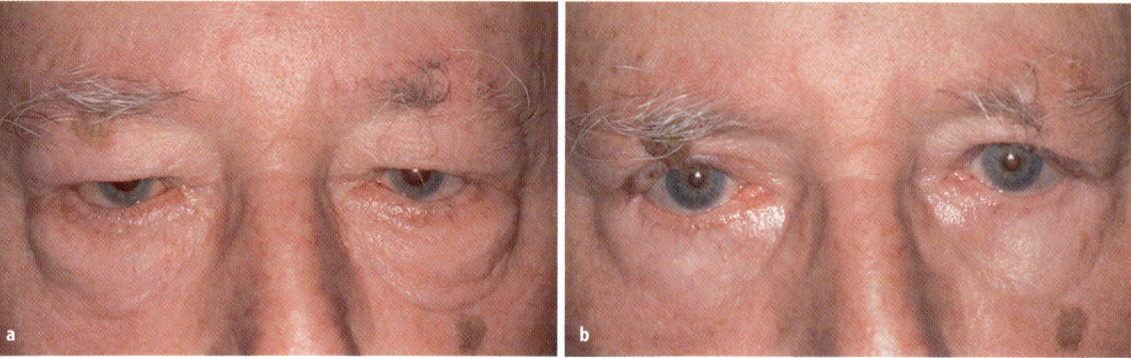

Fig. 3.1.18. Acquired dermatochalasis involving the upper and lower eyelids – blepharoplasty: **a** Preoperative appearance. **b** Appearance 3 months postoperatively

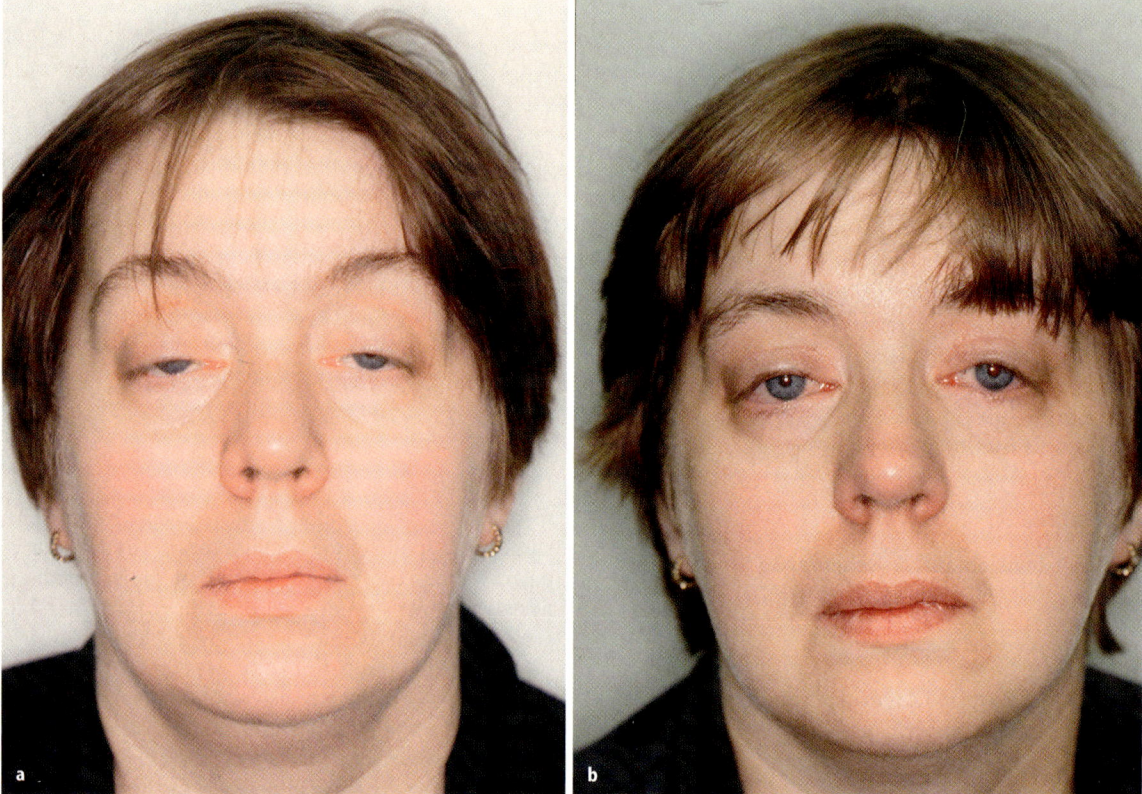

Fig. 3.1.19. Acquired myogenic blepharoptosis due to chronic progressive external ophthalmoplegia (CPEO) – brow suspension: **a** Preoperative appearance. **b** Appearance 12 months postoperatively

3.1.2.2
Eyelid Tumors

History and clinical examination using inspection, palpation and slit lamp biomicroscopy are important in the assessment of eyelid tumors. Ultrasonography, CT and MRI are rarely necessary to determine the borders of a lesion. Experienced clinicians are often correct (up to 90%) in the clinical diagnosis of basal cell carcinomas. Clinical diagnosis, however, requires histopathologic confirmation (Figs. 3.1.20–3.1.24). Knowledge about the frequency of individual benign and malig-

▷

Fig. 3.1.21. Sebaceous gland carcinoma of the eyelids: **a, b** Ulcerated sebaceous gland carcinoma involving the left upper eyelid in a 60-year-old woman (**a**). Histopathologic section (hematoxylin-eosin, original magnification ×50) of sebaceous gland carcinoma showing lobules of pleomorphic atypical tumor cells (*inset right*) with foamy cytoplasm strongly positive for fat using Oil Red O (*inset left*) (**b**). **c, d** Diffuse sebaceous gland carcinoma presenting as unilateral blepharitis of the left upper eyelid in a 55-year-old woman (**c**). Histopathologic section (hematoxylin-eosin, original magnification ×150) showing diffuse tumor invasion of the epidermis (pagetoid spread of sebaceous gland carcinoma cells contributing to the clinical appearance of diffuse blepharitis) (**d**). (From Conway et al. 2004)

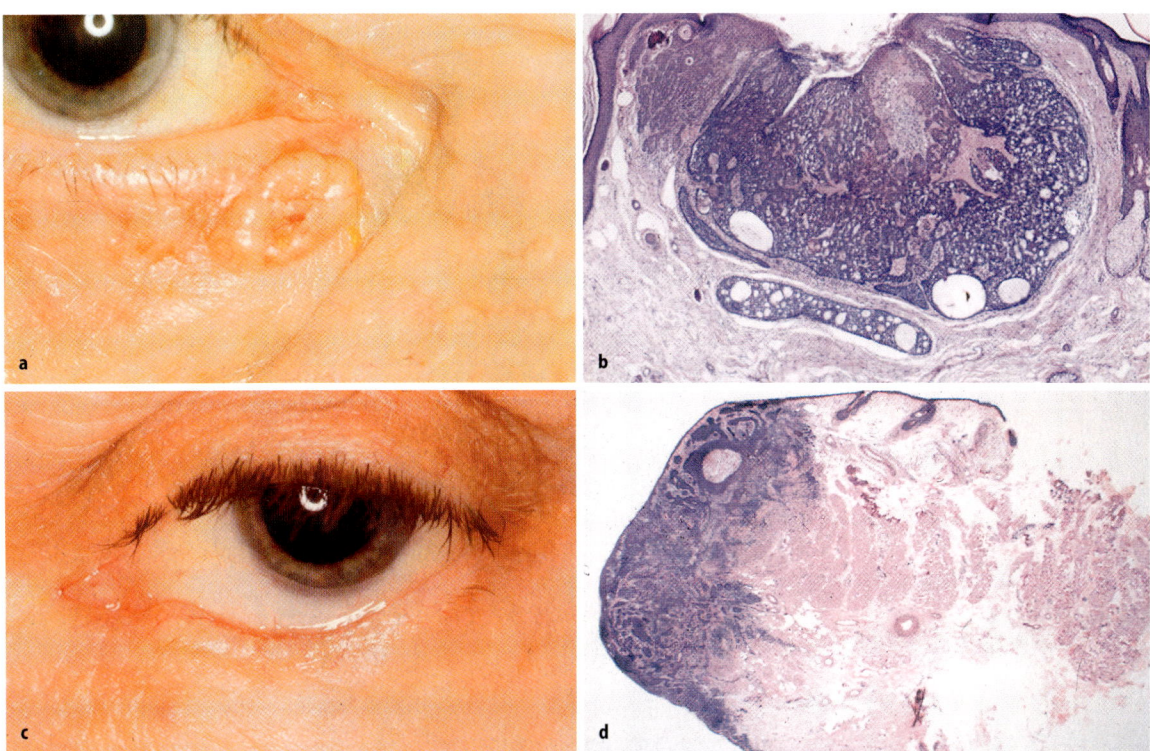

Fig. 3.1.20. Basal cell carcinoma of the eyelids: **a, b** Noduloulcerative basal cell carcinoma of the right lower eyelid in a 65-year-old man (**a**). Histopathologic section (hematoxylin-eosin, original magnification ×50) of noduloulcerative basal cell carcinoma showing closely compact basophilic nuclei and central crater (**b**). **c, d** Morpheaform (sclerosing) basal cell carcinoma involving the left medial lower eyelid in a 60-year-old woman (**c**). Histopathologic section (hematoxylin-eosin, original magnification ×25) of morpheaform basal cell carcinoma revealing tumor cell nests interspersed throughout the anterior and posterior portions of the eyelid margin (**d**). (From Conway et al. 2004)

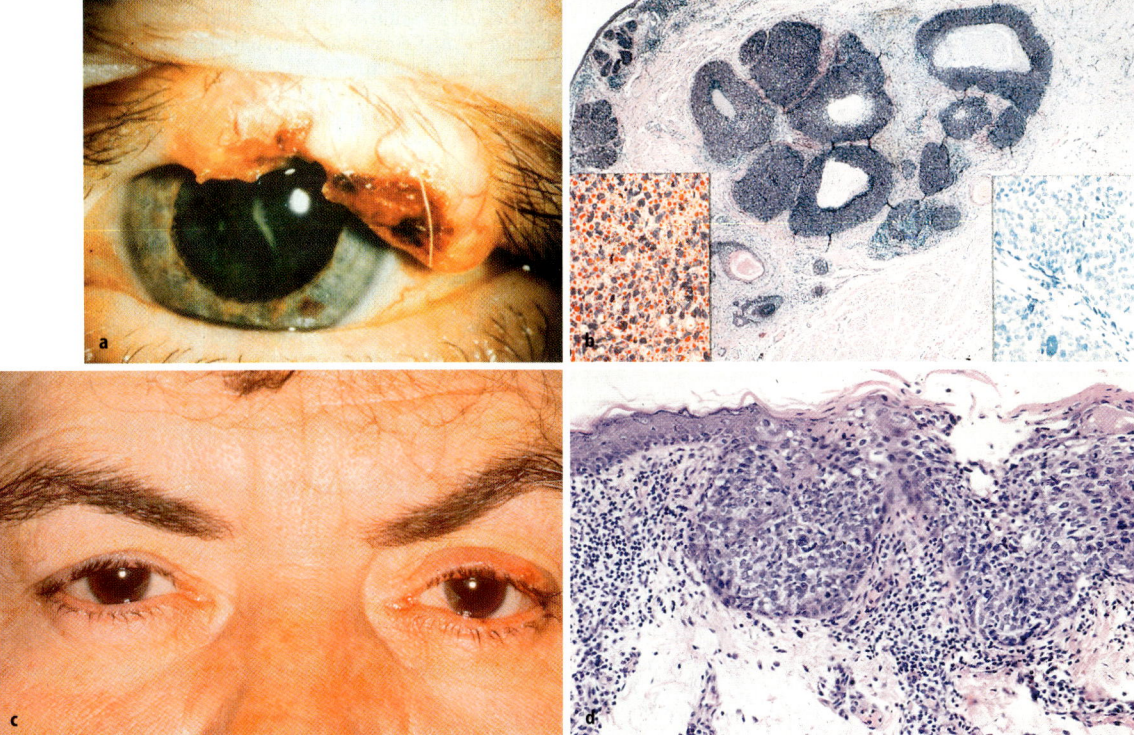

Fig. 3.1.21 (Legend see p. 40)

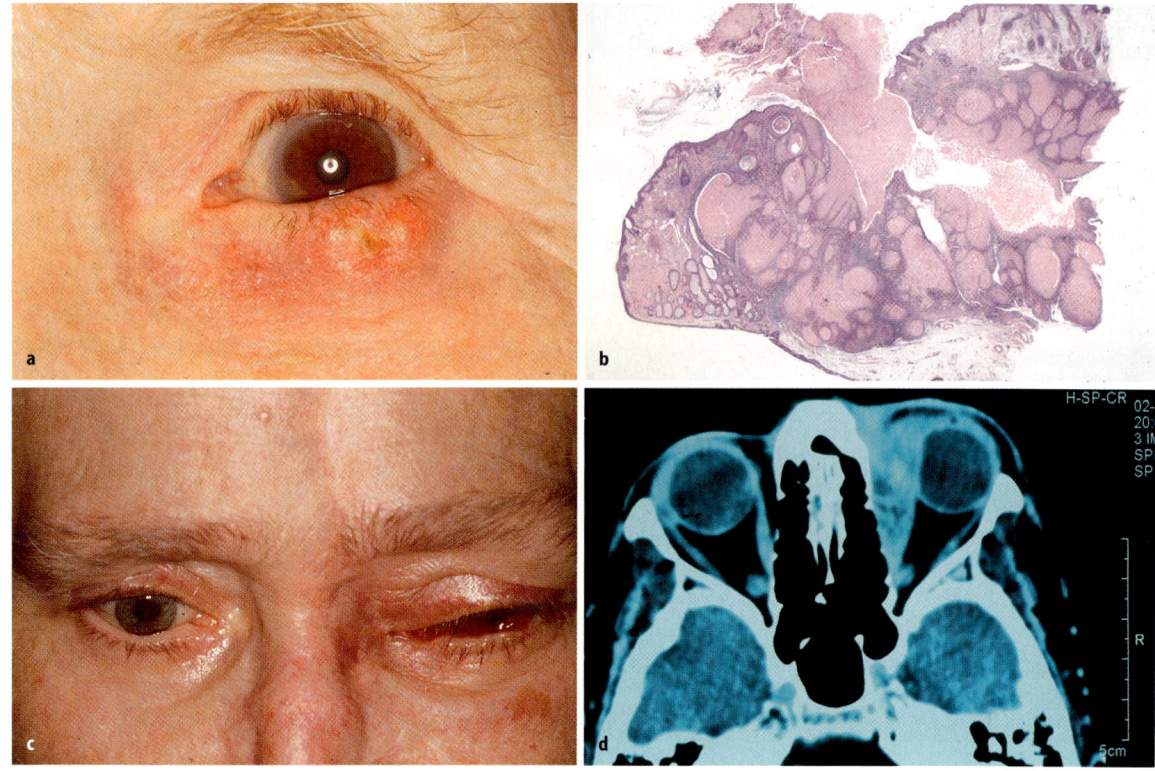

Fig. 3.1.22. Squamous cell carcinoma of the eyelids: **a, b** Squamous cell carcinoma of the left lower eyelid in an 80-year-old woman (**a**). Histopathologic section (hematoxylin-eosin, original magnification ×12.5) of full-thickness specimen of the lower eyelid showing portions of the squamous cell carcinoma involving both the anterior and posterior eyelid lamellae (note the central ulceration in the anterior eyelid lamella) (**b**). **c, d** Orbital invasion of an eyelid squamous cell carcinoma following incomplete excision previously in a 55-year-old woman (**c**). CT scan revealing marked orbital invasion of the squamous cell carcinoma (**d**)

Fig. 3.1.23. Malignant melanoma of the eyelids: **a** Nodular nonpigmented malignant melanoma of the upper eyelid in a 58-year-old man. **b** Histopathologic section (hematoxylin-eosin, original magnification ×200) showing typical melanoma cells in absence of pigment

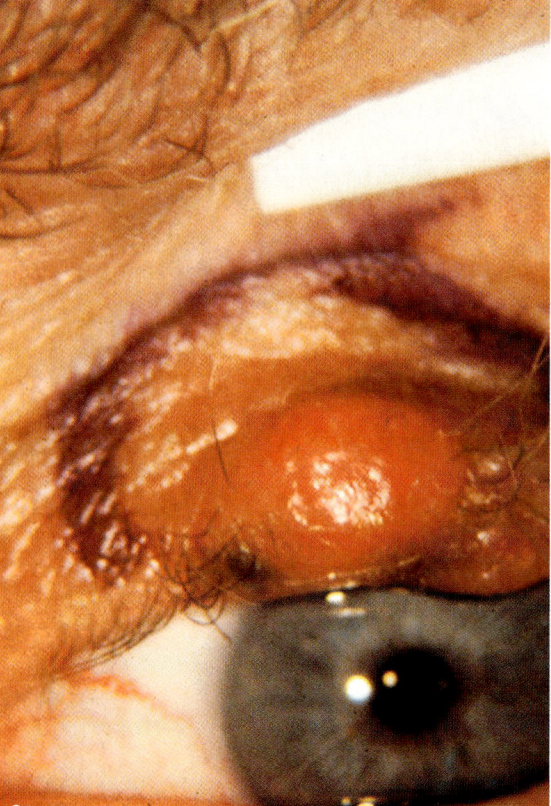

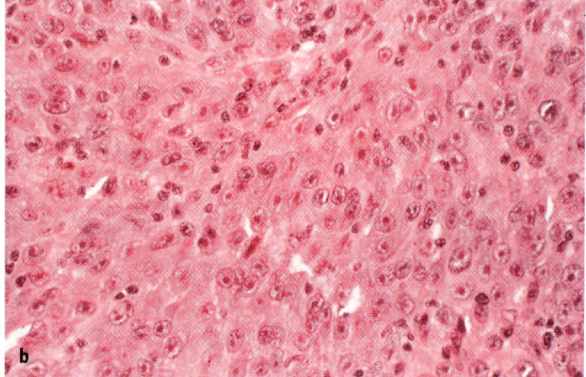

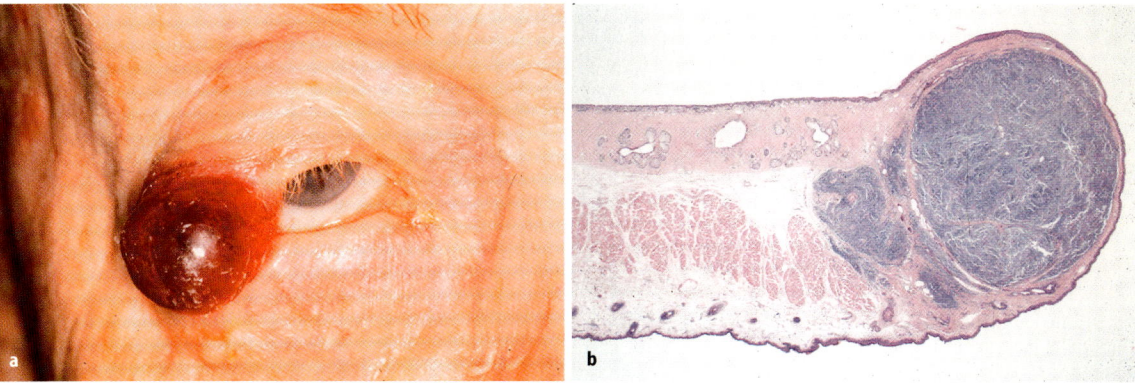

Fig. 3.1.24. Merkel cell carcinoma of the eyelids: **a** Merkel cell carcinoma of the right upper eyelid with typical cherry-red color, ball-shaped prominence and smooth surface. **b** Histopathologic section (hematoxylin-eosin, original magnification ×8) of the excised Merkel cell carcinoma showing subepithelial nests of basophilic tumor cells within both the anterior and the posterior eyelid lamellae. (From Colombo et al. 2000)

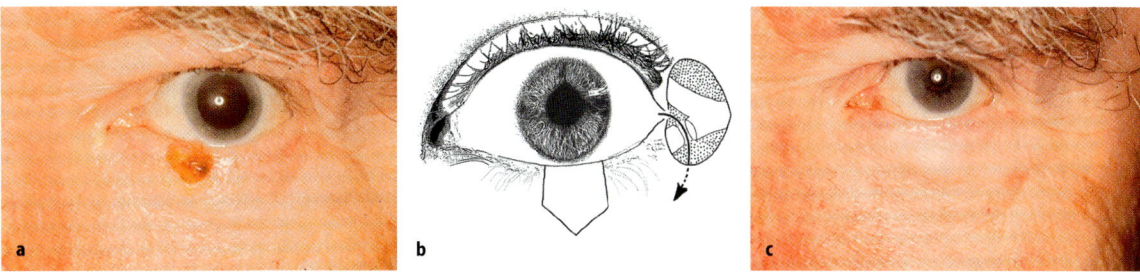

Fig. 3.1.25. Nodular pigmented basal cell carcinoma of the left lower eyelid – excision and direct closure procedure with inferior cantholysis: **a** Preoperative appearance. **b** Surgical technique (modified from Collin 2006). **c** Appearance 3 weeks postoperatively

nant lesions is helpful in their clinical differential diagnosis (Table 3.1.2). Histopathologic findings may be helpful to explain clinical findings. Moreover, they are essential in providing a microscopically controlled excision. Methods include conventional frozen section control, Mohs' surgery (frozen sections) and/or a two-step procedure using paraffin sections. The classification of the World Health Organization (WHO) provides guidelines for the diagnosis of eyelid tumors. The TNM classification (WHO and American Joint Committee of Cancer – AJCC) is helpful in determining the clinical and histopathologic stage of malignant eyelid tumors.

Depending on the extent of microscopically controlled tumor excision, the reconstruction of the eyelid must be performed with different techniques:

1. Partial defects only of the anterior eyelid lamella: direct closure (Fig. 3.1.25), flap, free graft
2. Partial defects only of the posterior eyelid lamella: tarsoconjunctival flap, periosteal flap, free grafts (tarsal graft, tarsomarginal graft, oral mucosa graft, nasal mucosa graft, auricular cartilage graft)
3. Full-thickness defects of both the anterior and posterior eyelid lamellae: flap combined with flap, flap combined with graft or vice versa (Figs. 3.1.26–3.1.28). (Do not combine two grafts!)

Table 3.1.2. Frequency of eyelid tumors (from Holbach et al. 2002a, b)

I. Benign eyelid lesions ($n=2,943$)	
1. Chalazion	32%
2. Seborrheic keratoses and inverted follicular keratosis	23%
3. Squamous papilloma	12%
4. Melanocytic nevus	12%
5. Cysts of sweat glands (apocrine and eccrine hidrocystoma)	5%
6. Epidermal inclusion cysts	4%
7. Granulomas (pyogenic, foreign body, paraffin)	4%
8. Dermoid cysts	3%
9. Keratoacanthoma	2%
10. Molluscum contagiosum	2%
11. Hemangioma	2%
12. Pilomatrixoma	1%
13. Phakomatous choristoma ("Zimmerman tumor")	<1%
II. Malignant eyelid lesions ($n=907$)	
1. Basal cell carcinoma	91%
2. Sebaceous gland carcinoma	3%
3. Squamous cell carcinoma	3%
4. Malignant melanoma	2%
5. Merkel cell carcinoma	0.5%
6. Metastatic eyelid disease	0.2%
7. Adenocarcinoma of sweat glands	0.2%

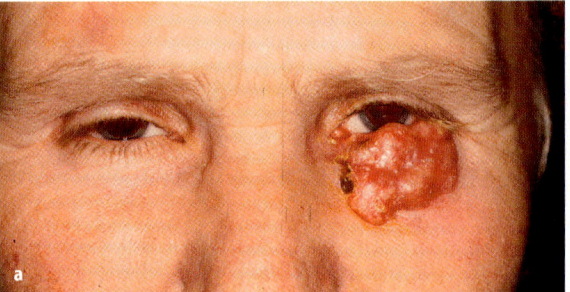 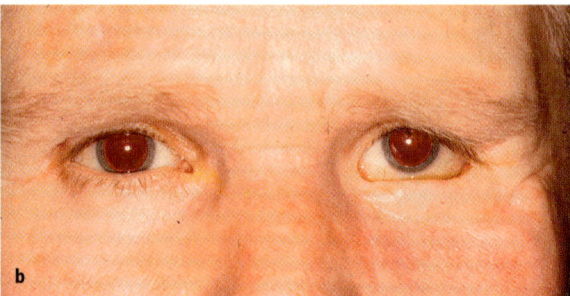

Fig. 3.1.26. Large nodular basal cell carcinoma of the left lower eyelid – full-thickness excision and eyelid reconstruction using a composite graft from the nasal septum for the posterior eyelid lamella and a transposition skin flap for the anterior lamella: **a** Preoperative appearance. **b** Appearance 3 months postoperatively

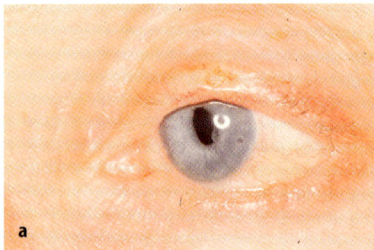 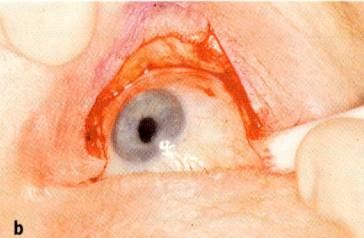 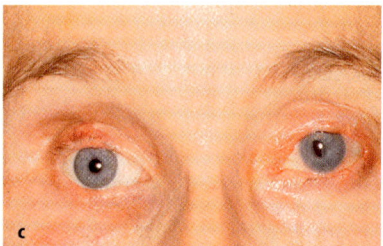

Fig. 3.1.27. Full-thickness defect of the left upper eyelid – eyelid reconstruction using two tarsomarginal grafts and a two pedicled myocutaneous flap from the ipsilateral upper eyelid: **a** Preoperative appearance. **b** Intraoperative situs. **c** Appearance 3 months postoperatively. (See Hübner 1999)

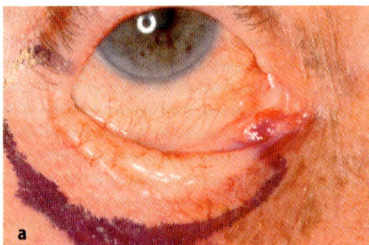 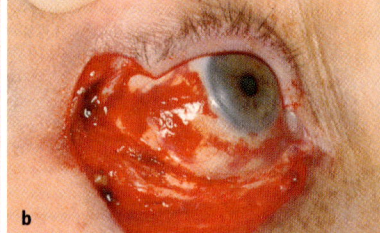 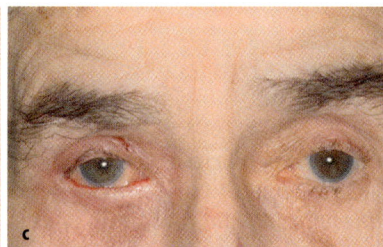

Fig. 3.1.28. Full-thickness defect of the right lower eyelid – eyelid reconstruction using a tarsoconjunctival flap from the upper eyelid (Hughes), a lateral periosteal flap and a transposition flap from the upper eyelid: **a** Preoperative appearance. **b** Intraoperative situs. **c** Appearance 1 day after opening of the Hughes plasty

References (see also page 379)

Adenis JP, Morax S: Pathologie orbito-palpébrale. Paris: Masson; 1998

American Joint Committee on Cancer: Carcinoma of the eyelid. In: AJCC: Cancer staging manual – sixth edition. New York: Springer; 2002: 349–354

Collin JRO: A manual of systematic eyelid surgery. London: Butterworth Heinemann; 2006

Colombo F et al: Merkel cell carcinoma: Clinicopathologic correlation, management, and follow-up in five patients. Ophthal Plast Reconstr Surg 2000;16:453–8

Conway RM et al: Frequency and clinical features of visceral malignancy in a consecutive case series of patients with periocular sebaceous gland carcinoma. Graefes Arch Clin Exp Ophthalmol 2004;242:674–8

Conway RM, Themel S, Holbach LM: Surgery for primary basal cell carcinoma including the eyelid margins with intraoperative frozen section control: comparative interventional study with a minimum clinical follow-up of 5 years. Br J Ophthalmol 2004; 88: 236–238

Font RL: Eyelids and lacrimal drainage system. In: Spencer WH (ed): Ophthalmic pathology. Vol. 4. Philadelphia, London, Tokyo: WB Saunders; 1996

Holbach LM et al: Differential diagnosis of lid tumors – Part 1 [in German]. Ophthalmologe 2002;99:394–413

Holbach LM et al: Differential diagnosis of lid tumors – Part 2 [in German]. Ophthalmologe 2002;99:490–509)

Hübner H: Chirurgische Therapie der Lidtumoren. I. In: Lommatzsch PK (ed): Ophthalmologische Onkologie. Stuttgart: Enke; 1999:48–61

Kröner B. Multiple ischemic infarction in the retina and uvea due to crystalline corticosteroid embolism following subcutaneous facial infections (in German). Klin Monatsbl Augenheilkd 1981; 178: 121–3

Kruse FE et al.: Konjunktiva. In: Naumann GOH et al.: Pathologie des Auges. Vol. 1. Berlin, Heidelberg: Springer;1997:398

Schlötzer-Schrehardt U et al: The pathogenesis of floppy eyelid syndrome – involvement of matrix metalloproteinases in elastic fiber degradation. Ophthalmology 2005;112:694–704

Shields JA, Shields CL: Atlas of eyelid and conjunctival tumors. Philadelphia: Lippincott Williams & Wilkins; 1999

Tyers AG, Collin JRO: Colour atlas of ophthalmic plastic surgery. London: Butterworth Heinemann; 2001:10–1;12

Lacrimal Drainage System

L.M. Heindl, A. Jünemann, L.M. Holbach

3.2.1 Surgical Anatomy

On lid closure tears are wiped to the nasal bulbar conjunctiva and tear meniscus and are then drained through the superior and inferior lacrimal puncta – which are open only with open eyes – and canaliculi into the lacrimal sac and by a sort of "lacrimal peristalsis" into the nose (Fig. 3.2.1). The canaliculi start with a 2-mm vertical component and continue with a horizontal portion 8–10 mm long. The common canaliculus, 1–2 mm long, leads into the lacrimal sac. Its entry into the sac at the internal ostium is often partially covered by a mucosal flap which is based anteriorly and also called "the valve of Rosenmüller." The lacrimal sac lies in the fossa between the anterior (frontal process of maxilla) and posterior (lacrimal bone) lacrimal crest and is surrounded by the anterior and posterior limbs of the medial canthal tendon. The body of the sac measures 10–12 mm in vertical height, and 3–5 mm of the sac (fundus) lie above the internal ostium. The suture line in the lacrimal fossa runs vertically between the thin lacrimal bone and the thicker frontal process of the maxilla. It is mostly located one-half of the way from the anterior to the posterior lacrimal crest. The sac leads into the bony nasolacrimal duct, which measures 12–15 mm in length and travels within the wall of the maxillary sinus and the lateral nasal wall. The duct extends for about 5 mm below the bony portion and opens beneath the inferior turbinate in the lateral wall of the nose. A mucosal valve (Hasner) usually prevents retrograde passage of mucus or air upwards. The nasal

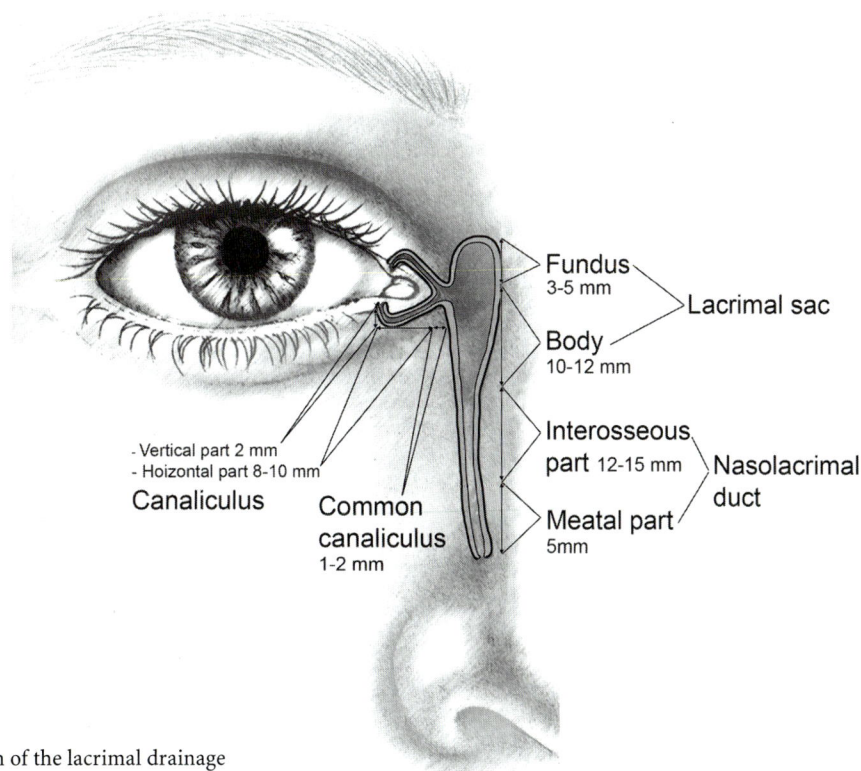

Fig. 3.2.1. Schematic illustration of the lacrimal drainage system with approximate measurements

entry site of a dacryocystorhinostomy lies at the anterior tip of the middle turbinate. The ethmoid sinus may extend to the lacrimal sac fossa. Bony removal of the lacrimal sac fossa may result in these situations in entry into the ethmoid sinus rather than into the nasal vault.

3.2.2
Surgical Pathology

The most common symptoms and signs indicating dysfunction of the lacrimal drainage system include epiphora, punctal discharge and medial canthal swelling.

Epiphora occurring in punctal, canalicular, lacrimal sac, nasolacrimal duct and nasal disorders (Table 3.2.1) is typically worse in the winter months and windy weather. The eye can be sticky due to an expressible mucocele or collected dried tears. The vision can be blurred secondary to an elevated tear meniscus (prismatic effect – especially on downgaze, for example when reading) or tear-splattered glasses. Chronic epiphora can induce red, sore lower-lid skin, with secondary anterior lamella (vertical) shortening (mild cicatricial ectropion). Excessive wiping away of tears can cause or exacerbate a medial ectropion.

Mucopurulent *punctal discharge* suggests stasis in the lacrimal sac or canaliculi, mostly secondary to nasolacrimal duct obstruction. Accumulation of inflammatory debris can result in *dacryolithiasis* seen in up to 15% of dacryocystorhinostomy surgeries. Lacrimal sac *stones* consist of dried mucus, lipid and inflammatory cells and are more likely to be found in chronically inflamed sacs.

Medial canthal swelling may be caused by an abscess, a dacryolith or a tumor in the lacrimal sac. But not all masses in the medial canthal area arise from the lacrimal sac (acute skin infection, acute ethmoiditis, ruptured dermoid cyst).

Actinomyces canaliculitis presents a characteristic clinical picture: epiphora and intense *itching*! This cannot be cured by local or systemic antibiotics: This is a "surgical entity" requiring internal slitting of the canaliculus – discharging a cotton-cheese like granula material. The sphincter muscle of Riolani controlling the punctum should be saved.

Swellings below the medial canthal tendon are typical of dacryocystitis. Differential diagnostic signs in favor of a tumor of the lacrimal sac (Fig. 3.2.2, Table 3.2.2) include a mass above the medial canthal ligament (absent in dacryocystitis), the presence of telangiectases in the skin overlying the mass (instead of the diffuse erythema of dacryocystitis) and the presence of serosanguineous discharge or a bloody reflux with atraumatic irrigation (both of which are not usually observed in dacryocystitis).

Table 3.2.1. Differential diagnosis of lacrimal drainage system disorders causing epiphora

Punctal causes of epiphora
Congenital punctal atresia
Punctal ectropion in eyelid malposition
Acquired punctal stenosis due to age-related atrophic processes, chronic inflammation, cicatricial conjunctival disease, systemic chemotherapeutic agents
Canalicular causes of epiphora
Congenital absence or fistula
Acquired intrinsic disorders: postherpetic infection (herpes simplex, varicella zoster), bacterial infection (e.g., actinomyces, chlamydia), trauma, postirradiation, pharmacological, intrinsic tumor (e.g., squamous papilloma, squamous cell carcinoma)
Acquired extrinsic disorders: compression and/or invasion and occlusion by adjacent tumor (e.g., basal cell carcinoma, squamous cell carcinoma, non-Hodgkin B-cell lymphoma)
Lacrimal sac causes of epiphora
Congenital diverticulum or fistula (from sac to nose or cheek)
Acquired intrinsic disorders: inflammation (extension of primary acquired nasolacrimal duct obstruction including dacryoliths, Wegener's granulomatosis, sarcoidosis, allergy, hay fever, atopy), trauma, intrinsic tumor arising within the sac and/or the sac walls (Table 3.2.2)
Acquired extrinsic disorders: adjacent tumor compressing and/or invading the sac from the outside (e.g., basal cell carcinoma, squamous cell carcinoma, non-Hodgkin B-cell lymphoma, neurofibroma)
Nasolacrimal duct causes of epiphora
Congenital nasolacrimal duct obstruction (delayed opening of valve of Hasner with/without dacryocele, craniofacial abnormality, rare nasolacrimal duct agenesis)
Primary acquired nasolacrimal duct obstruction (most common cause in adults)
Secondary acquired lacrimal obstruction, including trauma and tumors (as for sac and those extending from the maxillary sinus)
Nasal causes of epiphora
Allergic rhinitis, severe rhinosinus disease (e.g., polyps), previous nasal surgery
Tumors spreading from nasal space and/or adjacent sinuses

Table 3.2.2. Lacrimal sac tumors (from Font 1996)

I. **Epithelial tumors**
1. Squamous cell papilloma
2. Transitional cell papilloma
3. Mixed cell papilloma (exophytic or endophytic)
4. Oncocytic adenoma (oncocytoma)
5. Squamous cell carcinoma
6. Transitional cell carcinoma
7. Adenocarcinoma
8. Mucepidermoid carcinoma
9. Oncocytic adenocarcinoma
II. **Non-epithelial tumors**
1. Fibrous histiocytoma
2. Pyogenic granuloma
3. Neurilemmoma
4. Lymphoid tumors
5. Malignant melanoma
6. Angiosarcoma

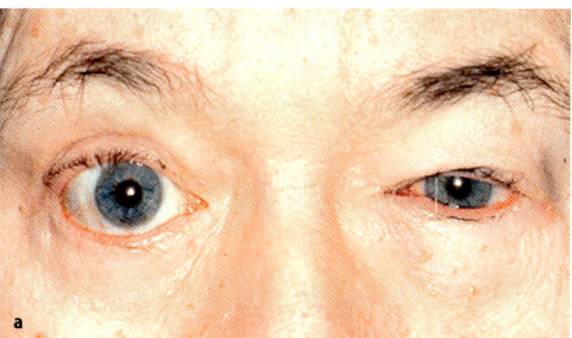
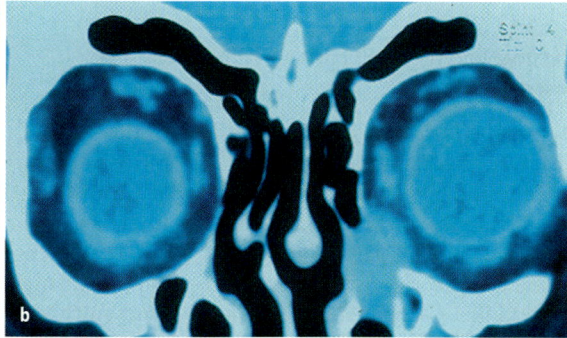

Fig. 3.2.2. Oncocytoma of the lacrimal sac: **a** Recurrent conjunctivitis and epiphora of the left eye for 6 years and left medial canthal swelling of 18 months' duration in a 66-year-old woman. **b** Coronal computed tomography scan revealing a non-calcified, soft-tissue, space-occupying process (*) in the region of the left lacrimal sac. **c** Histopathologic section (periodic acid–Schiff, original magnification × 100) showing a solid tumor with numerous cystic spaces filled with PAS-positive amorphous material surrounded by proliferating epithelial cells with granular cytoplasm. **d** Electron microscopy (*scale bar* 1 µm) demonstrating oncocytes densely packed with mitochondria of various sizes and shapes. (From Kottler et al. 2004)

3.2.3
Principles of Lacrimal Surgery

In lacrimal surgery the level of the obstruction revealed clinically by irrigation and probing of the nasolacrimal system is critical to the choice of operation:

1. Obstruction at or distal to the entry of the common canaliculus into the lacrimal sac: external dacryocystorhinostomy (with or without silicone tube intubation)
2. Obstruction at or beyond 8 mm from the punctum of one or both canaliculi, but proximal to the entry of the common canaliculus into the lacrimal sac: external canaliculo-dacryocystorhinostomy
3. Obstruction less than 8 mm from the punctum in both canaliculi: external dacryocystorhinostomy with bypass tube insertion.

3.2.3.1
External Dacryocystorhinostomy
(with or without Silicone Tube Intubation)

The principle is a *side-to-side anastomosis* between the lacrimal sac and nasal mucosa, effectively incorporating the lacrimal sac into the lateral wall of the nose. In order to prevent closure and scarring of the osteotomy or restenosis of the lacrimal outflow system, lacrimal canaliculi, common canaliculus, sac and anastomosis can be stented with fine silicone tubing.

Indications for external dacryocystorhinostomy include lacrimal mucocele (obstruction at the sac and nasolacrimal duct junction), dacryolithiasis, nasolacrimal duct obstruction in children not responding to probing and intubation, nasolacrimal duct obstruction in adults and functional lacrimal obstruction not responding to simpler methods of treatment such as horizontal lid tightening. Especially in the case of a common canalicular obstruction, a small scarred lacrimal sac or a repeat dacryocystorhinostomy, silicone tube intubation is indicated. The silicone tubing should be removed 2–4 months postoperatively, but earlier if the canaliculi are cheesewired by too tightly tied tubing.

3.2.3.2
External Canaliculo-Dacryocystorhinostomy

The principle is an anastomosis between the end of one or both canaliculi and the nose, using the lacrimal sac if present as a bridging flap.

Indications include canalicular obstructions with eight or more millimeters of remaining patent canaliculus, particularly in patients without any residual lacrimal sac following previous dacryocystorhinostomy.

3.2.3.3
External Dacryocystorhinostomy with Bypass Tube Insertion

The principle is an insertion of a bypass tube passed from the medial canthus through the soft tissues and the bony rhinostomy into the nasal cavity.

Indications include canalicular obstructions with less than 8 mm of patent canaliculus, a failed canaliculo-dacryocystorhinostomy and a functional lacrimal obstruction not helped by a routine dacryocystorhinostomy (as in a complete facial palsy).

Bypass tube surgery requires long-term aftercare by the ophthalmologist as well as the patient themselves, because complications such as migration, malposition or obstruction of the tube and granuloma formation may occur.

In addition to the external approach, *endonasal dacryocystorhinostomy* is widely in use. The nasal mucosa and lower lacrimal sac are approached via the nose using an endoscope for magnification and illumination. The mucosa is incised and surgically excised or laser ablated. The rhinostomy is usually smaller than that of external dacryocystorhinostomy. There are no sutured flaps. Tubes are usually used. Indications for endonasal (intranasal, transnasal) dacryocystorhinostomy include obstructions in the lower lacrimal sac and inferior to it.

References (see also page 379)

Busse H: Classical lacrimal apparatus surgery from the ophthalmological viewpoint [in German]. Ophthalmologe 2001; 98:602–6.

Emmerich KH, Busse H, Meyer-Rüsenberg HW: Dacryocystorhinostomia externa. Technique, indications and results (in German). Ophthalmologe 1994; 91:395–398

Font RL: Eyelids and lacrimal drainage system. In: Spencer WH (ed): Ophthalmic pathology. Vol. 4. Philadelphia, London, Tokyo: WB Saunders; 1996:2412–27

Hurwitz JJ (ed): The lacrimal system. Philadelphia: Lippincott-Raven; 1996

Iro H, Waldfahrer F: Endonasal lacrimal apparatus surgery from ENT specialist viewpoint (in German). Ophthalmologe 2001; 98: 613–616

Kottler UB et al: Epiphora und Konjunktivitis seit 6 Jahren. Ophthalmologe 2004;101:730–2

McNab AA: Manual of orbital and lacrimal surgery. Edinburgh: Churchill Livingstone; 1994

Olver J: Colour atlas of lacrimal surgery. London, Butterworth-Heinemann, 2002

Rose GE: The lacrimal paradox: toward a greater understanding of success in lacrimal surgery. Ophthal Plast Reconstr Surg 2004;20:262–5.

Struck HG, Weidlich R: Indications and prognosis of dacryocystorhinostomy in childhood. A clinical study 1970–2000. Ophthalmologe 2001;98:560–3

Thale A et al. Functional anatomy of the human efferent tear ducts: a new theory of tear outflow mechanism. Graefes Arch Clin Exp Ophthalmol 1998; 236:674–8

Orbit

L.M. Holbach, L.M. Heindl, R.F. Guthoff

3.3.1 Surgical Anatomy

In the upper eyelid the first structure encountered behind the septum is the *pre-aponeurotic fat pad*, which lies in the space between the septum and the levator aponeurosis. This is similar in the lower eyelid.

The *bony orbital walls* are of particular importance in relation to their adjacent structures (Fig. 3.3.1). The bony roof of the orbit has the anterior cranial fossa and the frontal sinus above. The medial bony wall has the ethmoid sinuses and posteriorly part of the sphenoid sinus lying medial to it. The maxillary sinus lies below the bony orbital floor. The anterior lateral wall has the temporal fossa with the temporalis muscle within it. More posteriorly, the lateral wall lies in front of the middle cranial fossa.

The medial wall of the orbit has the thin *lamina papyracea*, separating the ethmoid sinus from the orbit. The fossa lacrimalis lies anteriorly in the medial wall. It houses the lacrimal sac and is bounded anteriorly by the anterior lacrimal crest, posteriorly by the posterior lacrimal crest. The orbital floor is also very thin, in particular medially. The suture between the ethmoid and maxillary sinus forms the inferior border of the medial wall. This marks a thick strut of bone providing support for the inferomedial orbit. This *maxilloethmoidal* strut often remains intact following orbital trauma. It should be left intact anteriorly during inferomedial orbital decompression. The lateral wall has a thinner portion in its middle third between the orbital rim and the thicker bone of the greater wing of the sphenoid.

The orbit can be divided into three *surgical spaces*:

1. Extraperiosteal
2. Extraconal
3. Intraconal

The *extraperiosteal space* exists only when opened surgically or filled by a pathologic process. It provides surgical access in an easily dissected plane, and may harbor pathologic tissue such as blood and pus. The periosteum is an important barrier confining many pathologic lesions. To reach the extraperiosteal space, the periosteum is incised and elevated over the orbital rim where it is firmly adherent. Within the orbital walls, it strips from the bone more easily. It follows the contours of the bony orbital walls. There are, however, a number of structures passing through it which are encountered when dissecting this plane, e.g., during orbital exenteration or bony decompression of the lateral wall. These include the *zygomaticofacial nerve and artery* occurring a variable but short distance inside the rim closer

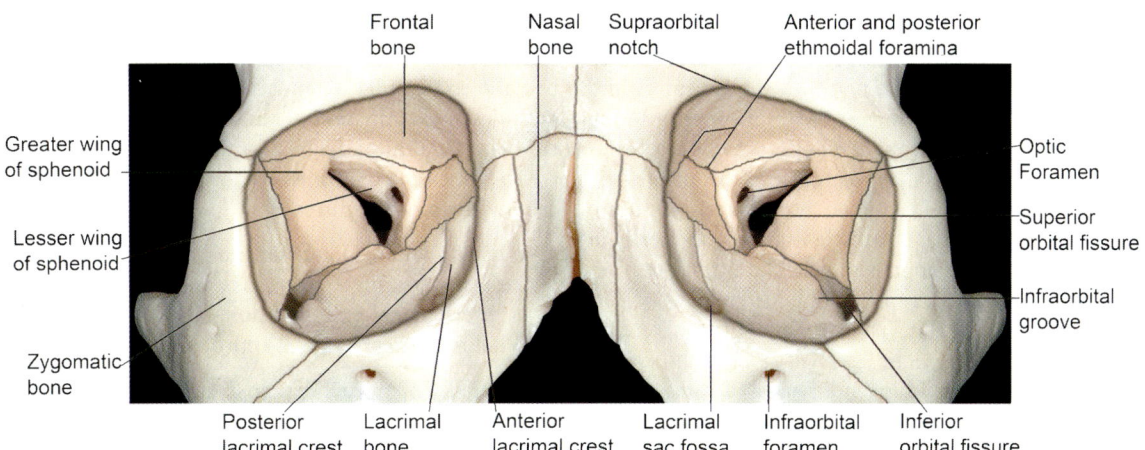

Fig. 3.3.1. Anatomy of the bony orbit

to the floor than the roof. Inferiorly, on the lateral wall, the lower edge of the greater wing and the smooth posterior wall of the maxillary sinus form the *inferior orbital fissure,* which does not contain as many important structures as the superior orbital fissure so that dissection after bipolar cautery, for instance in lateral decompression surgery, is justified. The origin of the *inferior oblique muscle* is on the medial part of the floor, just inside the orbital rim and lateral to the *nasolacrimal duct.* The *anterior and posterior ethmoidal vessels and nerves* are a useful landmark for the upper limit of the medial wall and the lower limit of the roof during bony decompression of the medial wall. The larger anterior ethmoidal bundle is found one-third to one-half the way back from the rim, and the posterior a variable distance behind, sometimes quite close to the orbital apex. The *supraorbital neurovascular bundle* may pass through a bony canal and pierce the periorbita anteriorly. It may also remain within the periorbita as it leaves the orbit in a notch. It is located along the superior orbital rim at the junction of its medial one-third. The *zygomaticofrontal suture* is on the lateral orbital rim at its superior one-fourth junction. It is a point of firm periosteal attachment and the most common location for dermoid cysts. The *superior orbital fissure,* which is located at the junction of the roof and lateral walls posteriorly, contains many important structures such as the oculomotor nerve with its superior and inferior divisions, the trochlear and abducens nerve, the first division of the trigeminal nerve, sympathetic fibers and veins connecting the orbit and the cavernous sinus. The orbital apex located between the roof and the medial wall contains the optic foramen with the optic nerve and ophthalmic artery.

The *extraconal space* contains the lacrimal gland and the extraocular muscles. The *lacrimal gland* lies in a bony fossa inside the orbital rim in the superotemporal quadrant. The larger orbital lobe of the lacrimal gland is only separated from the bone by the periorbita. It lies partly on the lateral horn of the levator aponeurosis. The palpebral lobe of the lacrimal gland lies laterally between the lateral horn of the levator aponeurosis and the conjunctiva. Lacrimal ductules from the orbital lobe pass through or around the palpebral lobe to empty into the lateral conjunctival fornix 4–5 mm superior to the tarsal border. The *extraocular muscles* provide a very obvious anatomic landmark as one dissects through the orbital fat. It may be helpful to use a traction suture through the lateral rectus muscle transconjunctivally in order to identify its course after lateral orbital wall removal. The four recti, superior oblique and levator palpebrae arise in the orbital apex (*annulus of Zinn*) and insert anteriorly on the globe (*spiral of Tillaux*) and eyelid.

The superior oblique tendon passes through the *trochlea* residing in a small bony fossa in the superomedial orbit inside the orbital rim. The trochlea can be safely lifted out of its fossa in extraperiosteal dissection. The recti and levator muscle receive their innervation from nerves entering the muscle bellies at the junction of the posterior and middle thirds. The trochlear nerve, however, enters the muscle belly on the superior surface of its posterior third. The inferior oblique muscle arises from the periosteum of the inferior orbital rim just lateral to the opening of the nasolacrimal canal. It passes beneath the inferior rectus towards the posterolateral aspect of the globe.

The *intraconal space* contains the orbital fat, which is structured by septa, as described by Koornneef (1979). These elements, partly forming pulleys, are leading to the sheath of the eye muscles, stabilizing and guiding their course during action. The ophthalmic artery and the optic nerve enter the orbit through the optic foramen. The first branch of the ophthalmic artery is the central retinal artery which arises near the orbital apex and runs forward beneath the optic nerve to pierce its dura about 10 mm behind the globe. The long posterior ciliary arteries (two to three) run forward within the adventitia surrounding the optic nerve and pierce the sclera laterally and medially to provide blood supply to the anterior segment of the eye. Fifteen to 20 short posterior ciliary vessels arise from the long posterior vessels in a ring around the optic nerve to supply the choroid and optic nerve head.

3.3.2
Surgical Pathology
3.3.2.1
Orbital Tumors

Clinical history (symptoms, duration) and examination findings (signs) are essential in the diagnosis of benign and malignant orbital lesions. Pain may be a prominent feature not only of inflammatory processes but also, e.g., adenoid-cystic carcinoma because of its tendency to infiltrate along sensory nerves. Imaging (orbital ultrasonography, computed tomography, magnetic resonance imaging) may provide additional information about location, size and extent of the mass, but allows no final diagnosis of tumor entity. Histopathologic examination is almost always necessary to confirm the clinical diagnosis in orbital diseases.

The following questions are to be addressed in a patient with an orbital tumor:

1. What is the most likely diagnosis? (benign versus malignant, infiltrative versus non-infiltrative)
2. Is an excisional or an incisional biopsy indicated?
3. What is the best surgical approach to the mass?

For clinical differential diagnosis the knowledge of the frequency of orbital lesions may be helpful (Tables 3.3.1, 3.3.2). The incidence varies with age. In childhood, dermoid cysts (Figs. 3.3.2, 3.3.3) and capillary hemangiomas are the most common benign lesions. In adults, thyroid-associated orbitopathy (Figs. 3.3.18, 3.3.19) is predominant, and the commonest benign tumors of the orbit are cavernous hemangiomas (Figs. 3.3.8, 3.3.9), requiring differential diagnostic distinction from hemangiopericytomas (Fig. 3.3.10), solitary fibrous tumors (Fig. 3.3.11) and neurilemmomas (Fig. 3.3.12). Malignant orbital disease, either primary or secondary, is rare, but can affect all ages. In childhood, rhabdomyosarcoma (Fig. 3.3.4) and metastatic

Table 3.3.1. Frequency of orbital tumors in children ($n=358$) (modified from Garner and Klintworth 1994, p 1525)

1.	Dermoid cysts	37%
2.	Hemangioma	12%
3.	Rhabdomyosarcoma	9%
4.	Optic nerve glioma	6%
5.	Neurofibroma	4%
6.	Metastatic neuroblastoma	3%
7.	Lymphangioma	3%
8.	Inflammatory pseudotumor	3%
9.	Leukemia and lymphoma	3%
10.	Lipoma	2%
11.	Meningeoma (orbital and sphenoid wing)	2%
12.	Schwannoma	2%
13.	Microphthalmus with cyst	1%
14.	Teratoma	1%
15.	Prominent palpebral lobe of lacrimal gland	1%
16.	Retinoblastoma	1%
17.	Sarcoma undifferentiated	1%
18.	Others	9%

Table 3.3.2. Frequency of orbital tumors in adults ($n=1,599$) (modified from Garner and Klintworth 1994, p 1524)

1.	Lymphoid tumors (lymphoid hyperplasia, non-Hodgkin lymphoma and others)	24%
2.	Vascular tumors (capillary and cavernous hemangioma, malformations, hemangiopericytoma, angiosarcoma)	16%
3.	Inflammatory lesions ("pseudotumor," sarcoid, fasciitis)	12%
4.	Lacrimal gland tumors (pleomorphic adenoma, adenocarcinoma, adenoid-cystic carcinoma, mucoepidermoid carcinoma, sebaceous gland carcinoma)	9%
5.	Secondary tumors (metastasis, local invasion)	8%
6.	Optic nerve tumors (meningeoma, pilocytic astrocytoma, malignant astrocytoma)	7%
7.	Dermoid cyst and other cysts	7%
8.	Peripheral nerve tumors (schwannoma, neurofibroma and others)	6%
9.	Myogenic tumors (rhabdomyosarcoma, malignant rhabdoid tumor)	5%
10.	Others (mucocele, cholesterol granuloma)	3%
11.	Fibrous tumors (fibrous histiocytoma, solitary fibrous tumor, fibrosarcoma)	1%
12.	Lipomatous tumors (pleomorphic lipoma, liposarcoma)	1%
13.	Histiocytic tumors (xanthogranuloma, Langerhans' cell histiocytosis)	0.5%
14.	Bony and cartilage-derived tumors (osteoma, chondroma, chondrosarcoma)	0.5%

Fig. 3.3.2. Orbital dermoid cysts located in different parts of the orbit and periorbita: **a, b** Subcutaneous mass (*) superotemporal to the right eye (near the zygomaticofrontal suture) in an 8-year-old girl (**a**). Appearance 2 months postoperatively following complete surgical excision through a superior eyelid crease incision (**b**). **c, d** Nasally located right periorbital dermoid cyst (*arrow*) in a 22-year-old female (**c**). Magnetic resonance imaging in T_2-weighted image showing a cystic lesion (*) with heterogeneous content (**d**)

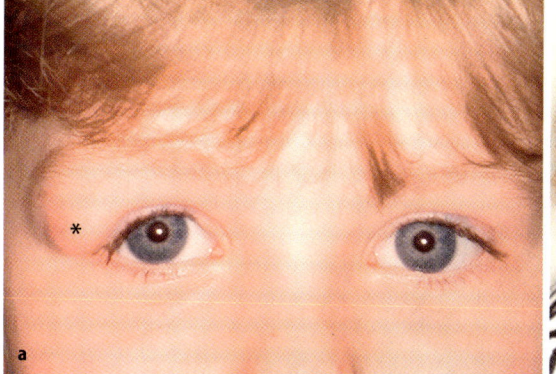
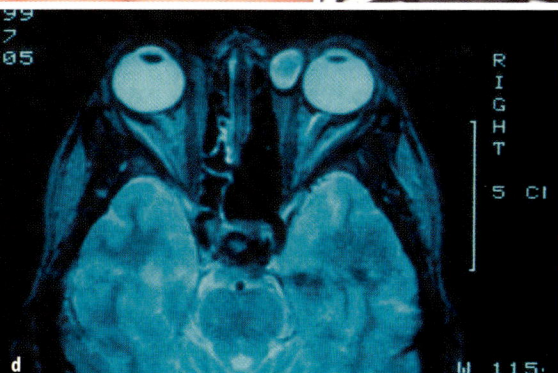
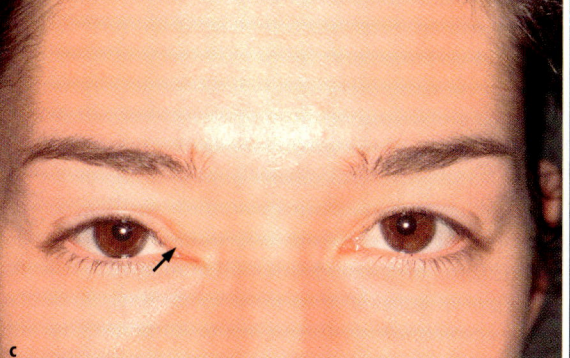

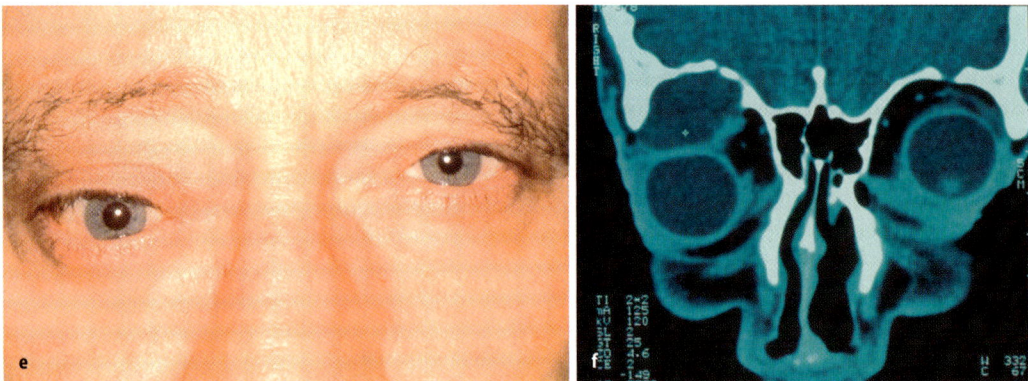

Fig. 3.3.2. e, f Large dermoid cyst located in the right orbit in a 57-year-old man (**e**). Coronal computed tomography scan showing a well-circumscribed cystic lesion (*) with bony fossa formation (**f**). (From Colombo et al. 2000)

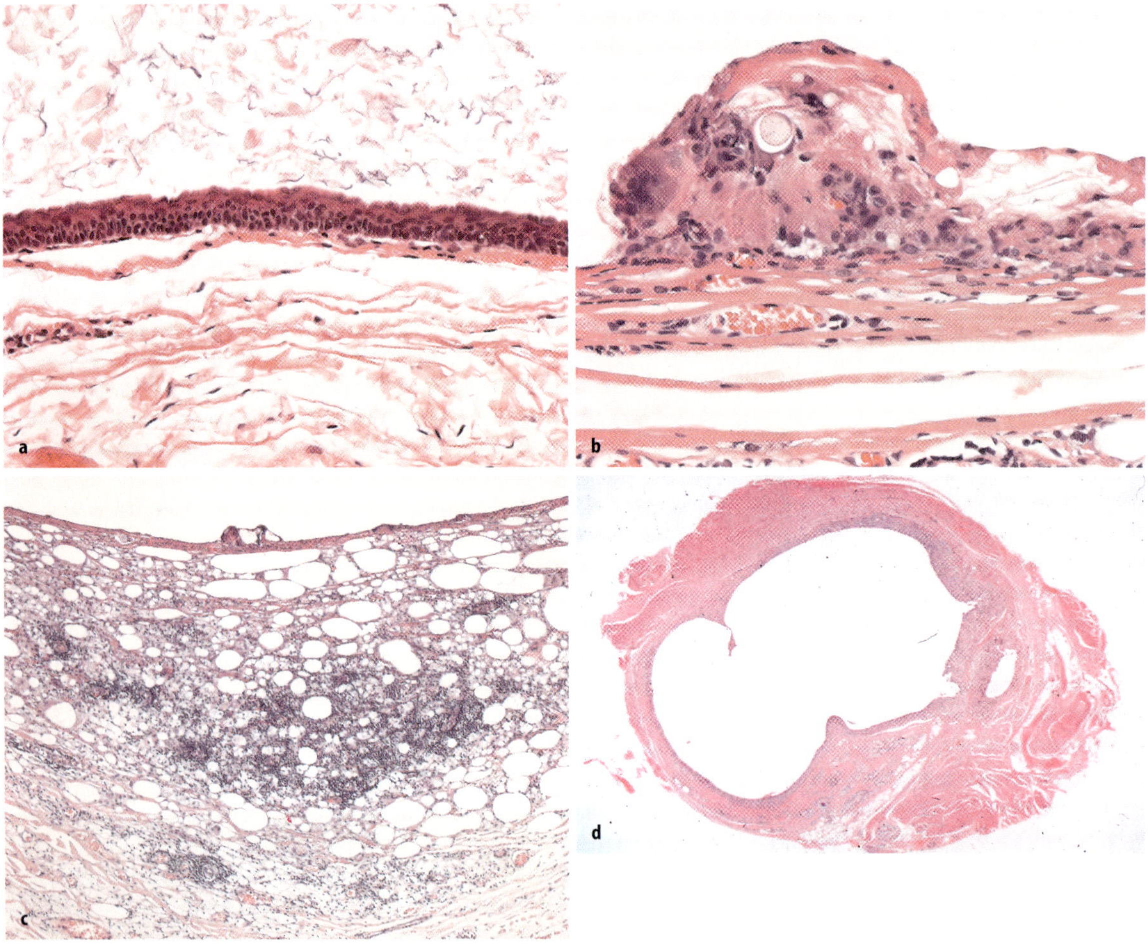

Fig. 3.3.3. Histopathology of orbital dermoid cysts: **a** Histopathologic section (hematoxylin-eosin, original magnification ×100) showing the epithelial lining of the dermoid cyst. **b** Granulomatous inflammatory infiltrate replacing the epithelial lining of the dermoid cyst. Notice a hair shaft (*arrow*) in the inflamed cyst wall (hematoxylin-eosin, original magnification ×200). **c** Presence of vacuoles of dissolved lipid within marked inflammatory infiltrate replacing the epithelial lining (hematoxylin-eosin, original magnification ×50). **d** Inflammatory infiltrate replacing the epithelial lining in its entire extent (hematoxylin-eosin, original magnification ×12.5). (From Colombo et al. 2000)

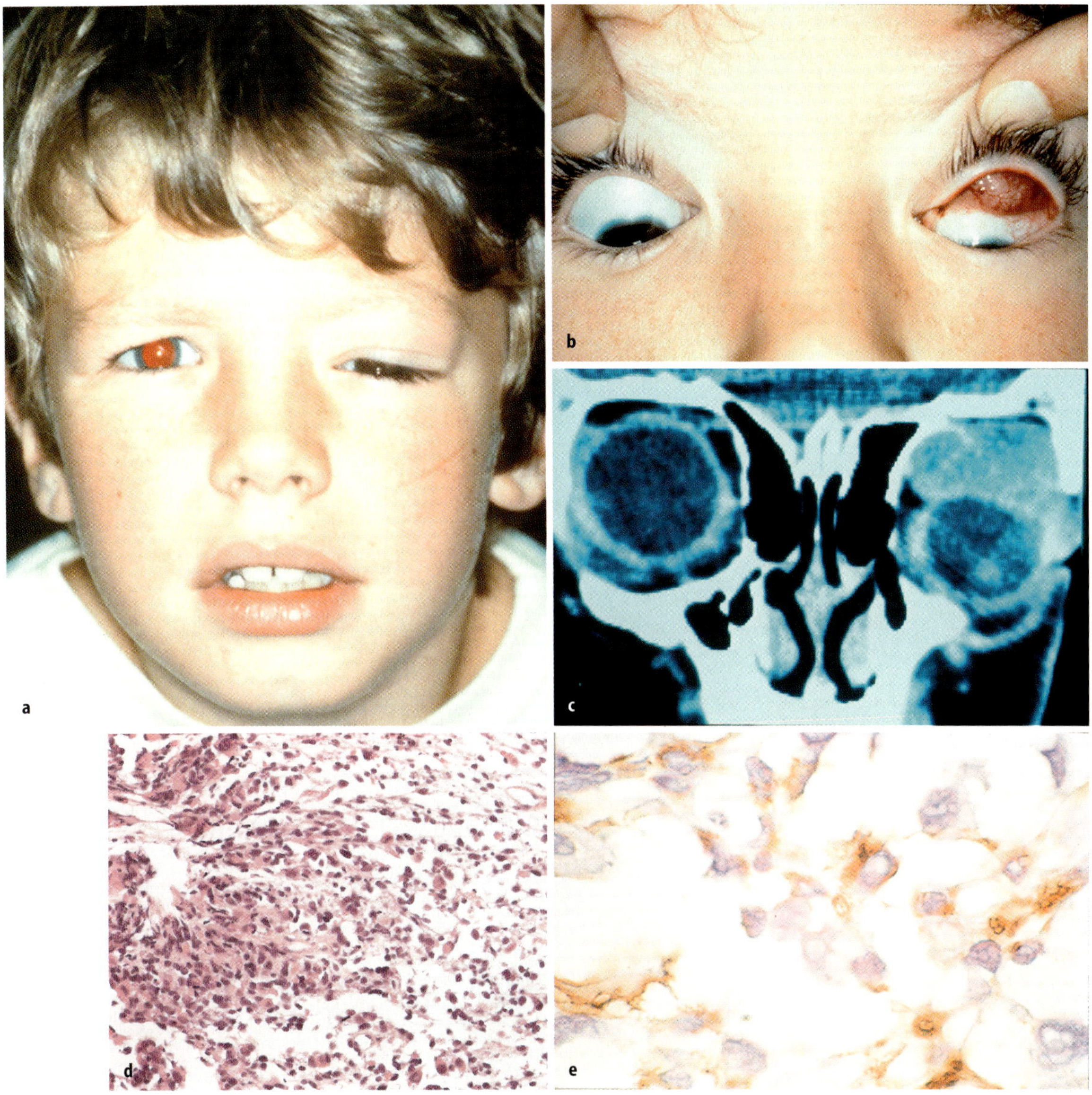

Fig. 3.3.4. Orbital rhabdomyosarcoma: **a** Progressive upper lid swelling and hypotropia of the left eye of 4 weeks' duration in a 9-year-old boy. **b** Subconjunctival mass of the left upper eyelid and anterior orbit. **c** Coronal computed tomography scan demonstrating a supra- and parabulbar mass (*) compressing the eyeball. **d** Histopathologic section (hematoxylin-eosin, original magnification ×100) showing malignant strap cells compatible with embryonic rhabdomyosarcoma of differentiated type. **e** Immunohistochemical profile of tumor cells showing strong positivity for desmin (peroxidase-antiperoxidase, anti-desmin, original magnification ×800). (From Holbach et al. 1989)

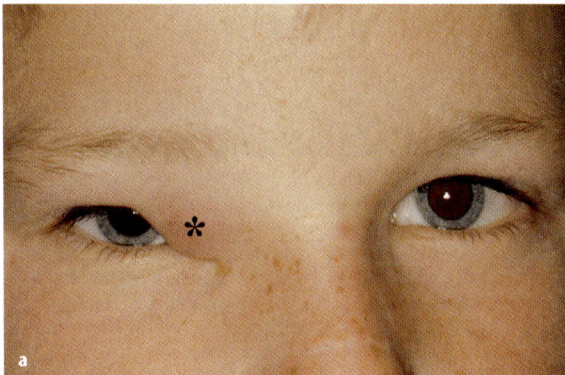

Fig. 3.3.5a (Legend see p. 54)

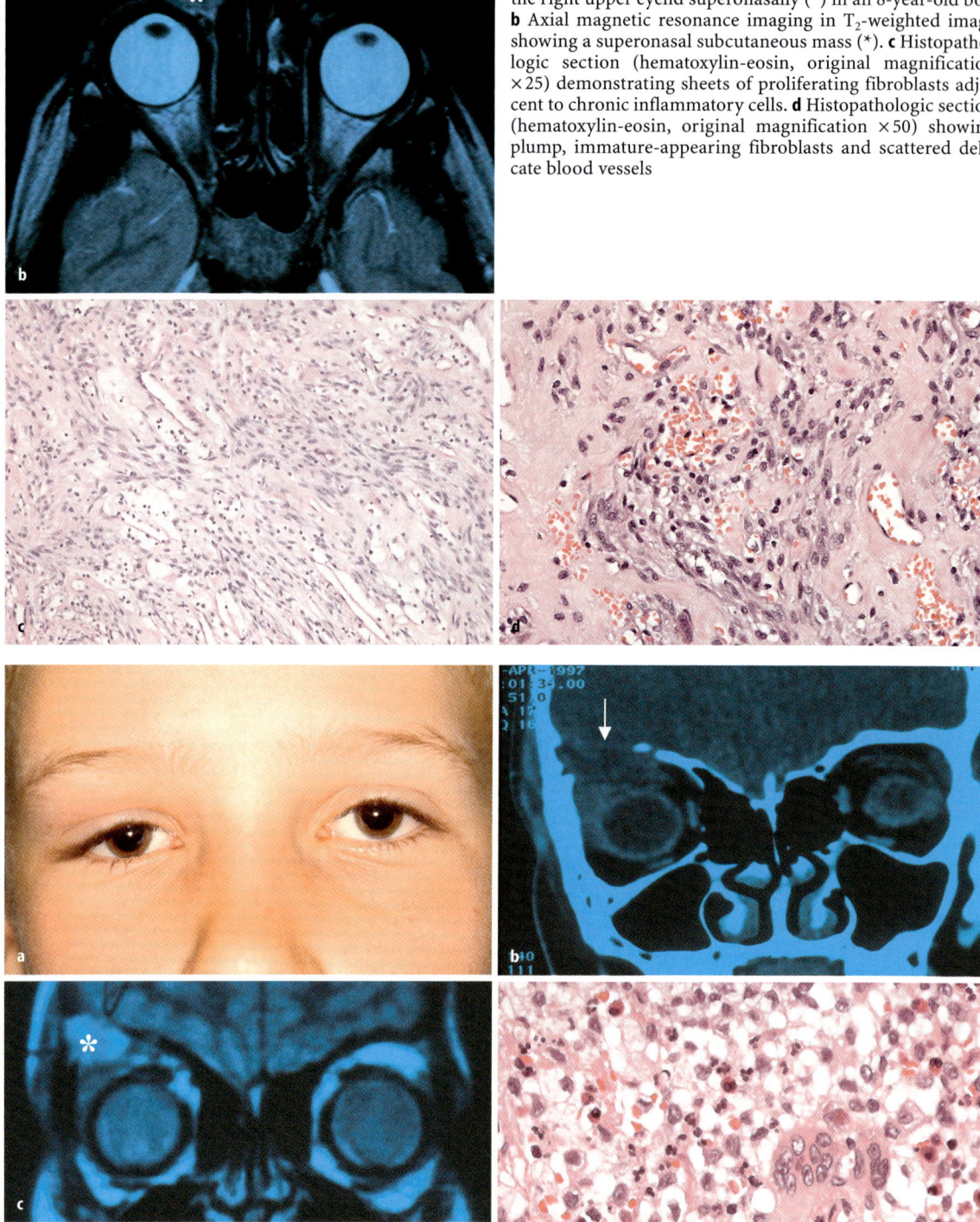

Fig. 3.3.5. Nodular fasciitis: **a** Acute swelling and redness in the right upper eyelid superonasally (*) in an 8-year-old boy. **b** Axial magnetic resonance imaging in T_2-weighted image showing a superonasal subcutaneous mass (*). **c** Histopathologic section (hematoxylin-eosin, original magnification ×25) demonstrating sheets of proliferating fibroblasts adjacent to chronic inflammatory cells. **d** Histopathologic section (hematoxylin-eosin, original magnification ×50) showing plump, immature-appearing fibroblasts and scattered delicate blood vessels

Fig. 3.3.6. Langerhans-cell histiocytosis of the orbit: **a** Painful reddish upper lid swelling of the right eye in a 9-year-old boy. **b** Coronal computed tomography scan showing a space-occupying lesion adjacent to a lytic defect (*arrow*) of the frontal bone laterally. **c** Coronal magnetic resonance imaging in T_2-weighted image revealing marked contrast enhancement of the superotemporal mass (*) close to the intracranial fossa. **d** Histopathologic section (hematoxylin-eosin, original magnification ×200) demonstrating admixture of histiocytes, eosinophils, lymphocytes and Langerhans' giant cells. (From Holbach et al. 2000)

Fig. 3.3.7. Orbital lymphangioma: **a** Rapidly progressive proptosis and downward displacement of the left eye in an 18-months-old boy. **b** Coronal magnetic resonance imaging in T_1-weighted image demonstrating a cystic mass (*) superonasal to the globe. **c** Sagittal magnetic resonance imaging in T2-weighted image revealing an extensive cystic lesion (*) involving most of the superior orbit. **d** Histopathologic section (hematoxylin-eosin, original magnification ×25) showing lymphatic vessels of different sizes, lined by endothelium and separated by thin, delicate walls. (See Cursiefen et al. 2001)

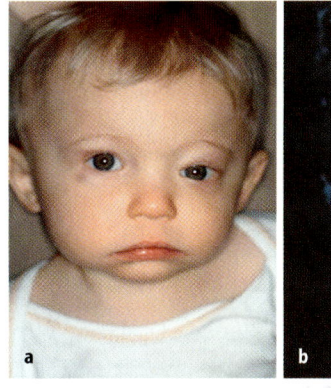
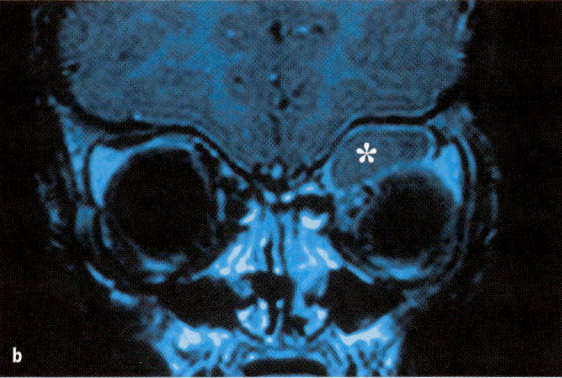
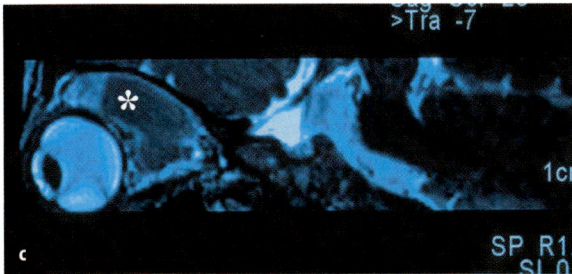
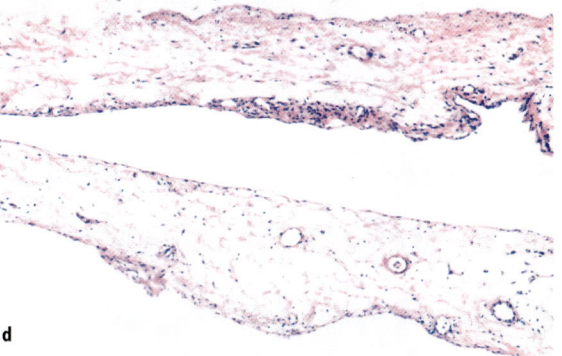

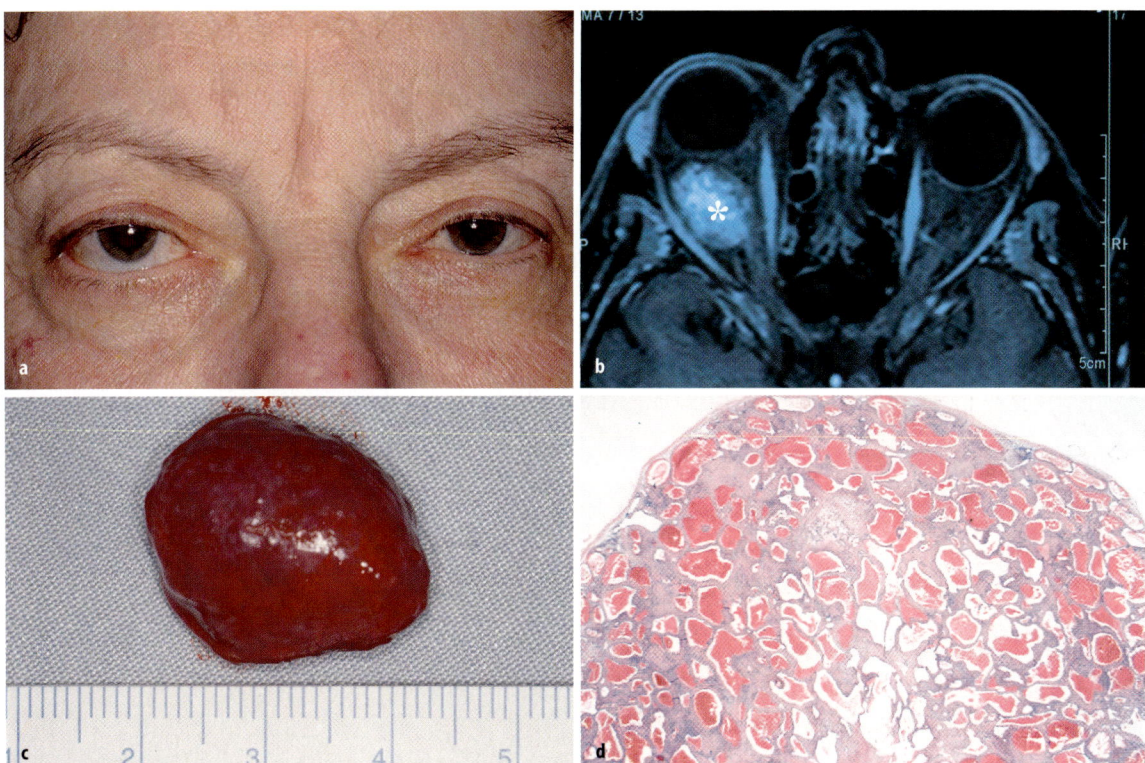

Fig. 3.3.8. Orbital cavernous hemangioma: **a** Slowly progressive proptosis of the right eye of 3 years' duration in a 62-year-old man. **b** Axial magnetic resonance imaging in T_1-weighted image revealing a spotted contrast enhancement of a large orbital mass (*) in the muscle cone. **c** Circumscribed reddish-blue tumor after surgical removal via a lateral orbitotomy. **d** Histopathologic section (hematoxylin-eosin, original magnification ×50) showing large congested cavernous vascular channels

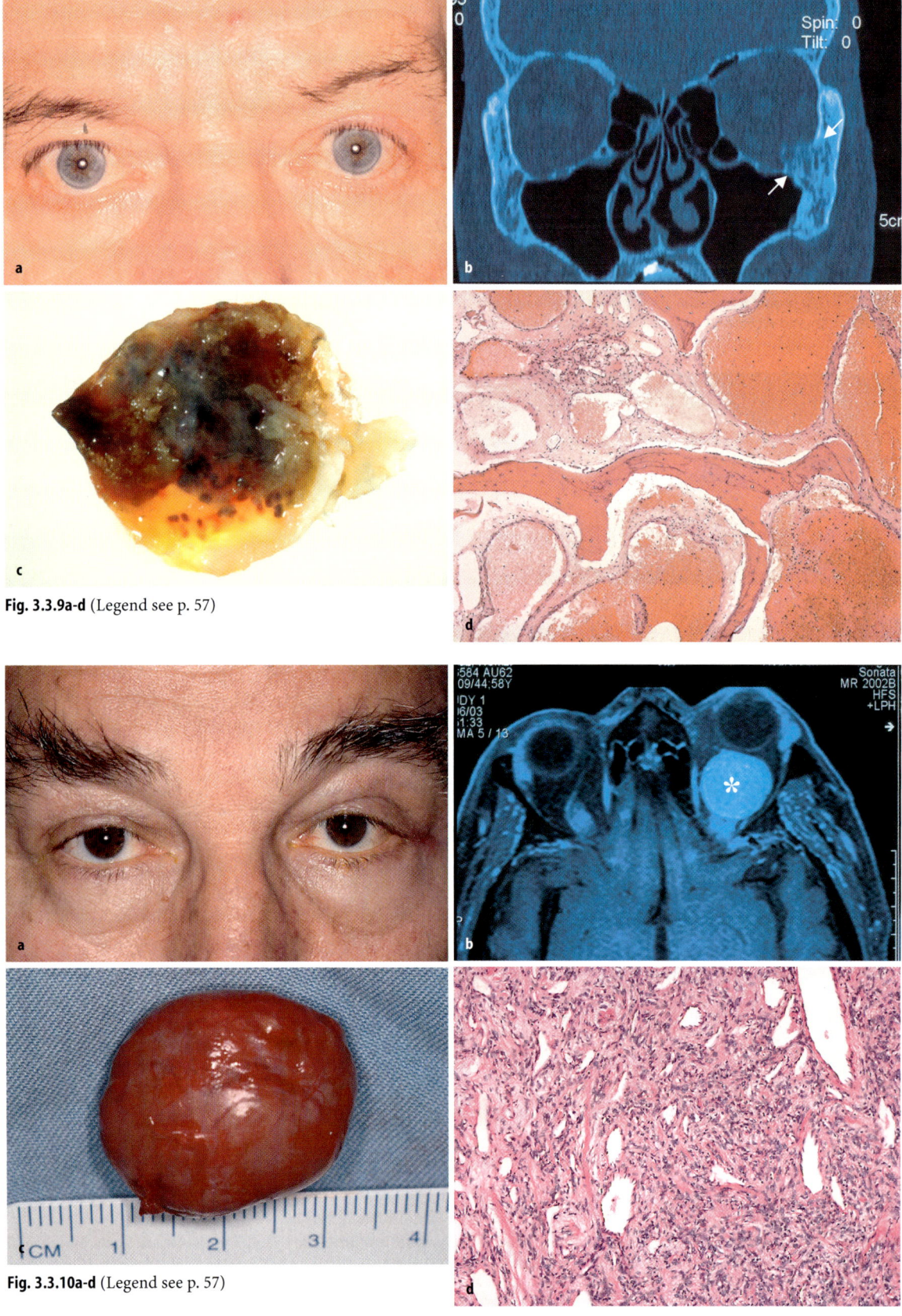

Fig. 3.3.9a-d (Legend see p. 57)

Fig. 3.3.10a-d (Legend see p. 57)

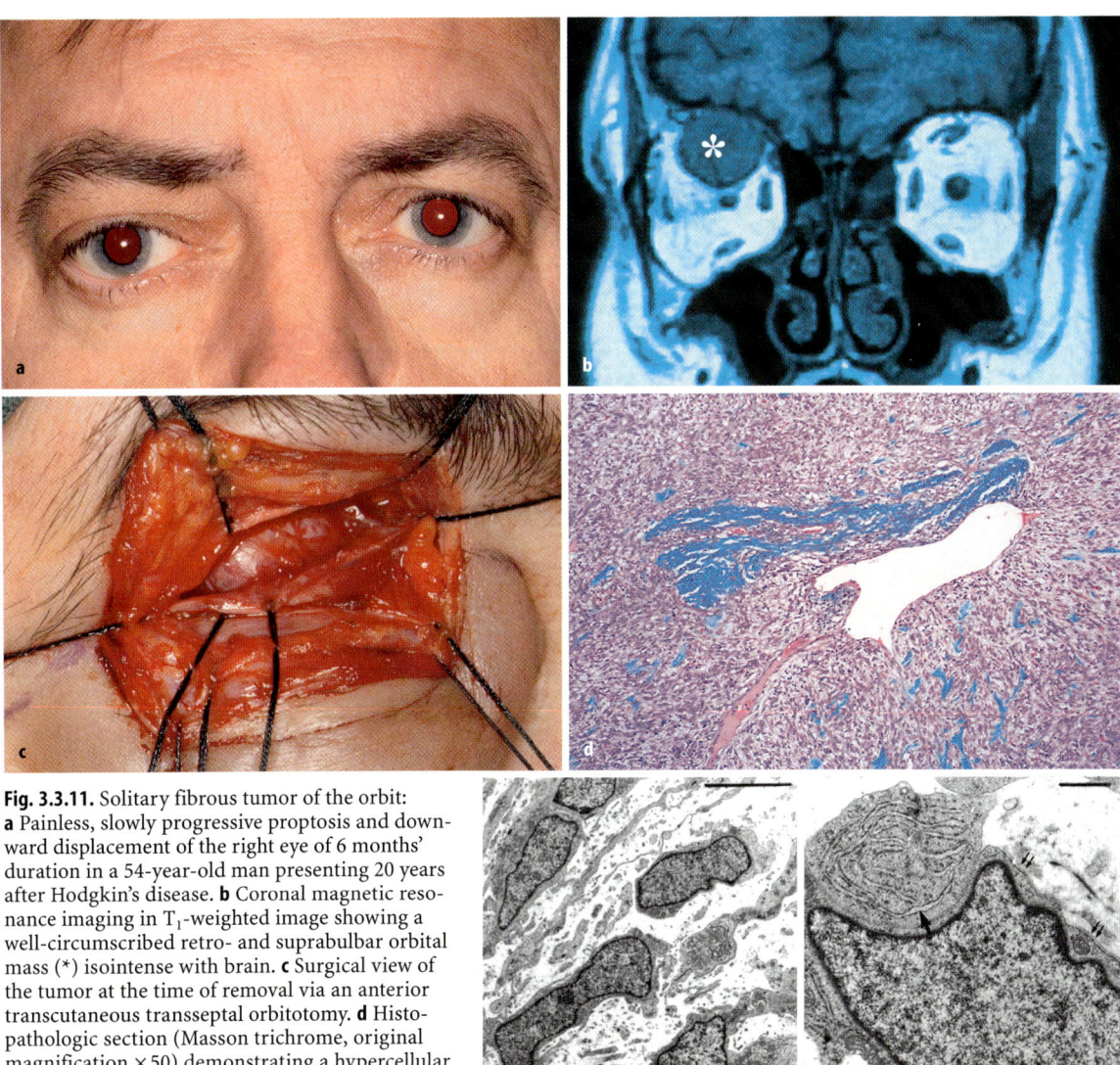

Fig. 3.3.11. Solitary fibrous tumor of the orbit: **a** Painless, slowly progressive proptosis and downward displacement of the right eye of 6 months' duration in a 54-year-old man presenting 20 years after Hodgkin's disease. **b** Coronal magnetic resonance imaging in T_1-weighted image showing a well-circumscribed retro- and suprabulbar orbital mass (*) isointense with brain. **c** Surgical view of the tumor at the time of removal via an anterior transcutaneous transseptal orbitotomy. **d** Histopathologic section (Masson trichrome, original magnification ×50) demonstrating a hypercellular tumor with multiple collagen bundles. **e** Electron microscopy (*scale bar* 5 µm) showing elongated tumor cells within a matrix of collagen. **f** Electron microscopy (*scale bar* 1 µm) revealing abundant, dilated rough endoplasmic reticulum in tumor cells (*single arrow*) and scanty fragments of basal lamina material adjacent to tumor cells (*double arrows*). (From Holbach et al. 2002)

◁
Fig. 3.3.9. Primary intraosseous cavernous hemangioma of the orbit: **a** Slight proptosis of the left eye in a 75-year-old man. **b** Coronal computed tomography scan revealing an intraosseous mass (*arrows*) in the left orbital rim inferolaterally with internal radiating trabeculations, a honeycomb pattern, and without signs of destruction of the surrounding tissue. The patient had undergone a nephrectomy for renal cell carcinoma 10 years previously. **c** Gross appearance after sectioning showing spongy, spiculated bone with blood cysts. **D** Histopathologic section (hematoxylin-eosin, original magnification ×50) demonstrating thin-walled, large, cavernous vascular channels filled with erythrocytes and surrounded by osseous trabeculae. (From Colombo et al. 2001)

◁
Fig. 3.3.10. Orbital hemangiopericytoma: **a** Progressive proptosis of the left eye of 6 months' duration in a 65-year-old man. **b** Axial magnetic resonance imaging in T_1-weighted image revealing a large, contrast enhancing, orbital mass (*) in the muscle cone. **c** Circumscribed red tumor after surgical removal via a lateral orbitotomy. **d** Histopathologic section (hematoxylin-eosin, original magnification ×50) showing typical "staghorn" branching of the blood vessels surrounded by small spindle-shaped pericytes with marked basal membrane

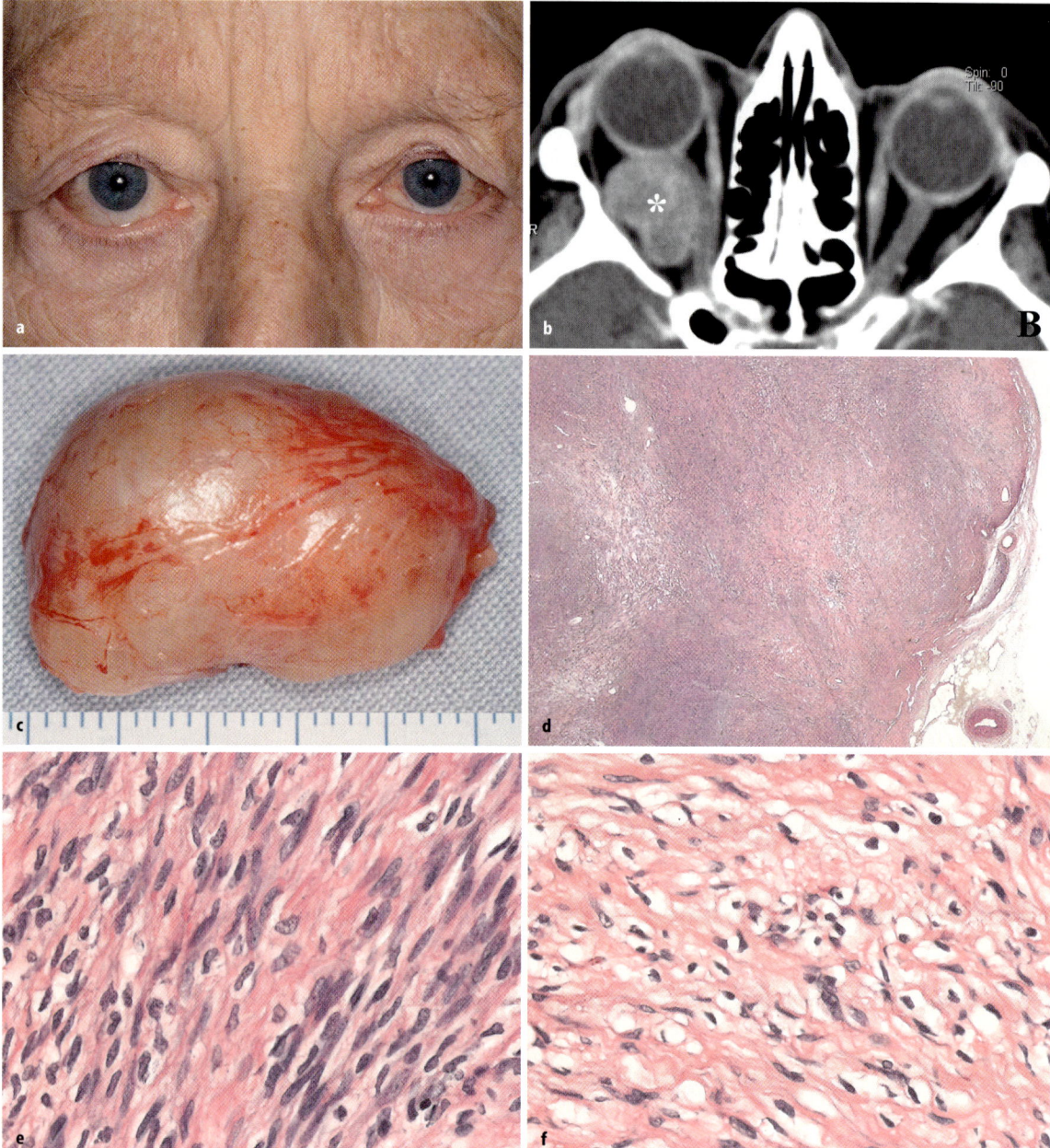

Fig. 3.3.12. Orbital neurilemmoma (schwannoma): **a** Proptosis and downward displacement of the right eye in a 63-year-old woman. **b** Axial computed tomography scan revealing a large circumscribed retrobulbar mass (*) occupying most of the posterior orbit. **c** Gross appearance of a well-circumscribed, encapsulated tumor after surgical removal via a lateral transosseous orbitotomy. **d** Histopathologic section (hematoxylin-eosin, original magnification × 25) showing a solid tumor surrounded by a pseudocapsule consisting of perineural tissue. **e** Histopathologic section (hematoxylin-eosin, original magnification × 200) demonstrating a tumor area of Antoni A pattern with fascicles of spindle-shaped cells. **f** Histopathologic section (hematoxylin-eosin, original magnification × 100) revealing an area of Antoni B pattern with more ovoid clear cells in another part of the tumor

▷

Fig. 3.3.14. Orbital involvement in multiple myeloma as the first sign of insufficient chemotherapy: **a** Sixty-year-old male presenting with left proptosis and chemosis 2 months after chemotherapy for multiple myeloma. **b** Axial magnetic resonance imaging in T_1-weighted image revealing a tumor (*) with homogeneous contrast enhancement filling the mediobasal part of the left orbit and compressing the eyeball. **c** Histopathologic section (hematoxylin-eosin, original magnification × 400) of the orbital tumor composed of monomorphic lymphoid cells with plasmacelloid aspect. Immunohistochemically, these cells were positive for plasma cell marker VS38c and negative for B-cell marker CD20. They showed monoclonality for IgG-λ-light chains and displayed a low proliferation rate (mitotic fraction below 1%). **d** Patient 3 months after incisional biopsy with surgical debulking, external beam radiation therapy of the orbit and repeated systemic chemotherapy. Note marked remission of orbital findings. (From Kottler et al. 2003)

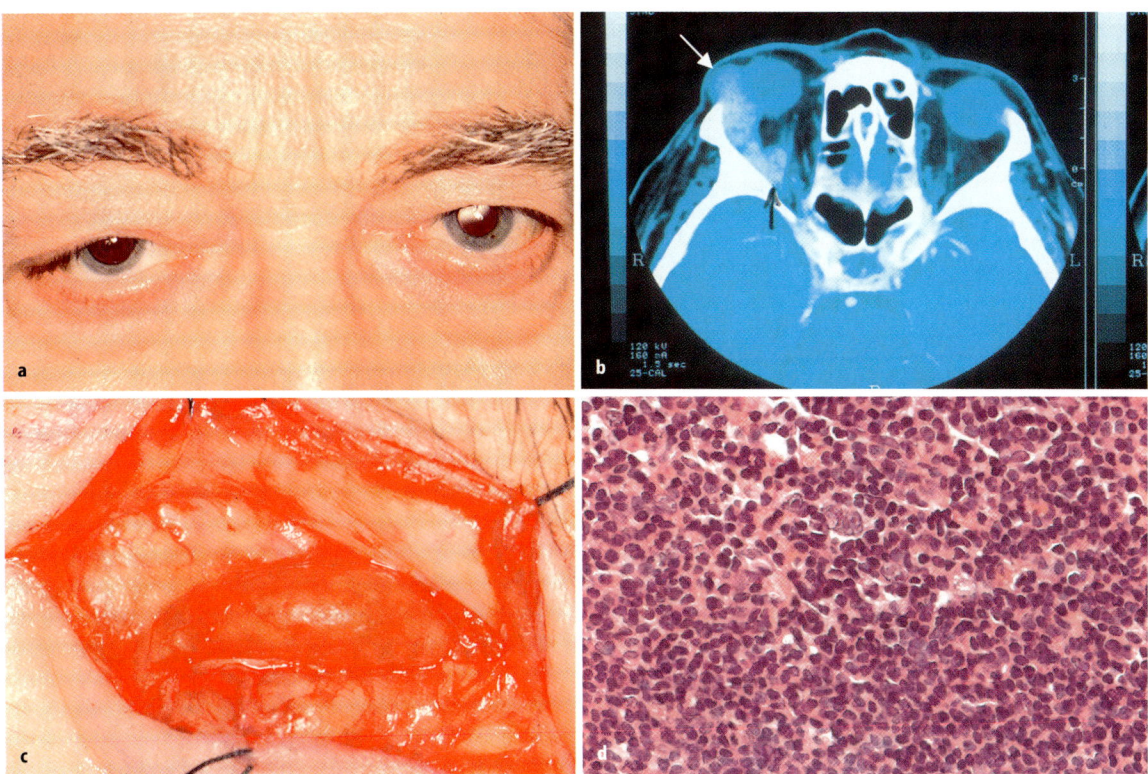

Fig. 3.3.13. Orbital marginal-zone B-cell lymphoma: **a** Slight proptosis and blepharoptosis of the right eye in a 72-year-old man with non-Hodgkin's B-cell lymphoma. **b** Axial computed tomography revealing a diffuse orbital mass that molds to the globe and involves the lacrimal gland and lateral rectus muscle. **c** Intraoperative appearance of the mass following anterior transcutaneous transseptal orbitotomy prior to biopsy and surgical debulking. **d** Histopathologic section (hematoxylin-eosin, original magnification ×100) showing extranodal marginal-zone B-cell lymphoma consisting of small lymphocytes and occasional blasts

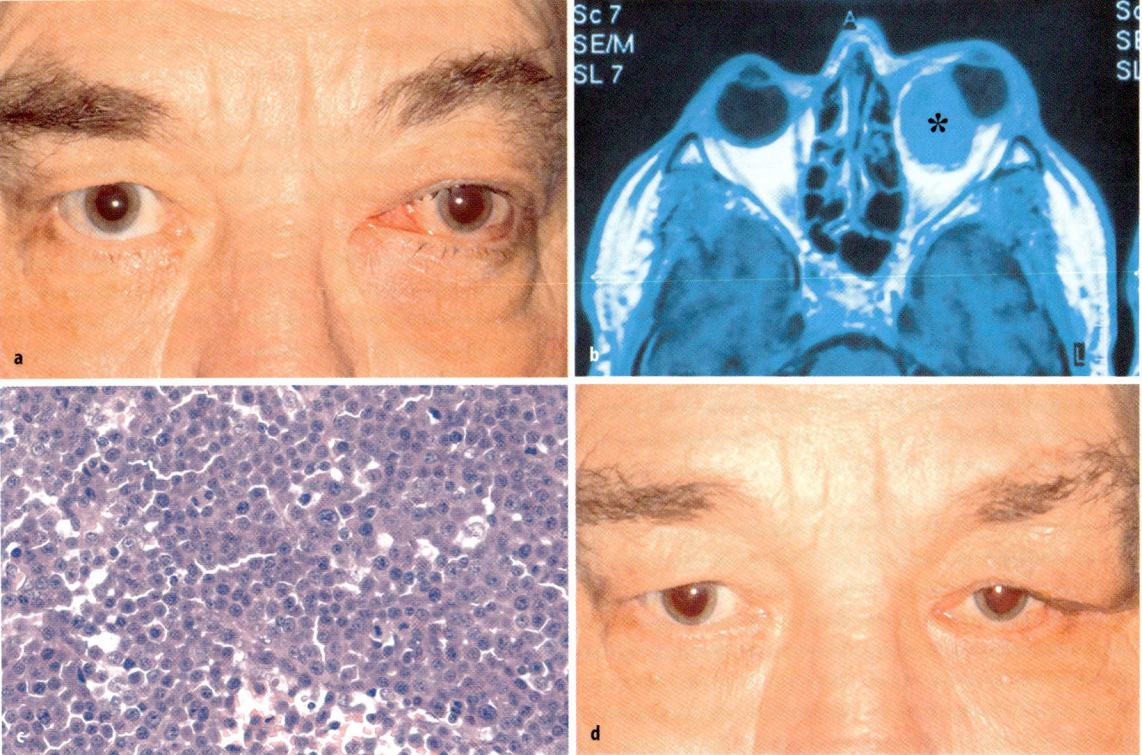

Fig. 3.3.14a-d (Legend see p. 58)

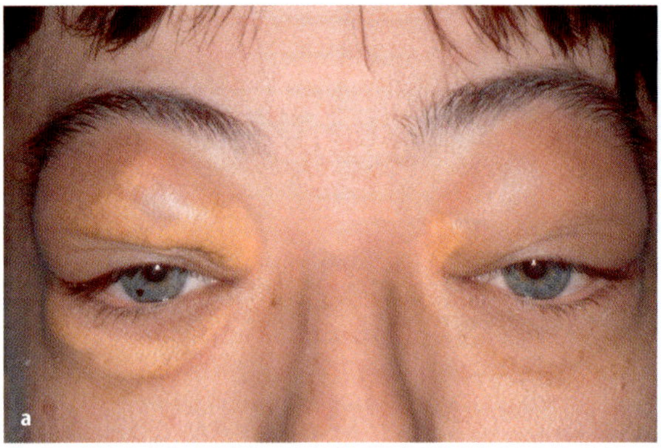

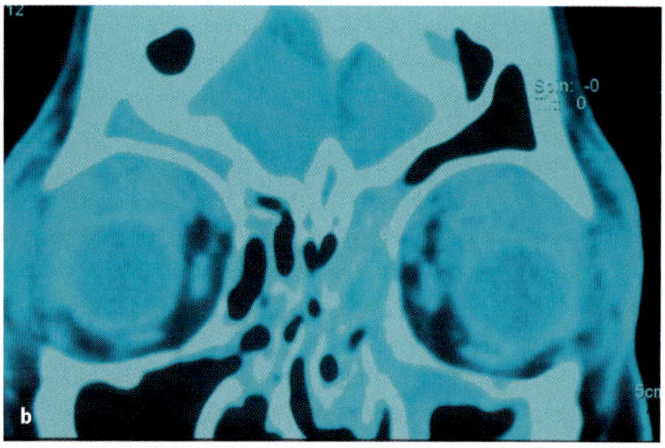

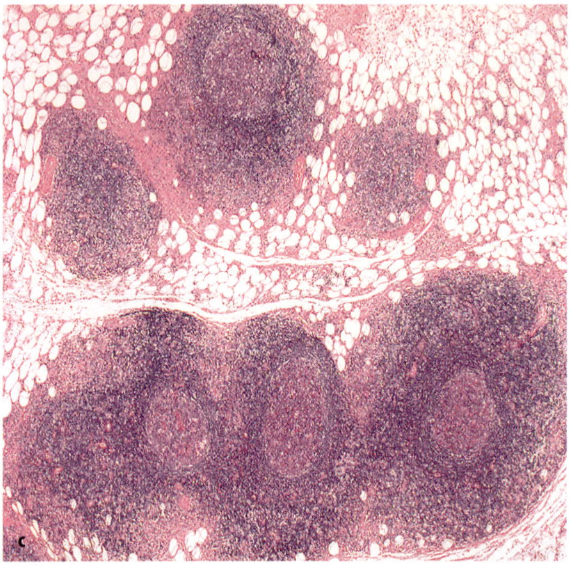

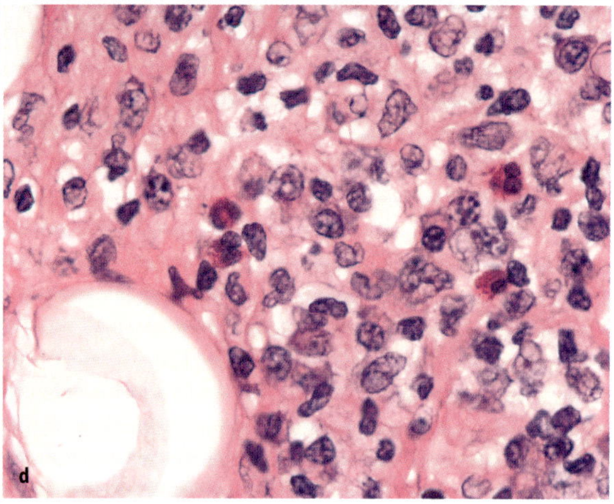

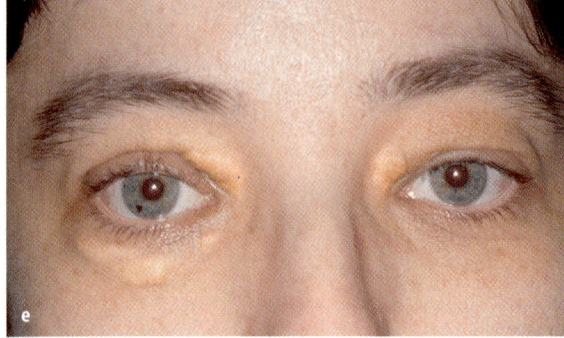

Fig. 3.3.15. Reactive polyclonal lymphofollicular hyperplasia of the orbit and periocular xanthogranulomas: **a** Thirty-one-year-old female with bilateral diffuse swelling and nodular tumefaction of the eyelids which had been slowly developing for 4 years. In addition, yellowish xanthomatous infiltrates are present in the anterior lid lamella. The patient also had allergic bronchial asthma. **b** Coronal computed tomography scan demonstrates infiltrative lesions in the upper orbit involving the rectus-superior-levator complex and the lacrimal gland. **c** Histopathologic section (hematoxylin-eosin, original magnification ×50) of the orbital lesion following anterior transseptal orbitotomy. It shows a polyclonal lymphofollicular hyperplasia. **d** In addition, eosinophils are present within the lesion (hematoxylin-eosin, original magnification ×400). **e** The findings improved dramatically following systemic steroids

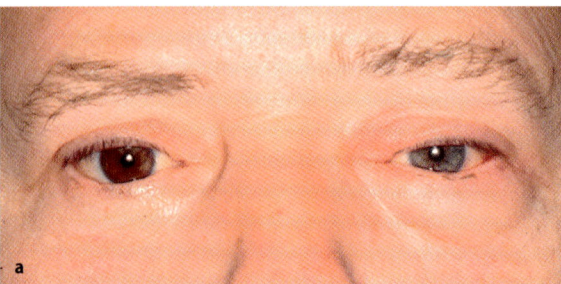

Fig. 3.3.16. Bilateral orbital metastases as the first presentation of breast adenocarcinoma: **a** Sixty-three-year-old female presenting with a 4-month history of bilateral lid swelling, chemosis and intermittent vertical diplopia

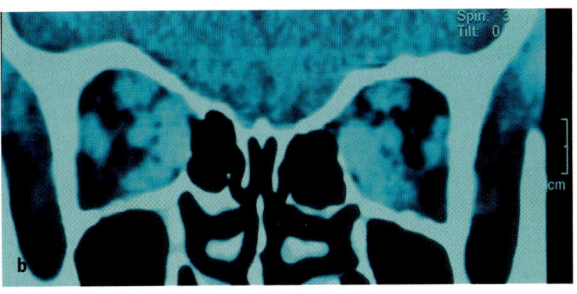
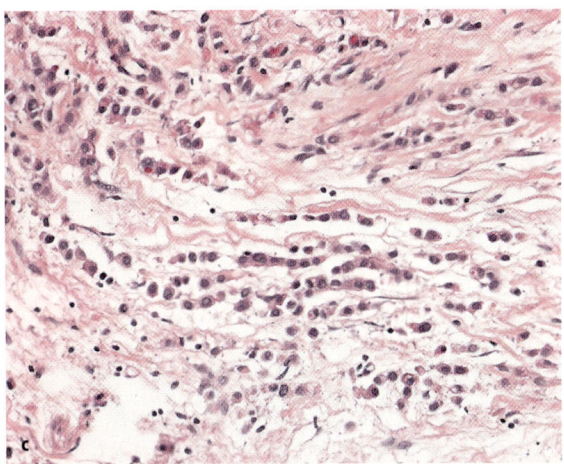

Fig. 3.3.16. b Coronal computed tomography scan revealing a peri- and retrobulbar infiltrative process with marked involvement of both extraocular muscles and orbital fat. **c** Histopathologic section (periodic acid-Schiff, original magnification ×50) showing desmoplasia with cords of malignant tumor cells ("Indian file"), compatible with metastatic adenocarcinoma of the breast

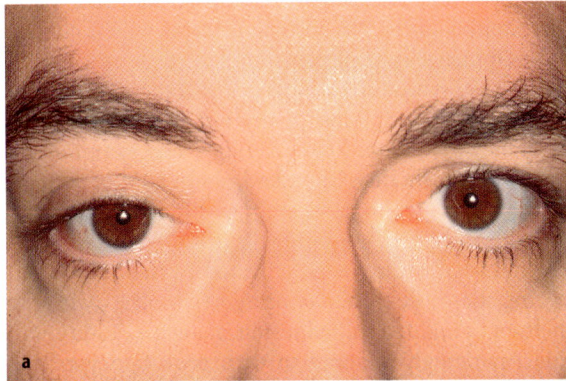
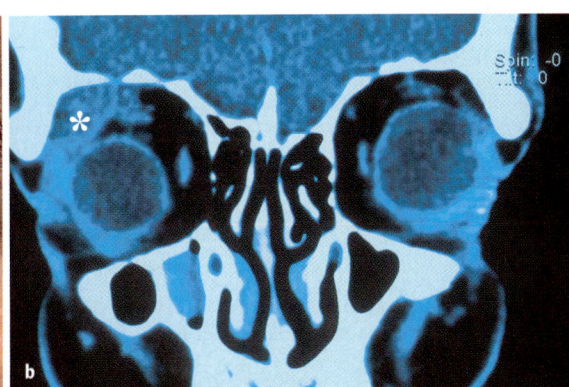
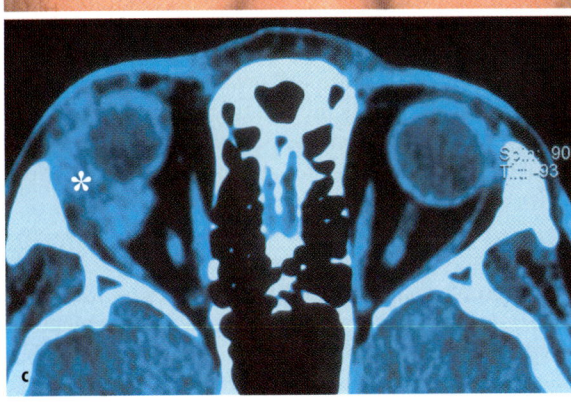
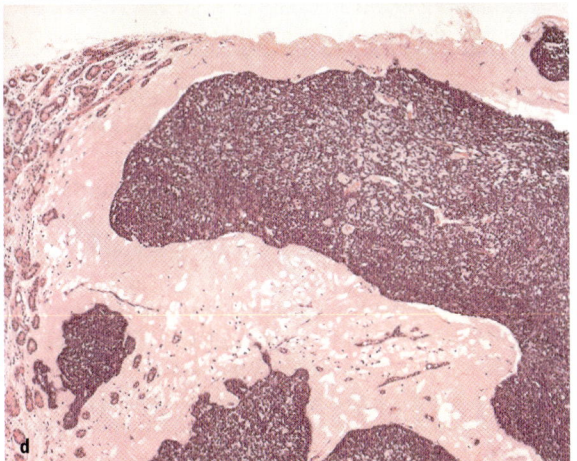

Fig. 3.3.17. Adenoid cystic carcinoma of the lacrimal gland: **a** Mild blepharoptosis of the right eye in a 46-year-old man. **b** Coronal computed tomography scan revealing an infiltrative orbital mass (*) involving the lacrimal gland and rectus-superior-levator complex. **c** Axial computed tomography scan demonstrating an infiltrative superotemporal process (*) with invasion of extraocular muscles. **d** Histopathologic section (hematoxylin-eosin, original magnification ×25) showing a prominent basaloid pattern associated with a worse prognosis than the non-basaloid type

neuroblastoma are common. The differential diagnosis of orbital rhabdomyosarcoma must include nodular fasciitis (Fig. 3.3.5), Langerhans-cell histiocytosis (Fig. 3.3.6) and lymphangioma of the orbit (Fig. 3.3.7). In adults, non-Hodgkin lymphomas (Figs. 3.3.13, 3.3.14) are most commonly encountered. Differential diagnostic considerations should include orbital lymphofollicular hyperplasia (Fig. 3.3.15), metastases (Fig. 3.3.16) and adenoid cystic carcinomas of the lacrimal gland (Fig. 3.3.17).

Table 3.3.3. Differential diagnosis of proptosis (modified from Hintschich and Rose 2005)

Acute onset (minutes to hours)
Orbital hemorrhage (due to trauma, vascular anomaly in children, arteriopathy with anticoagulation in adults)
Acute infective orbital cellulitis
Arteriovenous shunts

Subacute onset (days to weeks)
Childhood malignant orbital tumors (e.g., rhabdomyosarcomas)
Childhood capillary hemangiomas of the orbit
Adult orbital inflammation (granulomatous, xanthogranulomatous, lymphocytic)
Adult orbital infection by fungi, parasites, tuberculosis
Adult metastatic disease of the orbit

Chronic onset (over months)
Childhood benign orbital tumors (e.g., retrobulbar dermoid, optic nerve tumors)
Sinus mucoceles/tumors
Osseous disease of the orbit (e.g., fibrous dysplasia, osteoma, sphenoid wing meningeoma)
Adult benign orbital tumors (e.g., cavernous hemangiomas)
Some adult malignant orbital tumors (e.g., low-grade lymphomas, some carcinomas)
Adult low-grade orbital inflammation
Most adult vascular orbital lesions (arising from venous or arterial anomalies)

Acute-on-chronic onset (sudden acceleration of chronic condition)
Malignant transformation of benign orbital tumors (e.g., carcinoma in pleomorphic adenoma, sarcoma in fibrous dysplasia, lymphoma in Sjögren's syndrome)
Transformation of low-grade into higher-grade malignancy of orbital tumors (e.g., lymphomas, de-differentiation of sarcomas)
Spontaneous thrombosis in venous malformations of the orbit

Another differential diagnostic help for orbital lesions may be the onset of proptosis (Table 3.3.3). The possibility of malignant disease should be entertained wherever there is a rapidly or relentlessly progressive disease, an inflammatory picture or in atypical situations.

The decision whether to remove the whole lesion *(excisional biopsy)* or to obtain a representative biopsy *(incisional biopsy)*, the latter possibly combined with debulking surgery, depends on the most likely clinical diagnosis.

If the lesion is thought to be of chronic inflammatory origin, a lymphoma, a rhabdomyosarcoma or some other infiltrative lesion, then an incisional biopsy is indicated and possibly combined with debulking surgery. Only the histopathologic tissue diagnosis will allow a further plan of action to be drawn up, including, e.g., radiotherapy, chemotherapy or a combination of both or radical surgery such as orbital exenteration.

For circumscribed non-infiltrative lesions such as cavernous hemangiomas, hemangiopericytomas, neurilemmomas, solitary fibrous tumors, or dermoid cysts, complete excision (excisional biopsy) is the treatment of choice. If the clinical diagnosis is, e.g., pleomorphic adenoma of the lacrimal gland, then an excisional biopsy without tumor cell spillage is essential. In pleomorphic adenomas of the lacrimal gland, this always means a lateral orbitotomy. If the lesion is thought to be inflammatory, or a lymphoma or carcinoma, then an incisional biopsy via a direct transseptal anterior orbitotomy is preferred to obtain a histopathologic diagnosis.

3.3.2.2
Thyroid-Associated Orbitopathy – Endocrine Orbitopathy/Ophthalmopathy – Graves' Ophthalmopathy

Thyroid eye disease is the commonest cause of unilateral and bilateral proptosis in adults. The disease typically presents as Graves' disease – a multisystem, autoimmune, inflammatory disorder affecting thyroid gland, orbit, pretibial dermis and some periosteal loci – predominantly in the 3rd and 4th decades with a marked predominance in females.

The eye symptoms usually occur at the same time as the obvious symptoms of thyroid disease; however, they may precede or follow the signs and symptoms of thyroid abnormality. Untreated, about 80% of patients with Graves' orbitopathy are hyperthyroid, 5% hypothyroid and 15% euthyroid.

In Graves' orbitopathy, activated T-lymphocytes entering the orbit stimulate orbital fibroblasts with the help of cytokines and adhesion molecules to produce glucosaminoglycans and to turn pre-adipocytes into adipocytes, thus causing increased volume of extraocular eye muscles and retrobulbar fat contributing to eyelid swelling and proptosis. Formation of fibrosis in the altered tissues results in lid retraction and eye muscle restriction. Severe increase of soft tissue volume jeopardizes the optic nerve axonal flow and/or blood supply with consecutive loss of vision.

Therefore, the most important clinical signs and symptoms of Graves' orbitopathy include eyelid retraction, proptosis, eye motility impairment (with diplopia), swelling and redness of eyelids and conjunctiva, exposure keratitis and even corneal ulceration due to incomplete lid closure and reduced vision due to optic nerve compression. It is important to notice that only rarely is functional impairment combined with optic disc swelling (Figs. 3.3.18, 3.3.19).

Exact clinical classification of *disease severity* and *activity* is essential for the initiation of stage appropriate therapy.

Graves' orbitopathy can be divided into mild, moderate and severe disease based on the degree of proptosis, extraocular muscle involvement and the presence of optic neuropathy (Table 3.3.4). About 60% of the patients with thyroid eye disease have mild, 20% moderate and 10% severe orbitopathy.

Disease activity can be assessed by the clinical activity score (Table 3.3.5) based on four of the five classical

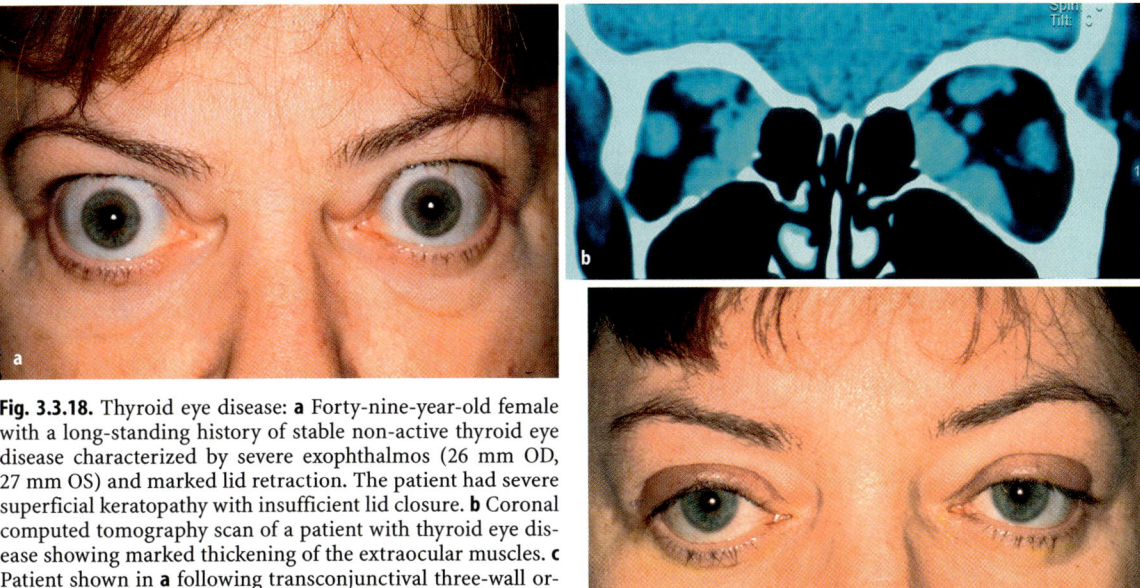

Fig. 3.3.18. Thyroid eye disease: **a** Forty-nine-year-old female with a long-standing history of stable non-active thyroid eye disease characterized by severe exophthalmos (26 mm OD, 27 mm OS) and marked lid retraction. The patient had severe superficial keratopathy with insufficient lid closure. **b** Coronal computed tomography scan of a patient with thyroid eye disease showing marked thickening of the extraocular muscles. **c** Patient shown in **a** following transconjunctival three-wall orbital decompression (swinging-eyelid approach) and upper blepharotomy in both eyes. Symptoms and signs showed marked improvement postoperatively

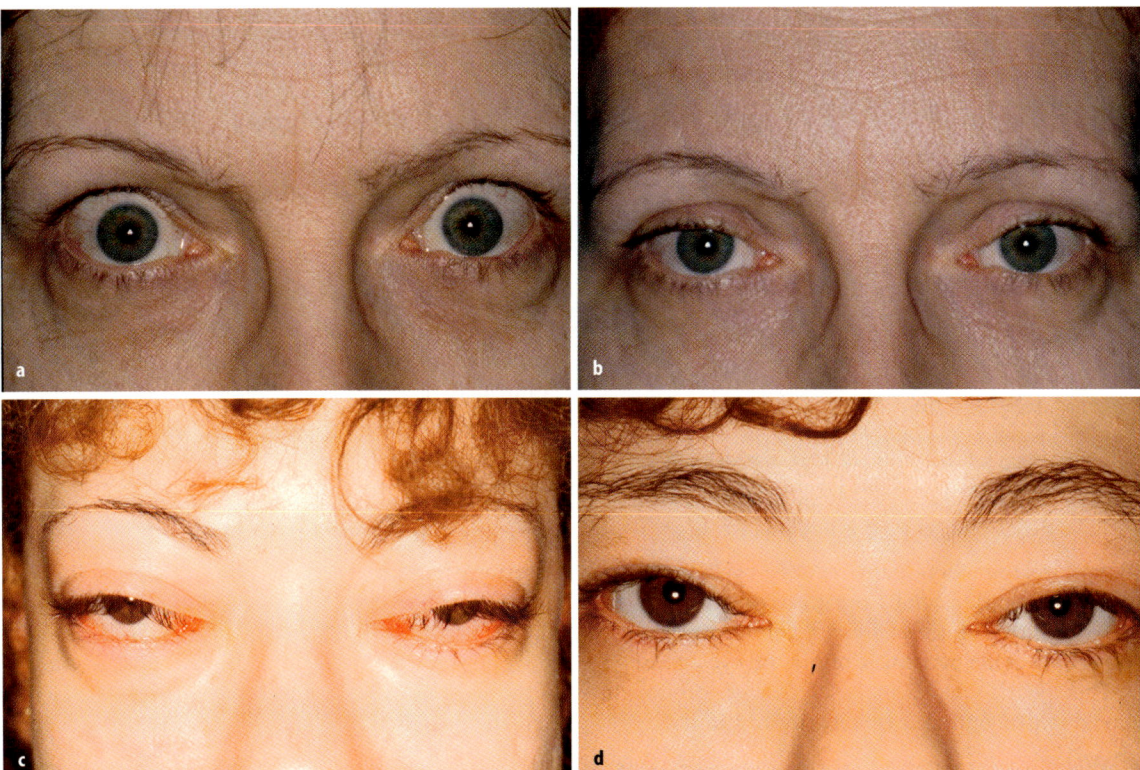

Fig. 3.3.19. Thyroid eye disease: **a** Forty-five-year-old female with non-active thyroid eye disease, marked upper lid retraction and superficial keratopathy due to corneal exposure. **b** Patient shown in **a** following upper blepharotomy and marked improvement of symptoms and signs. **c** Thirty-five-year-old female with exophthalmos, congestion and pseudoptosis due to thyroid eye disease. **d** Patient shown in **c** following transconjunctival three-wall orbital decompression (swinging-eyelid approach)

Table 3.3.4. Assessment of thyroid eye disease severity

Severity	Degree of proptosis[a] and other signs	Extraocular muscle involvement	Optic neuropathy
Mild disease	<3 mm ULN Mild soft tissue involvement	Intermittent diplopia (present only in fatigued patients)	No
Moderate disease	≥4 mm ULN Moderate soft tissue involvement	Inconstant or constant diplopia (present in secondary or primary gaze and reading positions)	No
			Visual acuity 8/10–5/10
Severe disease	Not applicable	Not applicable	Yes
			Visual acuity <5/10 Reduced visual field and color vision

[a] Degree of proptosis expressed in reference to the upper limit of normal (ULN) for the patient's ethnic group (18 mm in Asians, 20 mm in Caucasians, 22 mm in Afro-Americans)

Table 3.3.5. Clinical activity score of thyroid endocrine orbitopathy (from Mourits et al. 1997)

Criterion	Present
Pain:	
1. Painful, oppressive feeling on or behind the globe, during the last 4 weeks	1
2. Pain on attempted up, side or down gaze, during the last 4 weeks	1
Redness:	
3. Redness of the eyelid(s)	1
4. Diffuse redness of the conjunctiva, covering at least one quadrant	1
Swelling:	
5. Swelling of the eyelid(s)	1
6. Chemosis	1
7. Swollen caruncle	1
8. Increase of proptosis of ≥2 mm, during a period of 1–3 months	1
Impaired function:	
9. Decrease of eye movements in any direction ≥5°, during a period of 1–3 months	1
10. Decrease of visual acuity of ≥1 line(s) on the Snellen chart (using a pinhole), during a period of 1–3 months	1
Total score:	10
Total score ≥4: suggestive of active thyroid eye disease	

signs of inflammation (pain, redness, swelling and impaired function). A total score greater than or equal to 4 is suggestive of active Graves' orbitopathy seen in about 25% of the patients with thyroid eye disease.

Therapeutic management of Graves' orbitopathy should rely on both disease severity and activity:

1. *Mild disease:* supportive measures (stop smoking, artificial tears and ointments, sunglasses, correction of hyper- or hypothyroidism)
2. *Moderate disease:*
   a) *Active:* supportive measures, i.v. or p.o. prednisolone (60–100 mg/day tapered down over several months) and/or orbital radiotherapy (particularly in motility impairment and diplopia).
   b) *Inactive:* supportive measures, rehabilitative surgery (orbital decompression, extraocular muscle surgery, eyelid surgery).
3. *Severe disease:* supportive measures, i.v. methylprednisolone (1 g/day for three consecutive days in the first 2 weeks); in case of visual acuity improvement ongoing treatment with p.o. prednisolone, otherwise orbital decompression.

3.3.3
Principles of Orbital Surgery

3.3.3.1
Surgical Approaches to the Orbit in Orbital Tumor Surgery

3.3.3.1.1
Anterior Orbitotomy

Anterior Transseptal Orbitotomy

The principle is a direct approach through the eyelid and orbital septum to a process that is to be biopsied or completely removed.

Indications include incisional biopsies of any processes in the anterior half of the orbit including lacrimal gland biopsies.

In addition, excisional biopsies of selected processes in the anterior half of the orbit may be performed, e.g., anteriorly located cavernous hemangiomas, solitary fibrous tumors or dermoid cysts (not those placed laterally with an extension through the lateral orbital wall).

Contraindications include pleomorphic adenomas of the lacrimal gland except for the rare cases affecting only the palpebral lobe.

Anterior Transconjunctival Orbitotomy

The principle is an approach to a process via the conjunctiva for incisional or excisional biopsy.

Indications include any process that is visible subconjunctivally (e.g., incisional biopsy and debulking surgery in lymphoma of the conjunctiva and anterior orbit), in addition anterior intraconal processes in children and anteriorly placed intraconal processes for incisional biopsy.

Lacrimal gland biopsies should *not* be performed transconjunctivally as the lacrimal ductules will be damaged. Lacrimal gland biopsies of the orbital lobe should be performed transseptally.

Anterior Extraperiosteal Orbitotomy

The principle is an approach to a process via the extraperiosteal space without removal of bone. This is also valuable in the management of orbital fractures.

Indications include any process which has arisen from bone, invaded the bone or is confined to the extraperiosteal space, such as eosinophilic granuloma in Langerhans' cell histiocytosis, cholesterol granuloma, osteoma, intraosseous cavernous hemangioma, extraperiosteal hematoma or abscess.

Contraindications include incisional biopsies of potentially malignant processes which are confined to the orbit and do not involve the bone. This would open a surgical plane to a malignancy and jeopardize safe removal later if exenteration is required.

3.3.3.1.2
Lateral Orbitotomy

The principle is removal of the lateral orbital wall for better access to an orbital process.

The most common indications include intraconal processes for complete removal (excisional biopsy), e.g., cavernous hemangioma, hemangiopericytoma, schwannoma, in addition pleomorphic adenomas of the lacrimal gland (orbital lobe).

3.3.3.2
Surgical Management in Thyroid Eye Disease

Surgical treatment in Graves' orbitopathy including orbital decompression, extraocular muscle surgery and eyelid surgery is indicated for sight-threatening conditions like corneal exposure and/or optic nerve compression, but also for rehabilitative purposes. When indicated, orbital decompression should be performed as the first step prior to extraocular eye muscle and eyelid surgery.

3.3.3.2.1
Orbital Decompression

One common method is the partly transconjunctival, partly lateral canthal approach (swinging eyelid) for the decompression of one, two or three orbital walls.

Elective orbital decompression can be indicated in patients with aesthetically disfiguring proptosis and/or persistent orbital pain. Urgent indications include severe thyroid eye disease with optic neuropathy after the failure of glucocorticoid therapy, corneal ulceration due to severe proptosis and globe subluxation.

3.3.3.2.2
Extraocular Muscle Surgery

The aim of extraocular muscle surgery is to reduce diplopia in the primary gaze or reading position. It should be performed when Graves' orbitopathy has been *inactive* for 6–12 months. Most frequently the inferior rectus needs corrective surgery, followed by the medial rectus, the superior rectus and, rarely, the lateral rectus.

3.3.3.2.3
Eyelid Surgery to Prevent Lagophthalmus

Eyelid surgery represents the last step in surgical management of thyroid eye disease. Common surgical techniques for upper eyelid retraction are recession of Müller's muscle and the levator aponeurosis (blepharotomy) or the transpalpebral dissection of levator aponeurosis and Müller's muscle according to Koornneef.

3.3.3.3
Surgical Approaches in Anophthalmic Socket Surgery

Removal of the eye and/or orbital tissues may become necessary as a result of trauma, infection, inflammation, or neoplasia, as a consequence of a blind, painful and/or aesthetically disturbing eye. Depending on clinical diagnosis and the clinicopathologic concept of the underlying disease, the globe should be removed by *enucleation, evisceration* or *exenteration*. The absence or loss of an eye is of enormous psychological significance to any patient. Surgery of the anophthalmic socket is aimed at enabling the patient to wear a comfortable and aesthetically acceptable prosthesis which is stable and free from discharge.

3.3.3.3.1
Enucleation with Orbital Implants

The principle of enucleation is the removal of the entire globe by severing the attachments of the conjunctiva at the limbus, the extraocular muscles and optic nerve. An orbital implant (alloplastic or homologous, e.g., dermis-fat-graft) of adequate volume is usually inserted within Tenon's capsule or posterior to it.

The most common indications for enucleation include a *painful blind eye,* an intraocular tumor suspected to be malignant and not amenable to (brachy-)radiotherapy and the avoidance of sympathetic ophthalmia after ocular trauma. Enucleated globes allow reliable histopathologic examination.

3.3.3.3.2
Evisceration

The principle is the removal of the contents of the eye (i.e., uvea, retina, lens, vitreous) while leaving the sclera and extraocular muscles intact. The ocular remnant is fully mobile and there is less orbital fat atrophy. There are techniques in between evisceration and enucleation such as covering the implant with muscle pedunculated scleral flaps.

Contraindications include the *theoretical risk of subsequent sympathetic ophthalmia* although the incidence of these conditions appears *extremely low* following evisceration if uveal tissue is carefully removed.* Evisceration should not be performed when there is a risk of local tumor recurrence or when an intraocular tumor cannot be excluded. Histopathologic assessment of eviscerated specimens is difficult and not always reliable.

3.3.3.3.3
Exenteration

Exenteration of the orbit is a disfiguring procedure. Patients need careful counselling preoperatively. They should be aware of the profound differences between enucleation, evisceration and exenteration. In addition, there will often be a loss of sensation throughout the first division of the trigeminal nerve following this procedure.

Exenteration of the Orbit Sparing the Eyelids

The principle is to remove the contents of the orbit, sparing some or all of the eyelid skin.

Exenteration of the Orbit Including the Eyelids

The principle is to remove the eyelids and the whole of the orbital contents including the periorbita.

References (see also page 379)

American Joint Committee on Cancer: Cancer staging manual – sixth edition. New York: Springer;2002: 377–406

Colombo F, Naumann GOH, Holbach LM Chronic inflammation in dermoid cysts: a clinicopathologic study of 115 patients. Orbit 2000;19:97–107

Colombo F et al: Primary intraosseous cavernous hemangioma of the orbit. Am J Ophthalmol 2001;131:151–2

Cursiefen C et al: Orbital lymphangioma with positive immunohistochemistry of lymphatic endothelial markers (vascular endothelial growth factor receptor 3 and podoplanin). Graefes Arch Clin Exp Ophthalmol 2001;239:628–32

Garner A, Klintworth GK (ed): Pathobiology of ocular disease. 2nd ed (Part B). New York, Basel, Hong Kong, Marcel Dekker;1994

Guthoff R, Katowitz JA: Oculoplastics and orbit. Berlin, Heidelberg, New York: Springer;2006

Guthoff RF, Schittkowski MP, Klett A: Methods to improve prosthesis motility in enucleation surgery without pegging and with emphasis on muscle pedunculated flaps. In: Guthoff, Katowitz (Eds) Oculoplastics and Orbit, Essentials in Ophthalmology, Springer 2006;223–235

Hintschich C, Haritoglou C: Full thickness eyelid transsection (blepharotomy) for upper eyelid lengthening in lid retraction associated with Graves' disease. Br J Ophthalmol 2005; 89:413–6

Hintschich C, Rose G: Tumors of the orbit. In: Tonn JC, Westphal M, Rutka JT, Grossman SA (ed): Neuro-oncology of CNS tumors. Berlin, Heidelberg, New York: Springer; 2005: 269–90

Holbach LM et al: Immunocytochemical diagnosis of embryonic rhabdosarcoma of the orbit. Klin Monatsbl Augenheilkd 1989;195:190–5

Holbach LM et al: Langerhans-cell histiocytosis of the orbit; diagnosis, treatment and outcome in three patients – children and adults [in German]. Klin Monatsbl Augenheilkd 2000;217:370–3

Holbach LM et al: Solitary fibrous tumor of the orbit presenting 20 years after Hodgkin's disease. Orbit 2002;21:49–54

Jakobiec FA, Bilyk JR, Font RL: Orbit. In: Spencer WH (ed): Ophthalmic pathology. Vol. 4, Philadelphia, London, Tokyo: WB Saunders;1996

Kahaly GJ, Pitz S, Hommel G, Dittmar M. Randomized, single blind trial of intravenous versus oral steroid monotherapy in Graves' Orbitopathy. J Clin Endocrinol Metab. 2005 Sept; 90(9):5234–40)

Koornneef L Orbital septa: anatomy and function. Ophthalmology 1979;86:876–880

Kottler UB et al: Orbital involvement in multiple myeloma: first sign of insufficient chemotherapy. Ophthalmologica 2003; 217:76–8

McNab AA: Manual of orbital and lacrimal surgery. Edinburgh, London, Madrid, Melbourne, New York, Tokyo: Churchill Livingstone;1994

Mourits MP, Sasim IV: A single technique to correct various degrees of upper lid retraction in patients with Graves' orbitopathy. Br J Ophthalmol 1999;83:81–4

Mourits MP et al: Clinical activity score as a guide in the management of patients with Graves' ophthalmopathy. Clin Endocrinol (Oxf), 1997; 47:9–14

Paridaens DA, Verhoeff K, Bouwens D, van den Bosch WA: Transconjunctival orbital decompression in Graves' ophthalmopathy: lateral wall approach ab interno. Br J Ophthalmol 2000;84:775–81

Rohrbach JM, Lieb WE: Tumors of the eye and its adnexae [in German]. Stuttgart, New York: Schattauer;1998

Rootman J: Diseases of the orbit. A multidisciplinary approach. Philadelphia: Lippincott Williams & Wilkins, 2nd edn., 2003

Rose GE, Wright JE: Isolated peripheral nerve sheath tumours of the orbit. Eye 1991;5:668–73

Shields JA, Shields CL: Atlas of orbital tumors. Philadelphia, Baltimore, New York, London, Buenos Aires, Hong Kong, Sydney, Tokyo: Lippincott Williams & Wilkins; 1999

Wright JE, Rose GE, Garner A: Primary malignant neoplasms of the lacrimal gland. Br J Ophthalmol 1992;76:401–7

---

* However, the inner scleral layers and emissaria always contain uveal melanocytes – explaining the reports of sympathetic ophthalmia following evisceration.

Conjunctiva and Limbus Corneae

C. Cursiefen, F.E. Kruse, G.O.H. Naumann

3.4.1 Introduction

The role of the thin epithelium on the surface of the eye in the ocular adnexa is sometimes not sufficiently appreciated in its significance for normal vision. Similarly, the normal tear film is almost invisible but is of crucial significance for the optical qualities of the cornea. Its three main components are tears from the lacrimal glands, mucus from the goblet cells of the conjunctiva and the lipid layer from the meibomian glands. It not only constitutes the window to the outside world, but is also a prerequisite for free ocular motility and binocular vision. The corneal epithelium has recently been identified as being essential for maintaining the transparency of the corneal stroma (Cursiefen et al. 2006). The epithelium of the anterior segment of the eye and its adnexa therefore constitute one complex functional unit. Somewhat arbitrarily, we shall discuss the lids, the bulbar and tarsal conjunctiva and the cornea and limbus in separate chapters. For the microsurgeon the distinction between extra- and intraocular surgery is of practical importance. Conjunctival surgery does not carry the risks of intraocular surgery (see Chapters 2, 4).

3.4.2 Surgical Anatomy, Landmarks, Nerve Supply, and Vascular Supply with Blood Vessels and Lymphatics, Including Regional Lymph Nodes and Aqueous Episcleral Veins

The normal bulbar conjunctiva is very mobile against the underlying sclera; in contrast the tarsal conjunctiva and the caruncle are fixed. Unlike the intraocular space, the episclera and conjunctiva have a rich supply of lymphatic vessels connected to regional lymph nodes, both preauricular and submandibular (Cursiefen 2007; Gottschalk et al. 2006). Whereas conjunctival lymphatics are normally invisible at the slit lamp, they can be visualized histologically using novel specific markers of lymphatic endothelium [such as LYVE-1 (lymphatic vessel endothelial HA receptor); Fig. 3.4.1] (Gottschalk et al. 2006). Furthermore, conjunctival lymphatics become visible as distended sac-like structures when they become secondarily filled with blood, e.g., in conjunctival lymphangioma (see below) or surgical trauma to the lymphatics (Fig. 3.4.2). The outflow of the aqueous is visible with the slit lamp behind the limbus in the aqueous veins.

The normal conjunctiva is composed of a multilayered non-keratinized squamous epithelium, which is

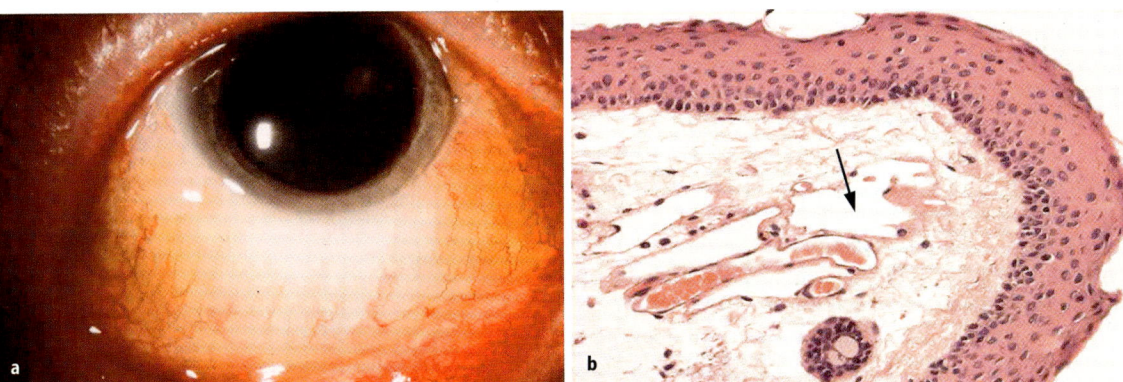

Fig. 3.4.1. Conjunctival lymphangioma which clinically manifested as chronic chemosis (*left panels*). Unequivocal diagnosis was made histologically with immunostaining using specific novel markers of lymphatic endothelium (LYVE-1, **d**). (Modified from Gottschalk et al. 2006). *Arrow* in **b** marks presumed lymphatic vessel in routine histology

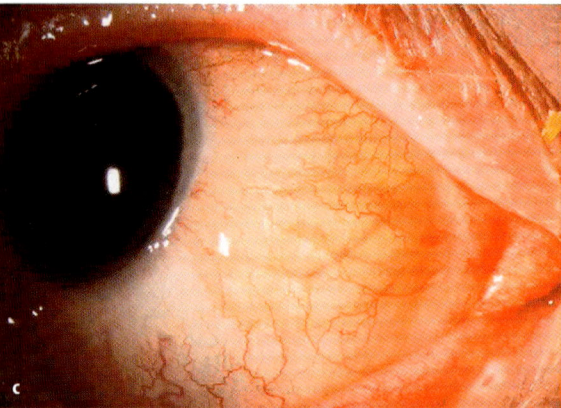

Fig. 3.4.1. (*Cont.*)

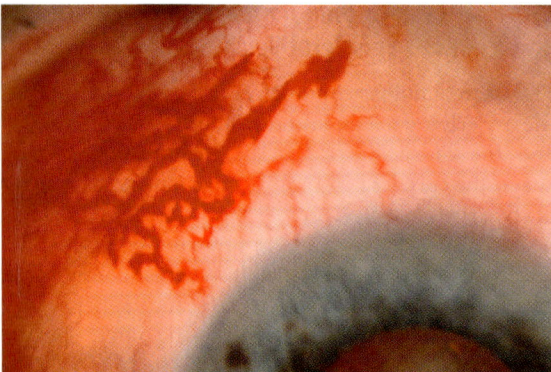

Fig. 3.4.2. Distended, normally invisible conjunctival lymphatics which become visible through iatrogenic trauma and secondary filling with erythrocytes during pterygium surgery. Note distended character of conjunctival lymphatics

Table 3.4.1. Differential diagnosis: follicular hypertrophy of the conjunctiva

A. Infectious
I. Acute
1. Viral
a) Adenovirus
– Type 8, 18 (keratoconjunctivitis epidemica; frequent)
– Type 3 (pharyngoconjunctival fever; frequent)
b) Herpes simplex
c) Newcastle disease
2. *Chlamydia oculogenitalis*
II. Chronic
1. Chlamydia
– Chlamydia trachomatosis
– Chlamydia psittacosis
2. Bacteria (e.g., *Moraxella*)
3. Spirochetes (e.g., *Borrelia burgdorferi*)
4. Virus (e.g., EBV, measles)
5. Molluscum contagiosum at lid margin
B. Non-infectious
I. Induced by drugs ("pseudotrachoma")
1. Iodine deoxyuridine
2. Eserine
3. Atropine
4. Different cosmetics
II. Immunologic reactions
1. Exogenic antigens: animal, plant, chemical
2. Hematogenous antigens: e.g., measles, German measles
III. Refractive anomalies

sitting on a densely vascularized conjunctival tissue. The conjunctiva contains numerous blood and lymphatic vessels. In addition, the extracellular matrix is composed of collagen fibrils, inflammatory cells and nerves. The non-keratinizing conjunctival epithelium also contains goblet cells, which are important for the production of the mucus layer of the precorneal tear film. Destruction of these goblet cells for example after chemical burns causes a goblet cell deficiency and goes along with a mucine deficiency causing dry eye syndrome.

The conjunctiva is immunologically a very active tissue and contains numerous lymphocytes which are organized in follicle form, a phenomenon which has been termed the "conjunctiva associated lymphatic tissue" (CALT). These inflammatory tissues are the anatomic substrate for follicular and papillary forms of conjunctival infections which allow differential diagnosis of a conjunctival inflammation (see Table 3.4.1, Fig. 3.4.3). Anatomically and functionally, the bulbar and tarsal conjunctiva intersect with the corneal epithelium at the limbus. (This is discussed in more detail in Chapter 5.1.)

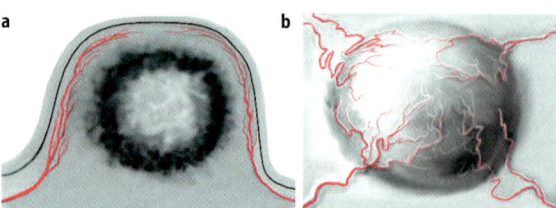

Fig. 3.4.3. Follicular form (**a, b**) and papillary form (**c, d**) of conjunctivitis. (modified after Völcker et al. 1980)

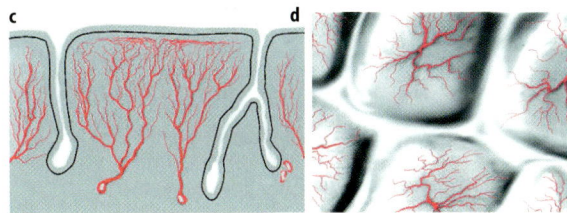

Fig. 3.4.3. (*Cont.*)

3.4.2.1
Limbal Stem Cells, Vogt's Palisades, Cornea Verticillata, Tear Film

These will be discussed in Chapter 5.1.

3.4.2.2
Langerhans Cells in the Limbal and Corneal Epithelium

This will be discussed in Chapter 5.1.

3.4.2.3
Bowman's Layer as Mechanical Barrier

This will be discussed in Chapter 5.1.

3.4.2.4
Keratocyte Distribution, Reaction to Trauma

These will be discussed in Chapter 5.1.

3.4.2.5
Nerve Supply of Superficial Cornea

This will be discussed in Chapter 5.1.

3.4.2.6
Anatomic Landmarks for Surgical Limbus: Edge of Bowman's Layer, Schlemm's Canal, Scleral Spur

This will be discussed in Chapter 5.1.

3.4.3
Surgical Pathology

Tumors of the conjunctiva rarely invade the underlying sclera. They respect Bowman's layer but may invade the corneal stroma peripheral to its edge (Fig. 3.4.4). Of interest to the ophthalmic microsurgeon are the prominent non-pigmented or pigmented processes. These include granulomatous inflammatory processes usually with involvement of the regional lymph nodes (Tables 3.4.2–3.4.4).

Table 3.4.2. Differential diagnosis of oculoglandular Parinaud conjunctivitis (modified after Völcker and Naumann 1980)

Frequent cause	
Cat scratch disease	(Gram-negative bacilla; *Afipia felis*)
Oculoglandular tularemia	(*Francisella tularensis*)
Sporotrichosis	(*Sporotrichum schenckii*)
Tuberculosis	(*Mycobacterium tuberculosis*)
Rare	
Lues I and II	(*Treponema pallidum*)
Coccidioidomycosis	(*Coccidioides immitis*)
Actinomycosis	(*Actinomyces israelii* or *propionicus*)
Blastomycosis	(*Blastomyces dermatosis*)
Yersiniosis	(*Yersinia pseudotuberculosis* or *enterocolica*)
Listeriosis	(*Listeria monocytogenes*)
Infection with *Pasteurella*	(*Pasteurella multocida*)
Infection with *Leptothrix*	
Infection with *Haemophilus*	(*Haemophilus ducrei*)
Infection with *Actinobacillus*	(*Actinobacillus mallei*)
Lymphogranuloma venereum	(*Chlamydia trachomatis* group L)
Rickettsiosis	(*Rickettsia conorii*)
Mumps	(Paramyxovirus)
Infectious mononucleosis	(Epstein-Barr virus)

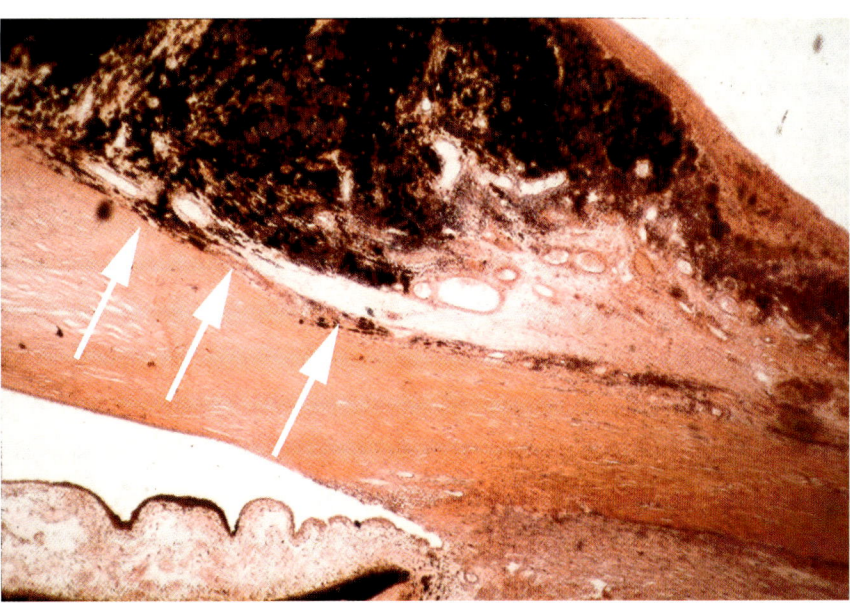

Fig. 3.4.4. Malignant melanoma of the conjunctiva extending onto the cornea, but respecting Bowman's layer as barrier. This has to be taken into account when removing tumors

Table 3.4.3. Etiology of symblepharon

1. **Immunologic diseases**
   - Pemphigoid caused by scars
   - Fuchs-Stevens-Johnson syndrome
   - Lyell syndrome
   - Dermatitis herpetiformis (Duhring)
   - Linear IgA disease
   - Acquired forms of epidermolysis bullosa
   - Keratoconjunctivitis atopica
2. **Bacteria**
   - *Borrelia burgdorferi*
   - *Corynebacterium diphtheriae*
3. **Chlamydia**
   - *Chlamydia trachomatis*
4. **Virus (rarely in heavy forms)**
   - Varicells
   - Adenovirus
5. **Chemical-physical noxa**
   - Lye burns
   - Burns
   - Pseudopemphigoid induced by medication (e.g., epinephrine, DFP, pilocarpine, timolol, etc.)

Table 3.4.4. Differential diagnosis of xerosis conjunctivae

A. **Malfunction of tear film**
  I. Lack of lipid phase
   - Blepharitis
   - Meibomitis
  II. Lack of watery phase (keratoconjunctivitis sicca)
   - Congenital
   - Hypoplasia of tear gland
   - Malfunction of innervation (e.g., Riley-Day syndrome)
   - Acquired
     – Involution of tear gland
     – Dacryoadenitis
     – Radiation/injury of tear gland
     – Systemic disease (e.g., Sjögren syndrome, sarcoidosis, rheumatoid arthritis)
     – Medication
     – Hormones
  III. Lack of mucus phase
   - Vitamin A deficiency
   - Medication
   - Pemphigoid/pseudopemphigoid
   - Erythema multiforme majus (Steven-Johnson syndrome)
   - Radiation

B. **Malfunction of function of lid**
   - Lagophthalmus
   - Incomplete lid closure
   - Anomaly of lid position (e.g., ectropium)
   - Symblepharon

C. **Malfunction of surface of epithelium**
   - Neurotrophic keratoconjunctivitis

Intraepithelial pagetoid growing sebaceous carcinomas originating from the lid or caruncle may present diagnostic problems. Chronic unilateral inflammatory processes require exclusion of sebaceous cell carcinoma.

Table 3.4.5. Differential diagnosis cystic/cystoid changes of the conjunctiva

A. **Conjunctival epithelium**
  I. Pseudocysts
   - Chronic recurrent conjunctivitis
   - Melanocytic nevi
  II. Implantation cysts after trauma or operation

B. **Retention cyst, accessory tear ducts**

C. **Moll cysts**

D. **Oncocytoma**

E. **Cystic dermoid (rare)**

F. **Lymphatic lesions**
   - Lymphangiectasia
   - Lymphangioma

Table 3.4.6. Differential diagnosis: leukoplakia of conjunctiva

I. **Benign**
   - Keratotic plaques – Bitot's spots
   - Keratoacanthosis
   - Pseudoepithelial hyperplasia
   - Hereditary benign intraepithelial dyskeratosis
   - Inverted follicular keratosis

II. **Precancerous**
   - Actinic/senile keratosis
   - Epithelial dysplasia – carcinoma in situ
   - Cancerous
   - Invasive carcinoma of the squamous epithelium
   - Mucoepidermal carcinoma

Processes originating from the subepithelial loose vascularized tissue containing lymphocytes are not salmon-colored and usually present a localized entity, but a systemic lymphoma must be ruled out (Table 3.4.5).

3.4.3.1
Hereditary Anomalies of the Conjunctiva: Conjunctival Lymphangioma

Whereas the normal cornea does not contain lymphatic vessels, there are abundant lymphatic vessels in the conjunctiva. These vessels sometimes become enlarged and may even fill with blood, thus causing blood-fluid levels, a phenomenon which can be easily diagnosed at the slit lamp (Leber's hemorrhagic lymphangiectasia; Fig. 3.4.2). Lymphatic vessels can be diagnosed unequivocally using special immunohistochemical stains, e.g., LYVE-1 (Figs. 3.4.1, 3.4.2).

3.4.3.2
Conjunctival Inflammations

There are numerous causes for conjunctival inflammations (see Table 3.4.6), which can cause specific or unspecific changes in the conjunctiva. Typical phenotypes are the follicular or the papillary forms of con-

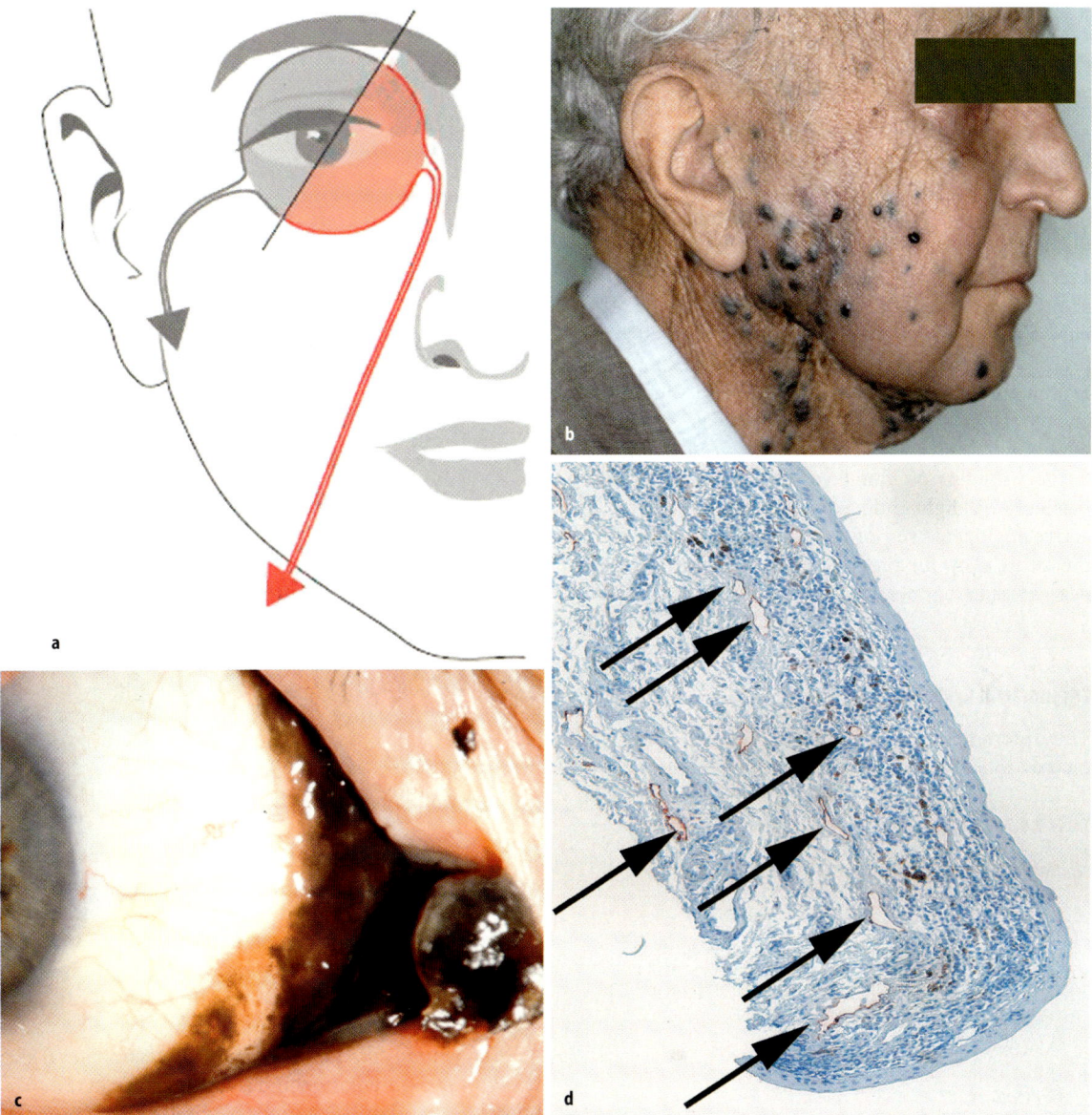

Fig. 3.4.5. a–c Lymphatic drainage to regional lymphatics in a patient with malignant melanoma of the conjunctiva (clinical pictures and histology stained for LYVE-1-positive lymphatic vessels: *arrows*). **a** Lymphatic drainage from the eye

junctival inflammation (Fig. 3.4.3). Lymphatic drainage from the conjunctiva goes to the preauricular and submandibular lymph nodes (Fig. 3.4.5).

3.4.3.3
Sarcoidosis and Conjunctival Involvement in Systemic Disease

The multisystem disease sarcoidosis often involves the conjunctiva. That can be useful for the diagnosis of the disease and to spare the patient more invasive histological diagnostic tests, e.g., in the lung. When conjunctival biopsy to establish the diagnosis sarcoidosis is planned, special attention should be paid to the lower fornix, where nodules can be detected most easily. These should be biopsied using topical anesthesia and without crushing the tissue to enable proper histological workup. Histologically these granules are characterized by a granulomatous inflammatory reaction, which is non-caseating, that is one can see macrophages, lymphocytes, epithelioid cells and giant cells.

3.4.3.4
Pterygium

Pterygium is a degenerative disease of the limbal conjunctiva in the lid cleft area, where a focal defect of limbal stem cells causes overgrowth of the densely vascularized conjunctival tissue onto the cornea. When this outgrowth causes higher astigmatism, reaches the center of the corneal tissue or causes other problems, for example cosmetic or tear film deficiency, pterygia should be excised. This should be done either in combination with a free conjunctival graft or amniotic membrane or a segmental limbal stem cell transplantation. Histologically, a pterygium is characterized by a multilayered non-keratinizing conjunctival epithelium, which sits on top of a densely vascularized conjunctival tissue with lots of blood vessels and degenerative – probably UV-light-induced – extracellular matrix. The active angiogenic response within a pterygium may in the future allow for antiangiogenic treatment strategies to treat recurrent pterygia.

3.4.3.5
Conjunctival Cysts

The differential diagnosis of conjunctival cysts is depicted (Table 3.4.7). These can be easily biopsied.

Table 3.4.7. Pigmented findings of conjunctiva and episclera

- A. **Melanosis acquired**
  - I. Bilateral racial epithelial
  - II. Unilateral acquired melanosis
- B. **Melanocytosis congenital uveal and episcleral**
  - I. Ocular
  - II. Oculodermal (nevus of OTA)
  - III. Oculofacial (nevus of ITO)
- C. **Melanocytic nevi**
  - Junctional
  - Dermal
  - Compound
- D. **Malignant melanoma**
- E. **Non-melanin:**
  - Ochronosis
  - "Senile" hyaline sclera plaques
  - Argyrosis
    - Endogenous
    - Exogenous
  - Metalloses

3.4.3.6
Conjunctival Tumors
3.4.3.6.1
Melanocytic Lesions

There are numerous reasons for melanocytic processes within the conjunctiva (Table 3.4.4). *Melanocytic nevi* usually are characterized by a cystoid appearance. This

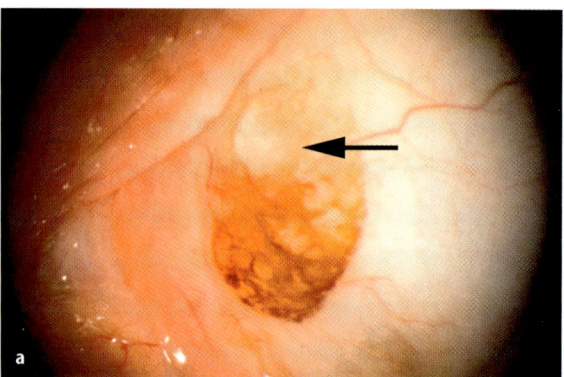
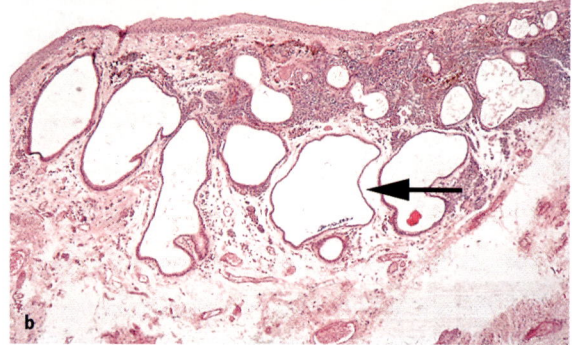

Fig. 3.4.6. Clinical (**a**) and histologic (**b**) appearance of conjunctival nevus with pseudocysts, which enable clinical diagnosis and can be clearly seen on histology ("naevus cysticus Fuchs")

comes from multiple pseudocysts which are usually located within the nevus (Fig. 3.4.6). Enlargement of the pigmented portions of the nevus and enlargement of the cysts may mimic malignant transformation of a nevus as well as by a collateral lymphocytic infiltration. Excisional biopsy assures the histological diagnosis.

Congenital, episcleral melanocytosis is unilateral and has a gray pigmentation and is located deep in the episcleral tissue, that is it cannot be moved by moving the conjunctiva, which can be done with conjunctival nevi. These lesions do not have to be excised, but have to be checked regularly, since they carry an increased risk of associated uveal malignant melanomas and of secondary open angle glaucomas.

3.4.3.6.2
Acquired Epithelial Melanosis

This has to be differentiated from secondary acquired melanocytic lesions, which may be induced by certain antiglaucoma drugs.

Primary epithelial acquired melanocytic lesions in contrast to conjunctival nevi are usually vaxing and varying in clinical appearance, may be multilocular and do not present intraepithelial cysts. These lesions are potentially premalignant and may develop into a

Table 3.4.8. Classification of primary acquired melanosis (courtesy of G.O.H. Naumann)

Stage I: Benign acquired melanosis
A. Minimal junctional activity
B. Intensive junctional activity

Stage II: Cancerous primary acquired melanosis
A. With minimal invasive growth
B. With intensive invasive growth

Table 3.4.9. Malignant melanoma of the conjunctiva: histologic classification

1. Microinvasion: basement membrane defect
2. Surface: invasion of the substantia propria without tumor nests
3. Deep invasion of the substantia propria with tumor nests
4. Invasion of the deeper structures: stroma of the conjunctiva, episcleral, sclera

Table 3.4.10. Reasons for "enlargement" of pigmented conjunctival nevus

1. Melanin deposition in preexisting nevus (puberty!)
2. Extension of preexisting pseudocysts
3. Collateral lymphocytic infiltrate and hyperemia
4. Malignant transformation

Table 3.4.11. Localized non-pigmented processes of the conjunctiva

I. Granulomatous inflammation with Parinaud syndrome
   Tuberculosis, syphilis
   Splendore-Hoeppli granuloma: organic foreign body material and parasites, e.g., onchocercosis

II. Epithelial processes
   Mild, moderate and severe dysplasia
   Corneal intraepithelial neoplasia (CIN), carcinoma in situ
   Mucoepidermoid carcinoma, pagetoid invasion from sebaceous carcinoma of the lid and caruncle
   Congenital: solid dermoid usually temporal inferior limbus
   Dermolipoma: usually temporal superior

III. Subepithelial tumors: tumors of the conjunctival stroma: myxoma, barium sulfate granuloma, fibrocystiocytoma

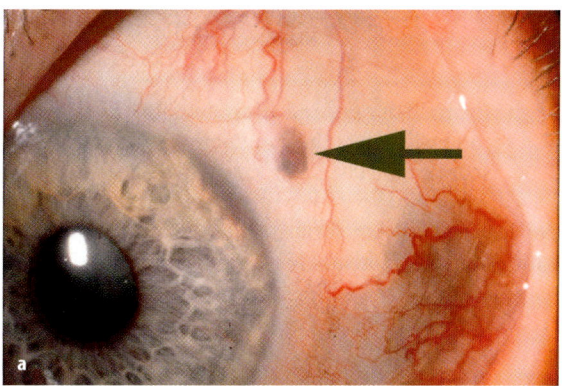
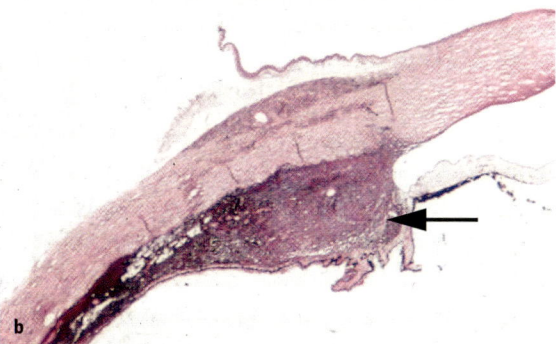

Fig. 3.4.7a, b. Extraocular extension of uveal melanoma presenting as brown epibulbar tumor

malignant melanoma. These have to be followed carefully clinically for any sign of enlargement or of change in pattern. Prominent areas should be biopsied and analyzed histologically.

Malignant melanomas carry a high risk for lymphatic metastases and may be classified analogously to those of the skin (Figs. 3.4.4, 3.4.5b). It seems that these malignant melanomas of the conjunctiva – as the malignant melanomas of the skin – do attract their own lymphatic drainage and thereby favor lymphatic metastases, which means that histologically by assessing the density of lymphatic vessels around a malignant melanoma of the conjunctiva, one can assess the risk of lymphatic metastases and enable specific anti-lymphangiogenic treatment.

Finally a brown pigmented lesion within the conjunctiva may also be an extraocular extension of an intraocular malignant melanoma in the uveal region (Fig. 3.4.7).

3.4.3.7
Amniotic Membrane Transplantation

Amniotic membrane transplantation is a useful tool for covering spontaneous or iatrogenic defects of the conjunctiva. Amniotic membrane consists of a cuboidal epithelium lying on a basement membrane layer, with an acellular matrix beneath. Amniotic membrane can be sutured into conjunctival defects, for example during fornix reconstruction, pterygium surgery or symblepharon surgery (see Chapter 5.1).

3.4.3.8
Limbal Stem Cell Transplantation

This is covered in more detail in Chapter 5.

3.4.3.9
Dry Eye

Severe forms of dry eye and all chronic forms of dry eye also secondarily affect the conjunctiva (Cursiefen et al. 2006; Jacobi et al. 2006). It is now widely accepted that the common final pathway of all forms of chronic dry eye leads to ocular surface inflammation, especially within the conjunctiva. There is upregulation of proinflammatory cytokines, upregulation of inflammatory cell receptors and inflammatory cell influx into the conjunctiva. This leads to increased apoptosis and especially destruction of goblet cells in the conjunctiva. This vicious circle of dry eye leading to ocular inflammation, which in turn leads again to dry eye, can be interrupted by anti-inflammatory treatment at the ocular surface, e.g., with topical cyclosporine eyedrops (cyclosporine 0.05%). In addition, *conjunctival folds*, especially at the temporal aspects, can be used for accurate diagnosis of dry eye (LIPCOF sign). Furthermore, *conjunctivochalasis*, that is the excessively loose nature of the temporal conjunctiva, can be associated with and a cause of certain forms of dry eye. Surgical excision of excess conjunctiva can be a method for alleviating symptoms in this form of dry eye.

3.4.3.10
Superior Limbal Keratitis (Theodore)

This special disease entity is characterized by foreign body sensation and itching and burning noticed at the superior limbal conjunctiva at the 12 o'clock position (Fig. 3.4.8). During inspection, the conjunctiva is thickened and slightly injected. The etiology of the disease is not completely understood, but it is associated with disturbances of thyroid gland function. Therapy can be by surgical excision of the affected conjunctiva, which histologically shows thickening of the epithelium, conjunctival hyperemia and increase of extracellular matrix in the subconjunctival space. Treatment options also include the use of contact lens and cautery of the affected area. Typically the affected area stains positive on bengal-rose staining.

3.4.3.11
Ligneous Conjunctivitis (Conjunctivitis Lignosa)

This rare entity is caused by a defect in plasminogen, thus causing excess deposition of fibrin in the conjunctival area. Clinically this disease usually affects children, which present with wood-like whitish membranes which are located at the tarsal conjunctiva and are composed of thickened amorphous tissue with lots of fibrin and mucopolysaccharides. Diagnosis nowadays is by cytology and molecular biological analysis of the underlying defect. Treatment requires substitution for plasminogen and excision.

3.4.4
Indications for Smear Cytology, Incisional or Excisional Biopsies, Autologous or Homologous Transplantation, Radiation, and Local and Systemic Chemotherapy

As the processes of the epithelium are easily accessible, cytologic smears may be helpful in chronic processes but usually cannot rule out oncologic entities. They are particularly useful in allergic conjunctivitis and in trachomas. Cytologic smears are also useful in the classification of dry eyes and limbus stem cell insufficiency (Cursiefen et al. 2006; Jacobi et al. 2006).

Depending on the extent of the lesion, excisional biopsy or selective incisional biopsies are performed. *"In case of doubt, take it out."* As the eye itself does not need to be opened, this procedure can easily be performed using local anesthesia. If a large defect results, this can be closed by autologous transplantation from the same or contralateral eye or by amniotic membrane transplantation. In the case of not curative excision of carcinomas or melanomas, local and systemic chemotherapy and sometimes radiation therapy may be indicated.

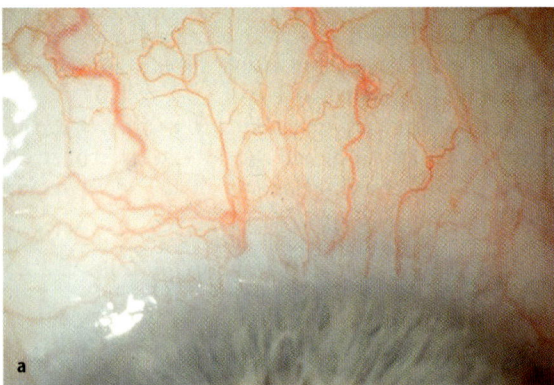
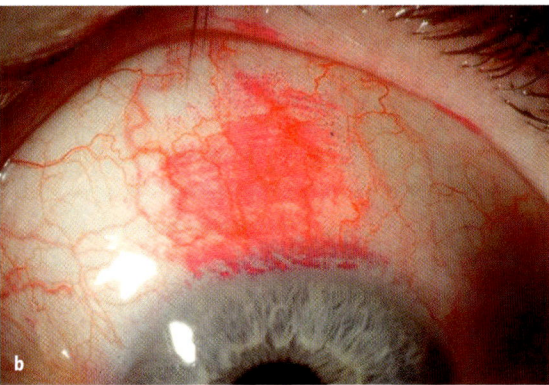

Fig. 3.4.8a, b. Theodore's superior limbal keratitis with typical rose bengal staining

Methods to cover large conjunctival defects after excision: Autologous conjunctiva may be used from the same or contralateral eye. After extensive necrosis following burns by heat, lye or acid, *nasal mucosa transplantation* may be superior to the transplantation of autologous buccal mucosa (Naumann et al., 1990). Amniotic membrane and cultured buccal epithelial transplantation have developed as a useful alternative option.

In view of the connection of the conjunctiva via the lacrimal sac to the nasal mucosa, consultation with the otolaryngologist should not be omitted if oncologic processes of the conjunctiva are diagnosed (Kruse et al. 2003).

3.4.4.1
Conjunctival Oncology: Melanocytic Processes

See above.

3.4.4.2
Limbus Stem Cell Insufficiency

See Chapter 5.

3.4.4.3
Amnion Transplantation

See Chapter 5.

3.4.5
Wound Healing: Influence of Basic Disease and Adjunct Therapy (Radiation, Chemotherapy)

Extensive conjunctival surgery may be complicated by the development of a dry eye syndrome, disturbance of the tear film and in addition normal ocular motility.

1. Processes of the temporal superior quadrant of the bulbar conjunctiva, e.g., dermolipoma and their excision, may unintentionally close the lacrimal ducts leading to a tear insufficiency, which may give rise to symptoms of dry eye syndrome.
2. Tear film stability may be disturbed by symblephara inhibiting the normal Bell phenomenon, which normally wipes the corneal surface and reestablishes the tear film regularly.
3. Excessive subconjunctival scarring: This may be induced by the surgical procedure or by the underlying disease process (e.g., ocular pemphigoid) – and may lead to diplopia by restricting the ocular motility.

References (see also page 379)

Cursiefen C, Chen L, Saint-Geniez M, Hamrah P, Jin Y, Rashid S, Pytowski B, Streilein JW, Dana MR. Nonvascular VEGF receptor 3 expression by corneal epithelium maintains avascularity and vision. Proc Natl Acad Sci USA. 2006; 103: 11405–10

Cursiefen C, Jacobi C, Dietrich T, Kruse FE. [Current treatment for dry eye syndrome]. Ophthalmologe 2006;103:18–24

Cursiefen C. Corneal immune and angiogenic privilege. In: Niederkorn J, Kaplan H. Immune privilege and the eye. Chem Immunol Allergy 2007;92:50–7

Gottschalk K, Rummelt C, Cursiefen C. [Conjunctival chemosis resistant to therapy] Klin Monatsbl Augenheilkd. 2006; 223:696–8

Jacobi C, Dietrich T, Cursiefen C, Kruse FE. [The dry eye. Current concepts on classification, diagnostics, and pathogenesis]. Ophthalmologe 2006;103:9–17

Kruse FE, Cursiefen C, Seitz B, Holbach L, Völcker H, Naumann GOH. [Classification of ocular surface disease. Part 1.] Ophthalmologe. 2003;100:899–915

Naumann GOH, Lang GK, Rummelt V, Wigand M. Autologous nasal mucosa transplantation in severe bilateral conjunctival mucous deficiency syndromes. Ophthalmology 1990; 97: 1011–1017

4 General Pathology for Intraocular Microsurgery: Direct Wounds and Indirect Distant Effects

G.O.H. Naumann, F.E. Kruse

All mechanical methods of intraocular surgery require perforation of the cornea and/or sclera. However, intraocular laser applications and transscleral diathermy or cryocoagulation are possible without creating an iatrogenic perforating wound of the eye wall. Only exceptionally diode laser coagulation may create a scleral defect. In order to choose the best access into the eye, the advantages and limitations of the principal options via the cornea, limbus or sclera need to be considered depending on the microsurgical objective (Table 4.1) (see also Chapter 2).

Three principal variants of intraocular microsurgery can be distinguished: (1) *wide-open sky;* (2) *minimally invasive;* and (3) *within* the intact eye. Elective microsurgical as well as traumatic openings of the eye have consequences beyond the entry site. Obviously a traumatic wound is more difficult to close and has a higher risk of infection (see Chapter 2).

All procedures adjacent to the limited space of the *anterior chamber* require a conscious awareness of the surrounding vulnerable tissues and cell populations. Free flow in the pupillary zone and free access through the trabecular meshwork must be preserved. The corneal endothelium, the significant structures of the iris as well as the lens capsule and anterior zonula insertion may be exposed to surgical trauma (Fig. 4.1).

The *vitreous cavity* in comparison to the anterior chamber is a much larger space. All manipulations need to respect the important vitreous attachments, the posterior lens capsule and posterior zonular insertion.

Certainly microsurgical manipulations of the sensory retina require special care and the potential "vagaries" of the retinal pigment epithelium must be kept in mind (see Chapter 5.6).

Any opening of the eye, be it in the anterior chamber or in the vitreous cavity, causes a more or less pronounced *acute ocular hypotony* and may lead to a choroidal effusion and/or hemorrhage, in extreme variants even to expulsive hemorrhage (see Chapter 2.2). The spectrum of the *size of the eye* beyond the range of the optical axis of 22–26 mm requires special attention.

Wound healing after intraocular surgery or trauma has essentially three aspects: (1) closure of the wound in the eye wall, (2) wound healing of the targeted tissue and (3) reversibility of the indirect distant effects. The latter will be discussed within the chapter on special surgical anatomy and pathology (Chapter 5). In view of the spectacular advances of intraocular microsurgery of both the anterior and posterior segment, a concept of a *"minimal eye"* will be proposed.

Indications for local or general anesthesia have been discussed (see Chapter 2, Sect. 2.3).

4.1. Access into the Eye: Principal Options and Anterior Segment Trauma

4.1.1 Direct Incisions and Wounds

4.1.1.1 Transcorneal Access

The state of Bowman's layer is of practical significance for the microsurgeon. If Bowman's lamella is absent, the method of suturing corneal wounds and corneal grafting must be modified (Figs. 4.2–4.4). Unsutured – located temporally – transcorneal incisions of 2,8 mm for extracapsular cataract extractions may be a risk for spontaneous leakage and insidious aspiration of surface fluids into the anterior chamber, including bacterial contamination, and may explain a "silent epidemic" (Peter McDonnell; see Taban et al. 2005) of postoperative endophthalmitis, up to 0.5%!

Table 4.1. Access into eye – principal options

1. *Transcorneal:* avascular wound healing
   a) Minimal mechanical opening for ECCE
   b) Laser trephination without wound deformation in PKP
2. *Limbal:* vascular wound healing
   a) Accelerated after cataract extraction (beneficial)
   b) Undesired after filtrating glaucoma surgery
3. *Transscleral:* vascular wound healing (including pars plana approach)

ECCE extracapsular catarct extraction, *PKP* perforating keratoplasty

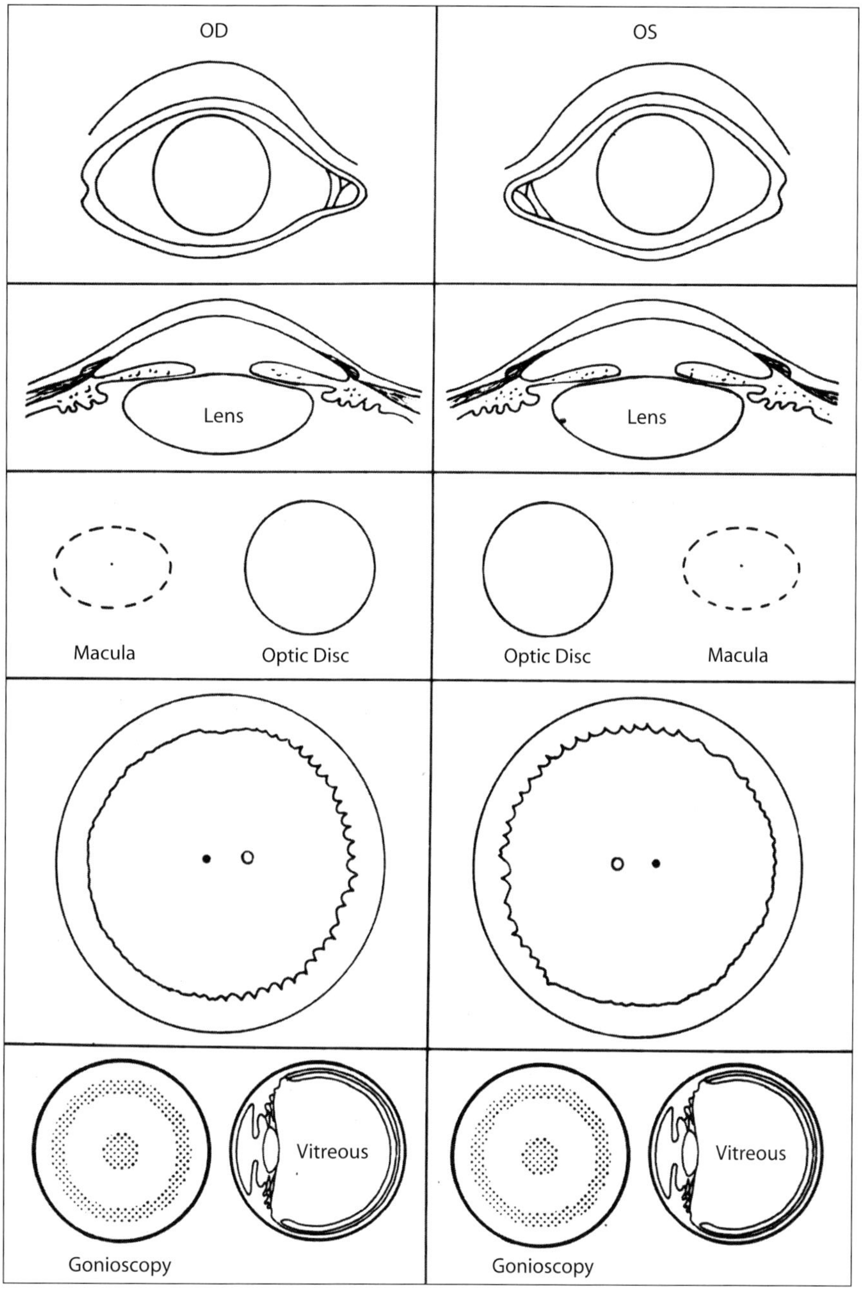

Fig. 4.1. "Erlangen sketch" for documentation of anterior segment and intraocular pathology

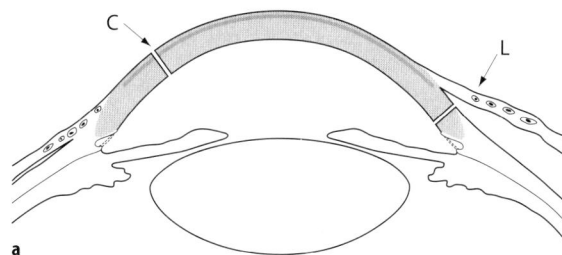
Fig. 4.2. a Access into the eye: corneal through Bowman's layer

In elective microsurgery of the lens and iris this approach has an obvious advantage due to the avascularity and biomechanics of the cornea. The lack of vessels and the low cellularity in the stroma are factors for a *delayed* avascular wound healing (Figs. 4.5–4.12). Both aspects and the "acquired anterior chamber immune deviation" privilege (ACAID) (Streilein et al. 2003; see Chapter 5.1) contribute to the relatively low incidence of immune reactions after perforating corneal grafts (see Chapter 5.1) in non-vascularized hosts.

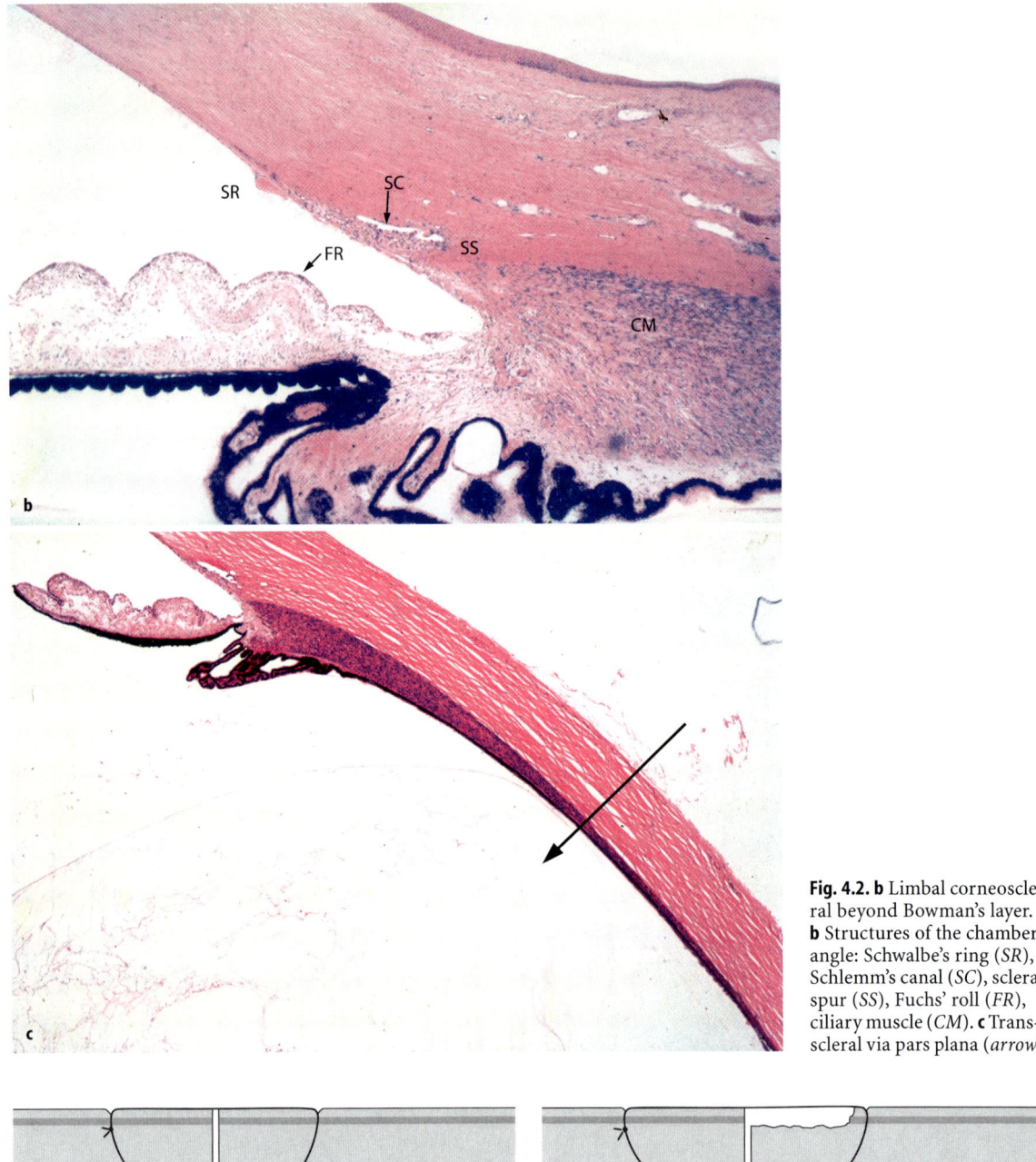

Fig. 4.2. b Limbal corneoscleral beyond Bowman's layer. **b** Structures of the chamber angle: Schwalbe's ring (*SR*), Schlemm's canal (*SC*), scleral spur (*SS*), Fuchs' roll (*FR*), ciliary muscle (*CM*). **c** Transscleral via pars plana (*arrow*)

Fig. 4.3. Bowman's layer is crucial for fixation of single and running sutures. **a** Normal corneal structure on host and graft: 10-0 nylon knot is buried below Bowman's layer. **b** Absence of Bowman's layer means risk of suture loosening. Wound closure should be modified by wider grip and interrupted suture preferred over running suture (see text)

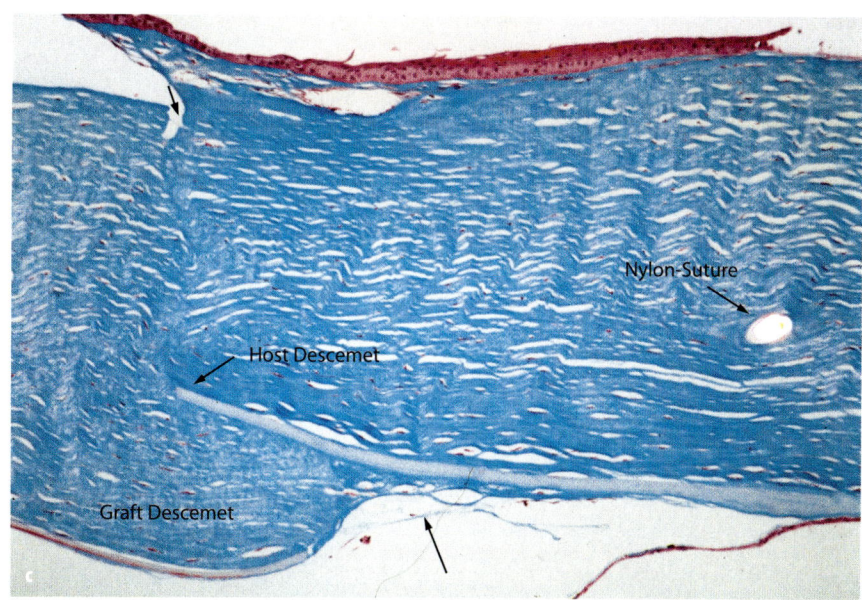

Fig. 4.3. c Host graft junction after penetrating keratoplasty following conventional trephination. Note deformation of scar (Masson staining)

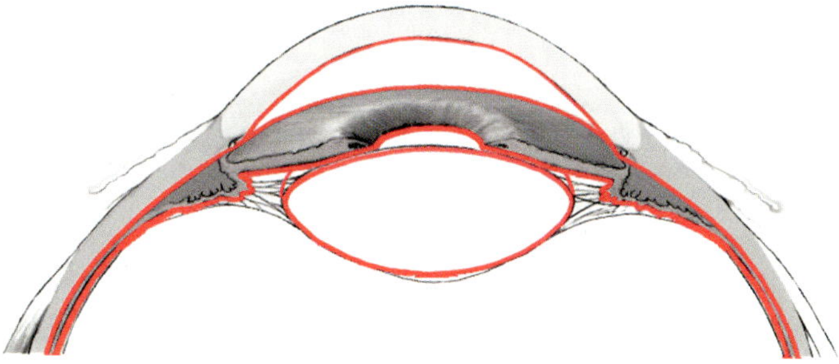

Fig. 4.4. Landmarks for the anterior segment surgeon: Bowman's layer, Descemet's membrane, scleral spur (*arrow*), lens capsule

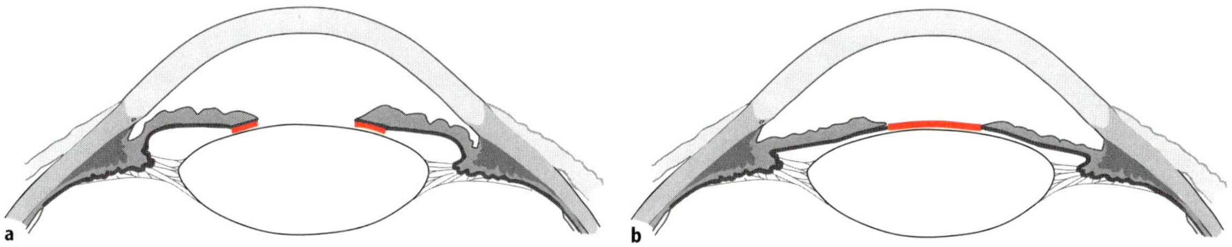

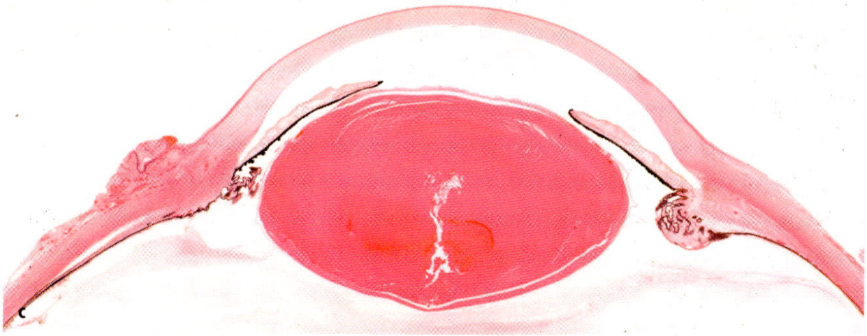

Fig. 4.5. a Seclusio pupillae: posterior synechiae. **b** Occlusio pupillae: posterior synechiae and fibrovascular membrane covering the pupil. **c** Intumescent cataract increases physiologic resistance of flow in pupillary area

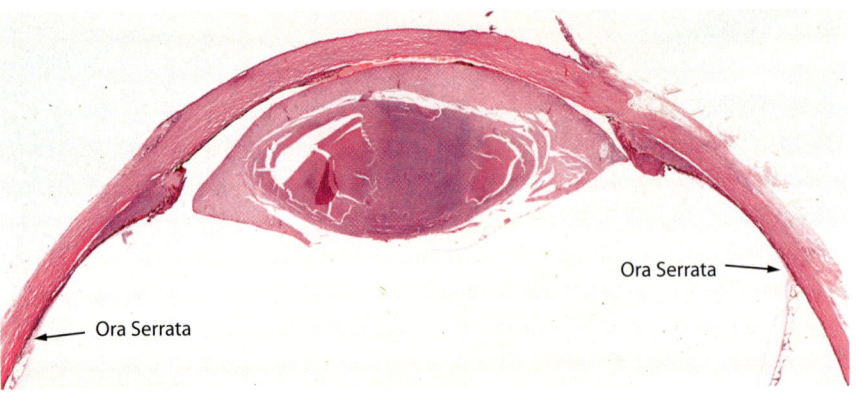

Fig. 4.5. d Ciliolenticular block pushing the lens and iris to the back of the cornea

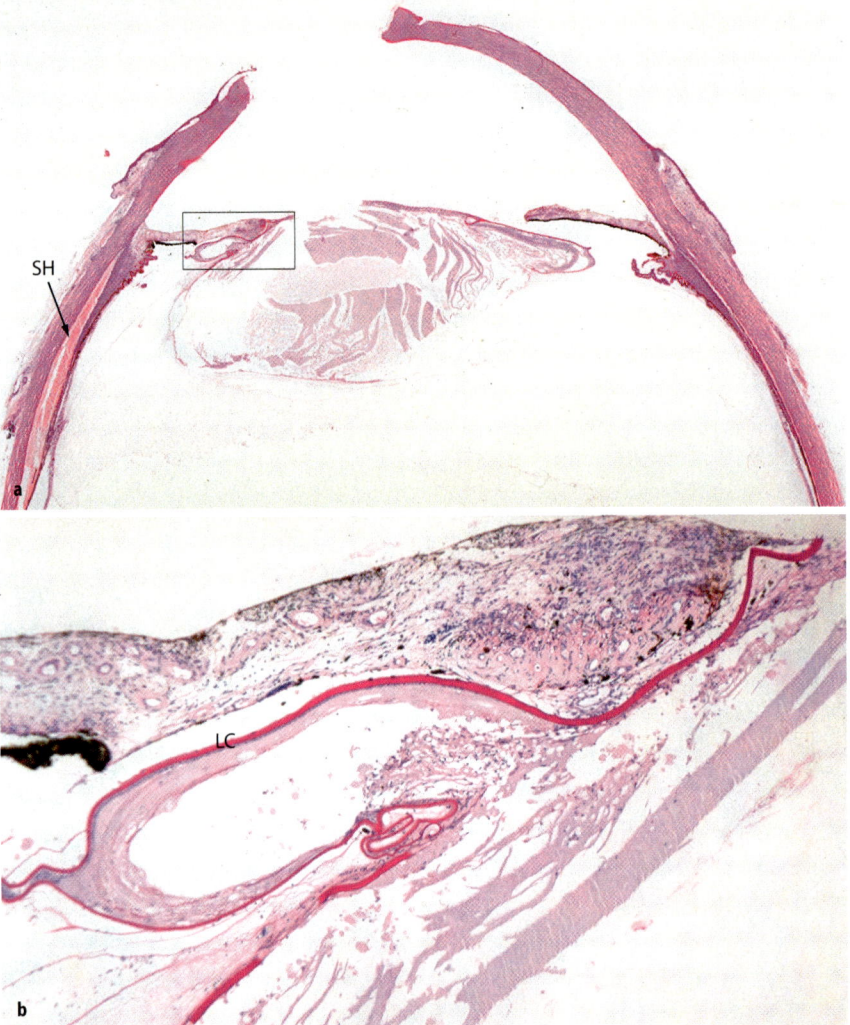

Fig. 4.6. Consequences of perforating injuries: **a, b** of cornea and almost complete resorption of lens, phakogenic uveitis 23 days after neglected trauma; no infection, supraciliary hemorrhage (SH). **b** Box from **a** at higher power. Lens capsule (*LC*) (PAS)

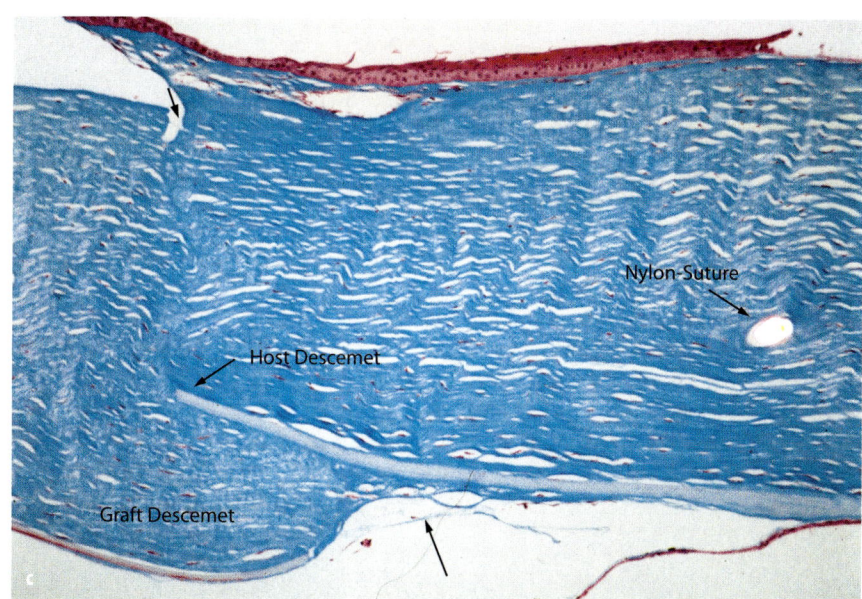

Fig. 4.3. c Host graft junction after penetrating keratoplasty following conventional trephination. Note deformation of scar (Masson staining)

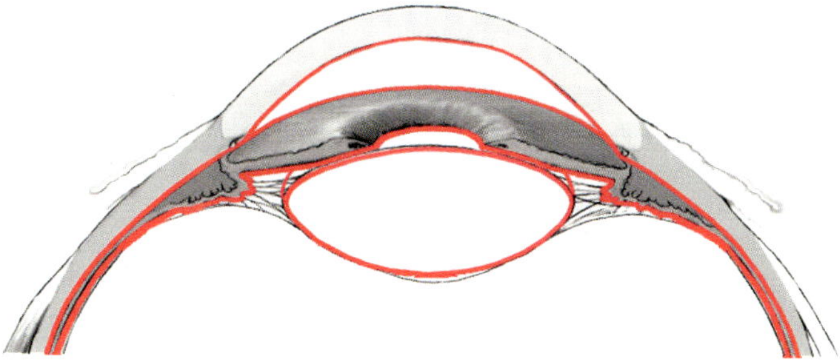

Fig. 4.4. Landmarks for the anterior segment surgeon: Bowman's layer, Descemet's membrane, scleral spur (*arrow*), lens capsule

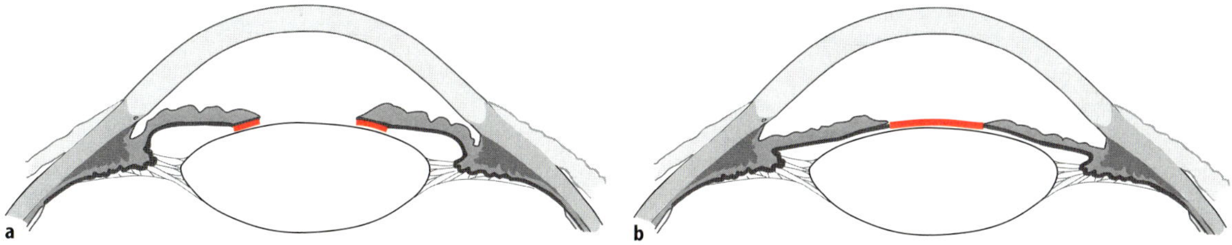

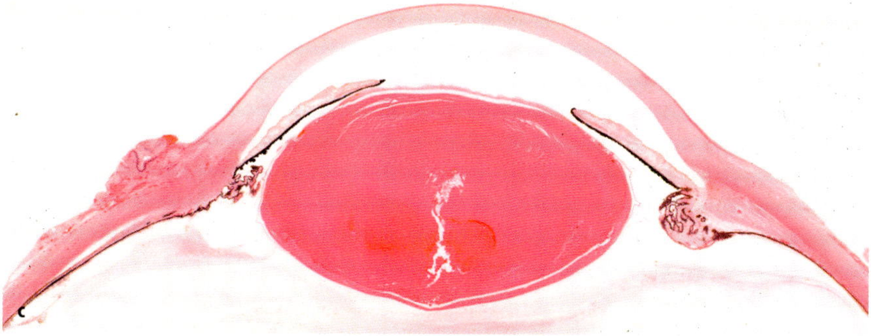

Fig. 4.5. a Seclusio pupillae: posterior synechiae. **b** Occlusio pupillae: posterior synechiae and fibrovascular membrane covering the pupil. **c** Intumescent cataract increases physiologic resistance of flow in pupillary area

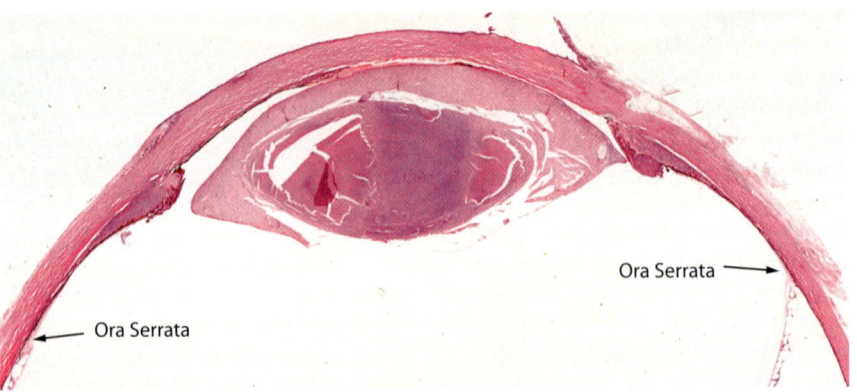

Fig. 4.5. d Ciliolenticular block pushing the lens and iris to the back of the cornea

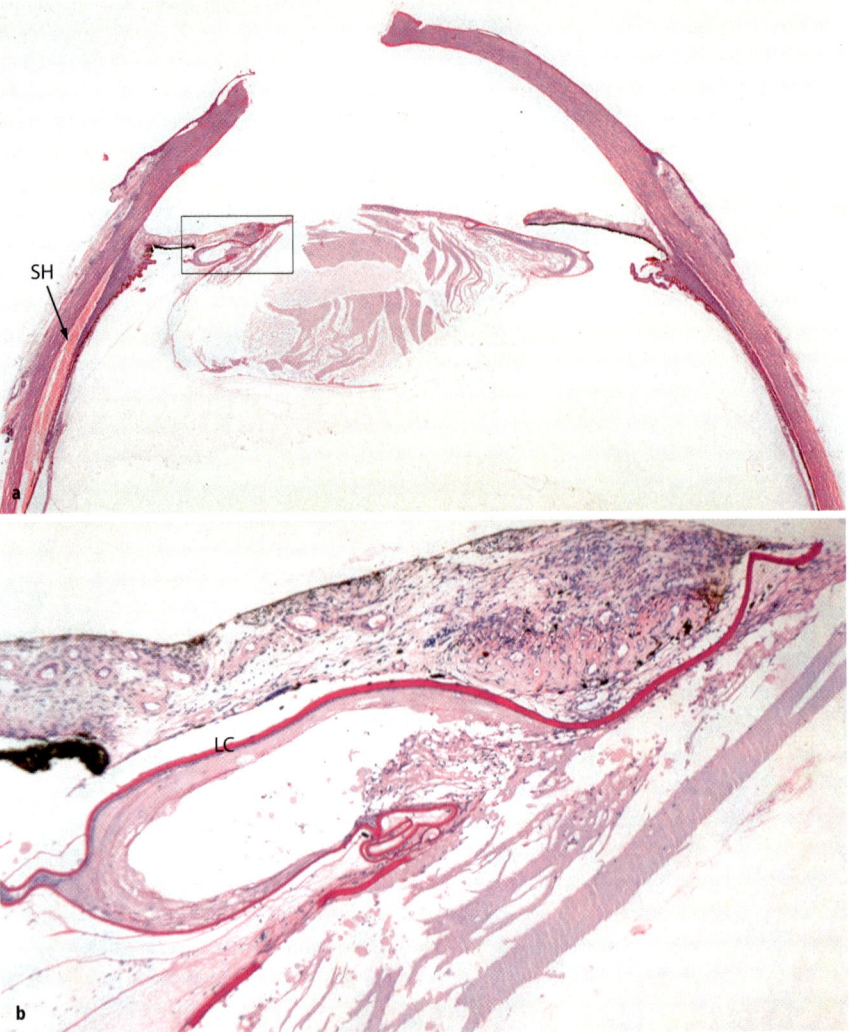

Fig. 4.6. Consequences of perforating injuries: **a, b** of cornea and almost complete resorption of lens, phakogenic uveitis 23 days after neglected trauma; no infection, supraciliary hemorrhage (SH). **b** Box from **a** at higher power. Lens capsule (*LC*) (PAS)

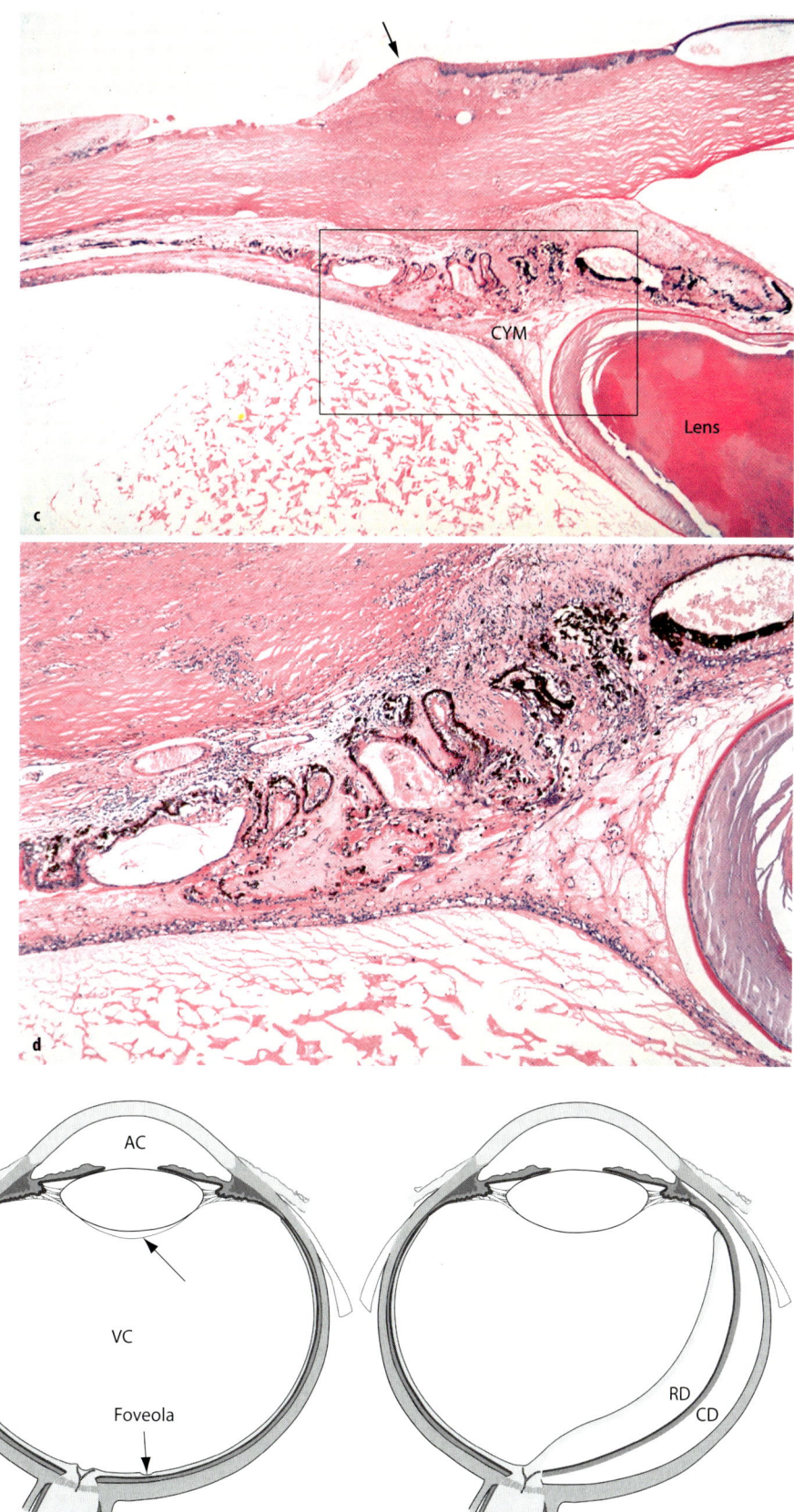

Fig. 4.6. c, d Limbal perforation (*arrow*) with consecutive cyclitic membrane (*CYM*) reaching up to the lens equator. **d** Box from **c** at higher magnification

Fig. 4.7. Obvious and potential compartments of the intraocular space. **a** Anterior chamber (*AC*), Berger's space (*arrow*), vitreous cavity (*VC*). **b** Sketch of choroidal (*CD*) and retinal detachment (*RD*)

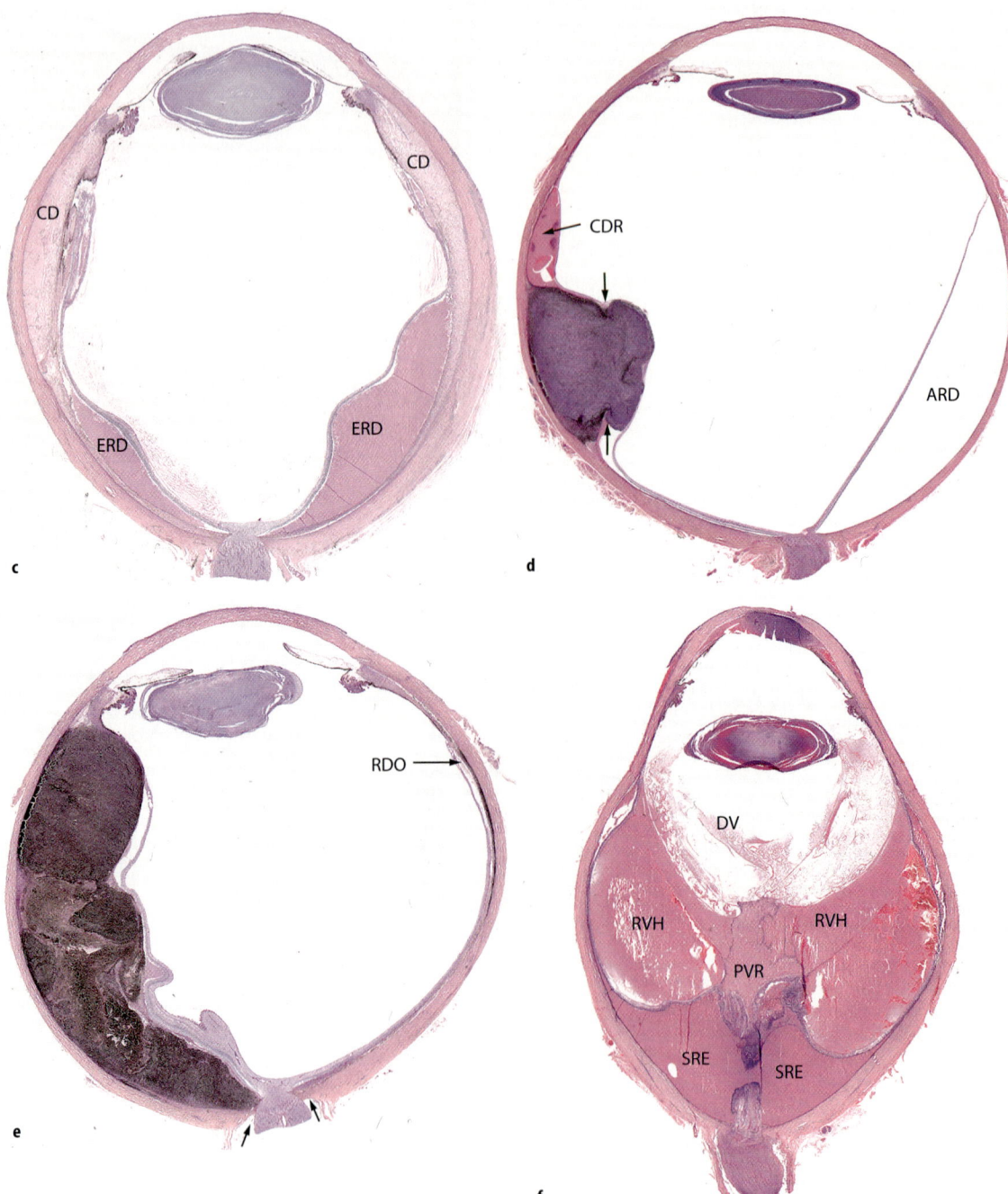

Fig. 4.7. c Choroidal (*CD*) and exudative retinal detachment (*ERD*); posterior scleritis (*arrow*). **d** Malignant melanoma of the choroid with collateral retinal detachment (*CRD*), perforation of Bruch's membrane (*arrows*); invading the sensory retina up to the vitreous cavity. Rønne type artificial retinal detachment (*ARD*). **e** Malignant melanoma of the uvea reaching from the ciliary body to the optic disc and beyond showing separate cell populations of the tumor. Note: tumor distant exudative retinal detachment at ora inferiorly (*RDO*). Juxtapapillary portion of the malignant melanoma in the *immediate* vicinity of the spinal fluid space behind the scleral ring of Elschnig (*arrow*). Malignant melanoma respects the structure of the sensory retina. **f** Necrotizing keratitis following secondary angle closure glaucoma with rubeosis iridis and massive proliferative vitreoretinopathy (*PVR*) in diabetes mellitus. Note: detachment of the vitreous (*DV*), retrovitreal hemorrhage (*RVH*), extensive retinoschisis, and subretinal exudate (*SRE*)

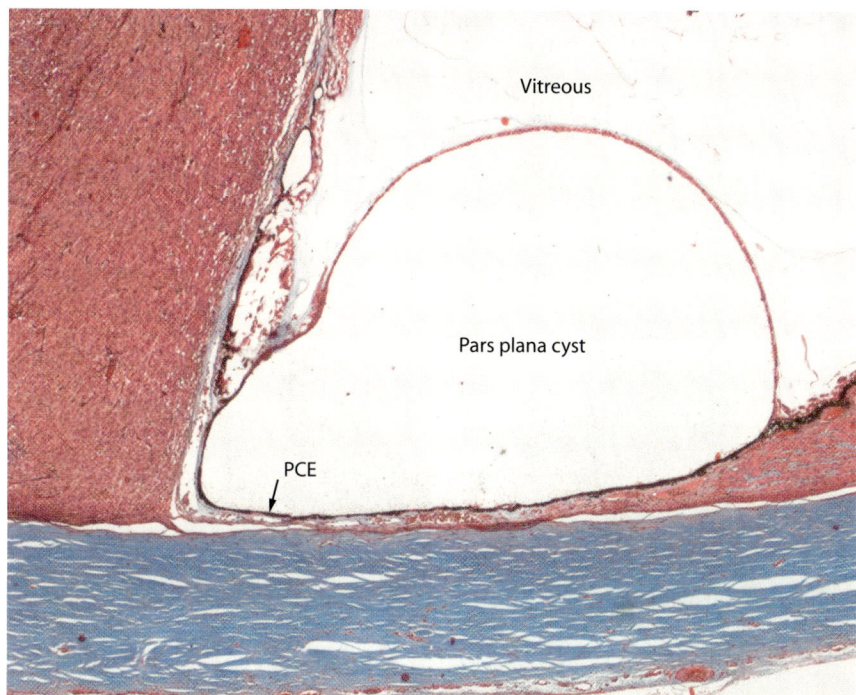

Fig. 4.7. g Pars plana cyst separating the non- from the pigmented ciliary epithelium (*PCE*): very common finding with aging (see Chapter 5.4) adjacent to large uveal malignant melanoma (MASSON)

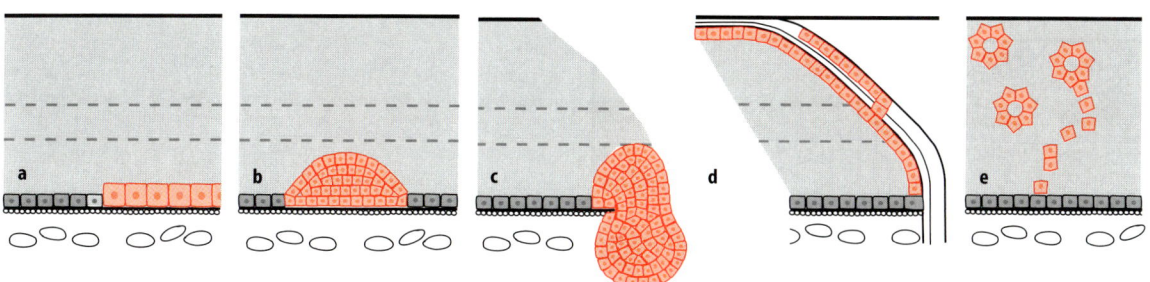

Fig. 4.8. "Vagaries" of the retinal pigment epithelium (RPE) in distinct pattern. **a** Hypertrophy of the RPE. **b** Focal hyperplasia of the RPE. **c** Hyperplasia into choroid. **d** Proliferation along axons. **e** Retinopathia sclopetaria: proliferation along the retinal capillaries

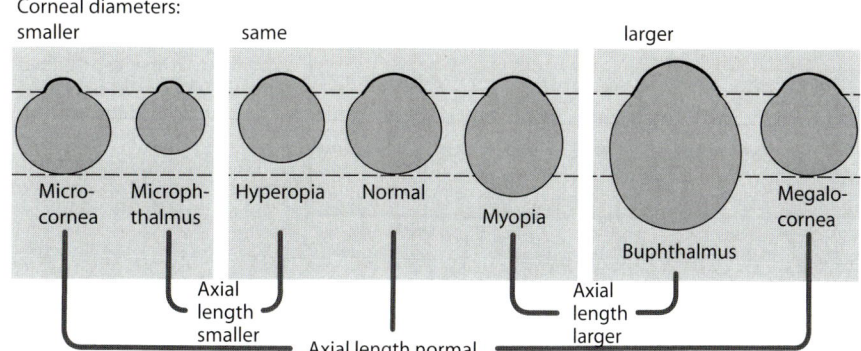

Fig. 4.9. Terminology of variation of the corneal diameter and the length of the optical axis in various congenital anomalies

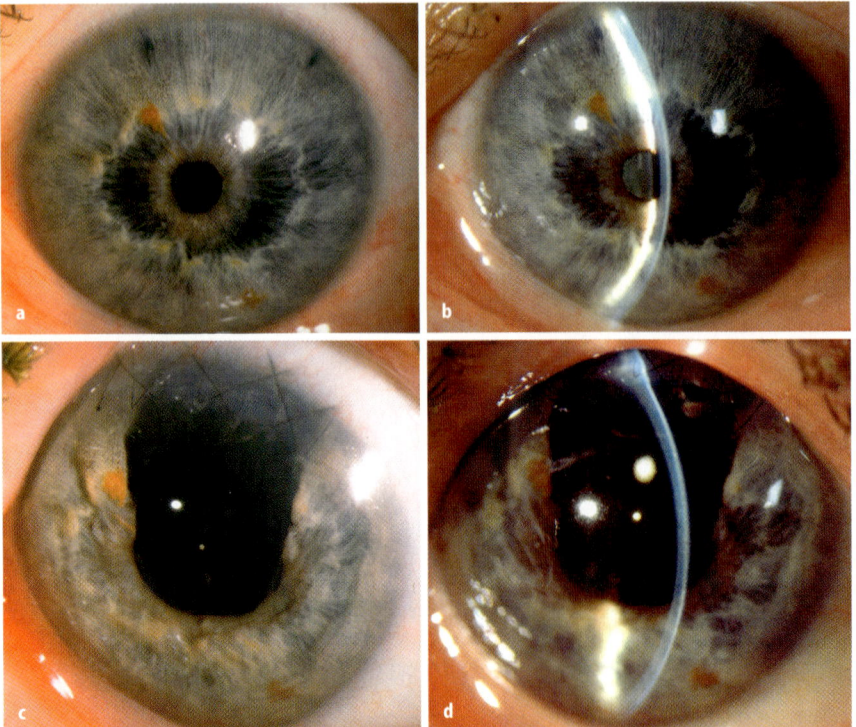

Fig. 4.10. Extreme nanophthalmus with microcornea and imminent angle closure glaucoma with extremely narrow anterior chamber and posterior subcapsular cataract. Axial length 16 mm, lens thickness 5.6 mm, corneal diameters 11 mm, corneal endothelial count 1,400 cells/mm^2; 51-year-old male. **a, b** After two YAG iridotomies. **c, d** Postoperatively after extracapsular cataract extraction. Implantation of 51 dptr. lens and sector iridectomy

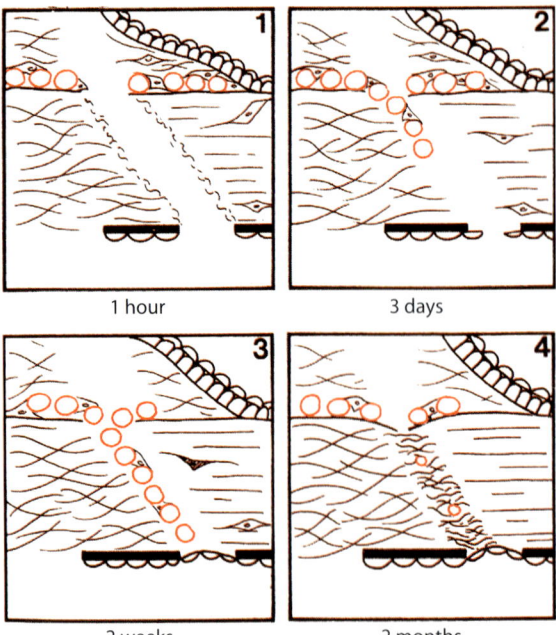

Fig. 4.11. a Limbal wound: *vascularized* wound healing. **1** The limbal wound with a conjunctival flap passes through episclera externally and enters the globe through Descemet's membrane and endothelium. Sclera is on the left and cornea on the right. Schwalbe's line (*SL*), trabecular meshwork™, Schlemm's canal (*SC*). The wound edge shows early disintegration. Neutrophiles and macrophages are omitted in this diagram. **2** Episcleral vessels and fibroblasts migrate down the wound. Some activity is present in the corneal fibroblasts. **3** Episcleral fibrovascular migration in the wound is stopped at the endothelium crossing the internal margin of the incision. **4** The number of vessels and their diameter decreases in the late stage of healing. Irregular collagen fibers and matrix fill the contracting wound. (Modified with kind permission of A.E. Grossniklaus (editor): Ophthalmic Pathology and Intraocular Tumors, Section 4, Basic and Clinical Science Course of the American Academy of Ophthalmology 2004).

▷
b Scar after perforating peripheral corneal wound with vascularization (PAS stain) **c** Interruption of Bowman's layer (*BL*); **d** defect in Descemet's membrane (*DM*) bridged by newly formed basement membrane produced by proliferating corneal endothelium

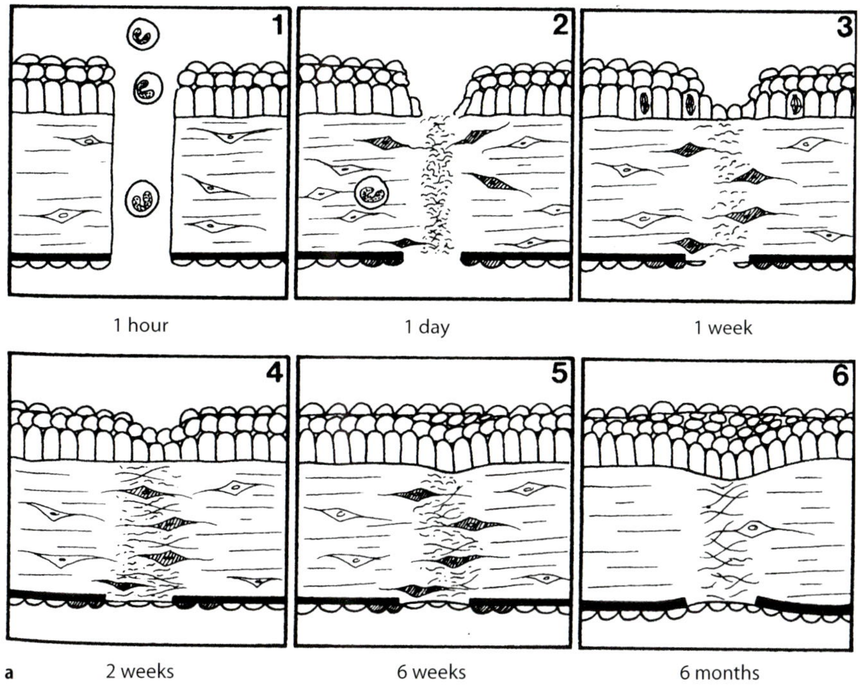

Fig. 4.12. Clear corneal wound: avascular wound healing. **1** The tear film carries neutrophils with lysozymes to the wound within an hour. **2** Within a day with closure of the incision, the wound edge shows early disintegration and edema. The glycosaminoglycans at the edge are degraded. The nearby fibroblasts are activated. **3** At 1 week, migrating epithelium and endothelium partially seal the wound; fibroblasts begin to migrate and supply collagen. **4** At 2 weeks fibroblast activity and collagen and matrix deposition continue. The endothelium, sealing the inner wound, lays down new (basement) Descemet's membrane. **5** At 6 weeks epithelial regeneration is complete. Fibroblasts fill the wound with type I collagen and repair slows. **6** At 6 months the final wound contracts. The collagen fibers are not parallel with the surrounding lamellae. The number of fibroblasts decreases. (Modified with kind permission of A.E. Grossniklaus (editor): Ophthalmic Pathology and Intraocular Tumors, Section 4, Basic and Clinical Science Course of the American Academy of Ophthalmology 2004)

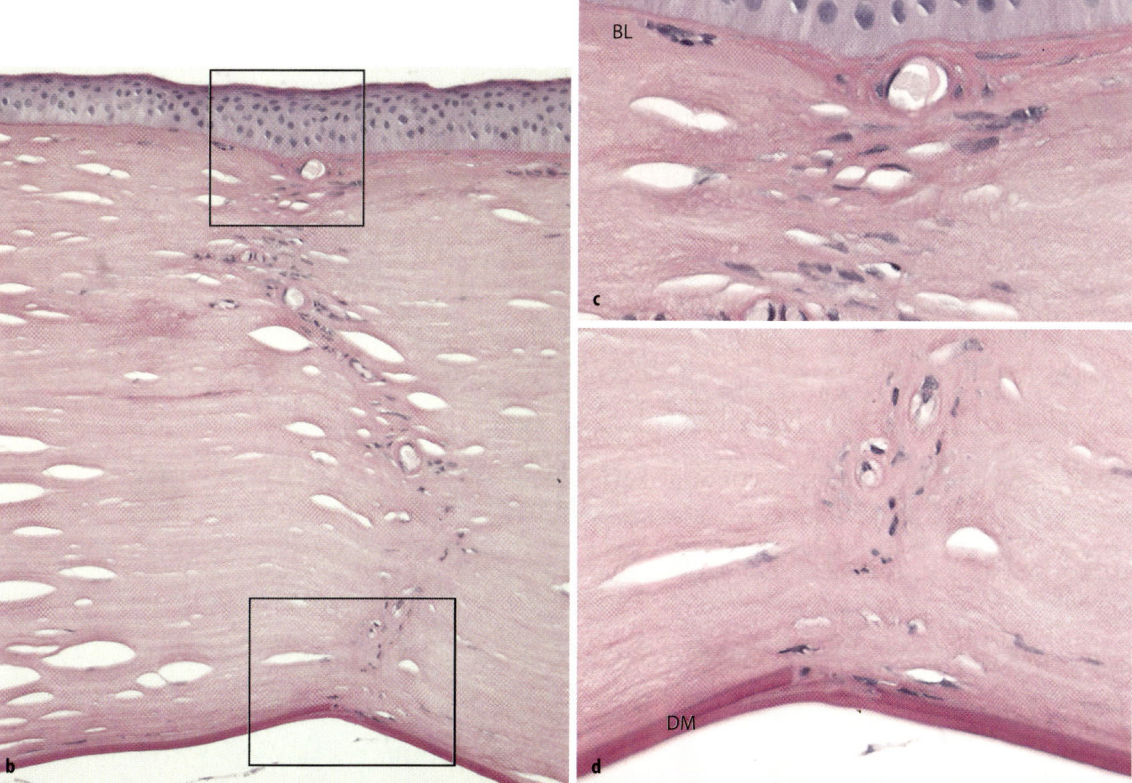

Fig. 4.11b–d (*Legend see p. 84*)

4.1.1.2
Access via Corneal "Limbus," Fornix and Limbus Based Conjunctival Flaps

Seen under the operating microscope, the term "*corneal limbus*" is rather vague. We suggest orienting along the landmarks visible directly under the operating microscope: the peripheral edge of Bowman's layer, Schwalbe's line, Schlemm's canal and the scleral spur. Schlemm's canal weakens the biomechanical resistance. The other areas with reduced *scleral thickness* are beneath the insertion of the straight extraocular muscles in the equatorial region, the lamina cribrosa and juxtapapillary between the retrobulbar meningeal subdural space and Elschnig's scleral ring (see Fig. 2.12). Severe contusions may lead to ruptures of the eye wall in these areas (Figs. 4.12–4.16).

The corneal limbus is one of the three mechanical "*loci minoris resistentiae*" of the scleral eye wall (Table 4.2), because in the corneoscleral transition zone wound

Table 4.2. Mechanical "loci minores resistentiae" of the eye wall-sclera

1. *Limbus corneae*: cornea-sclera transition including trabecular meshwork and Schlemm's canal: between scleral spur and Schwalbe's line
2. *Equatorial sclera*: insertion of four straight extraocular muscles reduces scleral thickness to less than 50%
3. *Lamina cribrosa*: exit of optic nerve fibers
4. *Juxtapapillary sclera*: relative gap between scleral ring of Elschnig and insertion of dura meninges (less than 50% scleral thickness elsewhere)

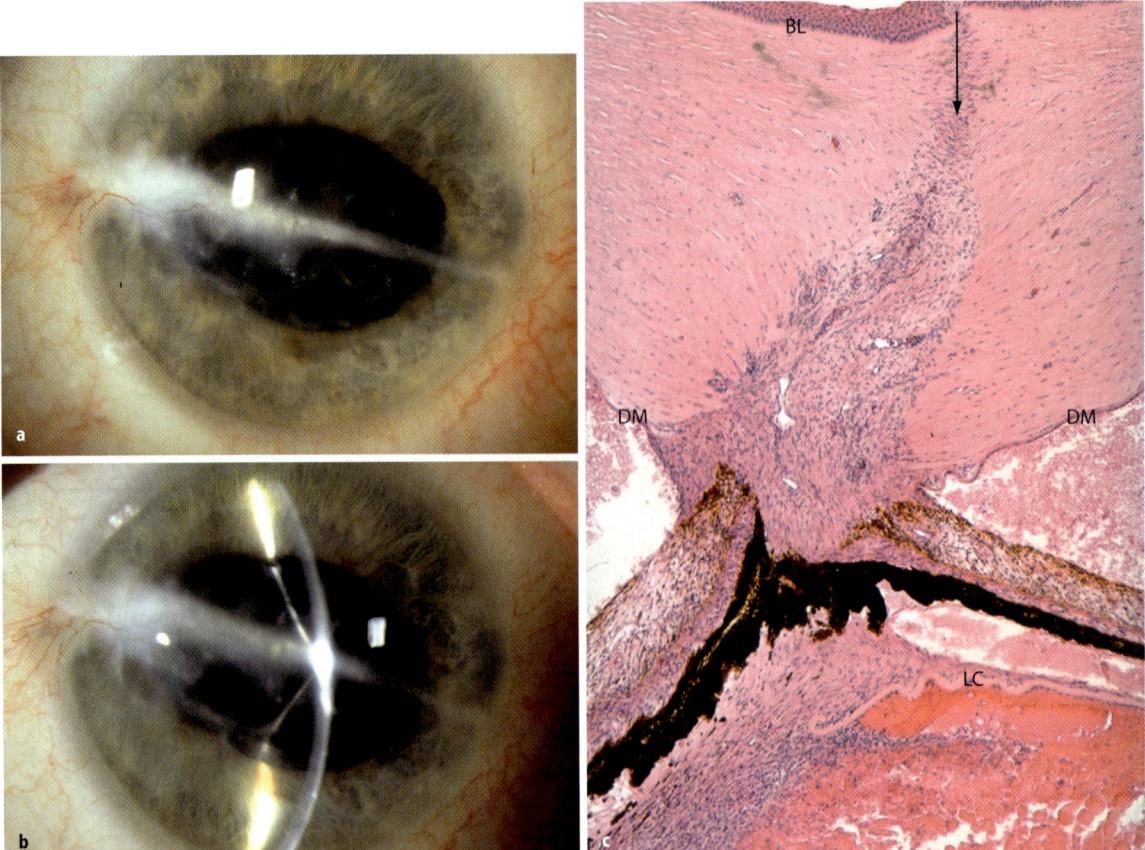

Fig. 4.13. Corneal scar, partially vascularized after penetrating injury and traumatic aphakia with incarceration of formed vitreous. **a, b** Slit lamp. **c** Iris incarceration into vascularized corneal scar (*arrow*) with traction on lens with "phacoanaphylactic endophthalmitis" by posterior synechiae. Descemet's membrane (*DM*), Bowman Layer (*BL*), Lens capsule (*LC*) such anterior synechiae need sharp dissection, blunt preparation may cause additional tauma

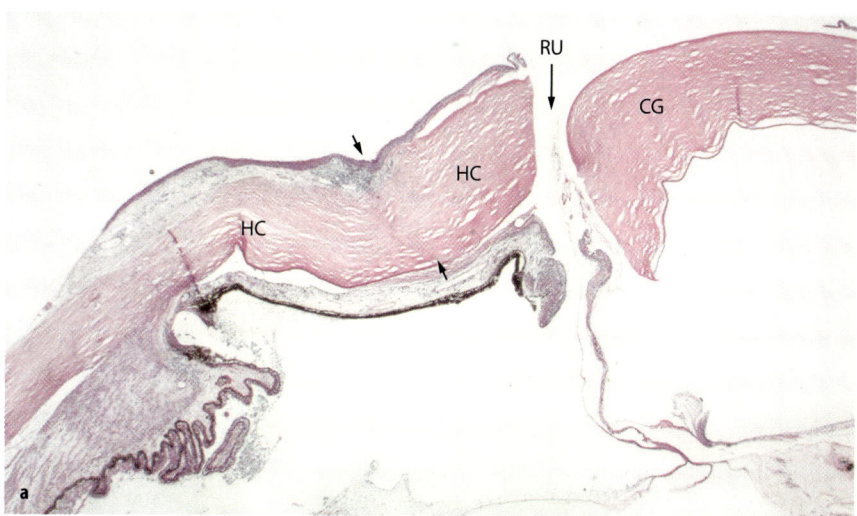

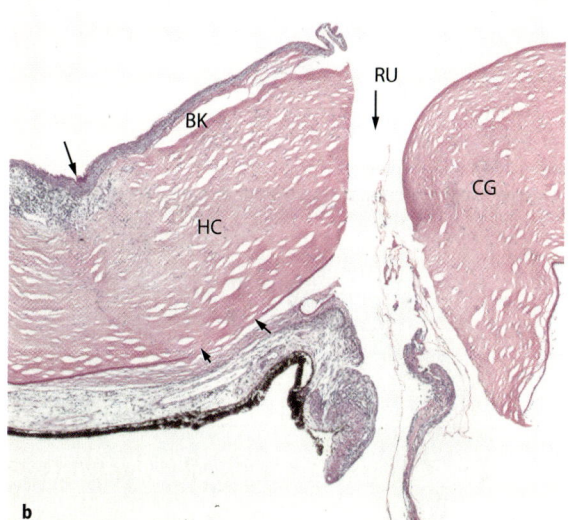

4.14. Wound rupture after cataract extraction and recent perforating keratoplasty with mycotic keratitis and epithelial invasion (PAS). Host cornea (*HC*), cornea graft (*CG*), Descemet's membrane (*DM*). **a** Blunt rupture of graft-host-cornea wound (*RU*) with vitreous and iris incarceration. Older partially vascularized corneal scar after cataract extraction with interruption of Descemet's membrane (*small arrows*). **b** Higher power shows vascularization from conjunctival limbus and fibrovascular tissue between the cornea and iris and of old scar with bullous keratopathy (*BK*) gap in Descemet's membrane (*small arrows*). **c** Opposite region of graft to a necrotizing keratitis on host and graft, granulomatous reaction against Descemet's membrane (*GRD*), purulent iritis and keratitis with mycotic elements (*arrow*), epithelial invasion (*EI*). **d** Higher power shows epithelial invasion (*EI*) along the edges of the old graft-host intersection. **e** Higher power shows edematous and vacuolated epithelium non-keratinizing epithelium growing over necrotic corneal edge. Descemet's membrane (*CM*), PAS stain

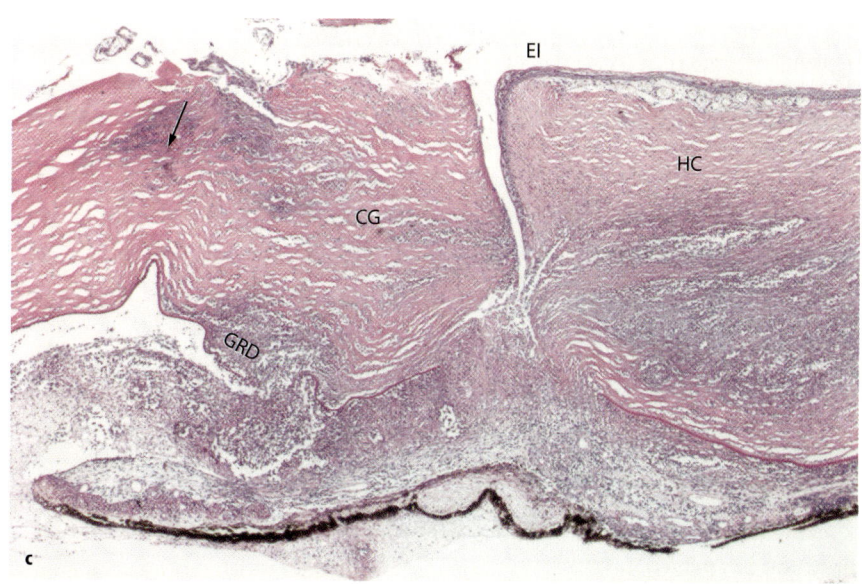

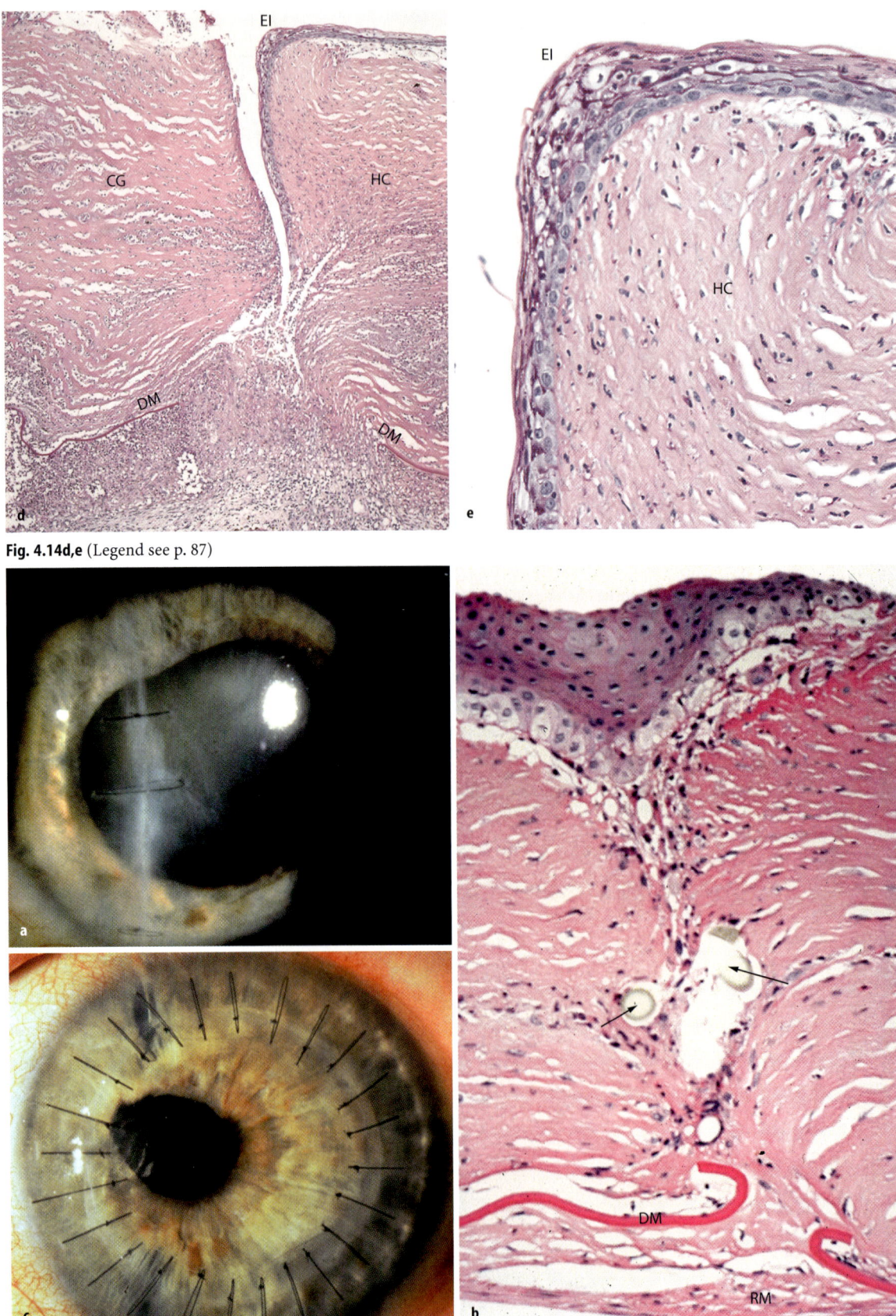

Fig. 4.14d,e (Legend see p. 87)

Fig. 4.15a-c (Legend see p. 89)

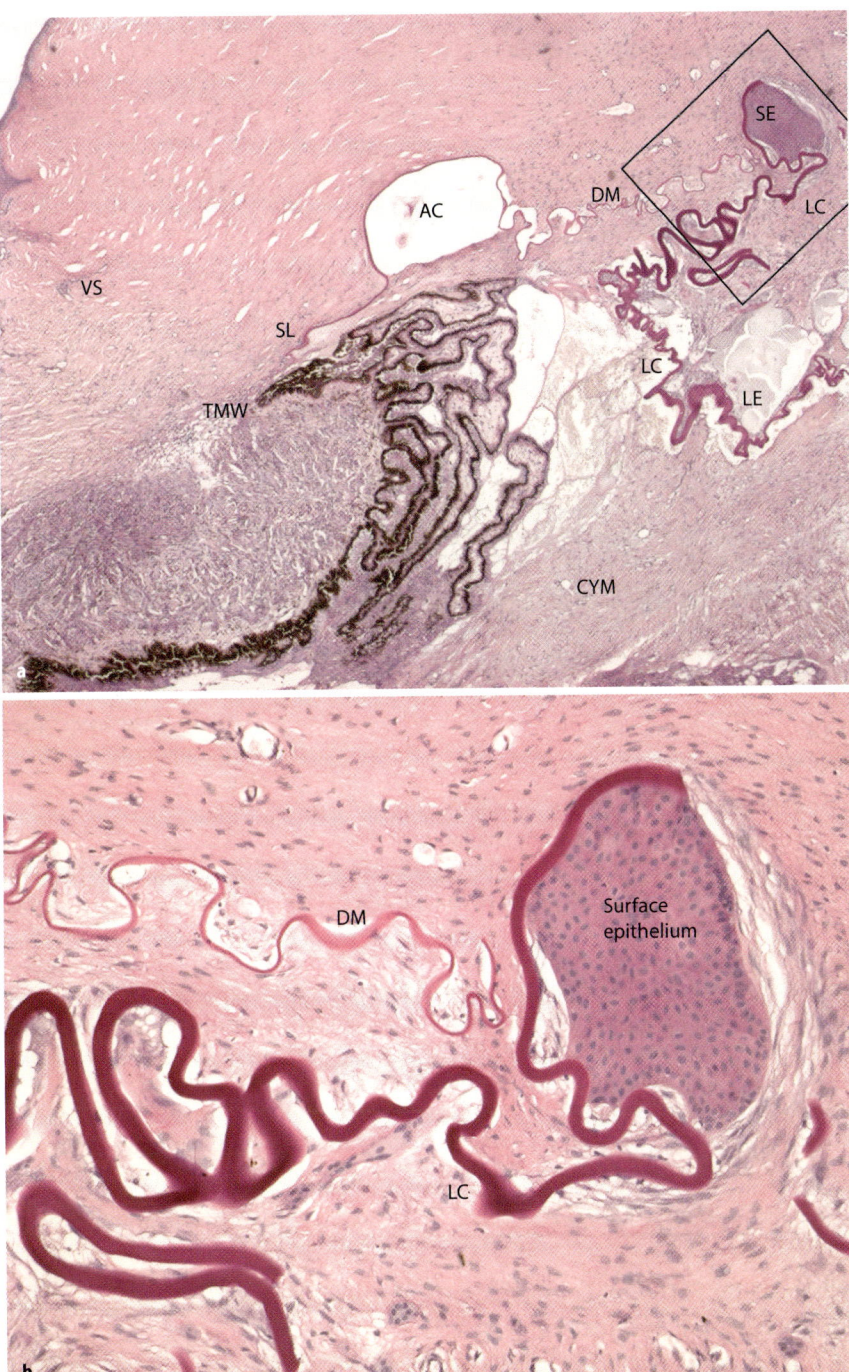

Fig. 4.16. Scars after severe perforating injury of the anterior segment: anterior chamber (*AC*) almost completely obliterated. Vascularized scar (*VS*) at limbus. Remnants of Descemet's membrane (*DM*) and lens capsule (*LC*) with lens epithelium (*LE*) enclose island of surface epithelium (*SE*). Cyclitic membrane (*CYM*), Schwalbe's line (*SL*), trabecular meshwork (*TMW*).
a Overview. **b** Box from **a** with higher magnification (PAS stain)

◁
Fig. 4.15. a Perforating corneal wound closed with two sutures with wound leakage. **b** Vascularized corneal scar with interrupted Descemet's membrane (*DM*) and suture track (*arrow*). Retrocorneal membrane (*RM*). **c** After elliptical corneal transplantation with excimer laser 193 nm trephination, cataract extraction and lens implantation

healing follows the *vascular pattern* originating from the conjunctival episcleral and scleral vessels (Fig. 4.12).

Both a transcorneal and limbus access potentially may be associated with invasion of the surface epithelium of cornea and conjunctiva into the eye, if the "contact inhibition" (Cameron et al. 1974) from the corneal endothelium does not work – particularly if the corneal rim is damaged by surgical trauma or preexisting disease, e.g., Fuchs' or PEX keratopathy (see chapter 6.3).

4.1.1.3
Pars Plana Transscleral Approaches

The transscleral approach overlying the pars plana of the ciliary body reduces the risk of hemorrhage from the ciliary processes and is sufficiently distant to the posterior pole of the lens to prevent its damage. Care must be taken to avoid that the inserting instrument is not caught in the pars plana uveal tissue and ciliary epithelial layer. Robert Machemer (1969) has opened a new era in vitreoretinal surgery using this venue.

4.1.2
Indirect Distant Effects

Manipulations in the *anterior chamber* associated with acute or chronic ocular hypotony may induce uveal effusion and choroidal detachment, and increase the risk of retinal detachment and age-related macula degeneration (see Chapter 2, 5.5 and 5.6).

Procedures within the *vitreous cavity* with implants and episcleral cerclage can lead to ciliary and pupillary block angle closure glaucomas or open angle glaucomas from silicone oil (see Chapter 5.2). All intraocular procedures cause a breakdown in the blood-ocular barrier leading to increased protein content in the aqueous and edema of the sensory retina – most pronounced as cystoid maculopathy.

4.2
Obvious and Potential Compartments of the Intraocular Space (Table 4.3) (Fig. 4.7)

The obvious *compartments* of the intraocular space are the anterior and posterior chamber and the vitreous cavity. A *potential* compartment of the intraocular space is the supraciliary space carrying the uveoscleral aqueous outflow. Dramatic ballooning as "*choroidal detachment*" may occur in acute and chronic persisting ocular hypotony (Fig. 4.6). This "cilioschisis" displaces the origin of zonular fibers inwards, allows subluxation of the lens anteriorly and reduces aqueous production – accentuating the persisting ocular hypotony.

Detachment of retinal pigment epithelium from

Table 4.3. Obvious and potential compartments of intraocular space

1. **Obvious:**
   Anterior and posterior chamber
   Vitreous space
2. **Potential spaces:**
   – Choroidal detachment: supraciliary and suprachoroidal space
   – Retinal detachment (rhegmatogenous, traction, exudative)
   – Separation of sensory retina from RPE
   – Disciform macula detachment
     a) Sensory retina RPE and
     b) RPE from Bruch's membrane
   – Ciliary body – pars plana cysts between ciliary epithelia
   – "Cysts" between layers of iris PE
   – Intraretinal cystoid degeneration/retinoschisis
3. **Iatrogenic: empty lens capsular bag**

Bruch's membrane and detachment of the sensory retina from the retinal pigment epithelium illustrate weak intercellular connections in the pathologic condition (Fig. 4.7, intraocular spaces) (see Chapter 2, 5.6, Sect. 5.6.1.4; Chapter 5.7).

"*Pars plana cysts*" are common and occur between the pigmented and non-pigmented ciliary epithelium (Fig. 4.7g).

4.3
Variants of Intraocular Microsurgery

Ideally – as a currently utopian goal – all intraocular microsurgery should be achieved within the intact closed eyeball. Today this is only possible with light and laser coagulation. Depending on the extent of the opening in the eye wall, the following three variants can be distinguished.

Considering the risk of *open eye surgery* we have to concentrate on three aspects:

1. The *direct wound* in the eye wall
2. The *target tissue*, e.g., iris, lens or vitreous
3. The indirect distant effects of the defect in the eye wall with consecutive hypotony, etc. (see Chapter 2.2).

4.3.1
Wide Open Sky Approach

Large defects in the eye wall require closure of the defect by corneal or corneoscleral grafts. Optical indications for *penetrating keratoplasty* require that the central region of the cornea is removed and the defect closed by a corresponding *corneal graft* fixed by sutures. In *non-vascularized cornea,* wound healing is slow, sutures are removed 1–2 years after penetrating keratoplasty and immune reactions are rare (less than 10%). In *vascularized corneal* scars, wound healing is less delayed, and immune reaction are more common. Absence of Bowman's membrane predisposes to loosening of 10-0 monofilament sutures (see above). *Corneoscleral defects* after excentric corneoscleral block excisions of tumors of the anterior uvea or of epithelial ingrowth and after removal of post-traumatic ectasies are covered by corneoscleral or *scleral grafts*. Wound healing in the area of the vascularized sclera is accelerated. Immune reactions occur almost *always* – earlier or later. The consecutive loss of the corneal endothelium and endothelial decompensation with graft edema is followed by consecutive vascularization and scarring of the edematous graft tissue including retrocorneal membrane formation (see Chapters 5.1, 5.4).

In *central corneal grafts* for optical indications, regrowth of the terminal branches of the trigeminal nerves is slow and may take years; in the corneoscleral tectonic graft this has not been studied yet.

Intracapsular cataract extraction today is infrequently performed in the industrialized countries. However, dislocated lenses with very hard brunescent, black or calcified lens nuclei with extensive fibrous metaplasia may require incisions of 180° at the limbus or transcorneally. These large wounds are usually not self-sealing and require wound closures with sutures.

Extracapsular cataract extraction with nuclear expression may be the preferred approach in countries where there are patients with far advanced mature and hypermature cataracts with a very hard nucleus. The corneoscleral wound may be structured in such a way that wound closure with sutures is not necessary (Albrecht Henning's "fish-hook technique").

4.3.2
Minimally Invasive Intraocular Microsurgery

Minimal *transcorneal*/transscleral wounds are self-sealing or can be closed with one single suture – reducing the risks of vis a tergo, paracentesis effects, etc. (see Chapter 2, Sect. 2.2). In the industrialized countries this is the preferred method of extracapsular cataract extraction with phakoemulsification (Kelman) and implantation of a foldable lens (see chapter 5.5).

Posterior sclerotomy overlying the pars plana of the ciliary body is necessary to release fluid from the supraciliary space and choroidal detachment in acute and chronic ocular hypotony syndromes. They may result from corneal perforation due to trauma or necrotizing keratitis or from excessive filtering bleb for chronic glaucoma or wound leaks. After closure of corneal wounds with some delay, release of the choroidal detachment may be a prerequisite for reformation of the anterior chamber at the end of the procedure.

Pars plana vitrectomy requires both a posterior sclerotomy and perforation of the uveal and epithelial pars plana of the ciliary body halfway between ora serrata and pars plicata approximately 4 mm behind the limbus.

Today it is the standard approach to enter the vitreous space. This entry through the pars plana permits introduction of illumination, irrigation and the cutting-suction instruments. Choice of the site of entry is between the four straight extraocular muscles to avoid encountering the anterior long ciliary arteries and nerves.

The principal advantage of minimally invasive intraocular microsurgery is that the *paracentesis effect and acute ocular hypotony phase of the surgical procedure are truly minimal in duration and extent*. The risk of direct infection from the periocular tissue of conjunctiva and lid through a wide open wound are minimized. But leakage of *unsutured* transcorneal stab wounds of 2,8 mm located temporally may be more common than assumed and *aspiration* of surface fluid into the anterior chamber can be easily observed if limbal capillaries are bleeding ("gulp phenomenon"). It may account for the "silent epidemic" of postoperative bacterial endophthalmitis following extracapsular cataract extraction with minimal corneal ports including implantation of foldable lenses (see Taban et al. 2005).

4.3.3
Intraocular Surgery Without Opening of the Eye Wall

Intraocular surgery without opening of the eye wall, particularly with lasers, excludes the risks of external infections, or "toxic anterior segment syndrome" (TASS), sympathetic uveitis, and epithelial ingrowth. However, damage is possible with contact lens delivery of lasers heating melanin granules in the central corneal endothelium that leads to decompensation. Laser coagulation of the periphery of the retina in addition to the corneal endothelial heating may also cause thermal damage to the "collarette" of the iris. Also the adjacent tissues of the iris such as lens capsule or posterior cornea may be damaged (see chapter 5.3).

Exact evaluation of the compartments within the untouched eye with non-invasive methods such as optical coherence tomography (OCT) define the iris position in the anterior segment without contact lens, helping to avoid unnecessary collateral damage.

Intraocular microsurgery within the *intact* closed eye: In 1949 the ophthalmologist Gerd Meyer-Schwikkerath (Fig. 1.1) introduced *"light surgery"* into medicine after unsuccessful attempts to use sunlight including a heliostat. He used xenon light with a similar spectrum of wavelengths. The replacement of the xenon lamp by lasers of various wavelengths 10 years later is only n important technical modification. The current concepts of diagnostic and therapeutic laser medicine originated from ophthalmology!

Thermic argon or krypton lasers are directed into the eye via three – mirror – and other contact lenses, to the trabecular meshwork or the root of the iris stroma peripheral to Fuchs' roll (laser iridotomy, see Chapters 5.2, 5.3). The sensory retina is involved via the *"oven" of the retinal pigment epithelium* (Fankhauser; Fig. 5.6.21).

YAG laser applications have made it possible to cut non-mechanically the secondary cataract after extracapsular cataract surgery. This is achieved both by the picosecond (Aron Rosa) and the nanosecond (Fankhauser) YAG lasers. However, only the nanosecond YAG laser of Fankhauser delivers enough energy for an iridotomy. Avoiding an opening into the eye wall also means avoiding all the inherent risks of open eye surgery, be it wide open sky or minimally invasive!

Transscleral coagulation by diathermy or cryoapplication is also performed without an opening in the eye wall – but with more scleral damage with heat!

Although the eye is not opened, laser coagulation of trabecular meshwork, iris, ciliary processes and fundus causes at least a *transitory* breakdown in the blood-ocular barriers.

4.4
Microsurgical Manipulations in the Anterior Chamber: Critical Structure and Vulnerable Cell Populations

The introduction of the operating microscope made it possible to perform precise microsurgical procedures within the anterior chamber and its adjacent structures. Awareness of the anatomy and histopathology is essential to prevent complications of these very vulnerable tissues.

4.4.1
Free Access to Trabecular Meshwork in Open Angle and Free Flow in the Pupillary Zone and Between the Pars Plicata and Lens Equator

The free flow of aqueous from the ciliary processes to the collector channels beyond Schlemm's canal is a prerequisite for equilibrium of the intraocular pressure. The flow of aqueous from the posterior ciliary processes to the retropupillary space depends on the clearance between lens equator and pars plicata of the ciliary body. The flow of aqueous through the pupil occurs in a "pulsating fashion" because the pupillary portion of the iris rests on the anterior lens capsule (Fig. 4.5).

This *"physiological pupillary resistance"* increases: (1) with *age*, due to an increased lens volume and the reduced pupillary mobility; (2) due to *increased viscosity* of the aqueous in inflammatory processes, after intraocular hemorrhage and early in pseudoexfoliation syndrome; and (3) by phacodonesis due to subluxation of the lens anteriorly or luxation in the anterior chamber. Free exit of aqueous requires direct access to the trabecular meshwork. Eighty-five percent of the aqueous drains via the transtrabecular route through Schlemm's canal to the collector channels to the episcleral aqueous veins and from episcleral vessels into the general circulation. Fifteen percent is handled by the uveoscleral outflow via the supraciliary space.

Primary and secondary glaucomas develop either with an *open* angle or by angle *closure* due to contact of the Fuchs' roll with Schwalb's line. In open angle glaucomas the obstacle to outflow is within the trabecular meshwork particularly close – juxtacanalicular – to Schlemm's canal or by proliferation of capillaries or corneal endothelium on its surface (see Chapter 5.2).

Only exceptionally do capillaries grow exclusively within the trabecular meshwork in herpetic keratouveitis (Lee syndrome) without neovascularization of the iris.

4.4.2
Corneal Endothelium

The depth of the anterior chamber varies between 1 and 3 mm depending on the size of the eye and the lens. Endothelial cell count decreases with age (Table 5.2.8); it is a structure most sensitive to surgical trauma. Endothelial proliferation is possible only to a limited degree. Extensive trauma to the corneal endothelium leads to mild and reversible or massive and irreversible endothelial decompensation and bullous keratopathy. Cornea guttata indicates abnormalities of the corneal endothelium and may be a precursor to Fuchs' endothelial dystrophy or PEX keratopathy. In pseudoexfoliation syndrome, hypoxia in the anterior chamber (Helbig et al. 1964; see Chapter 6.3) may additionally stimulate corneal proliferation (Zagorski et al. 1990) and migration over the trabecular meshwork (Fig. 4.4) (Schlötzer-Schrehardt and Naumann 2006; see also Chapter 6.3). The ophthalmic microsurgeon must make all efforts to avoid direct mechanical or thermal contact with the corneal endothelium. Also, light exposure from the operating microscope should be reduced if melanin granula are phagocytized by the corneal endothelium to avoid heating and necrosis of these cells. This may also occur both with laser trabeculoplasty and laser coagulation of the center or periphery of the fundus.

4.4.3
Iris Microanatomy

Central to the collarette, and peripheral to Fuchs' roll, the iris stroma is only half as thick as in the midportion!

Laser iridotomies are best performed *peripherally* to Fuchs' roll, exposed by a miotic pupil and therefore stretched iris (Fig. 4.10). The region of the lid fissure should – if possible – be avoided to prevent monocular diplopia.

If the iris dilates only poorly, laser coagulation of the peripheral fundus may easily (although unintentionally) involve the collarette and lead to focal thermal necrosis of iris stroma evident by collection of melanophages visible to the slit lamp at ×40 magnification ("Biocytology"). Trauma to the iris pigment epithelium by lasers or by mechanical instruments may lead to focal posterior synechiae. This risk is particularly high in *diabetic iridopathy* and *PEX iridopathy* (see Chapters 5.2, 5.3, 6.3) (Fig. 4.8).

In Asian eyes with brown irides, laser iridotomies for angle closure glaucoma may not infrequently be followed by progressive cataractous changes in the lens within 1 year (Arthur Lim 2005; Chapter 5.3). This has not been a problem in patients with blue or gray irides that are usually thinner and can be perforated with less energy.

4.4.4
Lens Capsule and Anterior Zonular Insertion

Any sharp or pointed instrument introduced into the anterior chamber may lead to unintentional defects in the anterior lens capsule and then to iatrogenic traumatic cataract. All instruments inserted into the anterior chamber should be handled with particular care in the pupillary zone of the anterior lens capsule where it is not protected by the iris. The anterior insertion of the zonular fibers needs to be particularly respected during capsulorrhexis in cataract surgery for children. Patients with pseudoexfoliation syndrome suffer from an instability of the zonular apparatus due to the peculiar PEX zonulopathy affecting origin, insertion and the free exposed zonules (see Chapters 5.5, 6.3).

Indirect distant effects are the result of ocular hypotony and paracentesis and other risks of intraocular surgery (see Chapter 2, 4.1.2).

4.5
Surgical Manipulation in the Vitreous Cavity: Critical Structures and Vulnerable Cell Populations

Microsurgery of the vitreous cavity has the goal to remove pathologic tissue from the vitreous, reduce traction on the sensory retina and thus facilitate reattachment of the detached retina. Accidental damage to the posterior portion of the lens, the sensory retina and the optic nerve head can be avoided by direct microsurgical observation and control.

4.5.1
Vitreous Attachments

The vitreous tissue is firmly attached to: (1) the vitreous base at the ora serrata involving the most anterior portion of the sensory retina and the posterior rim of the pars plana of the ciliary body; (2) Wieger's hyalocapsular ligament attached to the posterior capsule of the lens forming Berger's space; and (3) along the edge of the optic nerve head at Martegiani's ring (Fig. 4.7). Any traction on the lens capsule during extracapsular cataract extraction is transmitted from Wieger's ligament and the zonules to the vitreous base with the risk of creating peripheral retinal defects leading to retinal detachment.

4.5.2
Sensory Retina, Retinal Pigment Epithelium and Optic Nerve Head

Damage to these delicate and most important structures can occur by mechanical instruments, thermic argon or krypton laser or with the YAG laser. In addition "*phototoxic damage*" by blue light from the operating microscope is a theoretical possibility. Relative heating of the infusion fluid above room temperature may be an additional risk, whereas moderate cooling to 22 °C is perhaps protective (Rinkoff et al. 1986; Zilis et al. 1990).

Vitreoretinal surgeons are aware that the sensory retina in its physiologic stage is transparent. The internal limiting membrane (ILM) is the basement membrane of the Müller cells; its removal affects the Müller cells extending through the sensory retina to the so-called external limiting membrane, which is just a series of zonula occludentes between the Müller cells and photoreceptors. It is unknown, how removal of the ILM affects the significant role that Müller cells play in maintaining transparency of the inner retina via living optical fibers to the individual photoreceptors (Franze, Reichenbach et al. 2007, Reichenbach et al. 2007).

In normal constellations, *retinal pigment epithelium* (RPE) is a one-layered structure. If the contact inhibition by the photoreceptors is disturbed, "*vagaries*" of the individual RPE cells are seen. They spread throughout the sensory retina lining the retinal vessels and extending into the vitreous and participating in the proliferative vitreoretinopathy (PVR), causing contraction and irreversible changes in the vitreous (Fig. 4.8; see also Chapter 5.6).

4.5.3
Posterior Lens Capsule and Posterior Zonula Insertion

The posterior lens capsule is thinner than the anterior lens capsule and it is very vulnerable to mechanic trauma particularly in small eyes and with relatively large lenses. The posterior zonular insertions of the zonular apparatus attach peripherally to Wieger's ligament and may be selectively affected by pseudoexfoliation syndrome in addition to the weak anchorage in the ciliary epithelium and shearing of their insertion on the lens capsule.

4.5.4
Choroidal Hemorrhage

A vitreal approach to subretinal pathology such as pseudoepitheliomatous fibrous metaplasia of RPE in age-related macular degeneration with alterations of the choriocapillaries requires manipulations close to Bruch's membrane. The opening of this firm membrane poses the risk of a massive hemorrhage not only from the choriocapillaries but also from the larger choroidal vessels. If the intraocular pressure falls suddenly during vitreal surgery, the risk of a massive hemorrhage from the choroidal vasculature increases.

4.6
Role of the Size of the Eye

The size and details of the structures of every one of the eyes of the six billion people on this planet are unique. This allows biometric identification of a human being by the structure of the iris, the vascular tree of the retina and the pattern and the features of the optic nerve head (unless these are disturbed by surgical procedures). The optical axis of most eyes varies between 22 and 26 mm, with a mean of about 24 mm (Fig. 4.9). One may define eyes with a less than 22 mm optical axis as *nanophthalmus* or microphthalmus and those with more than 26 mm as *"high myopes."*

In *small eyes* the dimensions of the anterior chamber are narrower because of reduced corneal diameter and increased lens thickness. The risk of pupillary and ciliary block and angle closure is increased. The sclera tends to be thicker. Uveal effusion may develop because exit of the vortex veins is squeezed after opening the eye. The *"relative anterior microphthalmus"* (RAM) poses particular risks for intraoperative complications in intraocular microsurgery (Auffarth and Voelcker 2006) (see Chapters 5.2, 5.3, 5,5, 6.3).

High myopic eyes are characterized by a relatively deep anterior chamber and a wide open angle. Large myopic eyes often have a greater volume of vitreous cavity, and suffer earlier from vitreous detachment and increased risk of retinal detachment. If the liquefaction of the vitreous is advanced, the iris-lens diaphragm can "withdraw" deeper into the eye, at the moment the anterior chamber is opened. The sclera is thinner, and ectasias and staphylomata are more likely. This aspect must be considered if the mode of anesthesia is discussed with the patient. As the ciliochoroidal vasculature is distended and thinned, the risk of a rupture of the posterior ciliary artery at the entrance into the eye is increased leading to an expulsive choroidal hemorrhage particularly if the systemic arterial blood pressure is not compensated (see Chapter 2.2.3).

In short one could summarize: *small eyes have a more difficult anterior segment; large eyes are more prone to risks of posterial segment complications* (Tables 4.2, 4.3, 4.4).

Table 4.4. Principal options of intraocular surgery

1.	Wide open sky:	E.g., penetrating keratoplasty intracapsular cataract extraction
2.	Minimally invasive:	E.g., extracapsular cataract surgery with transcorneal opening or corneoscleral tunnel and foldable lenses; pars plana vitrectomy
3.	Within intact closed eye:	All intraocular laser application ("light microsurgery")

4.7
Wound Healing After Intraocular Microsurgery and Trauma

Wound healing after trauma and/or intraocular microsurgery has three essential aspects:

1. A *secure closure* of the wound in the eye wall to avoid persisting ocular hypotony and its consequences as distant effects. Depending on the location of the access into the anterior chamber in relation to Bowman's layer, an *avascular* wound healing (transcorneal) or a much faster *vascular* wound healing is expected via the subconjunctival limbus (see above). Both variants cross Descemet's membrane; the interruption of it remains visible for decades – although the proliferating and migrating corneal endothelium reforms a basement membrane bridging the defect in Descemet's membrane (Fig. 4.12b–d).

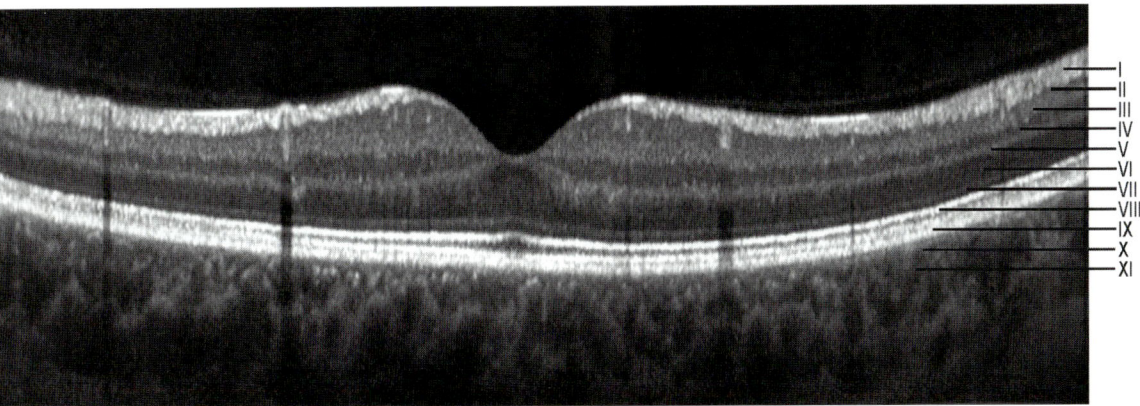

Fig. 4.17. Optic coherent tomography: vertical line scan (Spektralis ™HRA+OCT) through fovea centralis in a normal 39-year old male. *I* retinal nerve fibre layer, *II* ganglien cell layer, *III* inner plexiform layer, *IV* inner nuclear layer, *V* outer plexiform layer, *VI* outer nuclear layer, *VII* outer limiting layer, *VIII* border between inner and outer segments of photoreceptors, *IX* retinal pigment epithelium, *X* choriocapillaries, *XI* choroid. Vertical stripes from macular vessels (courtesy R. Laemmer, Dept. Ophthalmology, University Erlangen)

2. *Avoidance of excessive wound healing* and proliferation such as secondary cataract or proliferating vitreoretinopathy and scarring of filtering blebs. These will be discussed in the special pathology (Chapter 5).
3. *Cystoid maculopathy due to vitreous traction* from incarceration of formed vitreous and/or iris into perforating wound of the eye wall: "Hruby-Irvine-Gass syndrome." Before the introduction of ophthalmic microsurgery this was a common and devastating complication because the wound was closed without removing the vitreous strands.

Hruby (1951) was the first to describe "cystoid macular degeneration" 2 years before "macular degeneration" was seen by Irvine. Later Gass elaborated the differential diagnosis of "macular edema."

For reasons of history and precision, we suggest the term "*Hruby-Irvine-Gass syndrome*" be used instead of the term "Irvine-Gass syndrome" in the Anglo-Saxon literature. Since microsurgical methods allow proper cleaning of any wound from incarcerated vitreous and other ocular tissue, this syndrome has become rare.

It should not only be considered after penetrating wounds in the cornea and limbus but might also occur in partial pars plana vitrectomy and particularly after pars plana injections of medications into the vitreous cavity.

Cystoid maculopathy is a very common consequence of the paracentesis effect due to ocular hypotony following any intraocular procedure. It is easily overlooked unless postoperative fluoresceinangiography is used to detect the leakage of the perifoveolar capillaries. Recently high resolution non contact OCT approaching light microscopic dimensions is helpful to establish the diagnosis without exposing the patient to the risk (although minimal) of fluoresceinangiography (Fig. 4.17).

4.7.1
"Surgically Induced Necrotizing Scleritis" (SINS)

After initial uncomplicated wound healing this peculiar scleral necrosis can develop months after surgery. It is a rare event for reasons which are poorly understood (Fig. 4.18). Many of these patients suffer from "collagen disease".

4.7.2
Concept of a "Minimal Eye"

Due to the spectacular advances of anterior and posterior segment intraocular microsurgery, it is tempting to speculate on the minimal requirement for a modestly functioning eye: 4 mm clear central cornea; 180% open angle with access to the trabecular meshwork, to assure a sufficient outflow; 210% secreting pars plicata of the ciliary body to avoid insufficient inflow and ocular hypotony; transparent optical axis; and as much as possible 30–50% preserved sensory retina and 30–50% optic nerve axons (Table 4.5).

Table 4.5. Morphologic essential requirements for sustainable functioning "minimal eye"

1. *Cornea*: 4 mm clear in optical axis or excentric optical sector coloboma
2. *Angle of anterior chamber*: 180° open with access to intact trabecular meshwork
3. *Ciliary body*: 210° aqueous-secreting pars plicata
4. *Transparent* optical axis
5. *Retina/optic nerve*: as much as possible attached (depending on location)

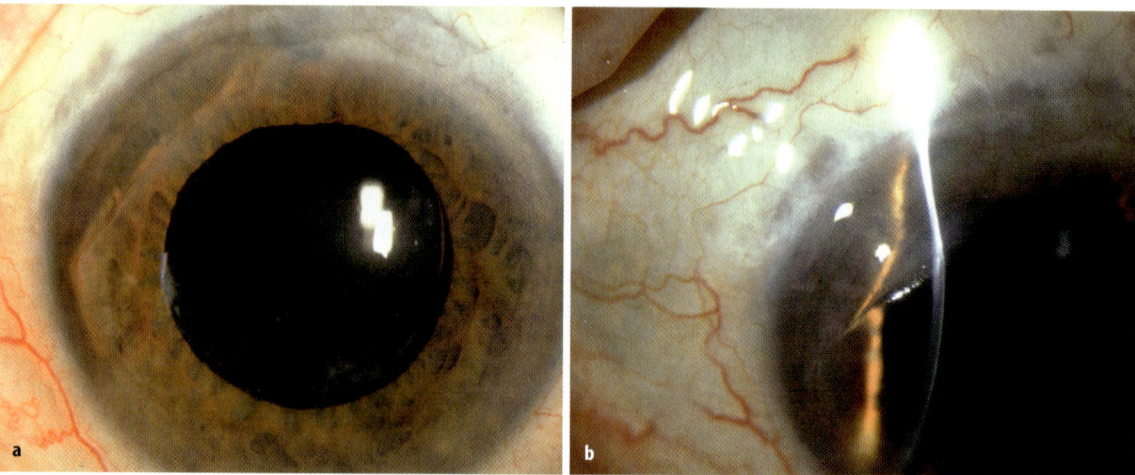

Fig. 4.18a, b. Surgically induced necrotizing scleritis (SINS) leading to limbal furrow and corneoscleral leakage forming filtering bleb after uneventful extracapsular cataract extraction with nuclear expression

References (see also page 379)

Auffarth GU, Voelcker H-E. Cataract surgery in 79 patients with relative anterior microphthalmus (RAM). A review of anatomy, associated pathology and complications. Klein Monatsbl Augenheilk: 2006;216(6):369

Cameron J, Flaxman B, Yanoff M. In-vitro studies of corneal wound healing, epithelial-endothelial interactions. Invest Ophthalmol Vis Sci 1974; 13:575

Franze K, Grosche J, Skatchkow SN, Schinkinger S, Foja C, Schild D, Uckermann O, Travis K, Reichenbach A, Guck J, Müller cells are living optical fibers in the vertebrate retina. Proc National Academy of Science (PNAS) 2007; 104:8287–8292

Grossniklaus AE (editor): Ophthalmic Pathology and Intraocular Tumors, Section 4, Basic and Clinical Science Course of the American Academy of Ophthalmology, 2004

Helbig H, Schlötzer-Schrehardt U, Noske W, Kellner U, Förster MH, Naumann GOH. Anterior chamber hypoxia and iris vasculopathy in pseudoexfoliation syndrome. Ger J Ophthalmol 1994; 3:148–153

Naumann GOH, Seibel W. Surgical Revision of Vitreous and Iris Incarceration in Persisting Cystoid Maculopathy (Hruby-Irvine-Gass Syndrome) – report on 27 eyes. Dev Ophthalmol 1985; 11:181–187

Reichenbach A et al.: Müller cells as players in retinal degeneration and edema. Graefe's Arch Clin Exp Ophthalmol 2007; 245:627–636

Rinkoff J, Machemer R, Hida T, Chandler D. Temperature-dependent light damage to the retina. Am J Ophthalmol 1986; 102: 452–462

Schlötzer-Schrehardt U, Naumann GOH. Ocular and systemic pseudoexfoliation syndrome. Am J Ophthalmol 2006: 141: 921–935

Taban M, Behrens A, Newcomb RL, Nobe MY, Saedi G, Sweet PM, McDonnell PJ: Acute endophthalmitis following cataract surgery. Arch Ophthalmol 2005; 123:613–620

Zagórski Z, Holbach CM, Hofmann C, Gossler B, Naumann GOH: Proliferation of corneal epithelial and endothelial cells in the trabecular region of human donor corneas in vitro. Ophthalmic Res 1990; 22:51–56

Zilis J, Chandler D, Machemer R. Clinical and histologic effects of extreme intraocular hypothermia. Am J Ophthalmol 1990; 109: 469–473

Special Anatomy and Pathology in Intraocular Microsurgery

Cornea and Limbus

C. Cursiefen, F.E. Kruse, G.O.H. Naumann

The cornea is more than just a transparent piece of collagen. All of its five anatomical layers are essential for maintaining an avascular, anti-inflammatory and transparent state of the cornea, thus enabling good visual acuity. Besides the five conventional layers of the cornea (i.e., epithelium, Bowman's layer, stroma, Descemet's membrane and corneal endothelium), there are several other (partly "invisible") structures and cell populations residing in and around the normal cornea. These include stromal and epithelial antigen-presenting cells (APCs: dendritic cells and macrophages), stromal and epithelial stem cells, limbal blood and – clinically invisible – lymphatic vessels as well as corneal nerves. All of these structures and cell populations are relevant for corneal microsurgeons in one or another aspect. In the following chapter, first *normal corneal anatomy* will be discussed briefly with respect to corneal surgery. Then selected *corneal pathologies* will be outlined with respect to surgical procedures of the cornea. Finally, pathologic aspects of certain *corneal surgical procedures* and aspects of *corneal wound healing* will be described.

5.1.1
Surgical Anatomy of the Cornea and Limbus

5.1.1.1
Corneal Epithelium

Corneal epithelium is a multilayered, non-keratinizing squamous epithelium of about 50–100 µm thickness. Epithelial cells are connected to the underlying basement membrane and Bowman's layer primarily by hemidesmosomes and anchoring fibrils. Defects in these anchoring complexes lead to recurrent corneal erosions such as in Cogan's map-dot-fingerprint dystrophy or after corneal trauma. Besides epithelial cells, there are numerous nerve endings in between the epithelial cells (400 times more than in the skin). These can be detected in vivo using confocal microscopy with the Heidelberg Retina Tomograph (HRT) II and Rostock cornea module (Fig. 5.1.1). Mechanical stress to these nerves such as in bullous keratopathy, e.g., in patients with Fuchs' dystrophy, can therefore cause tremendous pain (Fig. 5.1.2; see Sect. 5.1.1.12 below). Furthermore, there are specialized antigen-presenting cells (APCs) (Fig. 5.1.3) interdigitating in between epithelial cells. In contrast to normal APCs, the immunosuppressive microenvironment of the cornea leads to MHC class II negativity of these cells. Corneal inflammation leads to their activation thus causing higher rejection rates in inflamed high-risk recipient beds. In the limbal area in the so-called palisades of Vogt (Fig. 5.1.4) reside the epithelial stem cells which are responsible for epithelial regeneration and for maintenance of a corneal-conjunctival border. Furthermore they also explain the recurrence of corneal "stromal" dystrophies based on mutations in the keratoepithelin gene (granular and lattice dystrophy). Corneal epithelium itself exerts strong anti-inflammatory and antiangiogenic properties (Fig. 5.1.5). Transplantation of donor corneas without corneal epithelium, e.g., after abrasion, leads to increased post-transplantation neovascularization and inflammation.

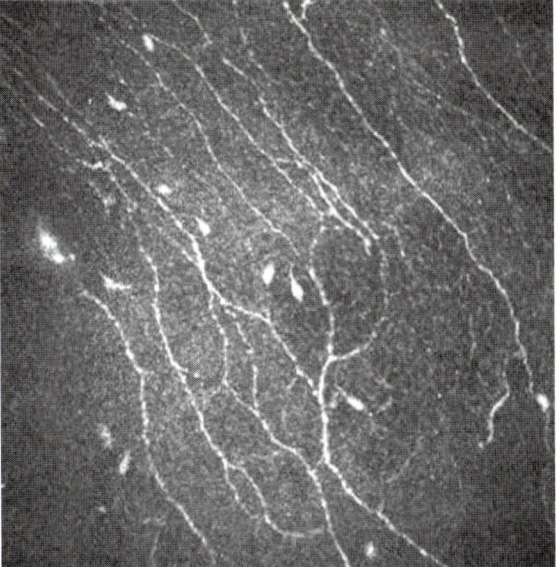

Fig. 5.1.1. In vivo confocal microscopy of subbasal corneal nerves (courtesy of K. Gottschalk)

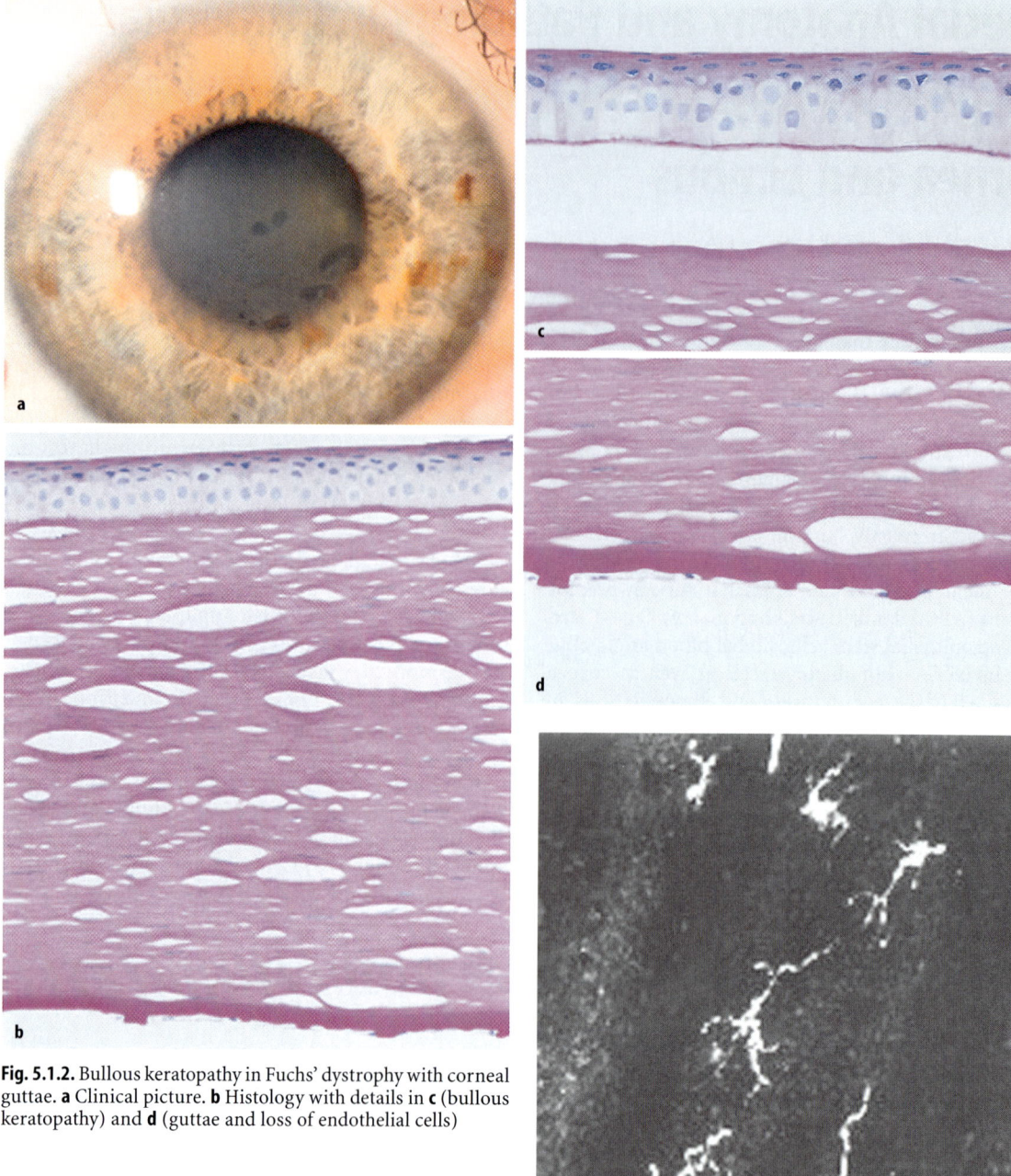

Fig. 5.1.2. Bullous keratopathy in Fuchs' dystrophy with corneal guttae. **a** Clinical picture. **b** Histology with details in **c** (bullous keratopathy) and **d** (guttae and loss of endothelial cells)

5.1.1.2
Bowman's Layer

Bowman's layer is an acellular section of the superficial stroma. In it resides most of the tensile strength of the cornea. Therefore diseases or surgical procedures (such as photorefractive keratectomy, PRK) leading to defects in Bowman's layer increase the risk for corneal ruptures and ectasias. On the other hand, sutures have to extend through Bowman's layer to ensure tight and effective suturing (important during repair of corneal wounds). Bowman's layer also is an important UV-

Fig. 5.1.3. Corneal Langerhans cells interdigitating in between corneal epithelium as visualized using in vivo confocal microscopy

shield protecting the inner eye. That has to be considered in patients having undergone PRK with partial or total destruction of this layer (UV protection via glasses!). In addition, an intact Bowman's layer is a nearly insurmountable barrier against the invasion of epithelial tumors into the corneal stroma. That means that during abrasion of conjunctival squamous cell carcinomas or melanomas of the conjunctiva which grow beyond the limbal barrier onto the cornea, care has be taken not to remove Bowman's layer (it does not need to be sacrificed).

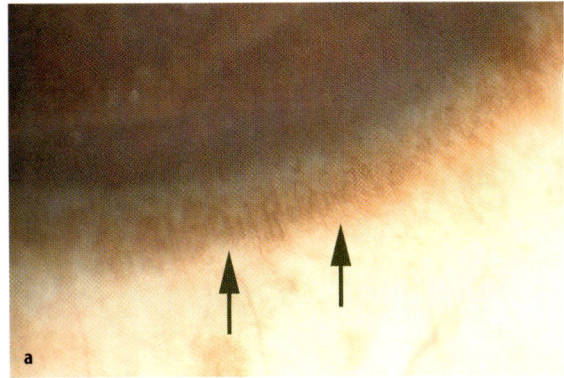

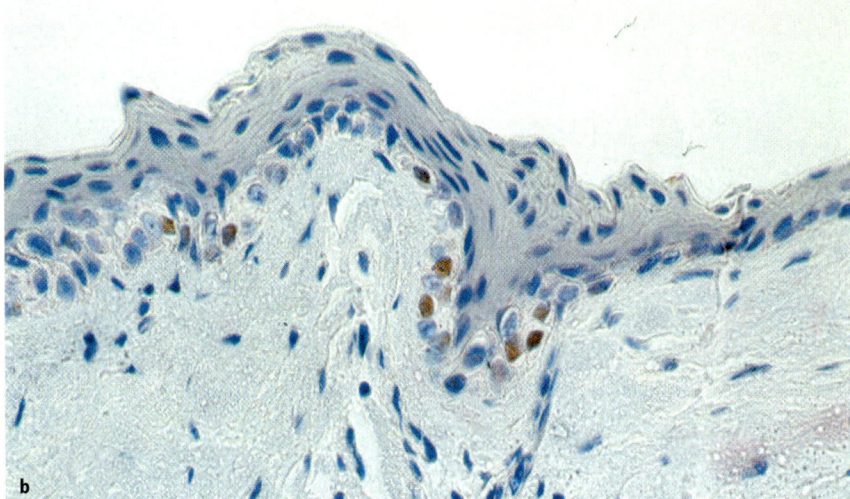

Fig. 5.1.4. Palisades of Vogt: localization of limbal stem cells: **a** Clinical picture. **b** Immunohistochemical staining with stem cell marker reacts positively at Vogt's palisades

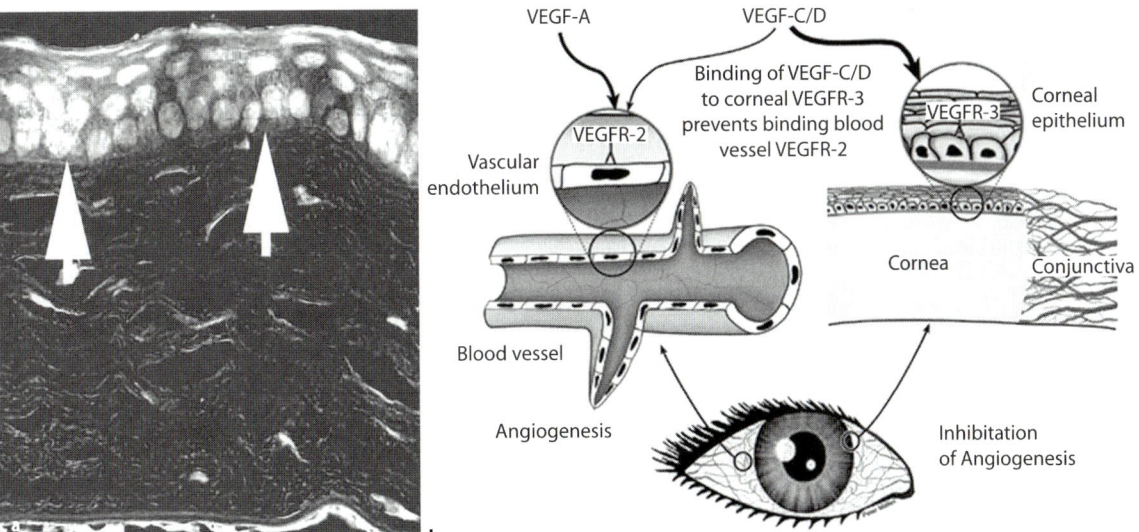

Fig. 5.1.5. Anti-inflammatory and antiangiogenic effects of corneal epithelium (modified from Cursiefen, Chen et al. 2006). An ectopically expressed receptor for proangiogenic and proinflammatory VEGF in the corneal epithelium (*arrows* in **a**) neutralizes VEGF in the cornea and prevents ligation of VEGF to limbal blood and lymphatic vessels. This natural cytokine trap thereby maintains normal corneal avascularity (**b**)

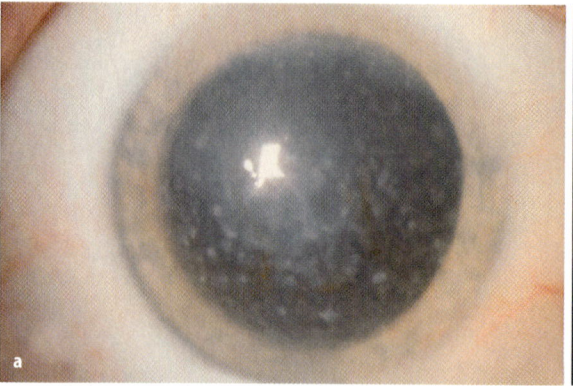
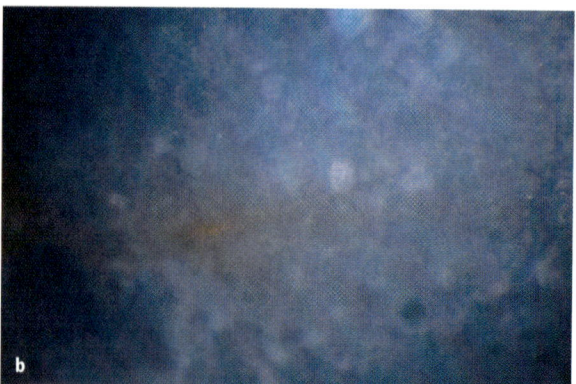
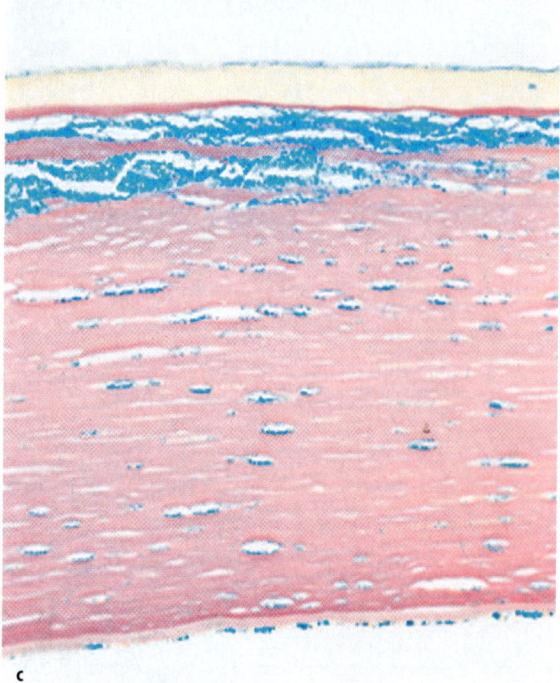

Fig. 5.1.6a–c. Macular corneal dystrophy: macular clouding of the whole cornea (in contrast to granular and lattice dystrophy) and positive staining for acid mucopolysaccharides. **b** Hudson-Stähli iron line (modified from Cursiefen, Hofmann-Rummelt et al. 2001)

5.1.1.3
Corneal Stroma

The corneal stroma consists of extremely regularly arranged bundles of collagen fibrils in a water-rich extracellular matrix composed of glycosaminoglycans. Disturbances of this fine-tuned arrangement cause corneal cloudiness. This can be due to changes in the extracellular matrix (such as deposition of unsulfated mucopolysaccharides in macular corneal dystrophy; Fig. 5.1.6) or the irregular arrangement of collagen fibrils in scars (such as "haze" after PRK). Besides these obvious components, the stroma contains corneal nerves (which are, e.g., cut during penetrating keratoplasty leading to a mild neurotrophic keratopathy after every keratoplasty), keratocytes, MHC class II⁻ antigen presenting cells (which seem to migrate out of the cornea during organ preservation thereby explaining the reduced rate of immune rejections of longer organ-cultured grafts) and stromal stem cells (role as yet poorly understood). The extremely regular and lamellar arrangement of corneal stroma enables a lamellar plane to be very nicely dissected in the deep stroma in deep anterior lamellar keratoplasty (DALK) as soon as the right plane is found.

5.1.1.4
Descemet's Membrane

Descemet's membrane is the basement of the corneal endothelium. It contains two components (anterior banded and posterior non-banded portion) and increases in thickness during life (thus enabling histological assessment of age using Descemet's membrane thickness). Defects in Descemet's membrane such as in acute keratoconus lead to influx of aqueous humor and stromal edema. This results in greatly reduced corneal tensile strength. Therefore, penetrating keratoplasty should never be performed in acute keratoconus, but rather after an interval of at least 3 months to allow endothelial cells to cover the defect and the cornea to regain a firmer, but scarred architecture (Fig. 5.1.7). A granulomatous reaction against Descemet's membrane signals an imminent or manifest leak and indicates urgent penetrating keratoplasty to avoid perforation of the ulcerated cornea. The differential diagnosis of Descemet's fold is depicted in Table 5.1.1. The differential

Table 5.1.1. Differential diagnosis of Descemet's folds

Delivery by forceps (vertical folds)
Buphthalmus (Haab's line)
Trauma, iatrogenic during surgery
Acute keratokonus
Parenchymatous keratitis

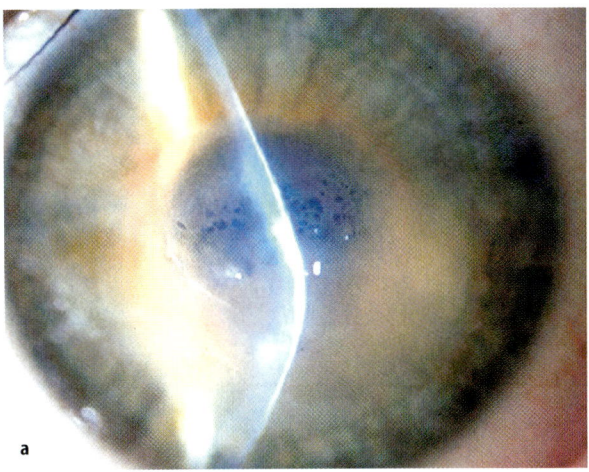
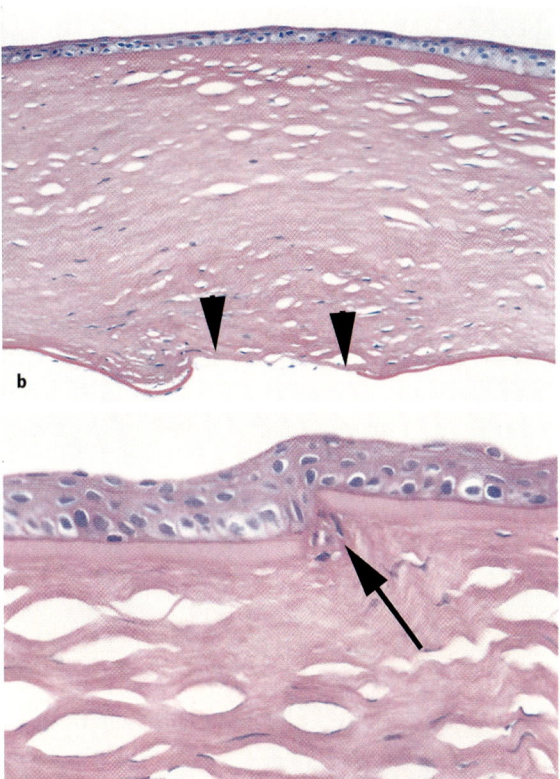

Fig. 5.1.7. Acute keratoconus. Typical clinical pictures with central stromal thinning and stromal edema causing secondary thickening. **b** Histology demonstrates defects in Descemet's membrane (*arrowheads*) leading to influx of aqueous humor into the cornea. **c** Typical defects of Bowman's layer which are pathognomonic for keratokonus on histology

diagnosis of "guttae," i.e., wart-like extensions of Descemet's membrane, include benign peripheral guttae ("Hassal-Henle warts"), central guttae in cornea guttata, guttae in Fuchs' endothelial dystrophy (combined with pigment inclusions in remaining endothelial cells and stroma edema) and secondary guttae (e.g., in macular corneal dystrophy). These represent unspecific responses of Descemet's membrane to as yet unknown stresses.

5.1.1.5
Endothelial Cells

Endothelial cells are the single layer of pump cells on the posterior aspect of the cornea responsible for constant dehydration of the cornea. These cells are postmitotic, decrease with age in numbers and are usually not able to regenerate (endothelial cell count at birth: around 4,000 cells/mm^2 and at age 50 around 2,500 cells/mm^2). But endothelial cells can migrate along a density gradient. Therefore in corneal diseases with severe loss of endothelium and necessity for keratoplasty, a graft diameter as large as reasonable from an immunological standpoint should be transplanted to allow migration of donor endothelium onto denuded recipient cornea. Endothelial cells have to be treated with great respect during cataract surgery to avoid postoperative edema and permanent corneal cloudiness. Especially in patients with risk factors such as pseudoexfoliation (PEX), corneal guttae, a preoperative endothelial cell count and pachymetry should be performed (see also Table 5.2.8 and Chapter 4.4).

5.1.1.6
Limbal Vascular Arcade

Whereas the normal cornea is free of both blood and lymphatic vessels (so-called "corneal antiangiogenic privilege"), there is an intense network of both blood and clinically invisible lymphatic vessels at the limbus (Fig. 5.1.8). This network extends circularly and respects a sharp transition into the avascular cornea. In case of corneal inflammation, here blood and lymphatic vessels start to grow out into the cornea (pathologic corneal hem- and lymphangiogenesis; Figs. 5.1.9–5.1.12). From here, APCs from the cornea or a corneal graft start migration via afferent lymphatics to the regional cervical lymph nodes to induce immune responses (Fig. 5.1.12). There seems to be a dynamic exchange between limbal macrophages and limbal lymphatic vessels with macrophages being able to transdifferentiate into lymphatic vascular endothelial cells. This enables rapid outgrowths of lymphatic vessels in case of severe corneal inflammation.

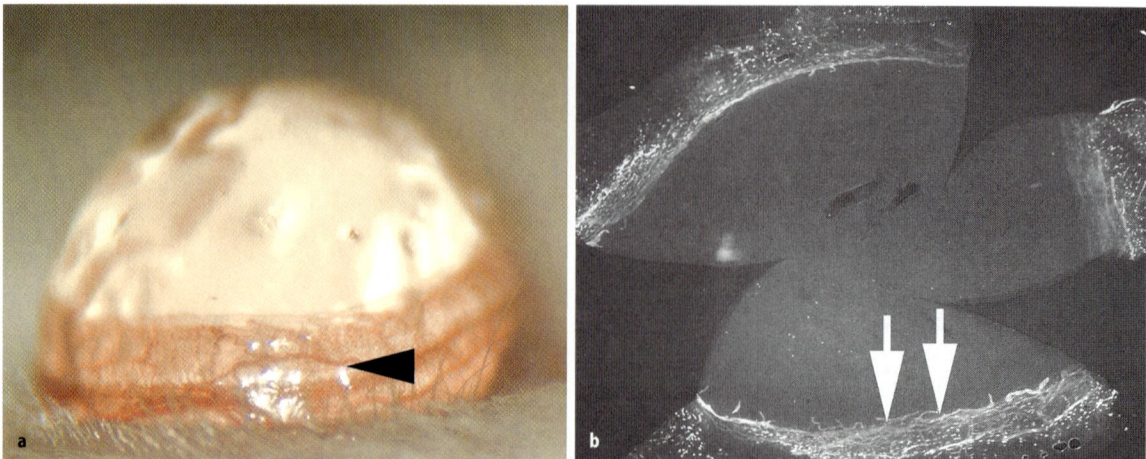

Fig. 5.1.8. Transition of avascular cornea into conjunctiva. The limbus demarcates a sharp border between hem- and lymphvascularized conjunctiva and avascular cornea (modified from Cursiefen, Chen et al. 2004). **b** Flatmount of cornea stained for blood vessels (*arrows*) mark limbus

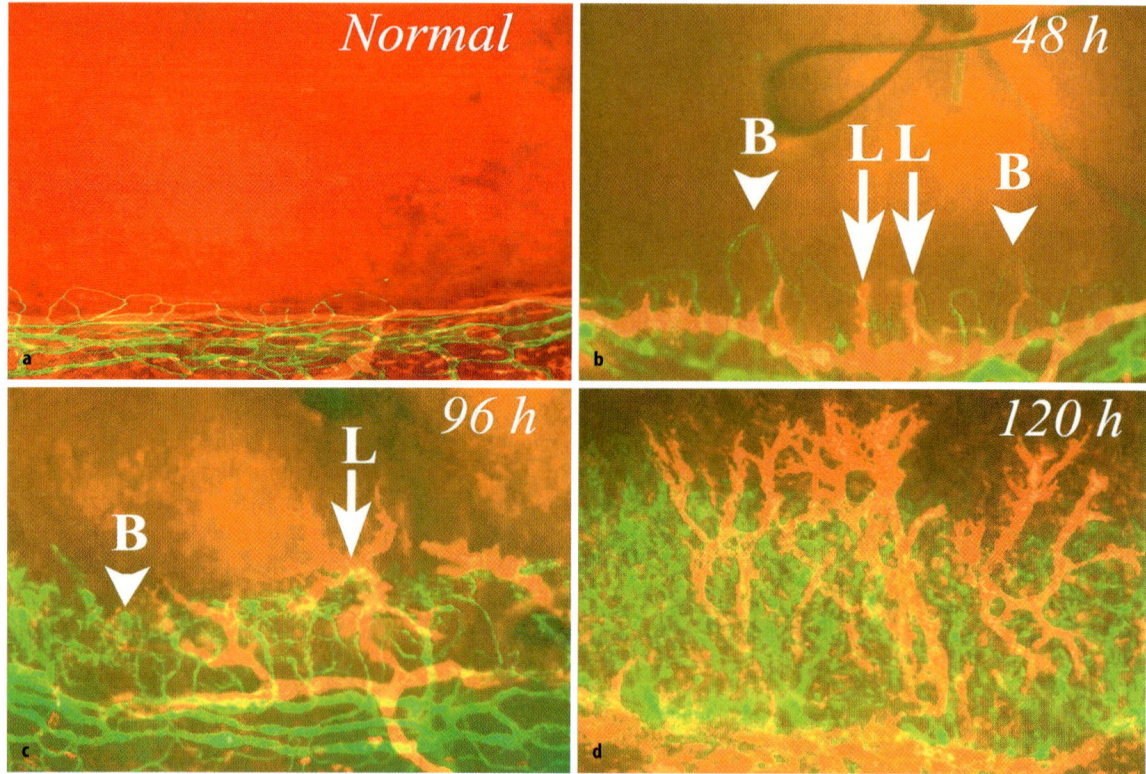

Fig. 5.1.9. After an inflammatory stimulus such as herpetic keratitis there are usually parallel ingrowths of both clinically *visible* blood and clinically *invisible* lymphatic vessels into the cornea as can be seen in these segments from murine corneal flat mounts (*B* blood vessels, *L* lymphatic vessels, blood vessels stained in *green*, lymphatic vessels stained in *red*) (from Cursiefen, Chen et al. 2004)

5.1.1.7
Tear Film

The precorneal tear film composed of the superficial lipid layer, a watery middle segment and a basal mucin layer is anchored to the corneal epithelium via epithelial glycocalyx and mucin interactions. An intact tear film is not only essential for good visual acuity (main refractive surface of the eye), but also for epithelial integrity and wound healing. Defects in the tear film, e.g., in neurotrophic keratopathy after laser in situ keratomileusis (LASIK), can cause wound healing problems. Furthermore, any form of "dry eye" causes surface in-

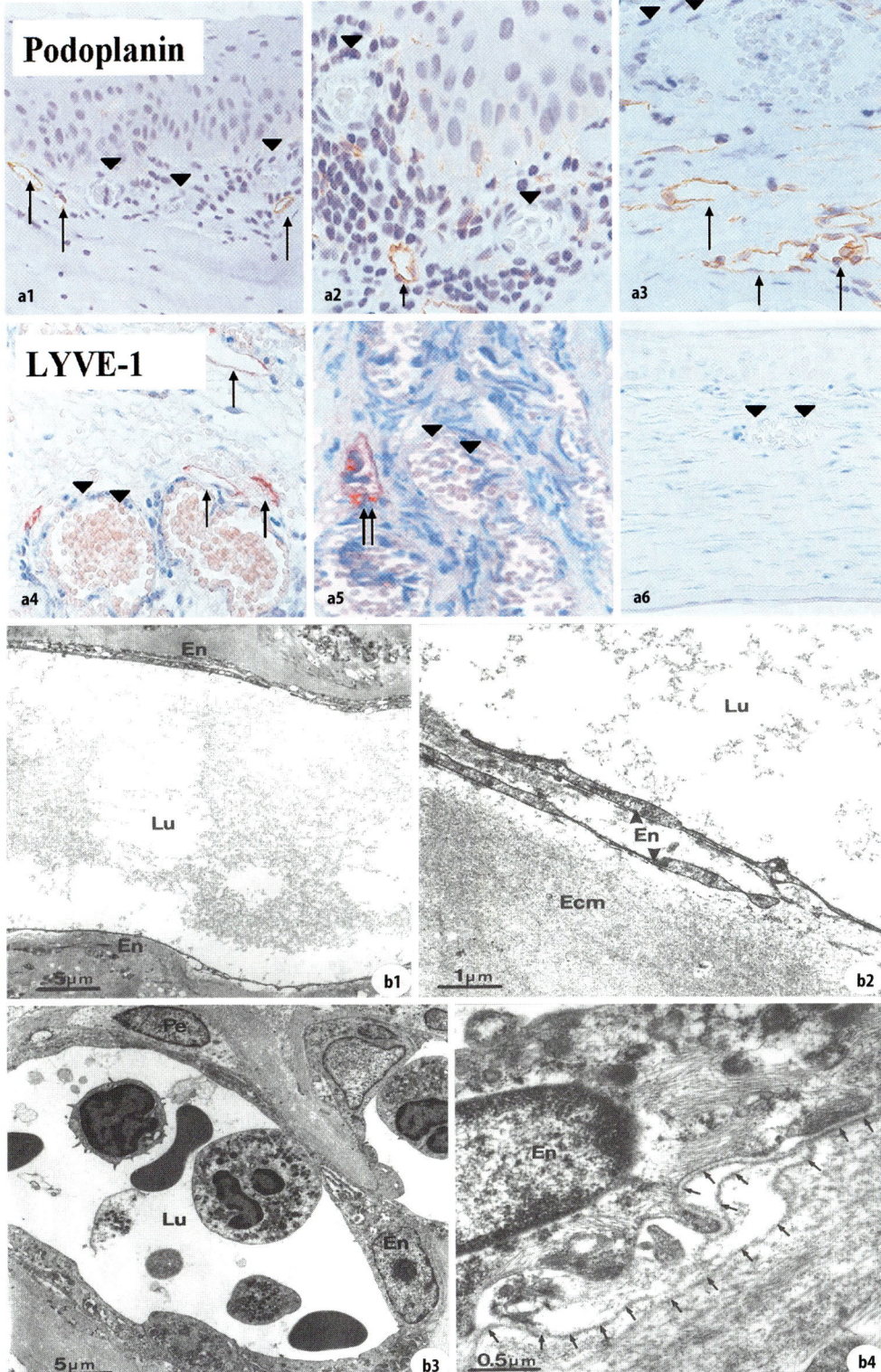

Fig. 5.1.10. Pathologic lymphangiogenesis in vascularized human corneas obtained after keratoplasty. Clinically invisible lymphatics are evidenced using novel specific markers in immunostaining (LYVE-1, Podoplanin) and electron microscopy (showing lymphatic vessels with empty lumen and absent vessel wall) (from Cursiefen, Schlötzer-Schrehardt et al. 2002). **b1, b2** Lymphatic vessels lack pericytes and basement membrane, which in contrast are present in blood vessels (**b3, b4**)

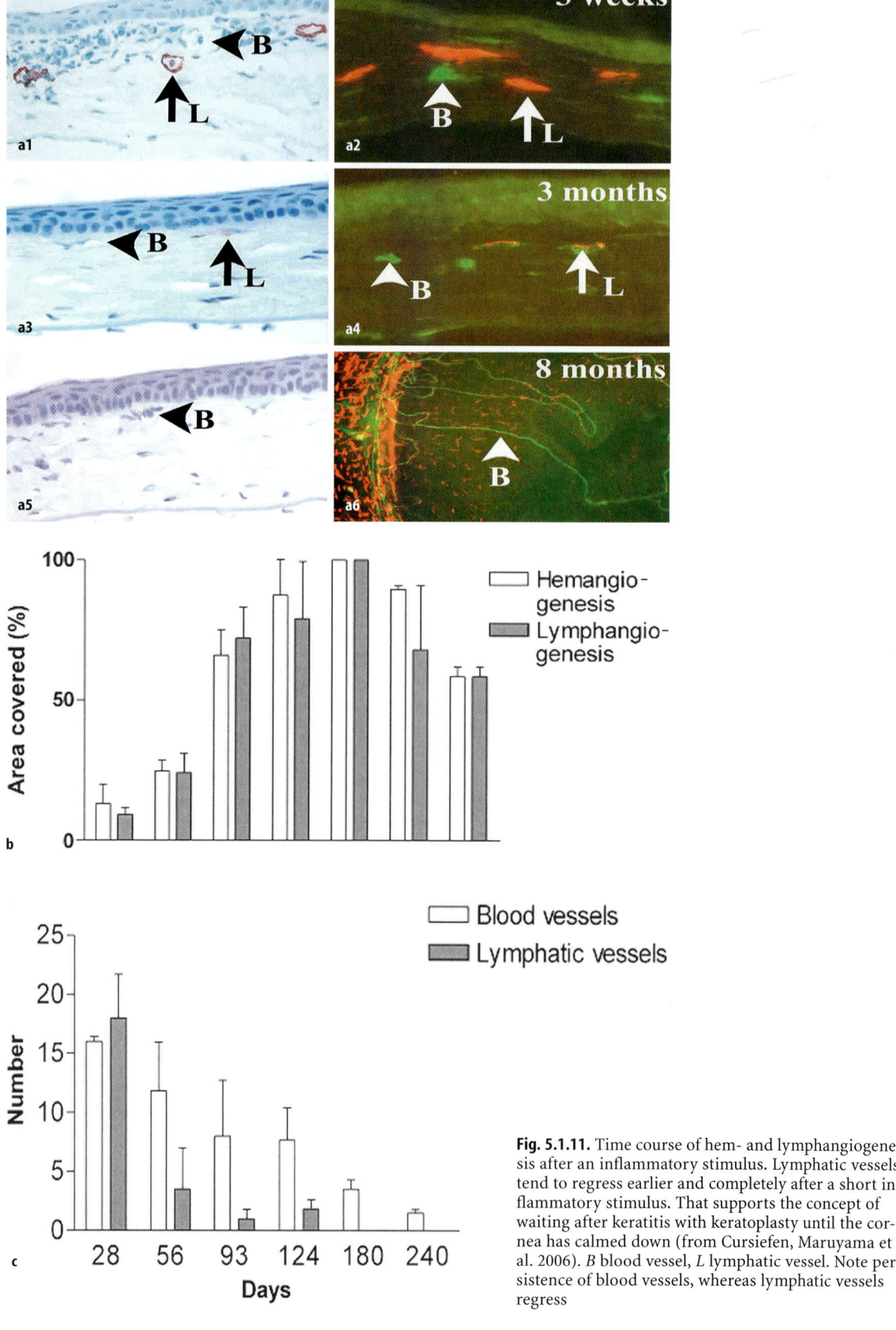

Fig. 5.1.11. Time course of hem- and lymphangiogenesis after an inflammatory stimulus. Lymphatic vessels tend to regress earlier and completely after a short inflammatory stimulus. That supports the concept of waiting after keratitis with keratoplasty until the cornea has calmed down (from Cursiefen, Maruyama et al. 2006). *B* blood vessel, *L* lymphatic vessel. Note persistence of blood vessels, whereas lymphatic vessels regress

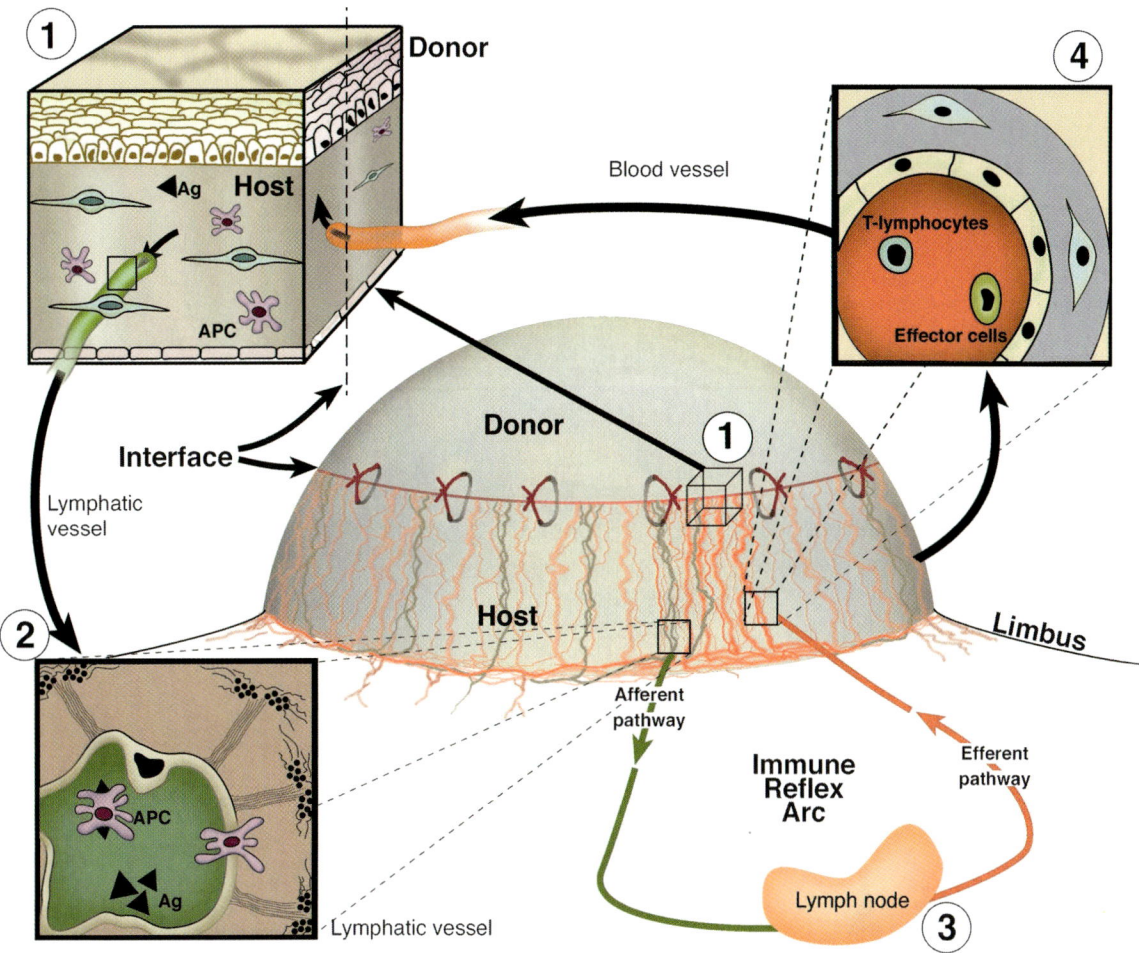

Fig. 5.1.12. Immune reflex arc leading to immune rejections after penetrating keratoplasty. Recent evidence suggests an important role of the afferent lymphatic arm in mediating immune responses. Blockade of the afferent lymphatic arm can promote graft survival even in vascularized high-risk eyes (modified from Cursiefen, Chen et al. 2003)

flammation leading to activation of corneal APCs. Therefore, thorough lubrication of the ocular surface after penetrating keratoplasty significantly reduces the risk of subsequent immune rejections.

5.1.1.8
Anterior Chamber Associated Immune Deviation (ACAID), Corneal Immune Privilege, Corneal Antiangiogenic Privilege

Corneal transparency is essential for good vision, an evolutionary highly conserved sensory function. Since blood vessels within the cornea are incompatible with good visual acuity, the cornea of higher animals has developed strategies to maintain the cornea avascular against the myriads of minor inflammatory and angiogenic stimuli the cornea is – due to its exposed anatomical position – constantly confronted with. This phenomenon has been termed "*corneal (anti)angiogenic privilege*" (Wayne Streilein). Several antiangiogenic factors in the cornea are strategically located at the inner and outer corneal barriers and are thought to be responsible for corneal avascularity. Corneal antiangiogenic privilege is redundantly organized [removal of one or more of the endogenous inhibitors of angiogenesis (such as thrombospondin) does not cause spontaneous angiogenesis] and already present very early during fetal development (Fig. 5.1.13). Besides antiangiogenic factors, the presence of soluble and fixed "decoy" receptors binding and inactivated angiogenic growth factors such as vascular endothelial growth factor (VEGF) is an important mechanism contributing to avascularity. These decoy receptors are also located at the inner and outer corneal barriers (epithelium and endothelium). Especially potent seems to be the strong ectopic expression on corneal epithelium of the VEGF receptor 3, which is normally only expressed on vascular endothelium (Fig. 5.1.5). Functional inactivation of

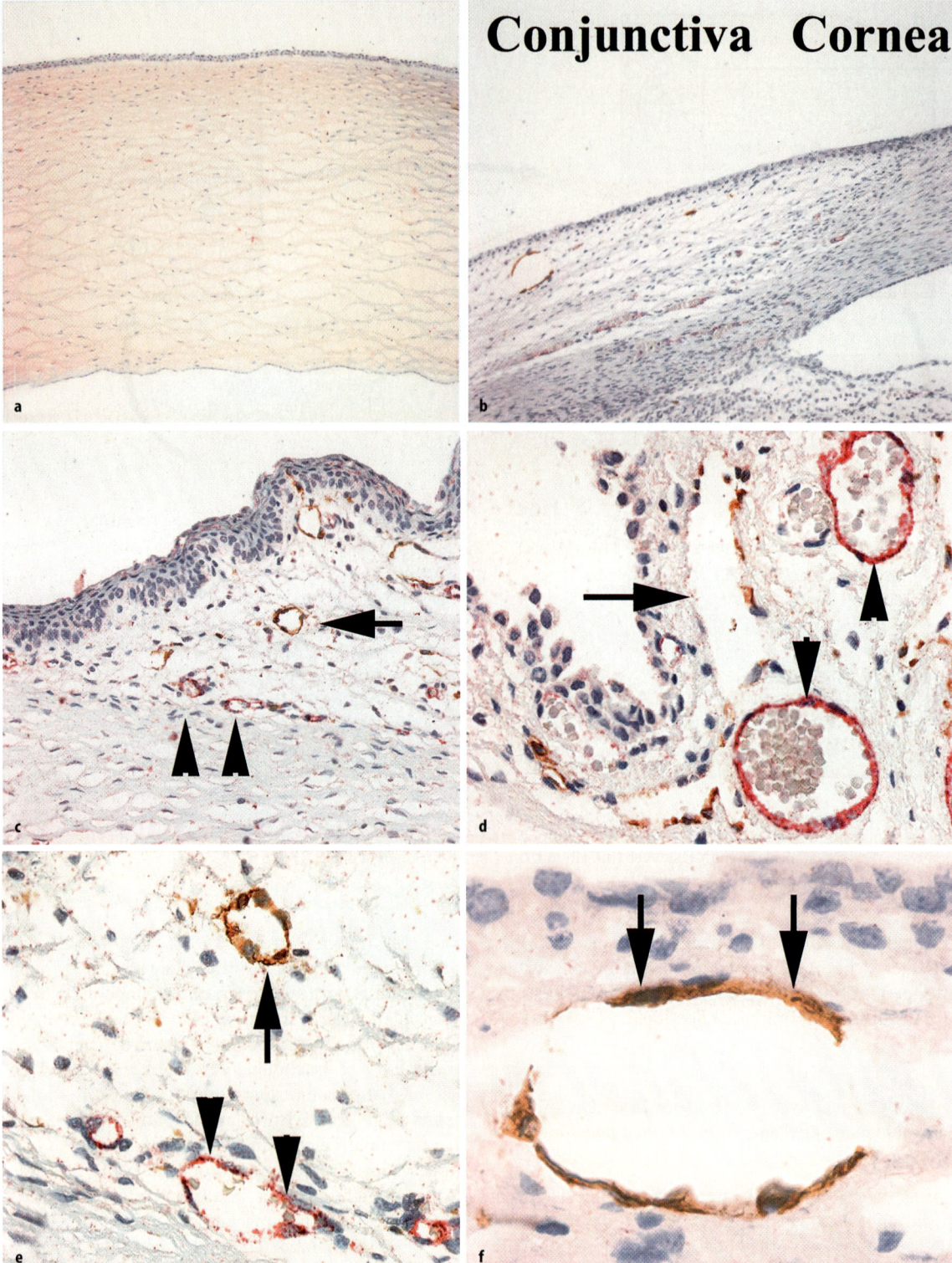

Fig. 5.1.13. Corneal angiogenic privilege is already in place during fetal development. Whereas conjunctiva contains blood and lymphatic vessels from week 13 onwards (**c–f**), the cornea (**a**) never contains blood vessels (stained *red*) or lymphatic vessels (stained *brown*) suggesting early and strong expression of antiangiogenic and antilymphangiogenic factors (modified from Cursiefen, Rummelt et al. 2006)

this receptor leads to significantly increased corneal neovascularization. The mechanisms of corneal anti-lymphangiogenic privilege, i.e., how the normal cornea maintains its freedom from lymphatic vessels, are as yet completely unknown.

Inflammatory processes within and behind the cornea can cause tissue destruction and scarring. Furthermore they can destroy the postmitotic corneal endothelial cells. Therefore, during evolution the cornea has developed several strategies to minimize inflammatory reactions in the cornea up to a point in severity where an immune response is essential for the survival of the whole organisms or the eye. This phenomenon has been termed *corneal immune privilege*. The phenomenal success of allogeneic corneal transplantation benefits from this "experiment of nature." The molecular mechanisms of corneal immune privilege seem to be closely connected to the ones maintaining corneal avascularity: Thrombospondin 1, e.g., is involved both in corneal avascularity and in corneal immune privilege. In contrast to corneal immune privilege, which is only acquired immediately prior to birth, corneal antiangiogenic privilege is already in place very early during fetal development (Fig. 5.1.13).

Another mechanism contributing to the extraordinary success of allogeneic corneal transplantation – even in the absence of HLA-matching and without systemic immunosuppression – is ACAID (*anterior chamber associated immune deviation*, Fig. 5.1.12). ACAID is defined as the systemic downregulation of a Th2 immune response against antigens injected into the anterior chamber of the eye. As a consequence, immune reactions against, e.g., donor endothelial antigens, are less destructive (fewer bystander effects). Furthermore, the cornea is not only an *immune privileged site* (allogeneic tissue transplanted into the cornea experiences unusually good and long survival), but also an *immune privileged tissue* in itself (corneal tissue transplanted heterotopically demonstrates an extended survival). Nonetheless, these privileges are not perfect and better understanding of the underlying mechanisms will therefore enable better therapy of defects.

5.1.1.9
Limbal Epithelial and Corneal Stromal Stem Cells
Ursula Schlötzer-Schrehardt

The corneal epithelium is a rapidly regenerating stratified squamous epithelium. Homeostasis of corneal epithelial cells is an important prerequisite for the integrity of the ocular surface and for visual function. Both under normal conditions and following injury, the maintenance of the corneal epithelial cell mass is achieved by a distinct population of unipotent stem cells (SCs) located in the basal epithelium of the corneoscleral limbus (Davanger and Evenson 1971; Schermer et al. 1986; Tseng 1989). These cells simultaneously retain their capacity for self-renewal and maintain a constant cell number by giving rise to fast-dividing progenitor cells, termed transit amplifying cells (TACs) (Lehrer et al. 1998), which can undergo only a limited number of cell divisions before they leave the proliferative compartment to become terminally differentiated (for review see: Tseng 1989, 1996; Dua and Azuara-Blanco 2000; Sangwar 2001; Lavker et al. 2004; Sun et al. 2004).

The limbus is a specialized region, which is highly vascularized, innervated, and protected from potential damage by UV light by the presence of melanin pigmentation. The concept of the limbal location of corneal SCs was first proposed by Davanger and Evensen (1971) suggesting that the highly undulating "palisades of Vogt" (Goldberg and Bron 1982) contained the proliferative cells that maintain the corneal epithelium. Clusters of small, roundish, densely packed cells are located throughout the basal cell layer at the bottom of the epithelial papillae separating the palisades. Within these clusters, one or few small, primitive appearing putative SCs and several larger, melanin-containing putative TACs can be distinguished. Limbal epithelial SCs are slow-cycling, have a high proliferative potential in vitro, lack the corneal epithelial differentiation-associated keratins K3/K12, and represent the predominant site of corneal tumor formation (Lavker and Sun 2000). From the percentage of radiolabeled thymidine retaining cells present in the limbal zone, it has been concluded that SCs may represent less than 10% of the total limbal basal cell population (Lavker et al. 1991). However, a major challenge in corneal SC biology is the ability to identify SCs in situ. Although a number of molecular markers for the limbal SC compartment has been proposed during the last few years, such as ABCG2, p63, keratin 5/14, keratin 19, α-enolase, vimentin, and integrin α9 (Daniels et al. 2001; Grueterich et al. 2003; Chen et al. 2004), their role in specifically identifying limbal SCs is still under debate.

Damage to or dysfunction of the limbal SC population results in partial or total limbal SC deficiency, which has severe consequences for corneal wound healing and ocular surface integrity (Huang and Tseng 1991; Chen and Tseng 1991; Dua et al. 2003). Limbal SC deficiency is characterized by conjunctival epithelial ingrowth, vascularization, chronic inflammation, recurrent erosions and persistent ulcer, destruction of the basement membrane, and fibrous tissue ingrowth leading to severe functional impairment (Puangsricharern and Tseng 1995; Holland and Schwartz 1996). In these cases, renewal of the SC population, e.g., by autologous or homologous transplantation of limbal tissue, is required for regeneration of the entire corneal surface and for restoration of visual function (Kenyon and

Tseng 1989; Kruse and Reinhard 2001). The procedures involve lamellar removal of 2 four-clock-hour limbal segments (usually superior and inferior) from the healthy donor eye and transplantation to the limbal-deficient eye after a complete superficial keratectomy and conjunctival peritomy to remove diseased surface epithelium. For patients with bilateral disease, the use of allogeneic limbal grafts, either as an intact annular ring or several segments of limbal tissue, is required. However, in both situations, donor site morbidity or immunologic rejection remain major complications. This has led to the recent development of therapeutic strategies such as ex vivo expansion of human limbal epithelial cells on amniotic membrane or fibrin gels for the purpose of transplantation (Lindberg et al. 1993; Tseng et al. 2002; Pellegrini et al. 1997; Schwab et al. 2000; Koizumi et al. 2001; Grueterich et al. 2002). For this procedure, only a small limbal biopsy of approximately 1–2 mm² is required, which minimizes potential damage to the healthy donor eye. Although the long-term results and safety of this procedure are yet to be determined, reasonable success of up to 1 year of follow-up has been achieved (Pellegrini et al. 1997). More recently, tissue-engineered strategies using autologous conjunctival epithelial or oral mucosal epithelial sheet transplantation have opened a new field for ocular surface reconstruction (Inatomi et al. 2005).

5.1.1.10
Corneal Innervation

The cornea is densely innervated by branches of the first trunk of the trigeminal nerve. These nerves enter the peripheral cornea unmyelinated and move centrally prior to moving through Bowman's layer and then spreading beneath and in between the corneal epithelium. Corneal nerves can now be visualized in vivo using confocal imaging techniques (Fig. 5.1.1).

5.1.1.11
Antigen Presenting Cells in the Cornea (Dendritic Cells and Macrophages)

Whereas historically the cornea has been thought of as being devoid of antigen-presenting cells (APCs) and as therefore being immune privileged, novel research has changed that picture. In recent years it became clear that in contrast the cornea is indeed endowed with significant numbers of resident inflammatory and antigen-presenting cells. This includes dendritic cells, and dendritic cells of the epithelium, i.e., Langerhans cells as well as macrophages. The difference to APCs at other locations and the reason for the long misconception of the cornea as a tissue missing APCs is the fact that central corneal APCs are immature and devoid of typical surface markers of APCs such as MHC class II and co-stimulatory molecules. These are only upregulated after inflammation (e.g., after penetrating keratoplasty). The central corneal epithelium and stroma therefore contains numerous dendritic cells, but these are class II negative. Langerhans cells increase in numbers after contact lens use (this has to be taken into account in keratoconus patients undergoing keratoplasty). Macrophages are only found in the corneal stroma. Towards the limbus these cell start to express typical markers of conventional mature APCs (Fig. 5.1.3).

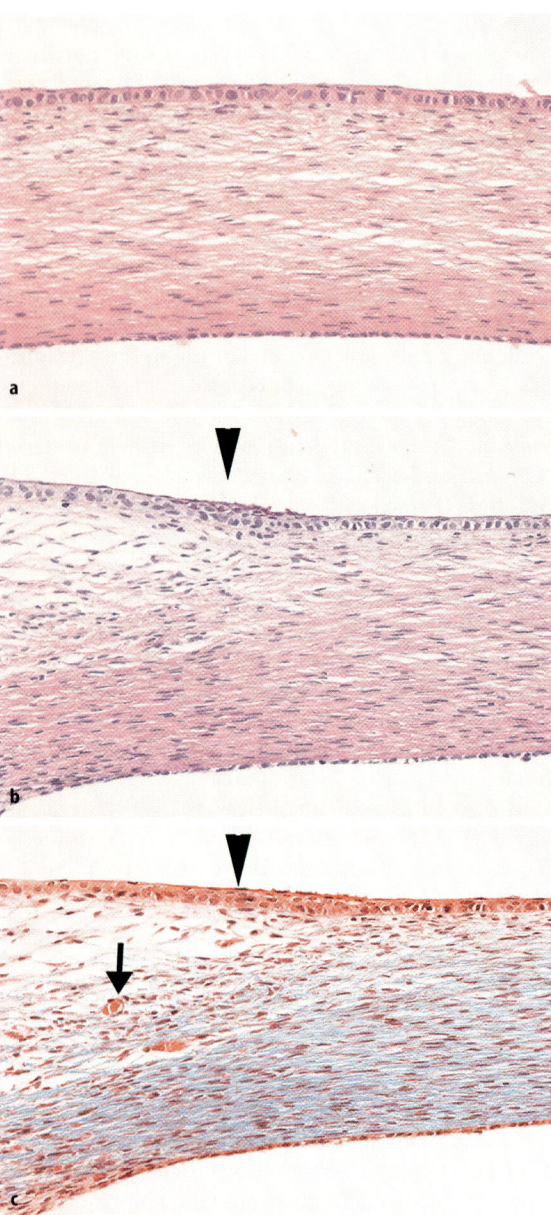

Fig. 5.1.14. Limbal transition zone in fetal human eyes (*arrow* limbus, *arrowhead* small blood vessel) (modified from Cursiefen, Rummelt et al. 2006)

5.1.1.12
Corneal Landmarks (Definition of Limbus)

The most important corneal landmarks relevant for the microsurgeon are at the limbus. There exists a surgical and an anatomical definition of this transition zone between vascularized conjunctiva and avascular cornea (Fig. 5.1.14): Anatomically the limbus is defined by a triangular segment between a vertical line from the end of Bowmann's layer to the end of Descemet's layer (Schwalbe's line) on the corneal side and a vertical line perpendicular to the surface above the scleral spur (Fig. 5.1.14). Clinically, the limbus most commonly is defined as the beginning of a clear cornea, for the corneal microsurgeon the peripheral edge of Bowman's layer. Due to the overgrowth of a vascular pannus (e.g., in contact lens wearing keratoconus patients) usually at the superior and less commonly at the inferior location, the surgical limbus is more centrally located than the true anatomical limbus at these locations. Based on

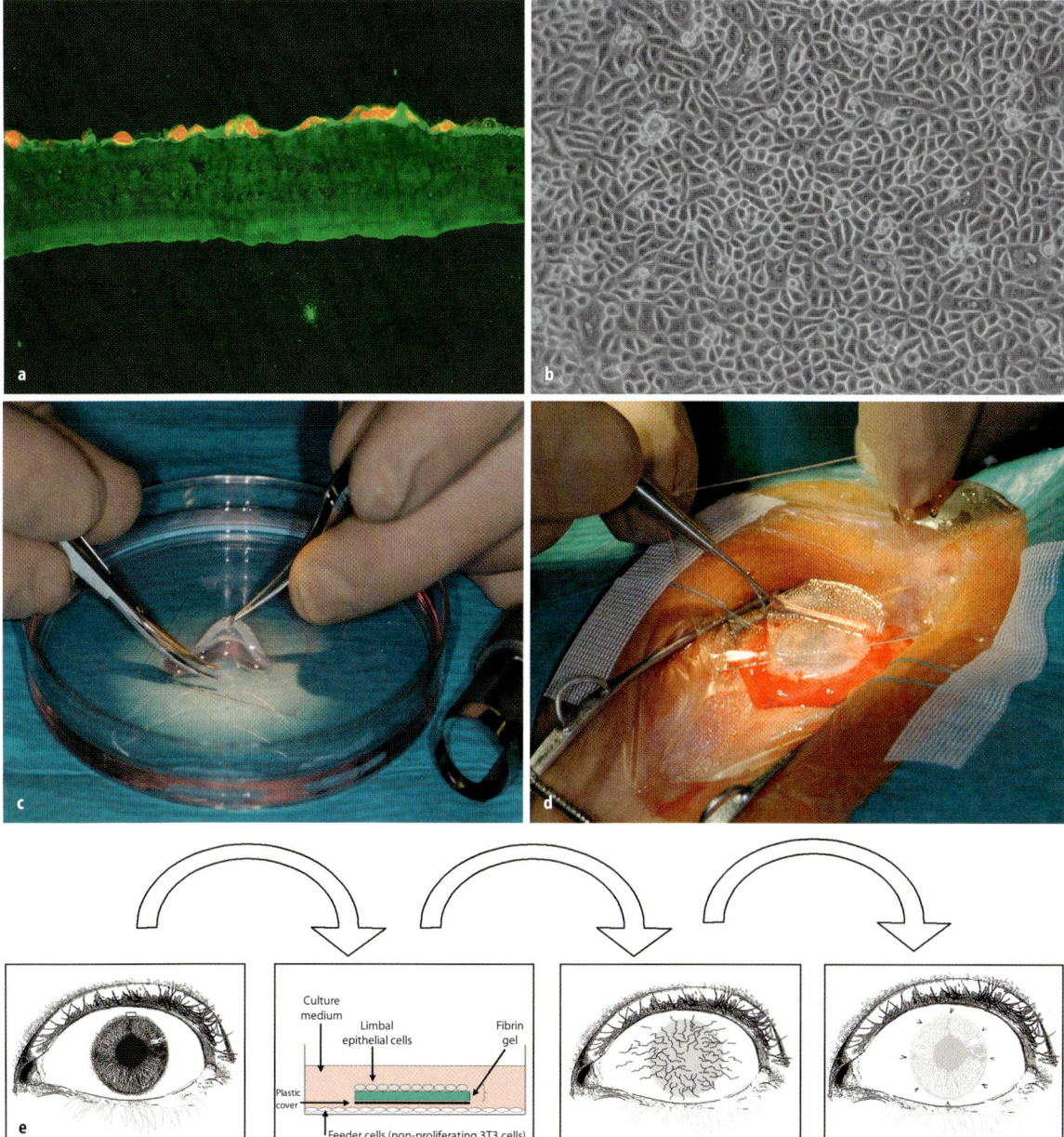

Fig. 5.1.15. Retrieval of healthy limbal stem cell tissue for ex-vivo amplification. **a** Cultured corneal epithelial stem cells on a fibrin gel (**b** view from above) are cut (**c**) and placed onto the recipient's eye (**d**) after they have been harvested from the contralateral healthy eye and have been amplified in culture (**e**) (modified from Cursiefen, Seitz and Kruse et al. 2004)

Table 5.1.2. Important corneal dimensions (modified from Rohen 1997)

Vertical diameter	10.6 mm
Horizontal diameter	11.7 mm
Thickness (central, peripheral)	550 μm (700 μm)
Curvature (anterior, posterior)	7.8 mm (6.5 mm)
Surface	1.3 cm²

identifying the limbus one can define the horizontal and vertical corneal diameters (normally 11 and 10 mm). Prior to penetrating keratoplasty, the diameter of donor tissue and recipient cornea to be removed has to be defined individually at the slit-lamp. A compromise has to be made between the pros and cons of a larger versus a smaller graft diameter: A larger graft diameter is beneficial for transplantation of as much viable endothelial cell material as possible and for lower postoperative astigmatism. On the other hand, the closer interface and suture material get to the limbal vascular arcade, the higher the chances are for corneal neovascularization, immigration of host APCs and subsequent immune rejections. In that respect, the surgical limbus is more important than the anatomical. Standard diameters for most non-keratoconus eyes are 7.5/7.75 (Barron trephine) and 8.0/8.25 for keratoconus; and 7.5/7.6 and 8.0/8.1 in excimer trephination, respectively. For retrieval of stem cell tissue from healthy contralateral eye in patients with unilateral limbal stem cell deficiency (e.g., after cautery) to be amplified ex-vivo in culture, it is important to realize the true anatomic limbus location is more peripheral so as to excise enough stem cell tissue including the palisades of Vogt (Figs. 5.1.4, 5.1.15).

5.1.1.13
Corneal Dimensions

Important corneal dimensions are outlined in Table 5.1.2.

5.1.2
Surgical Pathology of the Cornea

5.1.2.1
Hereditary Diseases of the Cornea

5.1.2.1.1
Corneal Dystrophies

Corneal dystrophies are inherited, bilateral diseases leading to reduced visual acuity and recurrent erosions usually early in life (in contrast to degenerative diseases with a later onset, and often unilateral pathology). Dystrophies in the cornea have traditionally been grouped according to the anatomical site predominantly affected. Recent progress in molecular biological analysis has greatly increased our understanding of the pathogenesis of corneal dystrophies. Several interesting and clinically relevant points will be discussed briefly here:

- The phenomenon of "**polyphenotypia**": Mutations in the same gene, e.g., the keratoepithelin gene on chromosome 5q31, cause plenty of dystrophies with clinically different phenotypes, such as granular dystrophies I, III, IV, lattice dystrophies I, III as well as Thiel-Behnke dystrophy.
- The phenomenon of "**polygeny**": On the other hand, clinically identical phenotypes can be caused by mutations in different genes. Mutations in the keratoepithelin gene on chromosome 5 as well as in the gelsolin gene on chromosome 9 can cause lattice corneal dystrophy.
- **Recurrences**: Since the gene defect, e.g., in all keratoepithelin mutation-based "stromal" (but in fact epithelial) dystrophies is not treated by performing conventional surgical treatments [lamellar or penetrating keratoplasty, phototherapeutic keratectomy (PTK), etc.], the original pathology will inevitably recur due to migration of new diseased epithelial cells from diseased limbal stem cells onto the cornea. Permanent cure can only be achieved by treating the underlying molecular defect in the limbal stem cells, e.g., by somatic gene therapy or by transplantation of healthy stem cells. Since deposition of pathologic keratoepithelin gene products starts from epithelial cells, it is not surprising that recurrences of granular and lattice dystrophy start around suture tracks with displaced epithelium and in the interface. Recurrences are most common after surgery for granular dystrophy, and less common for lattice and even less for macular dystrophy.
- **Inheritance**: Most corneal dystrophies are inherited in an autosomal-dominant pattern. Exceptions to the rule are, e.g., Lisch's dystrophy with an X-chromosomal pattern and macular corneal dystrophy with an autosomal recessive pattern (this follows the rule that recessive inheritance is initially associated with more severe disease than the dominant pattern).

A full discussion of the molecular pathogenesis and histopathology of all corneal dystrophies is beyond the scope of this chapter and we refer to recent reviews on these topics (for differential diagnosis of stromal dystrophies see Table 5.1.3). In contrast, we will briefly discuss surgically relevant points of selected corneal dystrophies grouped according to their anatomical site for didactical reasons although that does not reflect their pathogenesis.

Table 5.1.3. Differential diagnosis of the main stromal corneal dystrophies (Naumann 1997)

	Granular dystrophy	Lattice dystrophy	Macular dystrophy
Location	Center	Center	Center and periphery
Corneal layers involved	Epithelium and later stroma	Epithelium and later stroma	All layers
Mode of inheritance	Autosomal dominant	Autosomal dominant	Autosomal recessive
Staining	Masson	Congo red	Alcian blue
Reduced visual acuity	Late	Late	Early
Treatment	PTK and then PK	PTK and then PK	PK

Dystrophies Primarily Affecting Corneal Epithelium, Basement Membrane and Bowman's Layer

Cogan's map-dot-fingerprint dystrophy (Fig. 5.1.16) as well as Meesmann's dystrophy and less commonly Lisch's dystrophy can cause recurrent epithelial erosions. These entities therefore have to be ruled out in patients prior to undergoing refractive surgery. Histopathologically, a defect in epithelial basement membrane adhesion is causative for Cogan's dystrophy (resulting in recurrent epithelial detachment), whereas in Meesmann's dystrophy a defect in an intracellular intermediate filament (keratin) causes intracellular cyst formation. Lisch's dystrophy seems to be caused by an abnormal deposition of lipids in intracellular vacuoles. Reis-Bücklers dystrophy has meanwhile turned out to be a superficial subform of "stromal" granular dystrophy (type III). It can cause recurrent erosions as well. Due to its superficial location best initial treatment is with abrasion and PTK or lamellar keratoplasty and not with penetrating keratoplasty.

Stromal Dystrophies

Stromal dystrophies are characterized by deposition of abnormal material in the corneal stroma thereby interfering with corneal transparency and reducing visual acuity (see Table 5.1.3 for differential diagnosis). Traditionally this includes the "stromal" macular, granular and lattice dystrophies (plus rarer diseases such as Schnyder's crystalline dystrophy). Pathogenetically, granular and lattice dystrophy are primarily epithelial dystrophies caused by mutations of the epithelial keratoepithelin gene, whereas macular corneal dystrophy is a systemic defect of keratin sulfation affecting all layers of the cornea. Granular dystrophy is characterized by "granular" deposition of hyaloid and Masson positive material (Fig. 5.1.17). Important to mention is type II granular dystrophy, which affects people with a heritage from the Italian town of Avellino ("Avellino dystrophy"): Here both amyloid ("lattice") and hyaloid deposits can be found in the cornea. In lattice dystrophy, branching lattice deposits of amyloid cause corneal opacifications (histologically these stain with Congo red and have double fringency). Both dystrophies initially only affect the corneal center and leave clear tissue of cornea in between resulting in relatively pre-

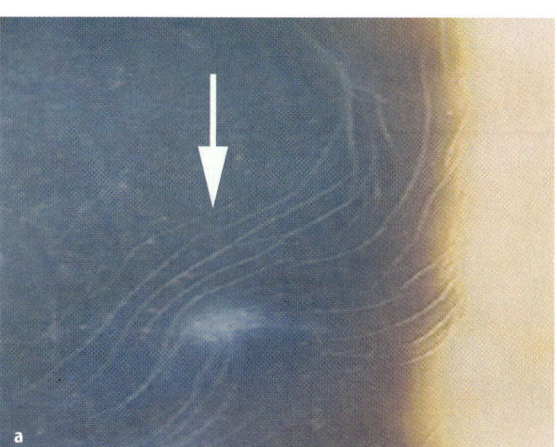
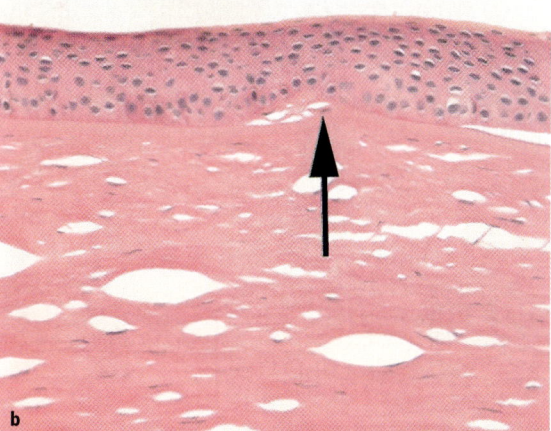
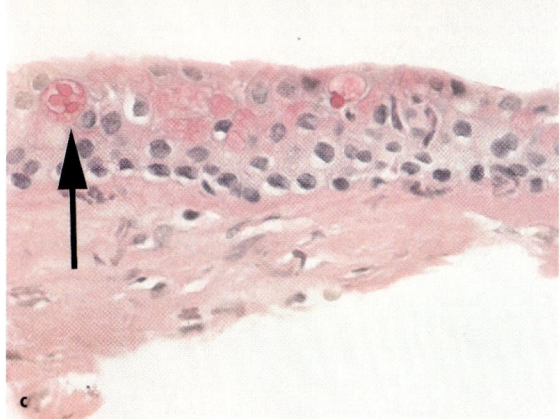

Fig. 5.1.16. Map-dot-fingerprint dystrophy (Cogan's dystrophy) with typical "fingerprint" lines in **a**, **b**, **c** Histology shows cysts and basement membrane duplications (PAS)

served good visual acuity (Fig. 5.1.18). Lattice dystrophy type II ("Meretoja" form) is not only a local amyloid deposition, but also part of a systemic amyloidosis causing a polyneuropathy. In contrast, in macular corneal dystrophy (MCD), macular like opacification coalesces early on resulting in early loss of vision. In contrast to the other two dystrophies, MCD also affects the corneal periphery. MCD is a systemic disorder of keratin sulfation based on chromosome 16, resulting in deposits of unsulfated keratan sulfate in the stroma (which stain with alcian blue; Fig. 5.1.6). MCD affects all layers of the cornea including corneal epithelium and can cause secondary corneal guttae. Treatment options here therefore are limited to full-thickness penetrating keratoplasty, whereas superficial forms of lattice and granular dystrophy can initially be treated by PTK or lamellar (possibly also deep lamellar) keratoplasty. Based on immunohistochemistry there exist two subforms of MCD: type I with an undetectable serum level of sulfated keratin sulfate (and no staining in the cornea) and a type II with normal serum levels and

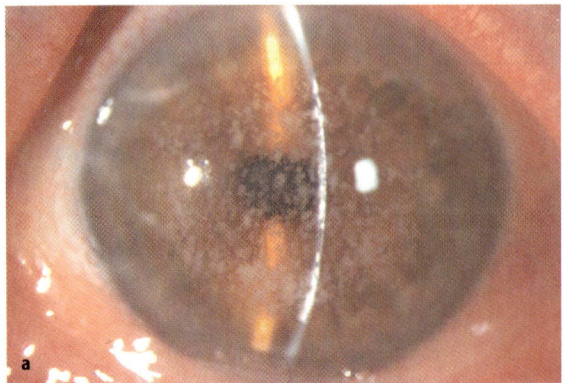

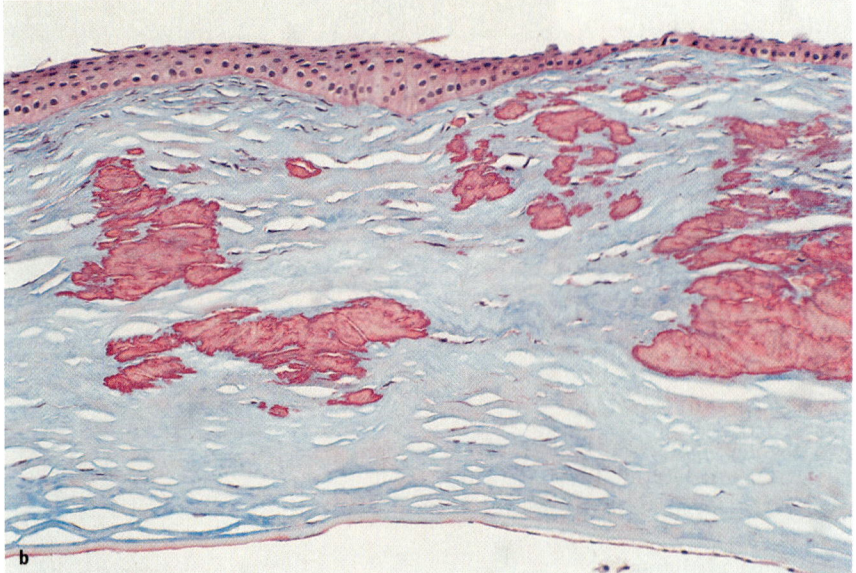

Fig. 5.1.17. Granular corneal dystrophy with "granular" deposits in the central corneal stroma (**a**), which stain positive with Masson (**b**)

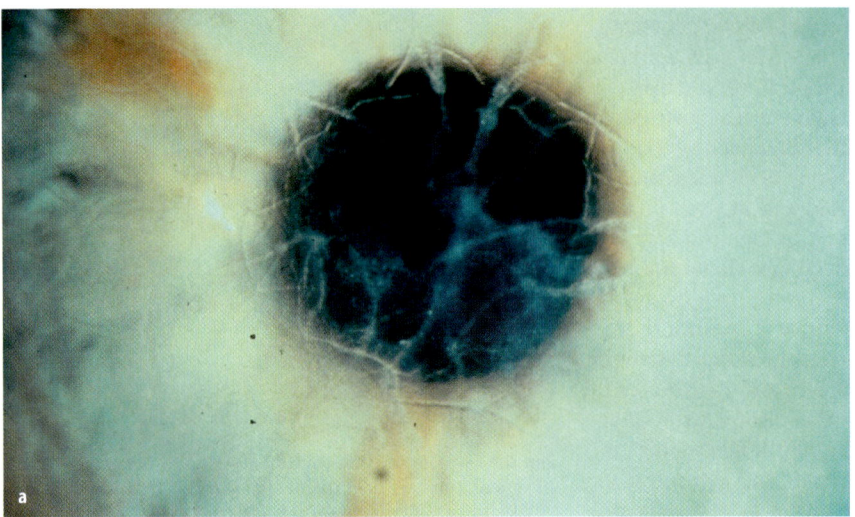

Fig. 5.1.18. Lattice dystrophy with fine tubes with double contour extending through central stroma (**a**), which stain positive on Congo red staining (*arrow*) for amyloid (**b**)

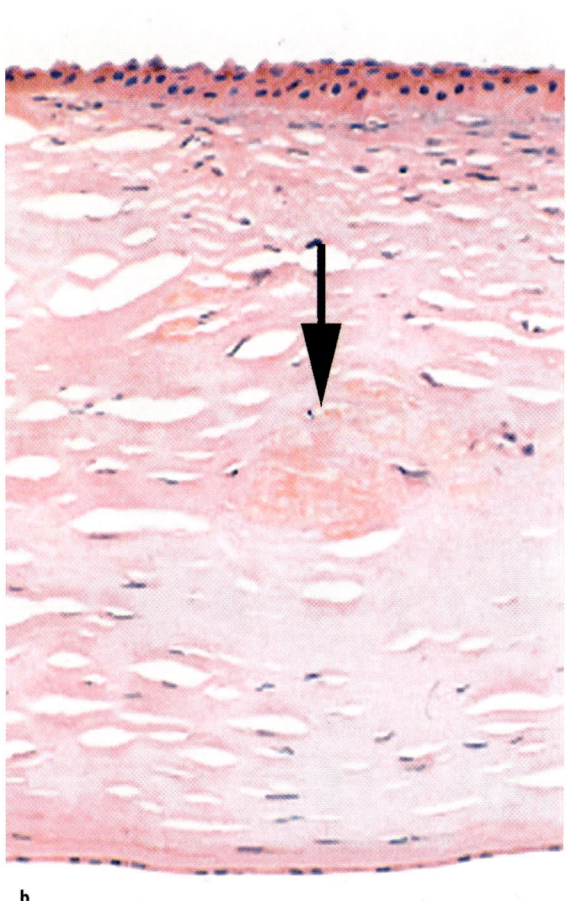

Fig. 5.1.18 (Cont.)

some staining for sulfated keratin sulfate in the cornea. Schnyder's crystalline stromal dystrophy is clinically characterized by a central glittering opacification, which on histology is defined by abnormal lipid deposits. In 50% of patients with Schnyder's dystrophy this is associated with a systemically elevated serum lipid profile.

Dystrophies of Corneal Endothelium

Fuchs' corneal dystrophy is the most common form of endothelial dystrophy and one of the most common causes for penetrating keratoplasty, too (Fig. 5.1.2). The etiology of this dystrophy is poorly understood. Mitochondrial mutations have been suspected to be causative. Loss of endothelial cells, formation of corneal guttae, phagocytosis of melanin by remaining endothelial cells and resulting predominantly central corneal stromal and epithelial edema are the slit-lamp and histologically visible sequelae. Reduced vision and painful bullous keratopathy are the consequences (Fig. 5.1.2). Symptoms are usually worse in the morning and get better during the day due to evaporation of stromal edema. It must be differentiated from "PEX keratopathy" (diffuse; see Chapter 6.3) and other causes of stromal edema [e.g., pseudophakic (central), etc.]. Treatment is by penetrating keratoplasty. CHED (congenital hereditary endothelial dystrophy, chromosome 20) causes stromal edema, but early on in life; it occurs in a recessive and a dominant form. In contrast to congenital glaucoma no Descemet-breaks develop. Schlichting's dystrophy is caused by an "epithelial transformation" of corneal endothelium, thus causing stromal edema. Care has to be taken to rule out a secondary open angle glaucoma in these patients. Treatment options for these diseases are full-thickness or posterior lamellar corneal transplantation.

5.1.2.1.2
Ectatic Disorders (Keratoconus, Keratoglobus, Keratotorus)

The cornea can be affected by several inherited ectatic disorders all leading to reduction of corneal thickness, corneal ectasia and subsequently reduced visual acuity due to high irregular astigmatism. The clinical and histological features of keratoconus are depicted in Fig. 5.1.7. Besides stromal thinning and ectasia, keratoconus is characterized by an epithelial Fleischer ring (ferritin iron ring at the base of the ectasia), prominent (myelinated) corneal nerves, Vogt lines (small vertical folds in Descemet's membrane) as well as an irregular astigmatism. Histologically, all are characterized by extreme corneal thinning with focal defects in epithelial basement membrane and Bowmans' layer (pathognomonic!; Fig. 5.1.7). Special care has to be taken during keratoplasty for ectatic disorders to suture graft and host surfaces at the same level to avoid outer steps; inner steps are unavoidable. Furthermore, care has to be taken to keep a distance as long as possible from the vascular pannus after contact lens use in keratoconus patients. For all patients undergoing refractive surgery it is imperative to rule out early forms of keratoconus to avoid postsurgical iatrogenic ectasias. Keratoglobus is thinning of the whole corneal stroma without an iron line. Keratotorus is a peripheral extreme thinning of the stroma with usually more centrally located outward bulging.

Acute Keratoconus

Acute keratoconus (hydrops) is caused by a rupture in Descemet's membrane in the course of stromal thinning. This leads to sudden influx of aqueous humor into the corneal stroma with resulting stromal edema and loss of vision. Irritation of corneal nerve endings due to resulting bullous keratopathy explains the pain often associated with acute keratoconus. The natural cause of acute keratoconus is characterized by slow migration of endothelial cells onto the denuded area on the posterior aspect of corneal stroma. A secondary thinner Descemet's membrane is layered down in the following months. The endings of ruptured Descemet's membrane show a characteristic inward rolling. With reendothelialization of the cornea, dehydration of the stroma sets in and the cornea slowly resumes its normal thickness usually with a residual central scar. The risk of spontaneous perforation in the course of hydrops is negligibly small. Nevertheless, intraocular pressure should be lowered to about 10 mm Hg and patients be advised not to traumatize the eye. Performing a keratoplasty in the acute phase is contraindicated due to weak biomechanical properties of the edematous cornea. Keratoplasty should be performed only after an interval of about 3–6 months when the cornea has resumed its normal thickness (Fig. 5.1.7).

5.1.2.2
Acquired Corneal Pathologies

5.1.2.2.1
Degenerations

Band Degeneration

Any systemic disease leading to elevated serum levels of calcium or phosphate (such as hyperparathyroidism, bone tumors, bone metastasis, sarcoidosis, etc.) as well as chronic ocular diseases (juvenile iridocyclitis, silicone oil tamponade, etc.; see Table 5.1.4 for differential diagnosis) can lead to abnormal deposition of calcium and phosphate in basement membrane, Bowman's layer and superficial stroma. Resulting visual acuity decreases can be corrected by corneal epithelial abrasion and EDTA application, since scarifying Bowman's layer by PTK is initially unnecessary.

Iron Lines

The location of different corneal irons lines is depicted in Fig. 5.1.19.

Table 5.1.4. Differential diagnosis of corneal band degeneration (modified from Naumann 1997)

Local diseases of the eye
Silicone oil tamponade
Juvenile rheumatoid arthritis
Ichthyosis
Systemic diseases causing increased serum levels of calcium and phosphate
Hyperparathyroidism (primary, secondary, tertiary)
Vitamin D intoxication
Sarcoidosis
Renal failure
Hyperphosphatemia
Bone tumors (multiple myeloma)
Bone metastases
Gout

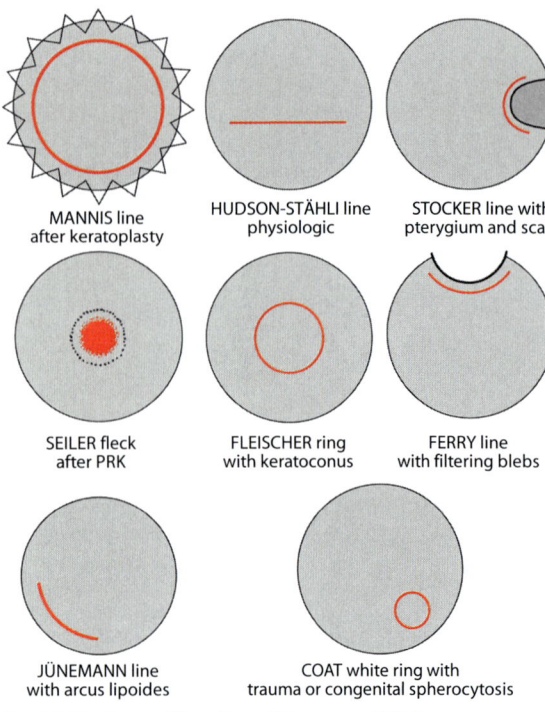

Fig. 5.1.19. Corneal iron lines (Naumann 1997)

5.1.2.2.2
Corneal Neovascularization (Angiogenesis and Lymphangiogenesis)

The normal cornea is devoid of both blood and lymphatic vessels. Corneal avascularity is of paramount importance for corneal transparency. Therefore, in all higher animals dependent on good vision, the normal cornea is avascular. In addition, the cornea tries to maintain avascularity even if challenged with minor angiogenic and inflammatory stimuli. That explains why angiogenesis, e.g., after refractive corneal surgical procedures, usually does not occur. The molecular mechanisms underlying this "antiangiogenic privilege" of the cornea are only partly understood. As with all privileges, corneal antiangiogenic privilege is not perfect. Severe inflammatory (e.g., in herpetic keratitis) and hypoxic (e.g., in contact lenses with low Dk value) stimuli as well as defects of limbal barrier function can cause ingrowths of blood vessels into the cornea (corneal angiogenesis). These blood vessels reduce corneal transparency also due to secondary opacifying changes in the corneal stroma such as deposition of lipid (lipid keratopathy), lipofuscin (Braun et al., 1997) fluid (stromal edema) and blood (hematocornea, Fig. 5.1.20).

In addition to the biomicroscopically visible blood vessels, biomicroscopically invisible lymphatic vessels grow into the cornea in inflammatory lesions (lymphangiogenesis). Novel markers of lymphatic vascular endothelium such as LYVE-1 (lymphatic vessel endotheli-

5.1.2 Surgical Pathology of the Cornea

surrounding connective tissue. Novel in-vivo confocal microscopical strategies (e.g., using the HRT II with cornea module) seem to allow the visualization of lymphatic vessels in vivo in human corneas. Lymphatic vessels are only found in association with blood vessels and are more common in the early phase after an inflammatory insult such as keratitis. Thereafter, lymphatic vessels regress much faster than do blood vessels. That explains the clinical observation that graft survival is better if keratoplasty is not performed in an acutely inflamed eye.

Besides reducing visual acuity, blood and especially lymphatic vessels have important implications for corneal transplant immunology. Corneal grafts placed into an avascular recipient bed (low-risk keratoplasty) are physically separated from the afferent (lymphatic) and efferent (blood vascular) arm of a so-called "immune reflex arc" leading to immune rejection. The excellent prognosis such grafts experience even without tissue matching is in sharp contrast to the high rejection rate when grafts are placed into prevascularized high-risk recipient beds. In the latter situation the graft has direct access both to lymphatic and blood vessels in the recipient rim. This means there is no longer a corneal immune privilege and the situation more closely mimics that of other solid tissue transplantations.

But not only preexisting, but (at least in animal models of low- and high-risk keratoplasty) also corneal neovascularization occurring only postoperatively significantly increases the risk for immune rejections. Novel antiangiogenic treatment strategies could significantly improve graft survival by inhibiting this postoperative neovascularization. Postoperative neovascularization is a common phenomenon in low-risk keratoplasty patients: it occurs in about 50% of patients and reaches the interface in about 10% of patients (Figs. 5.1.20, 5.1.21). The new blood vessels are usually oriented towards the suture material and then travel along the suture centripetally. Surgical risk factors for corneal neovascularization after keratoplasty are related to the distance between the inciting stimulus (wound healing in the interface and suture material itself) and the preexisting blood and lymphatic vessels at the limbus. Therefore a large graft diameter, small limbus-suture distance, small limbus-interface distance, a small inner suture angle (steep) and superior location of suture (vascular pannus) significantly increase the risk. If possible, sutures should therefore be placed as far away from the limbus as possible.

Treatment of corneal blood vessels is so far difficult. Novel topical antiangiogenic treatments provide new hope. These new drugs (such as topical antisense oligonucleotides or specific cytokine traps especially for growth factor VEGF) potently inhibit corneal neovascularization in animal models and first human patients. They primarily act on newly outgrowing and

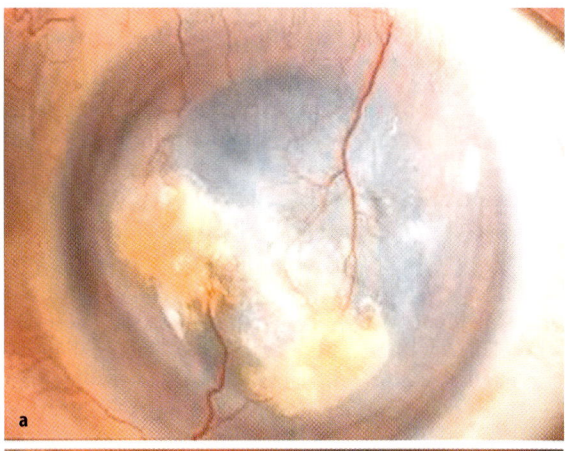
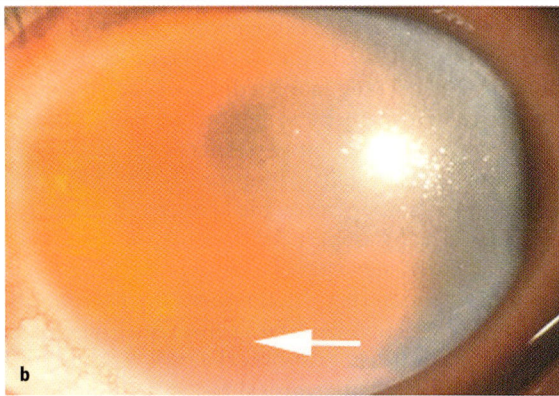
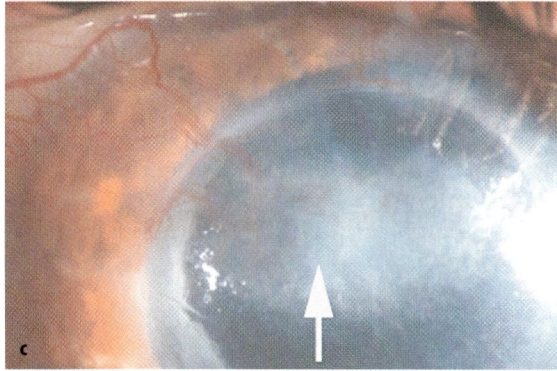

Fig. 5.1.20. Corneal neovascularization causes reduction in visual acuity primarily due to secondary opacifying changes in the corneal stroma such as deposition of lipid (lipid keratopathy), lipofuscin, blood (hematocornea) (**b**), fluid (stromal edema) (**c**) (modified from Cursiefen, Chen et al. 2003)

al HA receptor-1) made it possible to identify lymphatic vessels in excised vascularized human corneas (Figs. 5.1.9, 5.1.10). Electron microscopy of corneal lymphatic vessels (Fig. 5.1.10) demonstrates why these vessels are not visible at slit-lamp magnifications and in routine histology sections (Fig. 5.1.10): Lymphatic vessels do not contain red erythrocytes but rather have an empty lumen. In addition, they lack a normal vessel wall, thus minimizing the contrast between vessels and

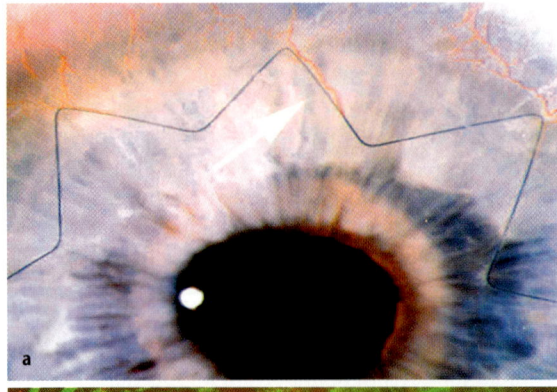

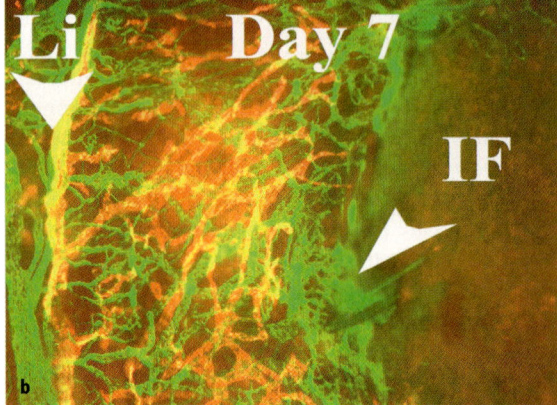

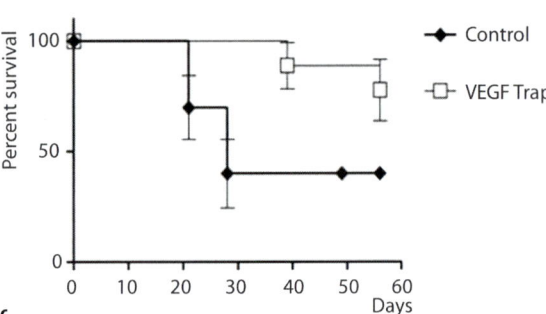

Fig. 5.1.21. Postkeratoplasty neovascularization is a common phenomenon after low-risk keratoplasty and predisposes to subsequent immune rejections. **a** Postkeratoplasty corneal neovascularization is usually directed towards suture material. **b** Animal models suggest that clinically visible blood vessels are associated with clinically non-visible lymphatic vessels (here stained in *red*, blood vessels in *green*, *Li* limbal vascular arcade, *IF* interface between donor and host tissue). **c** Inhibition of postkeratoplasty corneal neovascularization improves graft survival (modified from Cursiefen, Maruyama et al. 2004)

therefore immature blood vessels. Mature, long established and pericyte covered blood vessels are difficult to regress. The most promising approach here is the thermal cautery of the afferent blood vessels using cautery onto a 10-0 needle sutured through the vessel. Prior to refractive surgery or excimer laser penetrating keratoplasty, larger corneal blood vessels should temporarily be occluded using thermal cautery.

5.1.2.2.3
Neurotrophic Keratopathy

As outlined above, the cornea receives abundantly rich sensory innervations by branches of the first arm of the trigeminal nerve. The final branches interdigitate in between corneal epithelial cells. In recent years ample evidence has suggested that besides providing sensory innervations (and thereby maintaining tear film production via feedback to the autonomous innervations of tear glands) there is an intensive cross-talk between epithelial cells and nerve terminals. Terminal nerve endings secrete growth factors which the epithelium needs for regeneration and maintenance. On the other hand, do epithelial cells release neurotrophic factors essential for survival of nerve endings, such as nerve growth factor (NGF). Loss of corneal sensory innervations thereby not only causes a dry eye (due to reduced frequency of lid closure and reduced autonomic stimulation of tear glands), but also reduces epithelial healing capacity. This combination causes the disastrous clinical picture of neurotrophic keratopathy. Stage I is characterized by superficial punctate keratopathy, stage II by persistent epithelial defects and stage III by corneal ulceration (Fig. 5.1.22). Novel in vivo confocal imaging technology allows for in vivo visualization and quantification of subbasal corneal nerves, e.g., to quantify reinnervation after corneal transplantation or refractive surgery. Clinically, special care has to be taken to provide sufficient lubrication after keratoplasty or refractive surgical procedures (such as LASIK) being associated with corneal denervation. Fortunately, mild neurotrophic keratopathy after LASIK subsides usually within the first 6 months after surgery. Topical treatment with nerve growth factors such as NGF has proven to be principally helpful in patients with neurotrophic keratopathy.

5.1.2.2.4
Keratitis/Infections

Central keratitis may be caused by a variety of infectious agents (such as herpes virus, bacteria or fungi) or may be a sequela of neurotrophic keratopathy (or vernal keratoconjunctivitis leading to a "shield ulcer"). In case of uncertainty about the etiology of a central corneal keratitis, taking a corneal swab or tissue sample biopsy for histology can be helpful. That is especially true if *Acanthamoeba* keratitis is suspected. Clinical and histological features of several cases of infectious keratitis are depicted in Fig. 5.1.23.

Herpetic viral keratitis has both a distinct clinical picture and typical histological features. Clinically and histologically herpes infections which are epithelial (dendritiforme or geographic), stromal (necrotizing stromal keratitis) or endothelial (disciform keratitis)

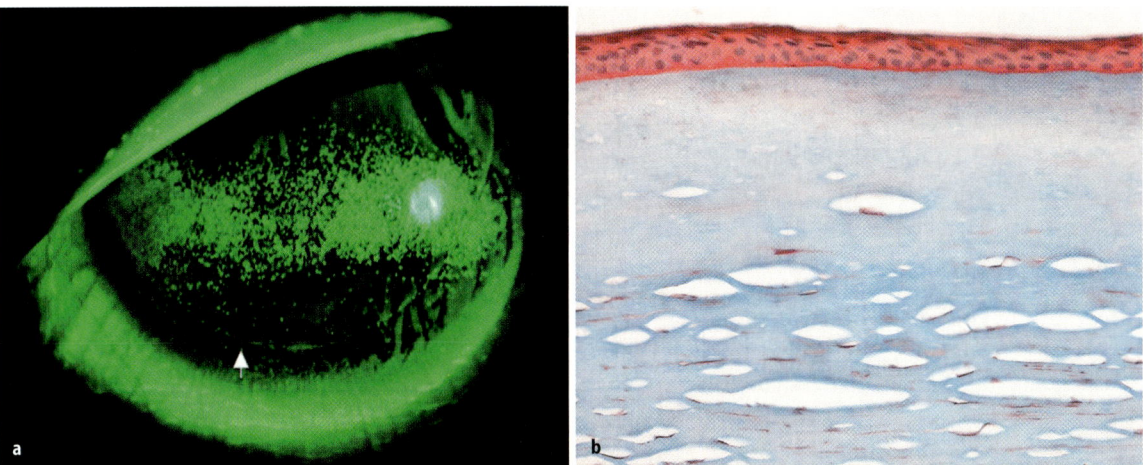

Fig. 5.1.22. Neurotrophic keratitis after refractive surgery (LASIK fluorescein staining). **b** Histological appearance of neurotrophic keratopathy with loss of keratocytes in the upper stroma (Masson) (modified from Cursiefen, Seitz et al. 2005)

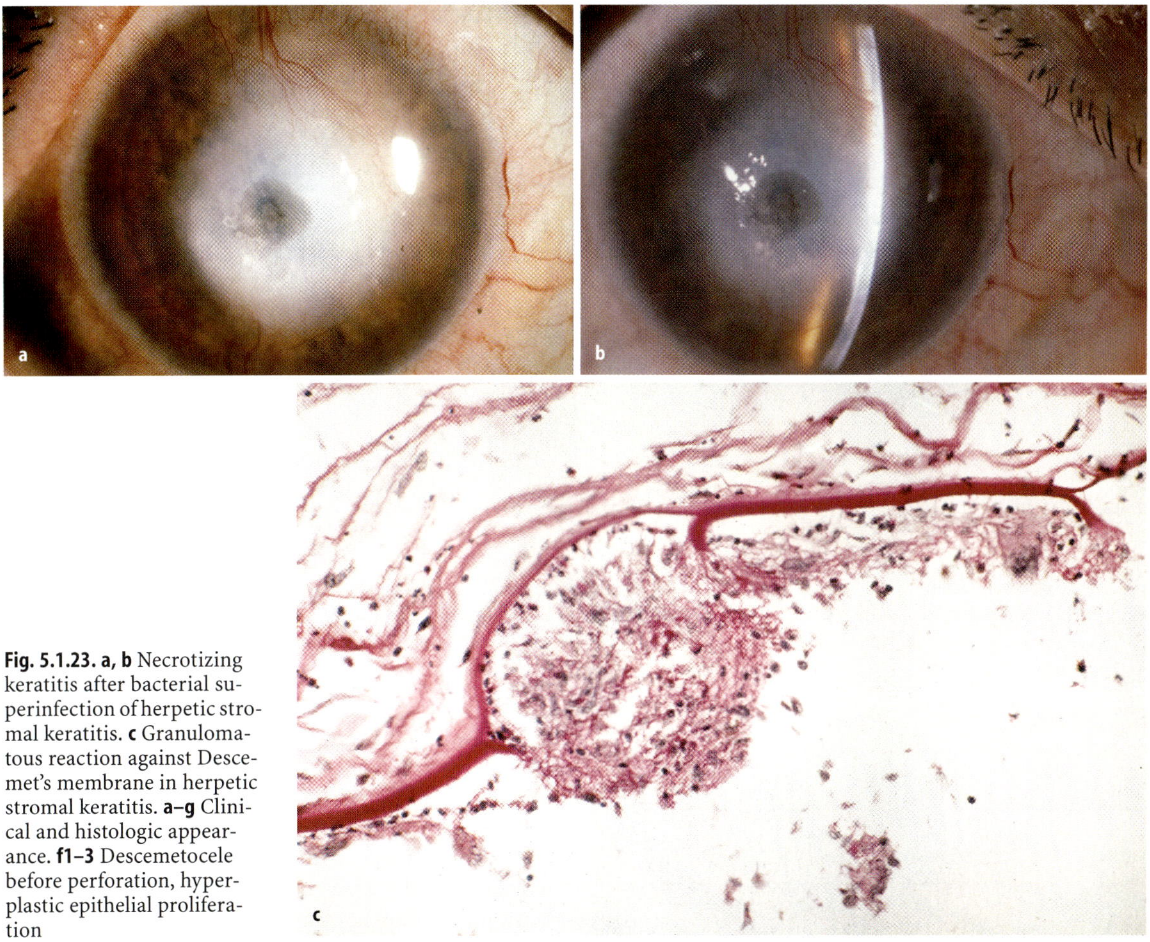

Fig. 5.1.23. **a, b** Necrotizing keratitis after bacterial superinfection of herpetic stromal keratitis. **c** Granulomatous reaction against Descemet's membrane in herpetic stromal keratitis. **a–g** Clinical and histologic appearance. **f1–3** Descemetocele before perforation, hyperplastic epithelial proliferation

can be differentiated. *Avascular* corneal lesions after herpes corneae more likely contain herpes simplex virus in the stroma. Following perforating keratoplasty (PKP) the risk of an infectious recurrence is increased. In contrast vascularized herpetic scars usually do not show virus persistence; after PKP an immune reaction is more likely (*"Holbach's rule"*; Holbach et al. 1991, 1992). If a granulomatous reaction against Descemet's membrane is suspected, imminent surgical action is necessary to avoid perforation.

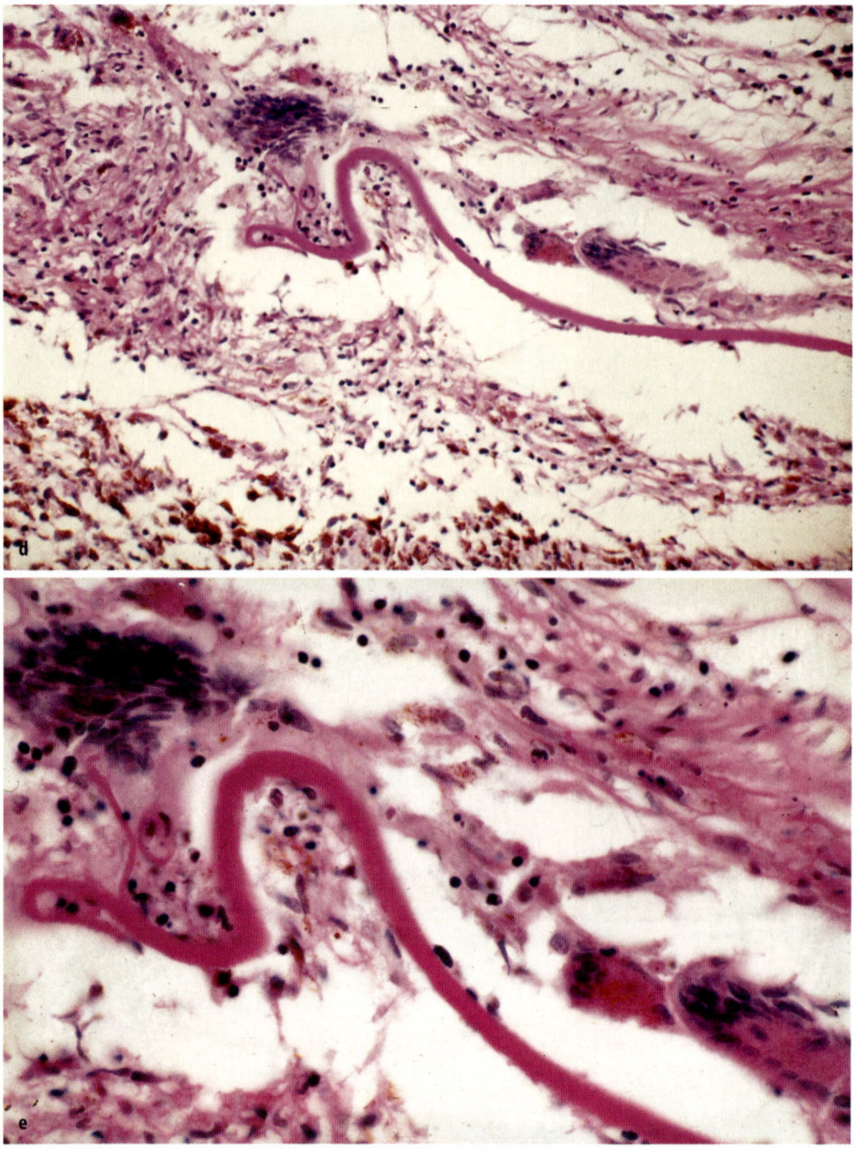

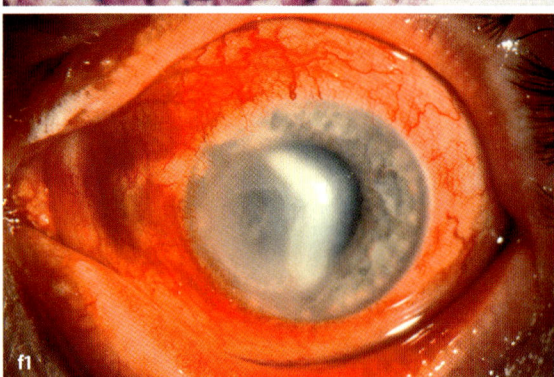

Fig. 5.1.23 (*Cont.*)

5.1.2.2.5
Trauma

Corneal wound healing is – since it is avascular – very slow. Therefore corneal sutures after traumatic lacerations should be left in place for at least 6 months. After keratoplasty we recommend performing the last suture removal only 18 months after grafting and only earlier if there is progressive corneal neovascularization (in the near future novel topical antiangiogenic eye drops may alleviate this problem). Figure 5.1.24 gives an example of avascular wound healing (keratoplasty).

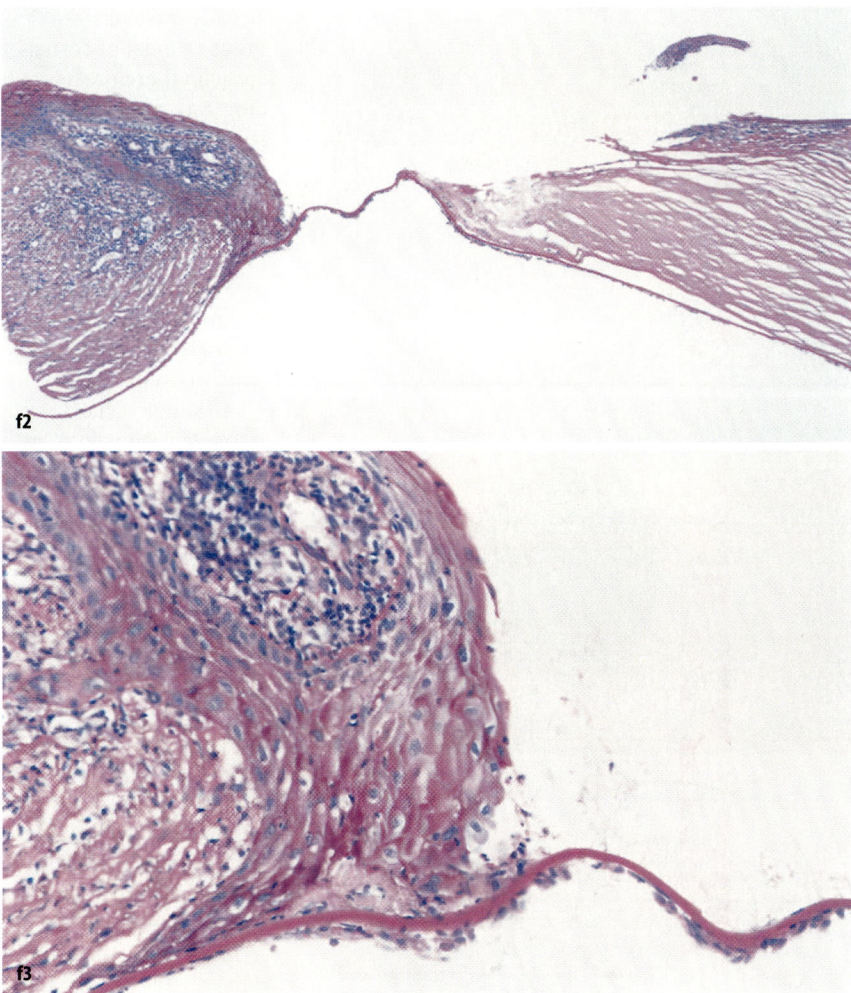

Fig. 5.1.23 (*Cont.*)

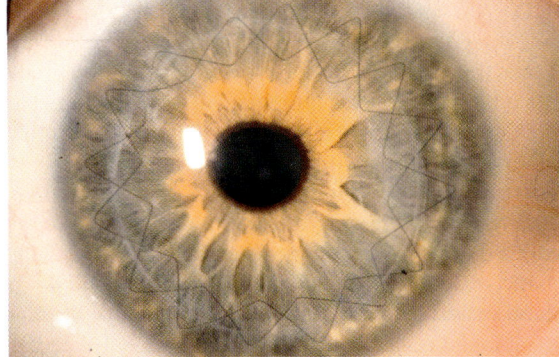

Fig. 5.1.24. Avascular wound healing after keratoplasty for keratokonus with both of the double-running sutures in place

5.1.2.2.6
Immune Reactions

Immune rejection is still the leading cause of graft failure after corneal transplantation. It occurs in roughly 20% of patients who have undergone normal-risk keratoplasty within the first 10 years, but is much more common after high-risk keratoplasty (about 50% after 5 years). Immune reactions can be directed against all three main layers of the cornea, but clinically the one against non-regenerating endothelium is the most common and relevant form. Immune rejections against the corneal endothelium can – in contrast to other solid tissue grafts – be visualized at the slit lamp. Clinically one can differentiate an *acute diffuse form* (80% of low-risk immune rejections) from a *chronic focal form* (Fig. 5.1.25). In both instances immune effector cells (macrophages, T-lymphocytes evading from iris vessels) attack the corneal endothelium causing "precipitates" (with resulting stromal edema), breakdown of the blood-aqueous barrier (clinically: cells, flare) and conjunctival injection. Breakdown of the blood-aqueous barrier nowadays can be quantified by laser tyndallometry and this allows "titration" of local and systemic anti-inflammatory therapy. Histologically, loss of corneal endothelium is the hallmark of immune reactions, having led to re-grafting because of graft failure. Recently, besides preexisting corneal blood and lym-

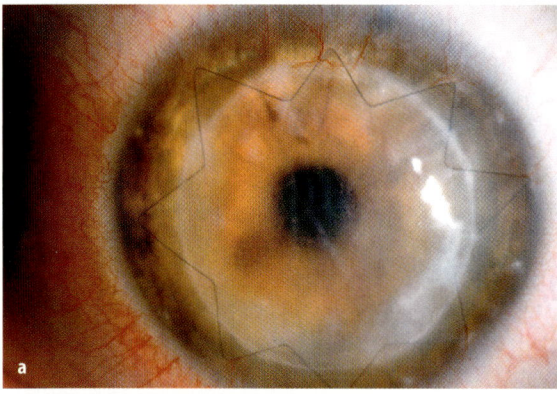

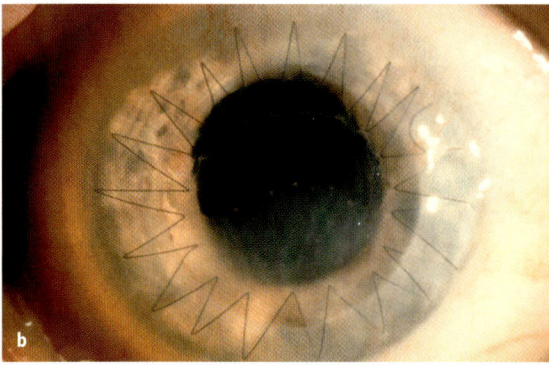

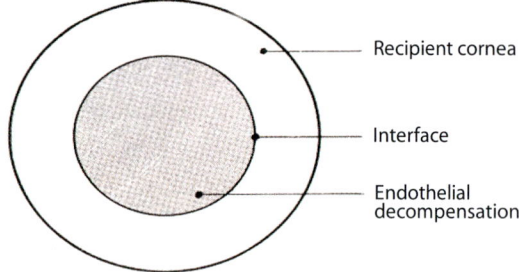

c1 Acute diffuse immune reaction

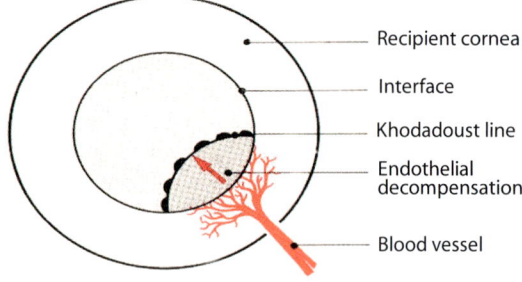

c2 Chronic focal immune reaction

Fig. 5.1.25. Different types of immune rejection can be classified from the slit-lamp appearance: acute diffuse (**a**) versus chronic focal immune rejection (**b**)

phatic vessels, corneal neovascularization occurring only *after* keratoplasty has been shown to significantly increase the risk of immune reactions. This was true for both preoperatively avascular as well as preoperatively already vascularized high-risk recipient bed (in the mouse model of corneal transplantation). The corneal surgeon therefore has to take care to minimize postkeratoplasty neovascularization, e.g., by less traumatizing surgical techniques (non-mechanical excimer laser trephination is associated with less trauma and less postkeratoplasty neovascularization compared to conventional mechanical trephination), suturing and surgical techniques (smaller graft diameter, increasing suture distance from limbus, placing the suture knot in the donor bed below Bowman's layer, etc.) or new antiangiogenic treatment options (such as VEGF trap or Avastin eyedrops).

Although it has been known for many decades that transplantation into an inflamed vascularized cornea carries an increased risk of subsequent immune rejection, whereas the prognosis is better if transplantation is performed only after the inflammation has calmed down, the molecular mechanisms underlying this phenomenon have only been unravelled recently. Blood and even more lymphatic vessels reaching the host graft junction and thereby physically connecting the graft to the host immune system greatly increase the risk of immune rejections. Inflammation is now known as the most potent inducer of hem- as well as lymphangiogenesis in the cornea. Local depletion of inflammatory cells in the cornea (e.g., macrophages by subconjunctival clodronate liposome injection) or the whole animal (by irradiation) nearly completely inhibits angiogenesis and lymphangiogenesis in the cornea. Inflammatory cells such as macrophages are key players in inducing corneal hem- and lymphangiogenesis. Not only do they release most of the known hem- and lymphangiogenic growth factors (such as VEGF A, C and D), but on the other hand macrophages also physically integrate into new corneal lymphatic vessels. That means that immature monocytic cells can differentiate into a blood and also a lymphatic vascular endothelial phenotype. Therefore it is appreciable that in acutely inflamed eyes, e.g., with a corneal ulcer, there are numerous blood and lymphatic vessels as well as activated APCs greatly increasing the risk of an immune rejection. When the inflammation has calmed down, lymphatic vessels very quickly regress and – in contrast to blood vessels – do not persist. This is related to the fact that lymphatic vessels do not have a vessel wall whereas corneal blood vessels are quickly covered by pericytes and thereby become independent of angiogenic growth factors for survival (Figs. 5.1.26, 5.1.27). Consequently lymphatic vessels in human corneas were much more common in the early phase of corneal inflammation and absent in all "blood" vascularized corneas with a history of more than 3 years after the inflammation. Therefore it is better not to transplant into freshly inflamed corneas if possible.

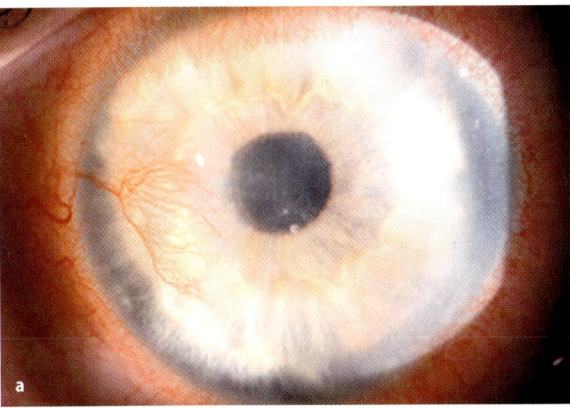
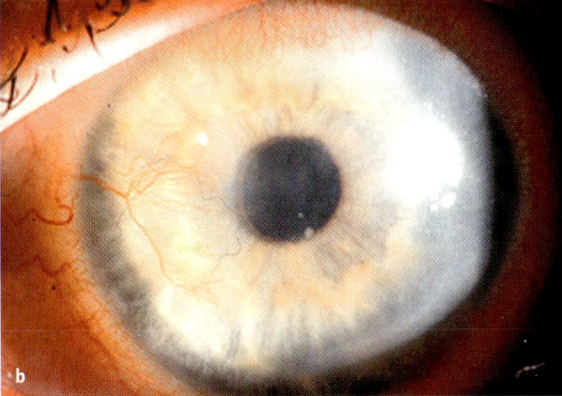
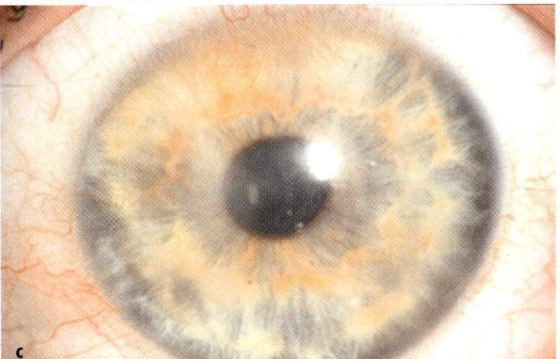

Fig. 5.1.26. Pathologic new blood vessels in the human cornea are quickly covered by pericytes and no longer depend on angiogenic growth factors (modified from Cursiefen, Rummelt et al. 2003). Novel antiangiogenic treatment strategies therefore are most promising in the early phase of corneal neovascularization: inhibition of neovascularization with antisense oligonucleotide against IRS-1. **a** Prior to and **b, c** after topical treatment 2× daily for 4 weeks

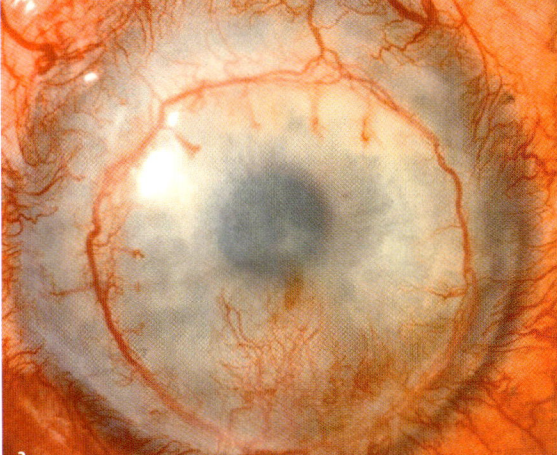
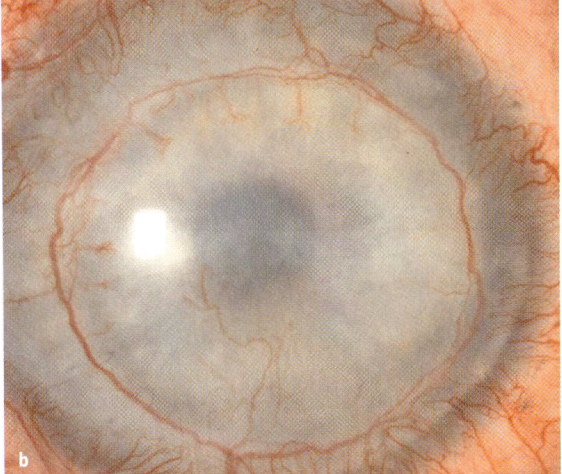

5.1.3
Surgical Procedures

5.1.3.1
Penetrating Keratoplasty

Penetrating keratoplasty is defined as the transplantation of a full thickness cornea into a recipient eye. *Lamellar keratoplasty* in contrast means transplantation of only parts of a cornea either as anterior lamellar keratoplasty (epithelium and varying parts of the stroma) or as posterior lamellar keratoplasty (corneal endothelium and varying portions of stroma). Several histopathologic aspects of corneal transplantation will be discussed below:

5.1.3.1.1
Surgical Technique

Trephination of donor and host tissue can be done with different instruments either mechanically or non-mechanically with the excimer laser (Fig. 5.1.28). Non-mechanical trephination has the advantage of less postoperative astigmatism and a less intensive wound healing response, thus also less postkeratoplasty neovascularization.

Fig. 5.1.27. Antiangiogenic therapy with bevacizumab eye drops (Avastin) potently inhibits corneal neovascularization after limbal stem cell deficiency (**a** prior to, **b** 4 weeks after additional Avastin eye drops ×5/day; modified from Bock et al. 2007; after limbal stem cell transplantation and perforating keratoplasty)

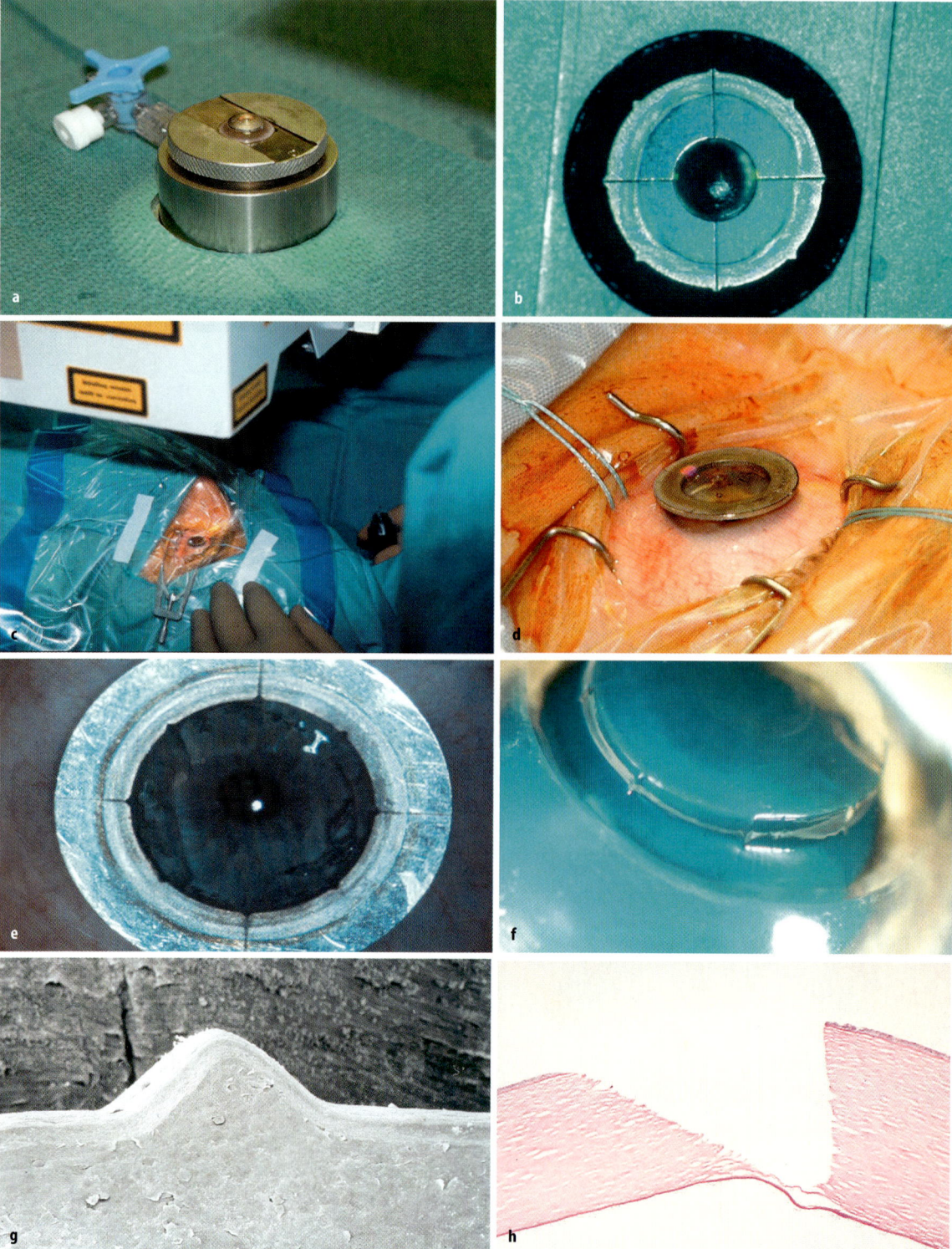

Fig. 5.1.28. Non-mechanical excimer laser keratoplasty yields lower postoperative astigmatism and better visual acuity. An artificial chamber (**a**) is used to cut out the donor tissue using a donor mask with eight orientation teeth (**b**). On the patient (**c**), a similar corresponding recipient mask (**d**) is used to cut out recipient tissue accordingly. The orientation teeth allow for correct positioning to avoid "horizontal torsion" and the excimer laser for very precise cutting of the interface reducing "vertical tilt" (**e–h**) Concept of Excimer Laser-Trephination (**i**)

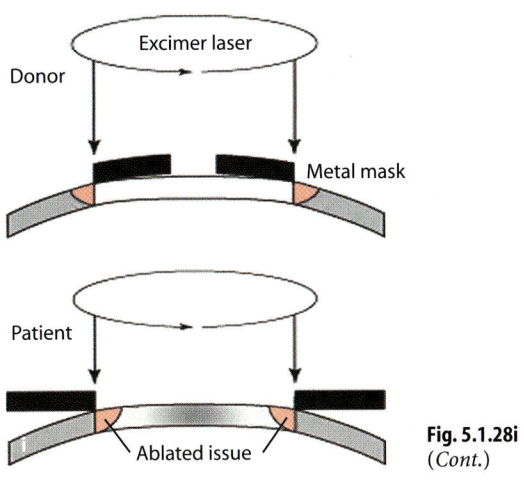

Fig. 5.1.28i (*Cont.*)

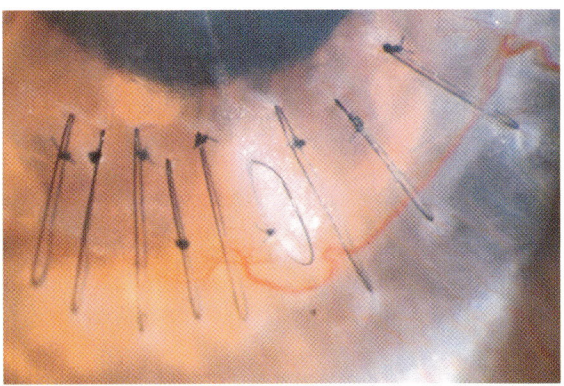

Fig. 5.1.29. A loose suture after keratoplasty attracts blood vessels, lymphatic vessels and antigen-presenting cells and induces immune rejections. Since loose sutures no longer contribute to mechanical stability, they have to be removed immediately

5.1.3.1.2 Suturing Technique

Suturing of the donor cornea into the recipient bed nowadays is usually done with 10-0 nylon sutures. These are placed as a double running cross-stitch diagonal suture according to Hoffmann or in vascularized high-risk eyes with defects in Bowman's layer and increased risk of suture loosening as single stitches. Due to the slow wound healing, sutures are usually left in place for at least 1 year. Although nylon sutures are relatively inert, they still cause subclinical inflammatory reactions in the surrounding corneal tissue and incite corneal neovascularization. UV-light-induced breakdown of nylon increases the irritation. Postkeratoplasty neovascularization in preoperatively avascular low-risk beds is always directed towards the outer suture turning points and follows the suture centripetally. A larger distance towards the limbus reduces the risk for neovascularization and therefore should promote graft survival.

5.1.3.1.3 Complications

Loose sutures and spontaneous breaks of nylon sutures usually after 2 years are a stimulus for inflammation and neovascularization and thereby greatly increase the risk for immune rejections. Since they do not have any tensile function anyway, they have to be removed immediately (Fig. 5.1.29).

Incongruence between the inner edges of host and donor cornea can lead to outgrowth of activated stromal keratocytes onto the posterior aspect of donor and host tissue. Such a *retrocorneal membrane* appears as a mildly opaque membrane posterior of Descemet's membrane. The accompanying destruction of corneal endothelium leads to overlying stromal edema and cloudiness.

Immune reactions, postkeratoplasty neovascularization and recurrence of *primary disease* are discussed above.

5.1.3.2 Lamellar Keratoplasty

Lamellar keratoplasty has several advantages over penetrating keratoplasty: the risks of surgery on the open eye are avoided (see Chapters 2, 4: expulsive bleeding), in the case of (deep) anterior lamellar keratoplasty the risk of an endothelial immune reaction is avoided and in the case of posterior lamellar keratoplasty where only endothelial cells plus are transplanted the risk of postkeratoplasty astigmatism is reduced because the anterior stroma and Bowmann's layer are left in place (DSAEK; Fig. 5.1.30).

Problems associated with lamellar keratoplasty include epithelial ingrowths and interface scarring today called haze. The latter is caused by deposition of acid mucopolysaccharides in the wound gap in between donor and host tissue. Deep anterior lamellar keratoplasty (DALK) with extremely smooth surfaces of the lamellae seems to reduce the risk of postoperative haze. Downgrowth of corneal and conjunctival epithelial cells into the interface can occur after all lamellar corneal procedures (including LASIK) as well as after clear-cornea cataract surgery. If epithelium invades into the interface gap, whitish drop like material can be observed. Surgical removal of the tissue is indicated when visual acuity drops or the cells immigrate for more than 1–2 mm (see Chapter 5.4).

Posterior lamellar keratoplasty opens new options for a less invasive treatment of endothelial corneal dystrophies together with a much faster visual rehabilitation and no need to suture the cornea (DSAEK; Fig. 5.1.30).

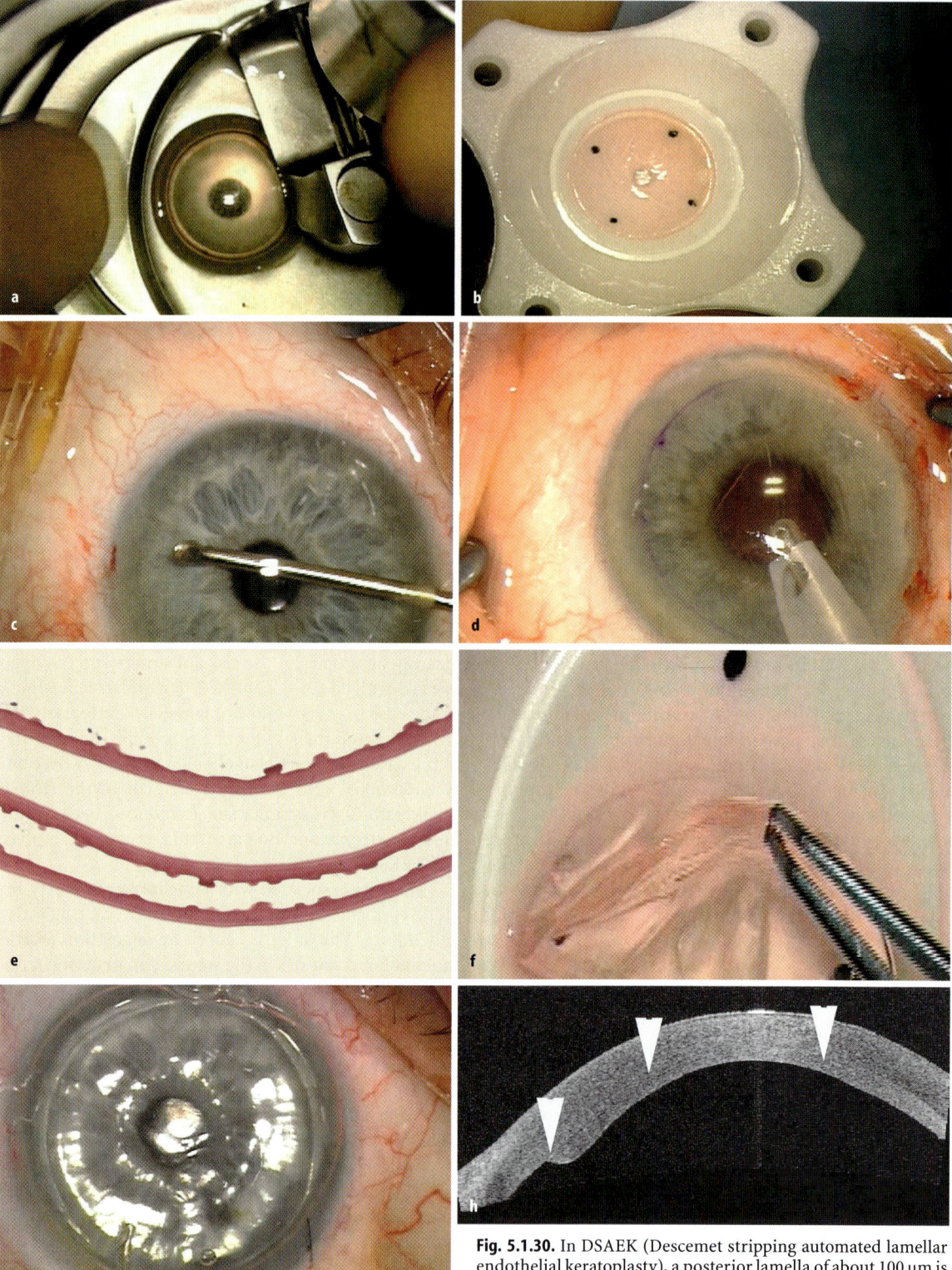

Fig. 5.1.30. In DSAEK (Descemet stripping automated lamellar endothelial keratoplasty), a posterior lamella of about 100 μm is cut with the microkeratome (**a**) from the donor cornea and punched out (**b**). In the patient, Descemet's membrane is removed from the cornea (**c**) and extracted from the eye (**d**). **e** Histology shows isolated removal of Descemet's membrane. The posterior donor lamellae is then placed behind the recipient's cornea (**f, g**) and fixed with air injection (to avoid pupillary block iridotomies are advisable). **h** Anterior segment OCT on day 7 demonstrates nicely adherent posterior lamellae (*arrows*) (from Cursiefen et al. 2007)

5.1.3.3
Refractive Surgery and Phototherapeutic Keratectomy

See section above.

5.1.3.4
Corneal Abrasion

Corneal abrasion means removal of corneal epithelium from the underlying basement membrane. Indications for corneal abrasion are: (1) recurrent corneal erosions secondary to dystrophies such as Cogan's or after trauma, and (2) conjunctival (pre)malignancies growing onto the cornea. This includes primary acquired melanosis with atypias, malignant melanomas of the conjunctiva, conjunctival intraepithelial neoplasia (CIN) and squamous cell carcinoma of the conjunctiva. During removal care has to be taken to remove all cells up to Bowmann's layer and beyond the limbal arcade. Bowman's layer should be left intact to act as a barrier against depth invasion. If histological workup suggests tumor infiltration up to the surgical excision margins, topical cytostatic treatment after surgery is recommended (such as mitomycin C 0.05% 5/daily for 2 weeks, then 2 weeks free interval and again 2 weeks treatment).

5.1.3.5
Amniotic Membrane Transplantation

Amniotic membrane transplantation has become a routine procedure for the treatment of persistent epithelial defects and stromal ulcers not amenable to conservative treatment. Amniotic membrane consists of a single epithelial layer, a basement membrane, and an acellular extracellular matrix (Fig. 5.1.31). The beneficial effect of amniotic membrane transplantation rests on several properties of this tissue: (1) amniotic membrane is anti-inflammatory (e.g., due to expression of interleukin-1 receptor antagonists) thereby dampening surface inflammation and promoting healing of the epithelial surface; (2) amniotic membrane is antiangio-

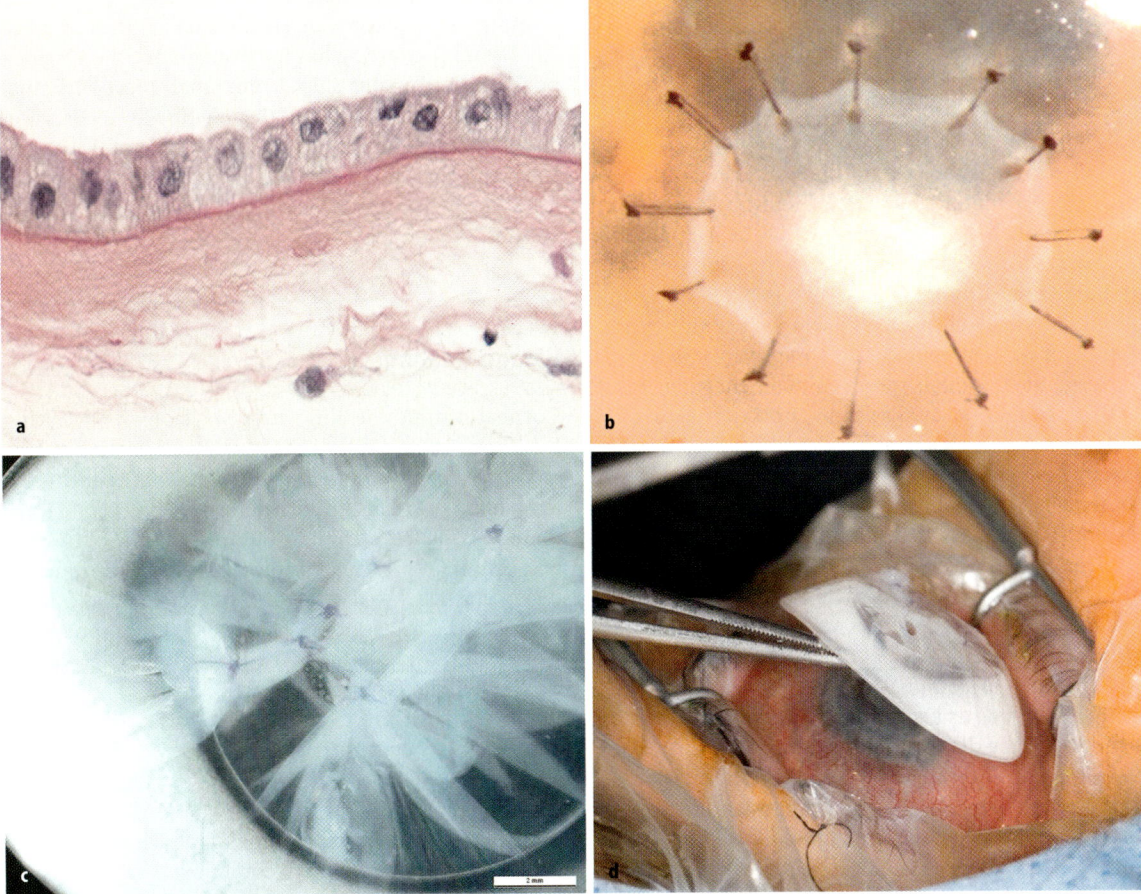

Fig. 5.1.31. Amniotic membrane consists of a single layer of epithelium with basement membrane and avascular stroma beneath (**a**). Amniotic membrane can be sutured directly onto the cornea (**b**) either as patch, graft or sandwich, or can be placed sutureless onto the cornea (**d**) after it has been sutured around an Illig device. **c** "Amniotic membrane covered bio-onlay" (from Cursiefen, Rummelt et al. 2007 and Seitz et al., 2005)

genic thereby reducing corneal neovascularization [e.g., by expression of pigment epithelium-derived factor (PEDF)]; (3) amniotic membrane can act as a basement membrane substrate for epithelial cells to grow out on; and (4) amniotic membrane integrates into the cornea intraepithelially, subepithelially and stromally and may thereby promote corneal biomechanical strength. Amniotic membrane can be used in three different surgical techniques: (1) as a biological contact lens (patch technique) when amniotic membrane is sutured above a persistent epithelial defect, e.g., in severe dry eye; (2) as a graft, when amniotic membrane layers are sutured into a corneal ulcer; and (3) in the sandwich technique, where patch and graft are combined. Amniotic membranes are quickly destroyed in acutely inflamed corneas sometimes within a few days; therefore it seems prudent to wait with amniotic membrane transplantation until corneal inflammation has calmed down. Restoration of epithelial hemidesmosomes on a basement membrane substrate is essential for permanent good epithelial adhesion. Amniotic membrane provides such a substrate and enables development of these adhesion structures.

5.1.3.6
Stem Cell Transplantation and Donor Limbal Stem Cell Procurement

Limbal stem cells are responsible for regeneration of corneal epithelium. They are located in a specialized "niche" at the limbus, clinically visible as the palisades of Vogt (Fig. 5.1.15). Histologically, the stem cell niche is characterized by melanin pigmented cells probably protecting stem cells from UV irradiation and by specialized basement membrane components (see Sect. 5.1.1.9 above). Limbal stem cell deficiency can result from hereditary (such as aniridia) or acquired diseases (most commonly chemical burns and autoimmune diseases). Destruction of the limbal epithelial cells has two consequences: loss of the normal barrier function of the limbal stem cells, that is loss of the sharp separation between vascularized conjunctiva and avascular cornea. This results in conjunctivalization of the corneal surface. Histologically, conjunctivalization is characterized by presence of goblet cells in the corneal surface and presence of conjunctival cytokeratins in corneal epithelium (such as keratin 19, loss of corneal keratins 3 and 12). If the diagnosis of conjunctivalization is not clear, the presence of goblet cells can clinically be detected using impression cytology and novel in-vivo confocal microscopically techniques. There seems to be a "cross-talk" between goblet cells, secreting the angiogenic growth factor VEGF, and stromal vascularization occurring in conjunctivalization. The other sequela of stem cell deficiency is persistent epithelial effects secondary to loss of normal epithelial regeneration. Based on the growing body of knowledge about limbal stem cells, recent years have seen a vast increase in therapeutic options for treatment of previously untreatable eyes with stem cell deficiency. Deficiency of limbal stem cells can be treated by limbal transplantation, either allogeneic or homologous. Second options are limbokeratoplasty procedures transplanting cornea and part of the limbus. The most recent and elegant therapy is the transplantation of ex-vivo cultivated limbal stem cells harvested either from the healthy contralateral eye or from donor eyes in case of bilateral diseases. This approach has the advantage of ex-vivo amplification of limbal stem cells, thereby minimizing the tissue which needs to be excised from the healthy eye and also allowing for storage of reserve tissue for later surgeries. Several potential media for transport of the cultivated stem cells exist: amniotic membrane, thermosensitive carriers and fibrin gels. The latter have the advantage of being more standardized than amniotic membrane and of easily dissolving on the ocular surface under local protease influence. Our own results and published data from the Pellegrini group suggest this approach to be effective in rehabilitating the ocular surface. Later penetrating keratoplasty can yield visual acuities of up to 1.0. Donor harvesting has to performed at the 12°clock position cutting out a 2×2 mm small piece of limbal tissue without damaging the healthy eye. Excision starts about 0.5 mm centrally to the edge of Bowman's layer and then moves posterior until about 1 mm behind it. Incision depth should not extend beyond 200 μm.

5.1.4
Wound Healing

Corneal wound healing after incisions penetrating Bowman's layer is different from wound healing at other sites of the body and much slower. That is due to the avascular nature of the cornea (lack of blood and lymphatic vessels), the immunosuppressed state of the cornea (immune privilege) and the tight interactions between epithelial and stromal cells ("cross-talk"). Most parts of the cornea such as Bowman' layer cannot be restored ad integrum. Special aspects of corneal wound healing will be discussed below:

5.1.4.1
Epithelial-Stromal Interactions

There is now ample evidence for an intensive molecular cross-talk between different components of the cornea. Stromal keratocytes, e.g., seem to depend on an intact corneal epithelium for survival. Experimental corneal abrasion causes apoptotic cell death of underlying keratocytes within minutes. This early response seems to be mediated via interleukin (IL)-1. Experimental PRK induces keratocyte apoptosis in underlying superficial stromal keratocytes, whereas LASIK causes apoptosis in keratocytes underlying the cut edge and along the stromal cut. This phenomenon can also be observed in patients with prolonged epithelial defects and after refractive surgical procedures. On the other hand, corneal epithelium does also play an important role in induction of myofibroblast differentiation of stromal keratocytes and haze development after refractive surgery. Fine-tuned pharmacologic interventions in this epithelial-stromal cross-talk may help minimize complications after refractive surgery in the future. Meanwhile special care has to be taken to avoid epithelial damage during surgery, also since corneal epithelium has potent anti-inflammatory and antiangiogenic properties. Interestingly, corneal epithelial regeneration after a stromal defect also "tries" to restore a smooth anterior corneal surface thereby partly regressing the effect of refractive surgery. The molecular mechanisms underlying this phenomenon are not understood.

Sufficient lubrication early postoperatively is nevertheless important to avoid epithelial wound healing problems. In contrast, in penetrating keratoplasty it takes up to 5 years for corneal nerves to reinnervate the central cornea so that moderate to severe forms of neurotrophic keratopathy with corneal ulceration can result. Central corneal sensitivity is usually not detectable until 18 months after surgery. To avoid neurotrophic complications and also to reduce corneal inflammation, which is caused by a dry ocular surface and which increases the risk for immune reactions by activating corneal antigen-presenting cells, sufficient lubrication at least until removal of the last sutures is mandatory.

Since it is now possible to visualize subbasal epithelial nerve bundles in vivo using confocal microscopy, it will be possible to individualize the hinge location during refractive surgery so that postoperative neurotrophic keratopathy can be minimized after LASIK (there are great interindividual variations in how subbasal corneal nerve bundles travel in each patient; see Sect. 5.1.1.10 above).

5.1.4.2
Epithelial Invasion (LASIK, Keratoplasty)

Any surgical procedure of the ocular surface and any traumatic displacement of epithelium into the eye can cause epithelial downgrowth into the anterior chamber or into the cornea. This can occur, e.g., after cataract surgery, keratoplasty or LASIK procedures. After LASIK, epithelium can invade into the flap bed. Epithelium has to be removed carefully surgically when invasion proceeds away from the surface or visual acuity drops. Risk factors include epithelial basement membrane dystrophies and type I diabetes.

Epithelial downgrowth into the anterior chamber may be either cystic or diffuse. Cystic epithelial downgrowth can be removed surgically completely by block excision (see Chapter 5.4; Fig. 5.4.31). Never try to laser these cysts since this can cause transformation into a diffuse epithelial invasion. Diffuse epithelial invasion usually is so extensive that it cannot be removed in toto; it invariably causes intractable rises of intraocular pressure (IOP). There is so far no curative treatment for extensive diffuse epithelial invasion.

5.1.4.3
Reinnervation After Penetrating Keratoplasty and Refractive Surgical Procedures

Corneal sensory innervations are cut completely during the process of penetrating keratoplasty and partly during LASIK. Consequently a mild neurotrophic keratopathy is common after both LASIK and keratoplasty. Fortunately, the keratopathy after LASIK usually is self-limited and disappears in most patients after 6 months.

5.1.4.4
Hem- and Lymphangiogenesis After Keratoplasty

The act of penetrating keratoplasty itself incites an angiogenic and lymphangiogenic response. After experimental penetrating keratoplasty in the mouse model of corneal transplantation, a combined outgrowth of both blood and lymphatic vessels can be observed starting at day 3 and reaching the donor-host interface at day 7 (Fig. 5.1.21). Since there is no significant difference in the angiogenic response after syngeneic versus allogeneic grafting, this early neovascularization after keratoplasty is not an early immune response, but rather a sequela of wound healing and surgical tissue destruction. The same phenomenon of postkeratoplasty neovascularization can be observed in patients – albeit to a lesser extent: About 50% of patients having undergone low-risk keratoplasty develop some mild neovascularization after low-risk keratoplasty. That this early postoperative neovacularization is related to wound healing and tissue destruction is nicely demonstrated by the observation that postoperative neovascularization is significantly greater after conventional mechanical versus non-mechanical excimer laser trephination (with less tissue destruction). Since postoperative neovascularization has been shown to be a risk factor for subsequent immune reactions, the surgical procedure itself and the surgical skills of the microsurgeon itself influence the postoperative neovascularization and postoperative rate of immune reactions.

5.1.4.5
Recurrence of Corneal Dystrophy

Since all surgical treatments available so far have not cured the diseased limbal epithelial stem cells themselves, recurrence of corneal dystrophies – especially the epithelial (and historically termed "stromal") ones caused by mutations in the keratoepithelin gene – is not surprising. Recurrences are most common after surgery for granular, then lattice and least common after surgery for macular corneal dystrophy. Nevertheless, we recently observed recurrence of a macular corneal dystrophy 49 years after initial penetrating keratoplasty. The former can often be treated with laser ablation of early superficial recurrence.

5.1.4.6
Replacement of Donor by Host Tissue After Keratoplasty

In contrast to other solid tissue transplantations and more like hematological transplants, most components of a donor cornea are replaced by recipient cells after keratoplasty. Whereas both clinical and experimental studies agree that corneal epithelium is quickly replaced by host epithelium, the rate and extent by which corneal stroma and endothelium is replaced by host tissue is very variable and depends on the primary cause of keratoplasty. Nonetheless both experimental and human studies demonstrate cases of a complete replacement of donor tissue by host cells. In contrast, late immune reactions occurring more than 10 years after keratoplasty indicate that depending on the primary cause, only incomplete replacement of donor tissue occurs.

References

Bock F, Dietrich T, Zimmermann P, Onderka J, Baier M, Cursiefen C. Antiangiogene Therapie am vorderen Augenabschnitt. Ophthalmologe 2007; 104:336–44

Bock F, Onderka J, Zahn G, Dietrich T, Bachmann B, Kruse FE, Cursiefen C. Bevacizumab is a potent inhibitor of inflammatory corneal angiogenesis and lymphangiogenesis. Invest Ophthalmol Vis Sci. 2007; 48:2545–52

Braun M, Holbach L, Naumann GOH. Die korneale Lipofuszinose – klinisch-pathologische Untersuchung von zehn Patienten. Klin Monatsbl Augenheilkd 1997; 210:121–123

Chen JJ, Tseng SC, 1991. Abnormal corneal epithelial wound healing in partial-thickness removal of limbal epithelium. Invest. Ophthalmol. Vis. Sci. 32, 2219–2233

Chen L, Hamrah P, Cursiefen C, Jackson D, Streilein JW, Dana MR. Vascular Endothelial Growth Factor Receptor-3 (VEGFR-3) mediates dendritic cell migration to lymph nodes and induction of immunity to corneal transplants. Nature Medicine 2004; 10:813–5

Chen Z, de Paiva CS, Luo L, Kretzer FL, Pflugfelder SC, Li D-Q, 2004. Characterization of putative stem cell phenotype in human limbal epithelia. Stem Cells 22, 355–366

Cursiefen C, Küchle M, Naumann GOH. Angiogenesis in corneal diseases: Histopathology of 254 human corneal buttons with neovascularization. Cornea 1998; 17: 611–613

Cursiefen C, Küchle M, Naumann GOH. Changing indications for penetrating keratoplasty: Histopathology of 1250 corneal buttons. Cornea 1998; 17: 468–470

Cursiefen C, Hofmann-Rummelt C, Schlötzer-Schrehardt U, Fischer DC, Küchle M. Immunphänotypische Klassifizierung der makulären Hornhautdystrophie: Erstbeschreibung des Immunphänotyps I A außerhalb Saudi-Arabiens. Klin Monatsbl Augenheilkd 2000; 217: 118–126

Cursiefen C, Rummelt C, Küchle M. Immunohistochemical localization of VEGF, TGFα and TGFβ$_1$ in human corneas with neovascularization. Cornea 2000; 19: 526–533

Cursiefen C, Schlötzer-Schrehardt U, Holbach M, Vieth M, Kuchelmeister K, Stolte M. Ocular findings in Fryns syndrome. Acta Ophthalmol Scand 2000; 78: 710–713

Cursiefen C, Hofmann-Rummelt C, Schlötzer-Schrehardt U, Fischer D-C, Haubeck H-D, Küchle M, Naumann GOH. Immunohistochemical classification of primary and recurrent macular corneal dystrophy in Germany. Subclassification of immunophenotype I A using a novel keratan sulfate antibody. Exp Eye Res 2001; 73: 593–600

Cursiefen C, Wenkel H, Martus P, Langenbucher A, Seitz B, Nguyen N, Küchle M, Naumann GOH. Peripheral corneal neovascularization after non-high risk-keratoplasty: influence of short- versus longtime topical steroids. Graefe's Arch Clin Exp Ophthalmol 2001; 239: 514–521

Cursiefen C, Martus P, Nguyen NX, Langenbucher A, Seitz B, Küchle M. Corneal neovascularization after nonmechanical versus mechanical corneal trephination for non-high-risk keratoplasty. Cornea 2002; 21: 648–652

Cursiefen C, Schlötzer-Schrehardt U, Küchle M, Sorokin L, Breitender-Geleff S, Alitalo K, Jackson D. Lymphatic vessels in vascularized human corneas: immunohistochemical investigation using LYVE-1 and Podoplanin. Invest Ophthalmol Vis Sci 2002; 43: 2127–2135

Cursiefen C, Chen L, Dana MR, Streilein JW. Corneal lymphangiogenesis: Evidence, mechanisms and implications for transplant immunology. Cornea 2003; 22: 273–81

Cursiefen C, Seitz B, Dana MR, Streilein JW. Angiogenese und Lymphangiogenese in der Hornhaut: Pathogenese, Klinik und Therapieoptionen. Ophthalmologe 2003; 100:292–9

Cursiefen C, Rummelt C, Küchle M, Schlötzer-Schrehardt U. Pericyte recruitment in human corneal angiogenesis. Br J Ophthalmol 2003; 87: 101–106

Cursiefen C, Chen L, Borges L, Jackson D, D'Amore PA, Dana MR, Wiegand SJ, Streilein JW. Via bone marrow-derived macrophages, VEGF A mediates lymph- and hemangiogenesis in inflammatory neovascularization. J Clin Investigation 2004; 113:1040–50

Cursiefen C, Maruyama K, Liu Y, Chen L, Jackson D, Wiegand S, Dana MR, Streilein JW. Inhibition of hemangiogenesis and lymphangiogenesis *after* normal-risk corneal transplantation by neutralizing VEGF promotes graft survival. Invest Ophthalmol Vis Sci 2004;45:2666–73.

Cursiefen C, Masli S, Ng TF, Dana MR, Bornstein P, Lawler J, Streilein JW. Roles of thrombospondin 1 and 2 in regulating spontaneous and induced angiogenesis in the cornea and iris. Invest Ophthalmol Vis Sci 2004; 45:1117–24

Cursiefen C, Ikeda S, Nishina PM, Smith RS, Ikeda A, Jackson D, Mo JS, Chen L, Dana RM, Pytowski B, Kruse FE, Streilein JW. Spontaneous corneal hem- and lymphangiogenesis in mice with destrin-mutation depend on VEGFR3-signaling. Am J Pathol 2005; 166: 1367–1377

Cursiefen C, Seitz B, Kruse FE. Neurotrophe Keratopathie: Pathogenese, Klinik und Therapie. Ophthalmologe 2005;102: 7–14

Cursiefen C, Seitz B, Kruse FE. 100 Jahre Hornhauttransplantation. Eine Erfolgsgeschichte mit Zukunft. Deutsches Ärzteblatt 2005:45: Seite A–3078

Cursiefen C, Chen L, Saint-Geniez M, Hamrah P, Jin Y, Rashid S, Pytowski B, Streilein JW, Dana MR. Nonvascular VEGF receptor 3 expression by corneal epithelium maintains avascularity and vision. Proc Natl Acad Sci U S A. 2006; 103: 11405–10

Cursiefen C, Maruyama M, Jackson DG, Streilein W, Kruse FE. Time-course of angiogenesis and lymphangiogenesis after brief corneal inflammation. Cornea 2006;25:443–7

Cursiefen C, Rummelt C, Neuhuber W, Kruse FE, Schroedl F. Absence of blood and lymphatic vessels in the developing human cornea. Cornea 2006; 25:722–6

Cursiefen C, Rummelt C, Kruse FE. Amniotic membrane covered bi-onlay. Br J Ophthalmol 2007; 91:841–2

Daniels JT, Dart JKG, Tuft SJ, Khaw PT, 2001. Corneal stem cells in review. Wound Rep. Reg. 9, 483–494

Davanger M, Evensen A, 1971. Role of the pericorneal papillary structure in renewal of corneal epithelium. Nature 229, 560–561

Dua HS, Azuara-Blanco A, 2000. Limbal stem cells of the corneal epithelium. Surv. Ophthalmol. 44, 415–425

Dua HS, Joseph A, Shanmuganathan VA, Jones RE, 2003. Stem cell differentiation and the effects of deficiency. Eye 17, 877–885

Goldberg MF, Bron AJ, 1982. Limbal palisades of Vogt. Trans. Am. Ophthalmol. Soc. 80, 155–171

Gottschalk K, Rummelt C, Cursiefen C. Therapierefraktäre Bindehautchemosis. Klin Monatsbl Augenheilkd 2006; 223: 696–8

Grueterich M, Espana EM, Touhami A, Ti SE, Tseng SC, 2002. Phenotypic study of a case with successful transplantation of ex vivo expanded human limbal epithelium for unilateral total limbal stem cell deficiency. Ophthalmology 109, 1547–1552

Grueterich M, Espana EM, Tseng SCG, 2003. Ex vivo expansion of limbal epithelial stem cells: amniotic membrane serving as a stem cell niche. Surv. Ophthalmol. 48, 631–646

Hamrah P, Liu Y, Zhang Q, Dana MR. The corneal stroma is endowed with a significant number of resident dendritic cells. Invest Ophthalmol Vis Sci. 2003;44:581–9.

Holbach LM, Font RL, Baehr W, Pittler SJ. HSV antigen and HSV DNA in a vascular and vascularized lesion of Hornhautstroma keratitis. Curr Eye Res 1991; 10 Suppl. 63–68

Holbach LM, Seitz B, Rummelt C, Naumann GOH. An increasing optical density of stromal lesions is associated with a decrease of detectable HSV antigen in HS-keratitis. Invest Ophthalmol Vis Sci 1992; 33: 482

Holland EJ, Schwartz GS, 1996. The evolution of epithelial transplantation for severe ocular surface disease and a proposed classification system. Cornea 15, 549–556

Huang AJ, Tseng SC, 1991. Corneal epithelial wound healing in the absence of limbal epithelium. Invest. Ophthalmol. Vis. Sci. 32, 96–105

Inatomi T, Nakamura T, Koizumi N, Sotozono C, Kinoshita S, 2005. Current concepts and challenges in ocular surface reconstruction using cultivated mucosal epithelial transplantation. Cornea. 24, S32–S38

Kenyon KR, Tseng SC, 1989. Limbal autograft transplantation for ocular surface disorders. Ophthalmology 96, 709–722

Koizumi N, Inatomi T, Suzuki T, Sotozono C, Kinoshita S, 2001. Cultivated corneal epithelial stem cell transplantation in ocular surface disorders. Ophthalmology 108, 1569–1574

Kruse FE, Reinhard T, 2001. Limbal transplantation for ocular surface reconstruction. Ophthalmologe 98, 818–831

Kruse FE, Cursiefen C, Seitz B, Voelcker HE, Naumann GOH, Holbach L. Klassifikation von Erkrankungen der Augenoberflaeche. Teil I. Ophthalmologe 2003; 100:899–915

Küchle M, Cursiefen C, Fischer D-C, Schlötzer-Schrehardt U, Naumann GOH. Recurrent macular corneal dystrophy type II 49 years after penetrating keratoplasty. Arch Ophthalmol 1999; 117: 528–531

Küchle M, Cursiefen C, Nguyen NX, Langenbucher A, Seitz B, Wenkel H, Martus P, Naumann GOH. Risk factors for corneal allograft rejection: intermediate results of a prospective normal-risk keratoplasty study. Graefe's Arch Clin Exp Ophthalmol 2002; 240: 580–584

Lavker RM, Dong G, Cheng SZ, Kudoh K, Cotsarelis G, Sun TT, 1991. Relative proliferative rates of limbal and corneal epithelia. Implications of corneal epithelial migration, circadian rhythm, and suprabasally located DNA-synthesizing keratinocytes. Invest. Ophthalmol. Vis. Sci. 32, 1864–1875

Lavker RM, Sun T-T, 2000. Epidermal stem cells: properties, markers, and location. Proc. Natl. Acad. Sci. USA. 97, 10960–10965

Lavker RM, Tseng SCG, Sun T-T, 2004. Corneal epithelial stem cells at the limbus: looking at some old problems from a new angle. Exp. Eye Res. 78, 433–446

Lehrer MS, Sun T-T, Lavker RM, 1998. Strategies of epithelial repair: modulation of stem cell and transit amplifying cell proliferation. J. Cell Sci. 111, 2867–2875

Lindberg K, Brown ME, Chaves HV, Kenyon KR, Rheinwald JG, 1993. In vitro propagation of human ocular surface epithelial cells for transplantation. Invest. Ophthalmol. Vis. Sci. 34, 2672–2679

Maruyama K, Li M, Cursiefen C, Keino H, Tomita M, Takenaka H, Jackson DG, Losordo DW, Streilein JW. Inflammatory lymphangiogenesis arises from CD11b+ macrophages. J Clin Invest 2005; 115: 2363–2372

Muller LF, Marfurt CF, Kruse FE, Tervo T. Corneal nerves: structure, contents and function. Exp Eye Res. 2003; 76: 521–42

Naumann GOH et al. Pathologie des Auges. Berlin: Springer 1980; 2. edition, 1997

Naumann GOH, Sautter H, (Mitwirkung von Bigar F) Surgical procedures of the Cornea, chapter 7 in: "Surgical Ophthalmology 1", Blodi FC, Mackensen G, Neubauer H. (eds.), Heidelberg-New York, Springer Verlag, 433–508, 1991

Naumann GOH. The Bowman Lecture Nr. 56, Part II: Corneal Transplantation in Anterior Segment Diseases. Eye 1995; 9:398–421

Nguyen NX, Langenbucher A, Seitz B, Graupner M, Cursiefen C, Kuchle M, Naumann GOH. Blood-aqueous barrier breakdown after penetrating keratoplasty with simultaneous extracapsular cataract extraction and posterior chamber lens implantation. Graefe's Arch Clin Exp Ophthalmol 2001; 239: 114–117

Nguyen NX, Seitz B, Langenbucher A, Wenkel H, Cursiefen C. [Clinical aspects and treatment of immunological endothelial graft rejection following penetrating normal-risk keratoplasty]. Klin Monatsbl Augenheilkd. 2004;221:467–72.

Pellegrini G, Traverso CE, Franzi AT, Zingirian M, Cancedda R, de Luca M, 1997. Long-term restoration of damaged corneal surface with autologous cultivated corneal epithelium. Lancet 349, 990–993

Puangsricharern V, Tseng SCG, 1995. Cytologic evidence of corneal diseases with limbal stem cell deficiency. Ophthalmology 102, 1476–1485

Sangwan VS, 2002. Limbal stem cells in health and disease. Biosci. Rep. 21, 385–405

Schermer A, Galvin S, Sun T-T, 1986. Differentiation-related expression of a major 64K corneal keratin in vivo and in culture. J. Cell Biol. 103, 49–62

Schlötzer-Schrehardt U, Kruse FE. Identification and characterization of limbal stem cells. Exp Eye Res. 2005;81:247–64

Schwab IR, Reyes M, Isseroff RR, 2000. Successful transplantation of bioengineered tissue replacements in patients with ocular surface disease. Cornea 19, 421–426

Seitz B, Grüterich M, Cursiefen C, Kruse FE. Konservative und chirurgische Therapie der neurotrophen Keratopathie. Ophthalmologe 2005;102:15–26

Streilein JW. Ocular immune privilege: therapeutic opportunities from an experiment of nature. Nat Rev Immunol. 2003; 3:879–89

Sun T-T, Lavker RM, 2004. Corneal epithelial stem cells: past, presence, and future. J. Invest. Dermatol. Symp. Proc., 1–6.

Tseng SCG, 1989. Concept and application of limbal stem cells. Eye 3, 141–157

Tseng SCG, 1996. Regulation and clinical implications of corneal epithelial stem cells. Mol. Biol. Rep. 23, 47–58

Tseng SC, Meller D, Anderson DF, Touhami A, Pires RT, Grueterich M, Solomon A, Espana E, Sandoval H, Ti SE, Goto E, 2002. Ex vivo preservation and expansion of human limbal epithelial stem cells on amniotic membrane for treating corneal diseases with total limbal stem cell deficiency. Adv. Exp. Med. Biol. 506, 1323–1334

Vinh L, Nguyen N, Martus P, Seitz B, Kruse FE, Cursiefen C. Surgery-related factors influencing corneal neovascularization after low-risk keratoplasty. Am J Ophthalmol 2006; 141:260–266

Glaucoma Surgery

A. Jünemann, G.O.H. Naumann

5.2.1 Principal Aspects of Glaucomas and Their Terminology

Glaucomas are a group of diseases that share as their main, but not only, risk factor an increased intraocular pressure leading to progressive and irreversible damage to the optic nerve head (Table 5.2.1). *Acute* glaucomas may develop sectorial iris necrosis and if the intraocular pressure is not relieved progressive ischemic infarcts of the prelaminar optic nerve disc are invaded by hyaluronic acid flowing from the vitreous cavity through the defective internal limiting membrane, so-called *cavernous optic atrophy*. In the acute phase the optic disc is prominent with indistinct borders – often invisible because of opaque optic media.

Chronic glaucomas develop a characteristic *excavation*, which can be documented by imaging techniques and quantified. Damage to the optic nerve head is the most important consequence of all glaucomas but the other intraocular tissues are also affected.

Primary glaucomas occur without obvious other intraocular disease, while *secondary* glaucomas follow other intraocular or extraocular diseases. The rise in intraocular pressure is almost always the consequence of an obstruction of the aqueous outflow either via the iris root covering the trabecular meshwork up to Schwalbe's line or due to obstacles in the trabecular meshwork in a gonioscopically open angle. Hypersecretion of aqueous is rare and not of practical significance.

Therapy for the *acute glaucomas* as a rule requires *immediate* microsurgical intervention to improve outflow. Therapy for the *chronic glaucomas* today usually starts with medications, most often applied locally but occasionally systemically. We shall discuss below both laser- and mechanical microsurgery for the improvement of aqueous outflow. If this is unsuccessful, cyclodestruction by various means has the aim of reducing aqueous inflow in the pars plicata of the ciliary body in order to balance the reduced outflow in acute and chronic glaucomas.

5.2.2 Surgical Anatomy

The intraocular pressure depends on a free flow of aqueous from the pars plicata of the ciliary body through the free space between the lens equator and ciliary body, the pupillary zone to the anterior chamber and the chamber angle. 85° continue through the trabecular meshwork to Schlemm's canal and 15% via the uveoscleral outflow following the supraciliary space. Flow from the secreting non-pigmenting ciliary epithelium through the narrow space between the lens equator and ciliary body is only rarely inhibited. Outflow through the normal pupillary zone has to overcome a *physiologic pupillary resistance*, which increases with age due to enlargement of the lens and rising rigidity of the iris sphincter. It is not continuous but intermitted and pulsatile. In comparison to other tissues the normal intraocular pressure is elevated. This is maintained by a physiologic resistance of outflow through the trabecular meshwork to Schlemm's canal and the collector channels leading to the aqueous veins visible at the limbus corneae (Fig. 5.2.1).

5.2.2.1 Landmarks for Gonioscopy

Landmarks for gonioscopy can only be recognized if the histopathology is kept in mind. Schwalbe's line or rim, corneoscleral and uveoscleral portions of the trabecular meshwork, scleral spur, and ciliary muscle insertion (Fig. 5.2.2) are gonioscopically the distinct parts of the anterior chamber angle (see also Chapter 5.3).

Table 5.2.1. Principal terminology of glaucomas

1. Clinical course:	Acute Chronic
2. Intraocular pressure:	High > 30 mm Hg "Ocular hypertension" 20 – 30 mm Hg "Normal tension" 10 – 20 mm Hg
3. Access to trabecular meshwork in anterior chamber:	Open angle ("narrow" variant and RAM) see Table 5.2.5 Closed angle

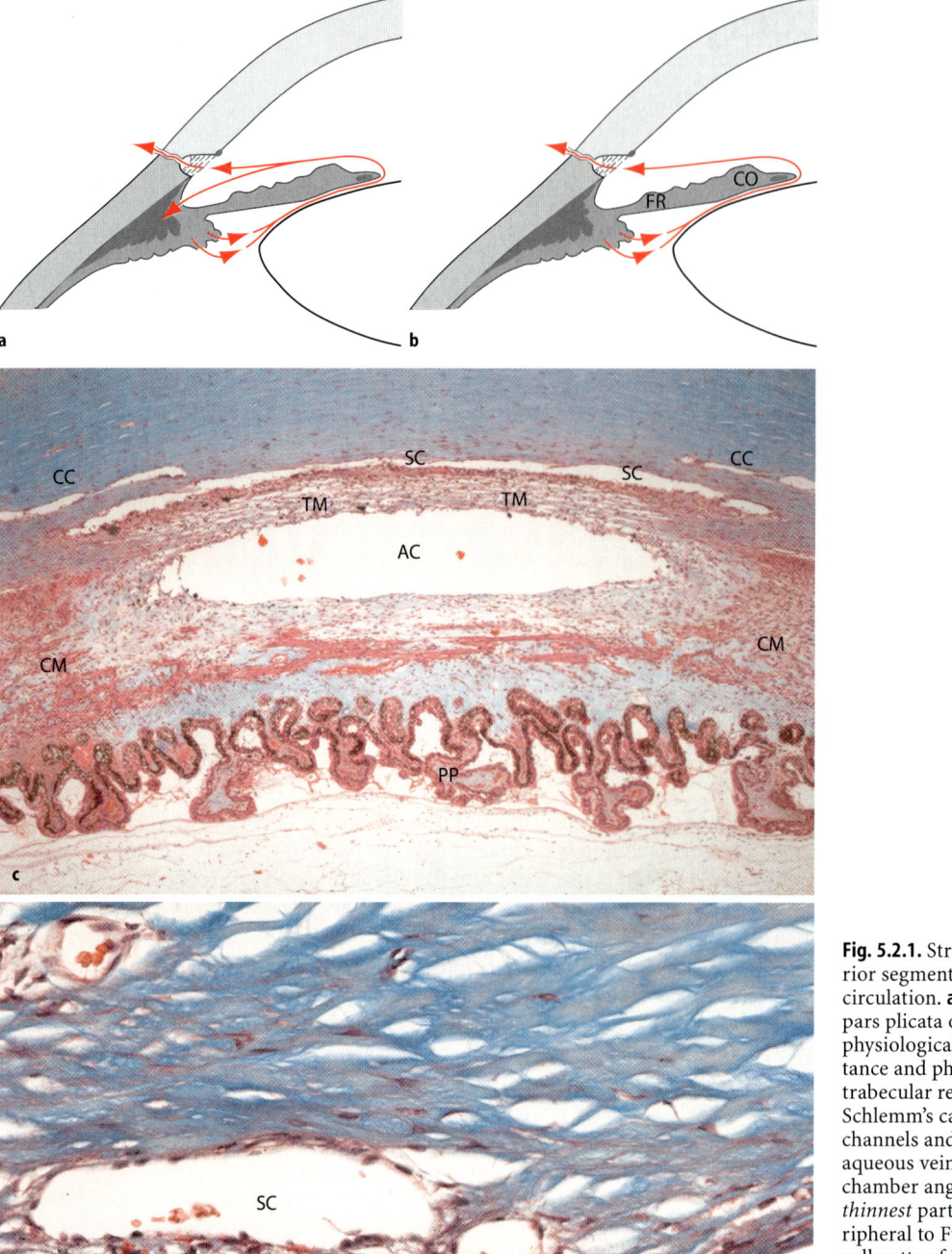

Fig. 5.2.1. Structures of anterior segment for aqueous circulation. **a** Secretion of pars plicata of ciliary body, physiological pupillary resistance and physiologic transtrabecular resistance to Schlemm's canal, collector channels and episcleral aqueous veins. **b** Normal chamber angle iris root as *thinnest* part of the iris, peripheral to Fuchs' roll (*FR*), collarette of iris (*CO*). **c** Section through Schlemm's canal (*SC*), trabecular meshwork (*TM*), most peripheral anterior chamber (*AC*), anterior portion of ciliary body with ciliary processes (*PP*). Ciliary muscle (*CM*) **d** Trabecular meshwork showing uveocorneal and scleral corneal portion of trabecular meshwork and Schlemm's canal with septae (Masson stain)

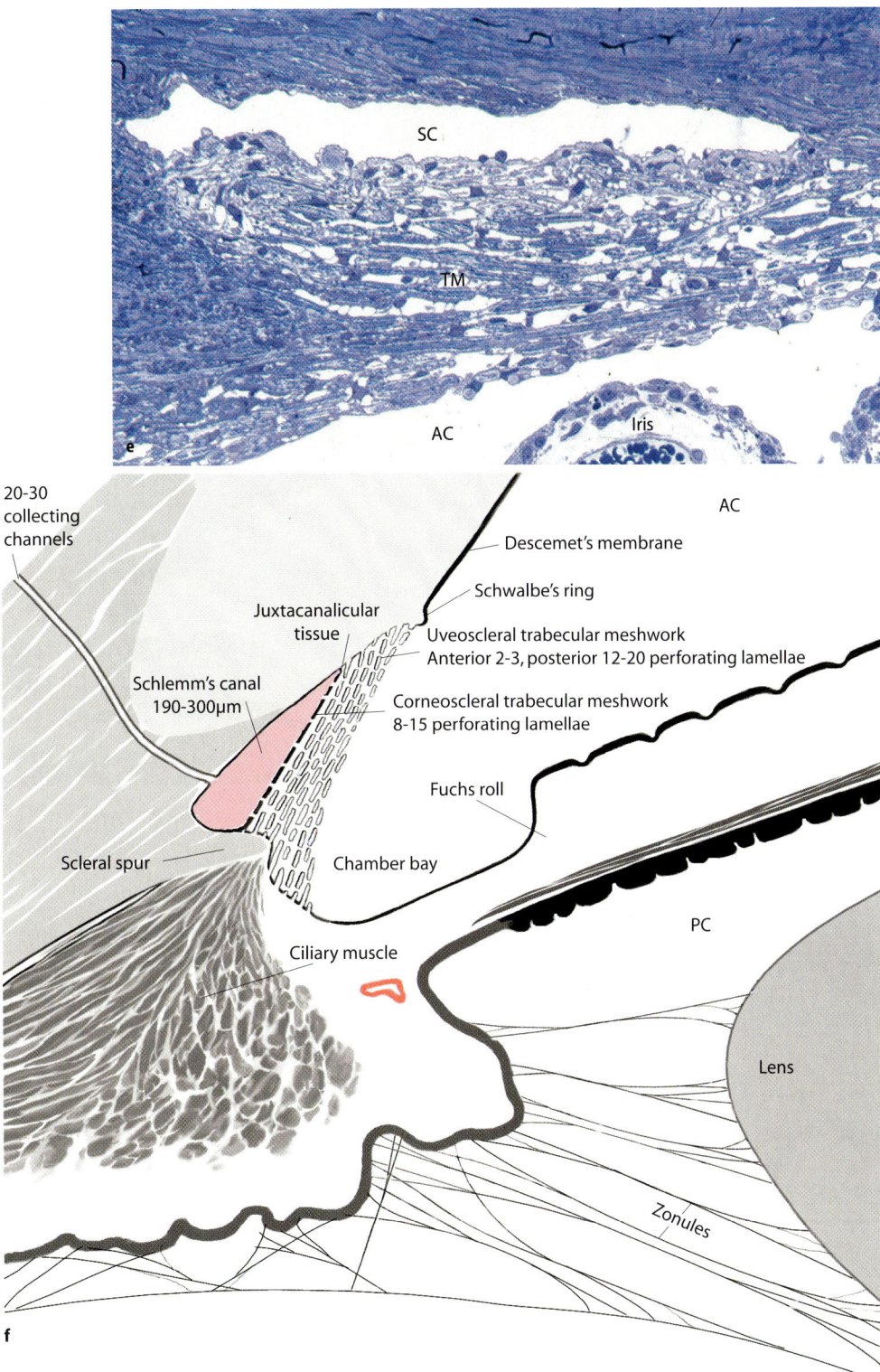

Fig. 5.2.1. e Trabecular meshwork (semi-thin section). (Courtesey of U. Schlötzer-Schrehardt). **f** Microanatomy of iris root, trabecular meshwork: Fuchs' roll (*FR*), uveocorneal (*UC*) and scleral corneal portion (*SC*) of trabecular meshwork, collector channels (*CC*), scleral spur (*SS*), ciliary muscle (*CM*), Schwalbe's line (*SL*), Schlemm's canal (*pink*); ciliary arterial circle of ciliary body (*red*) may be located in front of the ciliary muscle, but usually is embedded in the ciliary muscle. Note that the thinnest portion of the iris is located peripheral to Fuchs' roll

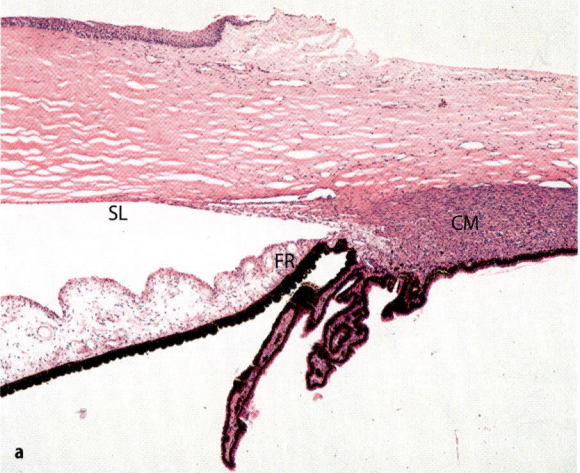
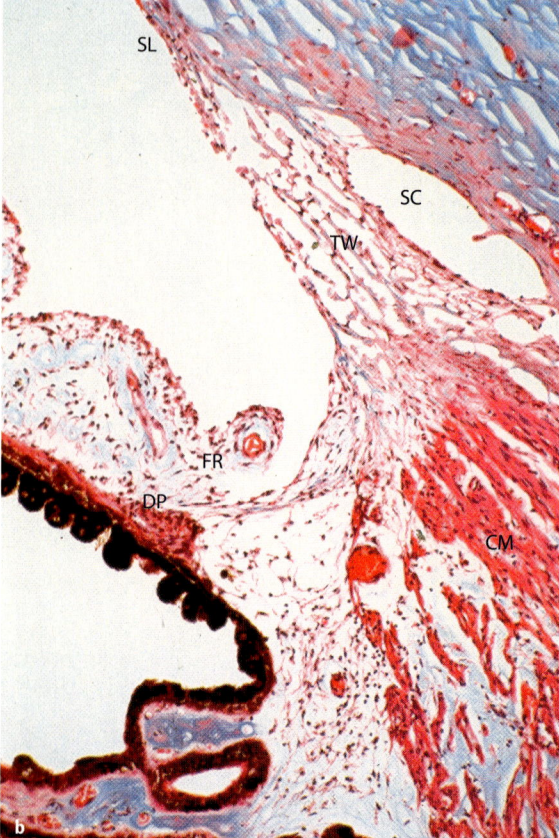

Fig. 5.2.2. Variation of chamber angle in unremarkable anterior segment. **a** Three-year-old child. **b** Structures of iris stroma covering anterior face of ciliary body extending to trabecular meshwork. Insertion of ciliary muscle (*red*) to scleral spur (*blue*) (Masson stain). **c** Different sections through chamber angle arranged from age 26 years up to age 71 years (PAS) Schwalbe line (*SL*), Schlemm canal (*SC*) Trabecular meshwork (*TW*), Ciliary muscle (*CM*), Dilatator pupillae (*DP*)

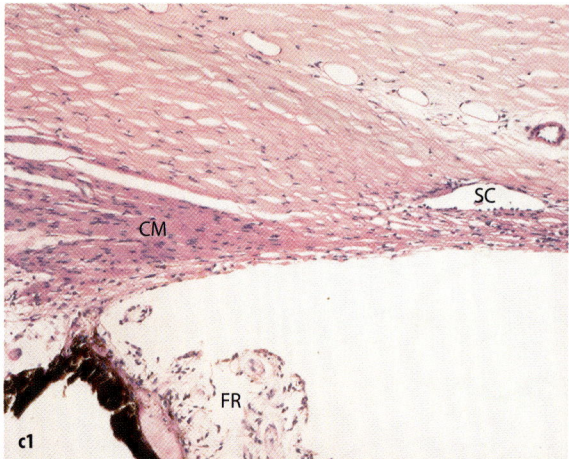
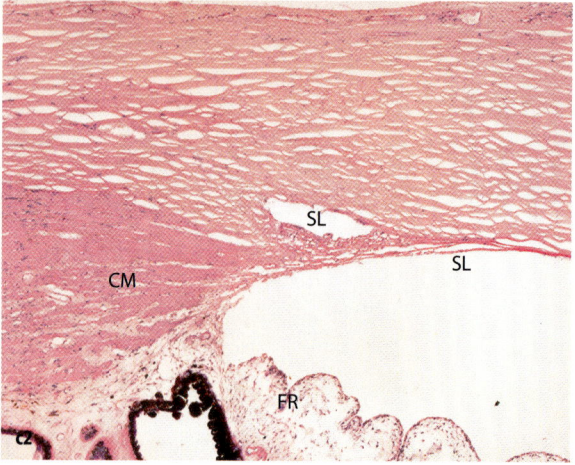

As persisting pathologic increased intraocular pressure originates from changes in the chamber angle, this region deserves special attention. The normal chamber angle really forms not an angle but rather a rounded *bay* and shows considerable variation in the degree of the angle between iris and cornea and also in the amount of uveal tissue connecting the iris stroma and scleral spur with strands up to Schwalbe's line (Fig. 5.2.1f).

Orientation is facilitated with aging as phagocytized melanin granules in the trabecular endothelium by their contrast allow easier recognition of the landmarks. Schlemm's canal is not directly visible, but retrograde blood filling from the aqueous veins to the collector channels into Schlemm's canal may help to locate this critical structure particularly in relatively young individuals – melanin dispersion and phagocytosis in the trabecular meshwork are usually not yet obvious. The relationship between Fuchs' roll and Schwalbe's ring must be kept in mind. Again, the position of the lens equator in relation to structures of the trabecular

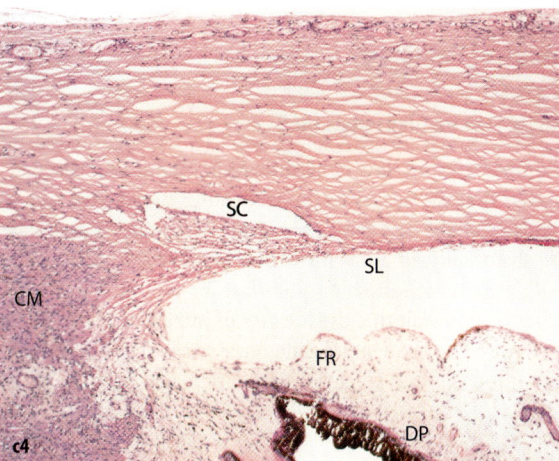

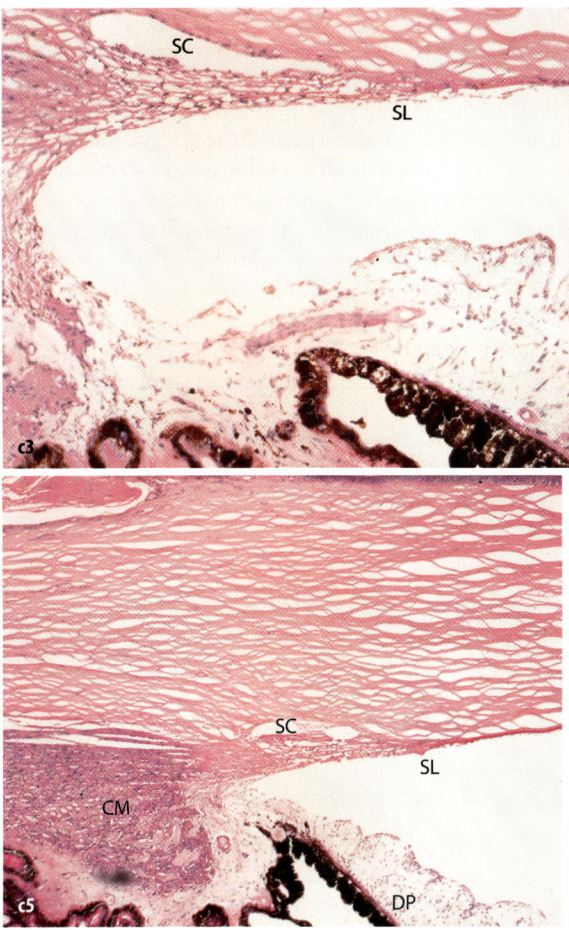

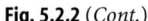

Fig. 5.2.2 (*Cont.*)

meshwork and pars plicata of the ciliary body individually vary widely. Asian eyes often are characterized by their relatively narrow anterior segment, which plays a role in the more common variants of angle closure glaucoma – also with a chronic course.

5.2.2.2
Landmarks for Surgical Corneal Limbus

Obviously this is the second most important region in glaucoma surgery: Current microsurgical procedures focus on the region of the limbus corneae, a relatively vague term. The *landmarks for the microsurgeon* working under a conjunctival flap are the peripheral *edge of Bowman's layer* and after creating a thick limbus based scleral flap the *scleral spur, Schlemm's canal* and *Schwalbe's line or rim*.

The anatomical limbus is situated where the peripheral cornea meets the sclera externally. The conjunctiva and Tenon's fascia insert separately within about 0.5 mm; the conjunctival epithelium covers the peripheral insertion of Tenon's fascia.

The limbus is a broad area of transition about 1 mm in width. The microscopic structure of the central border of the limbus towards the cornea is the end of Bowman's lamella and the end of Descemet's membrane, respectively. The peripheral border of the limbus is the scleral spur. Macroscopically a bluish-gray nacre-like appearance, due to the extension of the deeper corneal lamellae beyond the external margin of the peripheral cornea, constitutes the *surgical limbus* (see Fig. 5.2.14).

Posterior to the deep extending corneal lamellae in the scleral bed the sclera shows a more whitish and nacre-like appearance within a small area. This is the external landmark of the scleral spur. Anterior to this landmark, Schlemm's canal and trabecular meshwork appear as a grayish band. Retrograde blood filling of Schlemm's canal, i.e., following paracentesis, marks it as a reddish gray band. Additional landmarks can be aqueous veins, lymphatic channels (see Chapter 5.1) and surrounding capillaries along the canal of Schlemm. The scleral spur extends slightly posterior to this junction. It is important to recognize these landmarks, particularly when performing trabeculotomy of "non-penetrating" filtration surgery. The ciliary body is attached to the uveocorneal junction of the trabecular band and the sclera at the scleral spur.

Dissection through the sclera posterior to this junction will expose the ciliary muscle behind the pars plicata. Dissection of the scleral spur in trabeculotomy due to the false position of the trabeculotomy probe may result in cyclodialysis with persistent ocular hypotony (Chapter 5.4).

5.2.3
Surgical Pathology

5.2.3.1
Angle Closure Glaucomas (ACG)

Gonioscopy or low magnification light microscopy shows that the access to the trabecular meshwork is occluded by the iris root in contact with the trabecular meshwork up to Schwalbe's line (Figs. 5.2.3, 5.2.4a–d). Angle closures following *pupillary* or *ciliary block* (see Chapter 2) result in a drastic rise of intraocular pressure and the signs of an *acute* glaucoma: corneal endothelium decompensation, sectorial ischemic iris-necrosis with immobile distorted pupil and massive conjunctival and ciliary hyperemia of the episcleral vessels and multiple focal necrosis of the lens epithelium ("*Glaukomflecken*") (Fig. 5.2.5a–d). The cavernous atrophy of the optic disc usually is not visible because of the opaque media.

Patients from Asia also develop a *chronic* type of glaucoma due to progressive closure of the angle caused by *iris plateau syndrome* in the narrow anterior chamber with ciliary processes crowded behind the iris root.

Secondary ACGs most often develop rubeosis iridis following central retinal vein occlusion (CRVO), diabetic retinopathy and persisting retinal detachment (see Chapter 5.6). Insufficient restoration of the anteri-

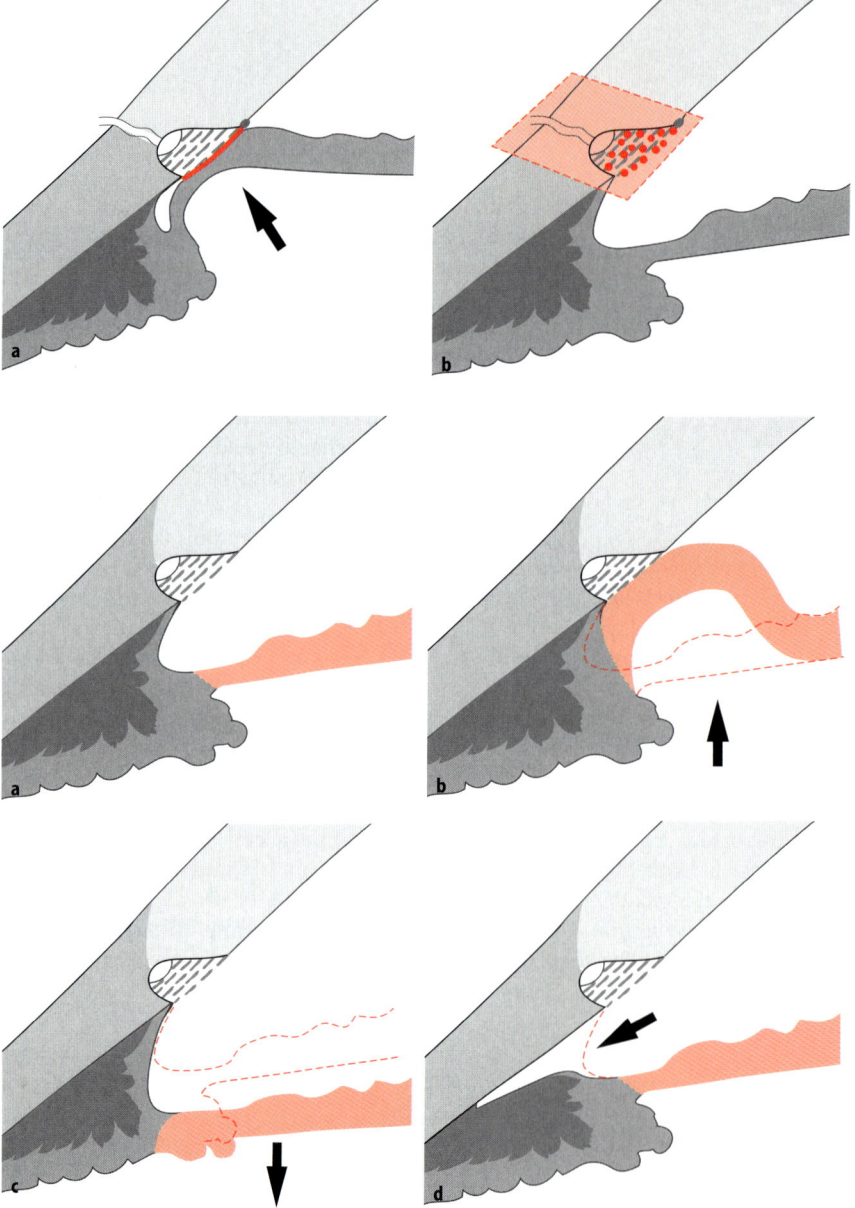

Fig. 5.2.3. Fundamental glaucoma patterns: **a** Angle closure glaucomas; **b** open angle glaucomas

Fig. 5.2.4. Chamber angle pattern by gonioscopy: **a** Wide open angle does not allow differentiation between normal and primary open angle glaucoma. **b** Angle closure glaucoma: iris root covering trabecular meshwork up to Schwalbe's line. **c** Contusion deformity of the anterior angle from displacement of the inner ciliary body tissue posteriorly. **d** Cyclodialysis following contusion

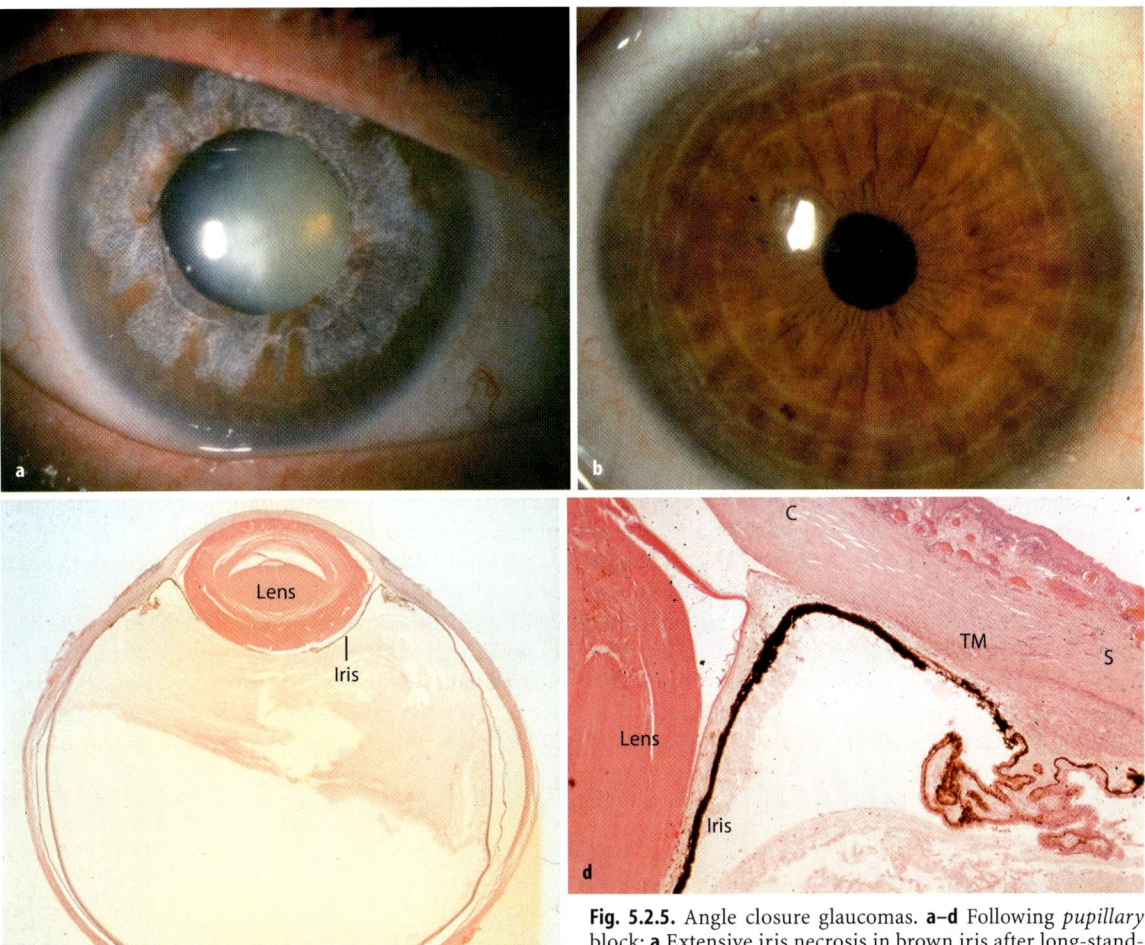

Fig. 5.2.5. Angle closure glaucomas. **a–d** Following *pupillary* block: **a** Extensive iris necrosis in brown iris after long-standing pupillary block. **b** In comparison to the uninvolved eye. **c, d** Anterior pupillary block by lens luxation in anterior chamber. Intumescent cataract. Trabecular meshwork (*TM*). Cornea (*C*), Sclera (*S*)

Table 5.2.2. Classification of primary and secondary angle closure glaucoma

Pupillary block
Primary "classic acute angle closure glaucoma"
Secondary: often with iris bombé

By ciliary block
Primary (very rare)
Secondary: ciliolenticular block: "malignant glaucoma": ciliovitreal block: seen in aphakia (rare)

Without pupillary or ciliary block
Primary: plateau iris (rare in Caucasians)
Secondary: due to peripheral synechiae without rubeosis iridis (e.g., associated with uveitis or after perforating injury)

With rubeosis iridis (associated with proliferative retinopathy) (e.g., diabetes mellitus, central vein occlusion and corneal endothelial overgrowth)

Table 5.2.3. Differential diagnosis of angle closure glaucomas

Parameter	After pupillary block	After ciliolenticular block
Distance between lens and cornea	Unchanged (lens in place)	Lens displaced anteriorly
Site of blockage of aqueous flow	Posterior to pupil	Posterior to lens
Conservative therapy	Miotics	Cycloplegia
Surgical therapy	Iridectomy (shunt between anterior and posterior chamber)	Lens extraction (with or without posterior pars plana sclerectomy and vitrectomy)

or chamber after perforating trauma or surgery also leads to angle closure. All variants may be associated with corneal endothelial proliferation and migration across the iridocorneal zone of contact in front of Schwalbe's line forming a pseudo-angle. More persons are found to have closed angles with anterior segment no-contact OCT than with gonioscopy in Asian eyes (Nolan et al., 2007; He et al, 2006).

5.2.3.2
Open Angle Glaucomas (OAG)

Gonioscopically and by light microscopy we cannot distinguish the appearance of the angle in a normal and in a primary open angle glaucoma (POAG) (Fig. 5.2.6a, b). Electron microscopically an increased number of Rohen plaques in the juxtacanicular region of the trabecular meshwork is supposed to distinguish the normal aging of trabecular meshwork from the pathology of primary open angle glaucoma. The number of trabecular endothelial cells decreases with age by 0.5% (Alvarado 1981) to 0.8% (Grierson 1984) per year. Primary open angle glaucomas show a trabecular endothelial cell count of *half* of the age norm (Tables 5.2.7, 5.2.8; see also Quigley, 2005; Jonas et al., 1999).

5.2.3.3
Secondary Open Angle Glaucomas (SOAG)

In contrast to primary, secondary open angle glaucomas reveal morphologic findings to illustrate the cause of the obstruction: Coagulated blood clot and black ball hyphema; *macrophagocytic* open angle glaucomas with hypermature cataract (*phacolytic*); and hemolytic, melanolytic and silicophagic glaucomas, which are in fact *acute* glaucomas requiring immediate microsurgical attention (Fig. 5.2.7, Tables 5.2.4, 5.2.5). In contrast to the elevated outflow resistance at the inner wall of Schlemm's canal, the pathology in SOAG due to dilated episcleral veins (Radius-Maumenee syndrome) is located outside Schlemm's canal (Fig. 5.2.8a–c). This entity requires a different surgical approach; sinosotomy (Ruprecht and Naumann, 1984) (see Fig. 5.2.14).

The most common type of chronic secondary open angle glaucoma is associated with *pseudoexfoliation syndrome*, demonstrating the typical microfibrillar deposits within the trabecular meshwork particularly juxtacanalicularly to Schlemm's canal (see Chapter 6.3). The more pseudoexfoliation (PEX) material is deposited the more likely ocular hypertension

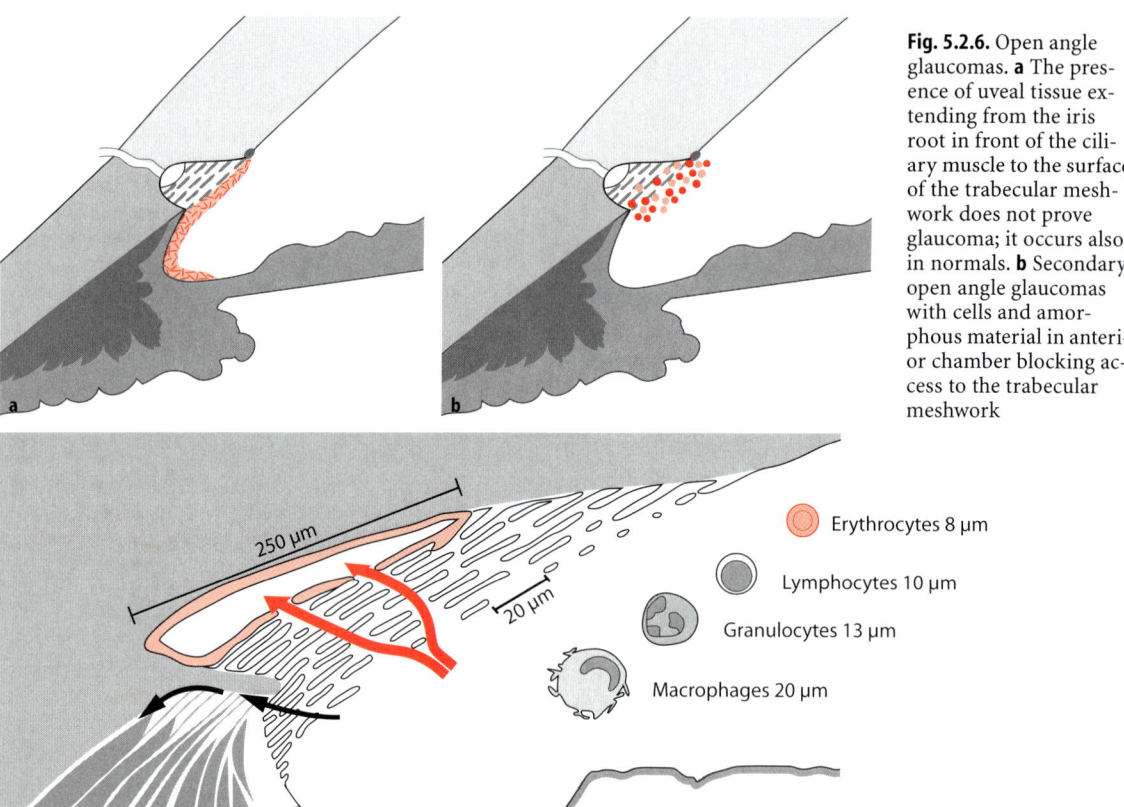

Fig. 5.2.6. Open angle glaucomas. **a** The presence of uveal tissue extending from the iris root in front of the ciliary muscle to the surface of the trabecular meshwork does not prove glaucoma; it occurs also in normals. **b** Secondary open angle glaucomas with cells and amorphous material in anterior chamber blocking access to the trabecular meshwork

Fig. 5.2.7. Pattern of macrophagocytic glaucomas (phacolytic, hemolytic, siliconophagic and melanophagic glaucomas): 20-μm macrophages block access to the pores of the trabecular meshwork towards the anterior chamber

Table 5.2.4. Classification of primary and secondary open angle glaucoma

A. Primary:
1. Primary open angle glaucoma (POAG) (chronic simplex glaucoma)
2. Special forms
   a) Congenital, juvenile and adolescent glaucoma
   b) Glaucoma associated with high myopia
   c) Pigmentary glaucoma (melanin dispersion syndrome)
   d) Glaucoma associated with diabetes
   e) Cortisone glaucoma

B. Secondary:
1. With pseudoexfoliation syndrome (PEX)
2. Uveitis
   a) Fuchs' heterochromic iridocyclitis
   b) Kraupa-Posner-Schlossman syndrome
   c) Keratouveitis: herpes simplex, herpes zoster ophthalmitis
3. α-Chymotrypsin-induced glaucoma (Kirsch)
4. Induced by blood or blood products
   a) Hyphema, incomplete or early
   b) Total hyphema and black-ball hemorrhage (coagulated blood-clot)
   c) Hemolytic glaucoma
   d) Ghost cell glaucoma after hemorrhage
   e) Hemosiderin-induced glaucoma
5. Associated with contusion-angle deformity
6. Macrophagocytic glaucoma
   a) Hemolytic
   b) Phacolytic
   c) Melanophage glaucoma, associated with malignant melanoma or after contusion injury
   d) Siliconophagic
7. Associated with intraocular tumors: juvenile xanthogranuloma, retinoblastoma, uveal malignant melanoma
8. Associated with epithelial ingrowth
9. Associated with orbital diseases [increased episcleral venous pressure (Radius-Maumenee), arteriovenous fistulas, and orbital inflammatory processes]

Table 5.2.5. Differential diagnosis: open but "narrow anterior chamber angle" – relative anterior microphthalmia (RAM)

Diagnosis	Increased tension	Angle closed due to pupillary block during mydriasis	Therapy
Individual variant	–	–	–
Threatening recurrent angle closure glaucoma	–	+	Iridectomy/iridotomy
Primary open angle glaucoma	+	–	Filtering operation
Primary open angle and threatening recurrent closed angle glaucoma	+	+	Iridectomy Filtering operation, urgent (one or two step)

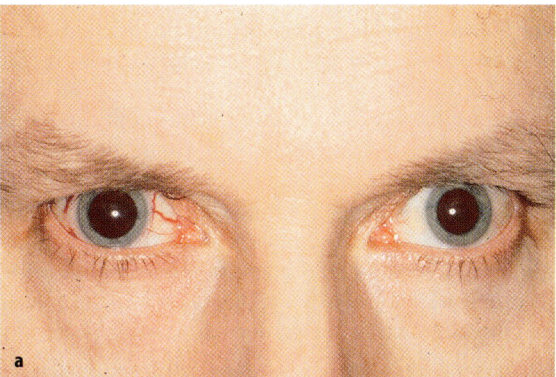
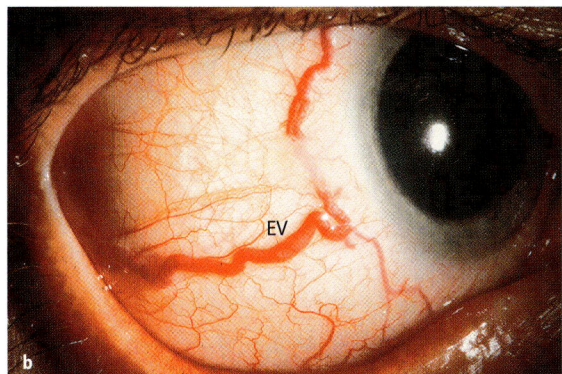
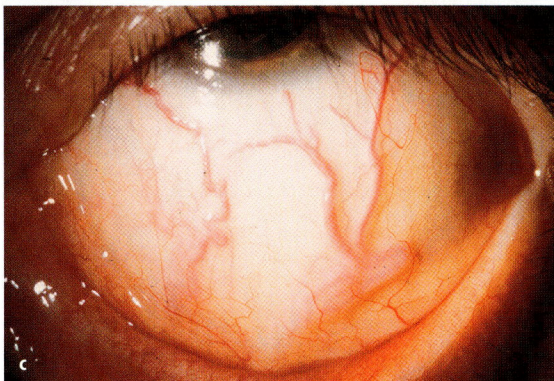

Fig. 5.2.8. Secondary open angle glaucoma due to idiopathic dilated episcleral veins (*Ev*) (Radius-Maumenee syndrome). The opening of the outer wall of Schlemm's canal (sinosotomy) is the chosen surgical procedure (see Fig. 5.2.14)

develops. However, the endothelial counts of the trabecular meshwork in PEX are comparable to those in age-marked controls (Schlötzer-Schrehardt et al. 1995).

5.2.3.4
Congenital Open Angle Glaucomas

The malformations of the main elements of the trabecular meshwork include malposition of the iris root, extension of the ciliary muscle up to Schwalbe's line and distorted layering of the trabecular meshwork (Table 5.2.6).

In simple buphthalmos, embryotoxon and Axenfeld syndrome, Schlemm's canal is usually present but intraoperatively is often hard to find. With malformation of the anterior segment in *anterior segment cleavage syndromes* (Rieger's anomaly, Peters' anomaly; Fig. 5.2.9a–d), Schlemm's canal may be absent as, e.g., in familial or sporadic aniridia (Fig. 5.2.10a, b, Table 5.2.6).

Trabeculotomy ab externo and goniotomy ab interno aim to dissect the abnormal tissue obstructing Schlemm's canal from the anterior chamber. Medical therapy is not a realistic option. Microsurgery is indicated as soon as the diagnosis is made. Trabeculotomy requires localization of Schlemm's canal and following its course with a probe before turning it into the anterior chamber tearing the trabecular meshwork. Really atraumatic manipulation of a trabeculotomy is impossible by the septations within Schlemm's canal and also because of its variable course (Fig. 5.2.11).

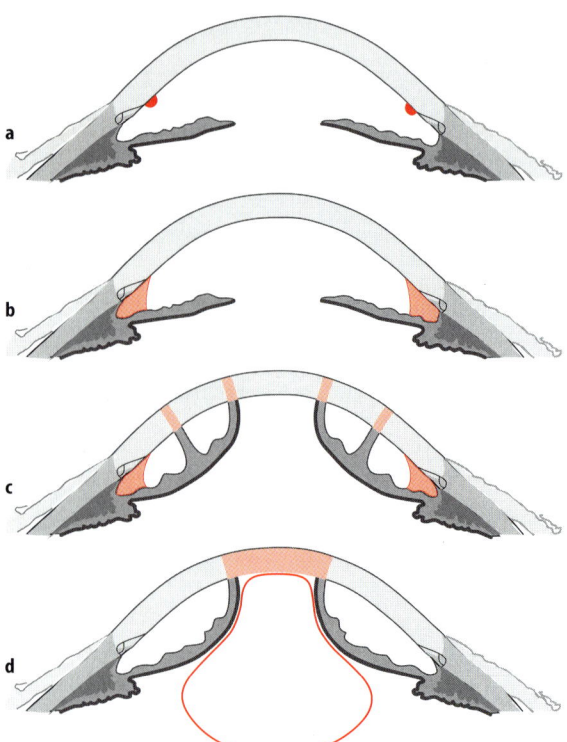

Fig. 5.2.9. Anterior chamber cleavage syndromes. **a** Embryotoxon posterior: prominent Schwalbe's rim or line. **b** Axenfeld anomaly: iris stroma covering the trabecular meshwork up to Schwalbe's line. **c** Rieger's anomaly: in addition to **b** several iridocorneal attachments more centrally. **d** Peters' anomaly: lens and central iris stroma attached to posterior cornea with defect in Descemet's membrane

Table 5.2.6. Congenital/infantile glaucoma (buphthalmos) with ocular and systemic diseases

1. Ocular (primary)
   - Isolated
   - Associated with Axenfeld's and Rieger's syndromes
   - Associated with Peters' anomaly
   - Associated with cornea plana (?)
2. Associated with systemic diseases
   - Phakomatoses: neurofibromatosis, Sturge-Weber syndrome
   - Pierre Robin syndrome
   - Rubinstein-Taibi syndrome
   - Lowe's syndrome
   - Trisomy 13
3. Secondary buphthalmos
   - Trauma
   - Juvenile xanthogranuloma of the iris
   - Retinoblastoma and pseudoglioma
   - Lymphangioma of the orbit

Table 5.2.7. Critical cell populations in open angle glaucomas

1. Endothelial: trabecular meshwork, Schlemm's canal; cornea (capillaries)
2. Elements in "aqueous"
   - Cells in aqueous: erythrocytes, leukocytes, macrophages
   - Melanin granules after opening of iris pigment epithelium and iris melanocytes
   - Extracellular pseudoexfoliation material
3. Non-pigmented ciliary epithelium
4. Ganglion cells
   - Retina
   - Uvea
5. Pseudoexfoliation syndrome: all tissues of anterior segment

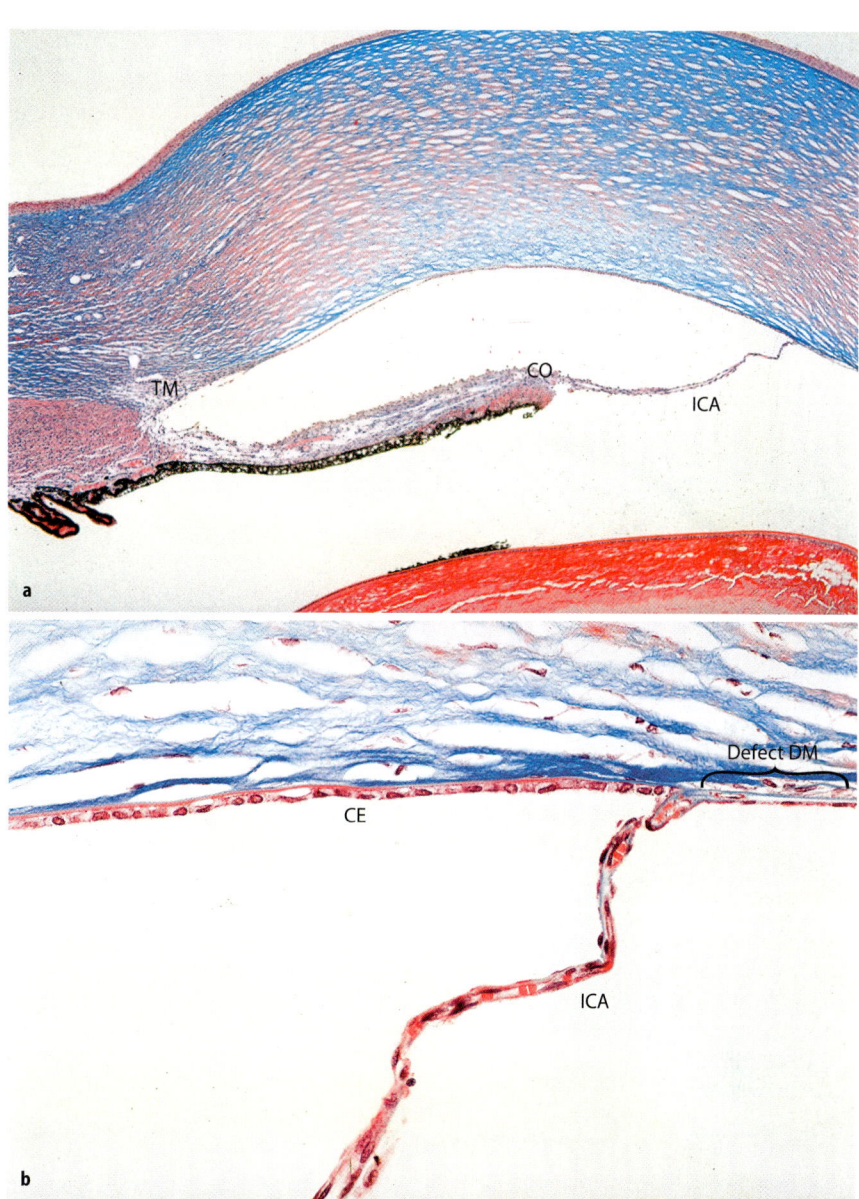

Fig. 5.2.10a, b. Peters' anomaly: Irido corneal adhesions (*ICA*) from collarette in contact with posterior central cornea adjacent to defect in Descemet's membrane (*DM*), Corneal endothelium (*CE*), trabecular meshwork (*TM*)

Table 5.2.8. Critical cell population with aging and open angle glaucoma (Alvarado, Grierson, Jonas et al. 1990, 1992; Knorr et al. 1991; Schlötzer-Schrehardt et al. 1991–2007)

	Trabecular endothelium syncytium	Cornea endothelium	Axons of retinal ganglion cells
With 20 years	750,000	3,000/mm²	1.2 × 10⁶
With 80 years	400,000	2,100/mm²	800,000
Normal aging/year	6,000 (= 16/day)	15/mm²/year	5,000 (≈12/day)
Cell loss/year	≈ 0.5% (Alvarado)	≈ 0.5%	0.4%
	≈ 0.8% (Grierson)		
POAG	*Half* of age norm	Approx. 1,600/mm²	Variably reduced
PEX	*Same* as norm	Reduced	

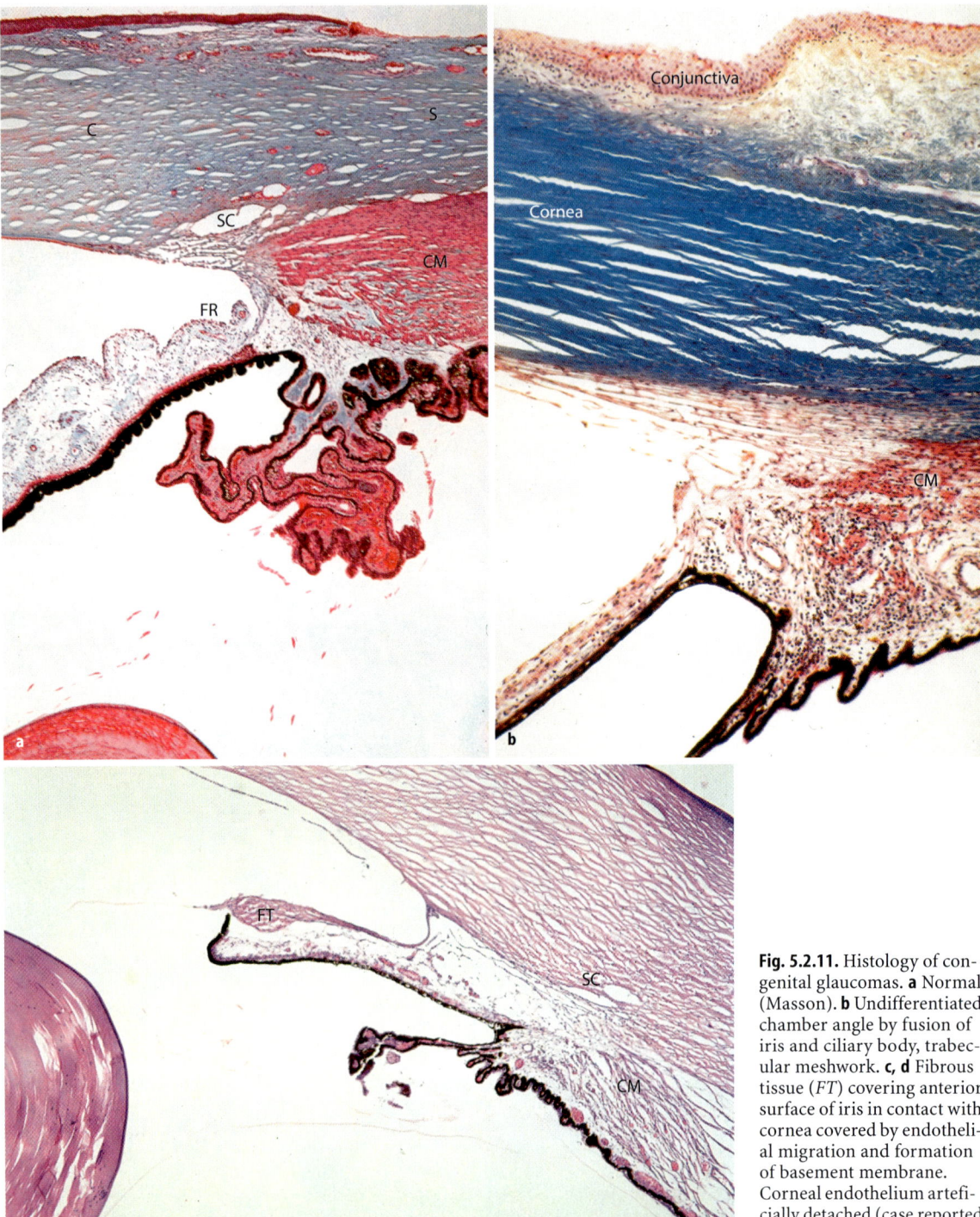

Fig. 5.2.11. Histology of congenital glaucomas. **a** Normal (Masson). **b** Undifferentiated chamber angle by fusion of iris and ciliary body, trabecular meshwork. **c, d** Fibrous tissue (*FT*) covering anterior surface of iris in contact with cornea covered by endothelial migration and formation of basement membrane. Corneal endothelium artefically detached (case reported by Karlsberg 1979).

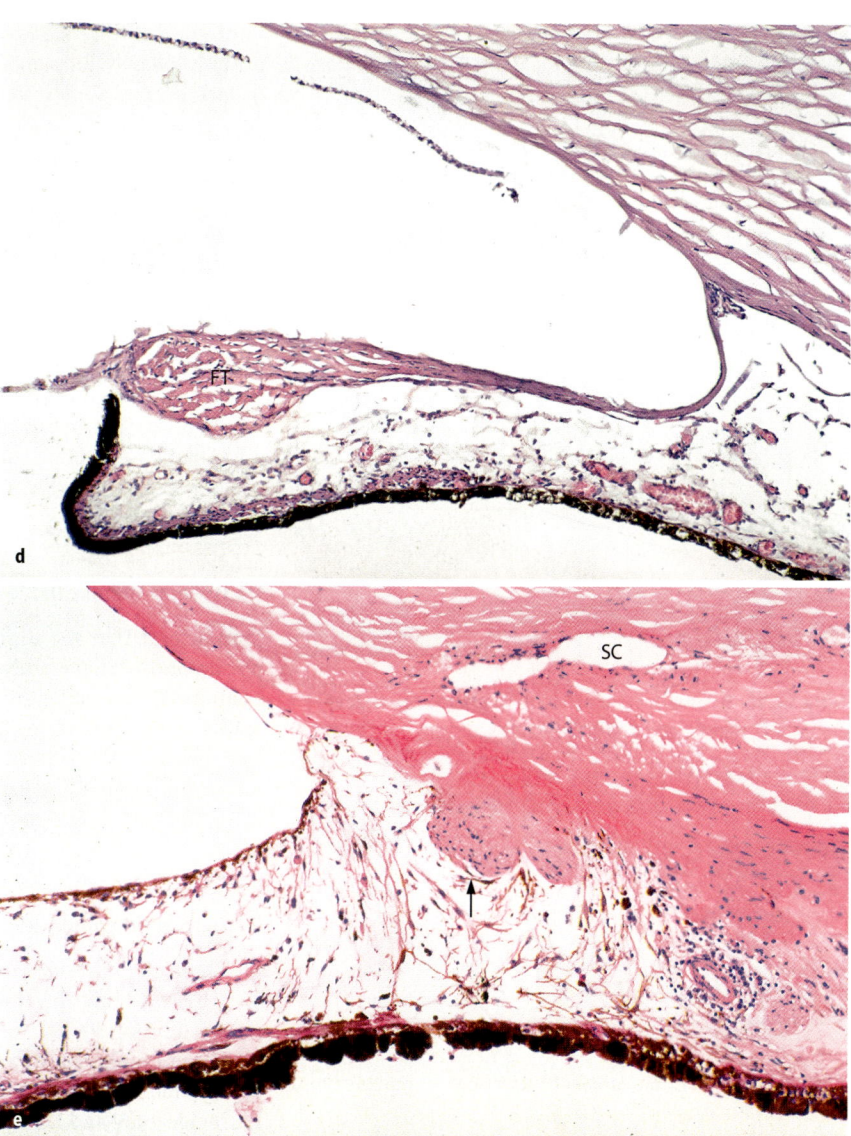

Fig. 5.2.11 (*Cont.*) **e** Atypical smooth muscle in front of Schlemm's canal (*arrow*) (PAS stain) (from the collection of Ashton, Maumenee, Green and Lee)

5.2.4
Indications and Contraindications for Microsurgery of Glaucomas

Laser (argon, neodymium-YAG, diode) mechanical microsurgery as well as cryo- (or dia-)thermy for cyclodestruction is used. Laser application focuses on the iris, the trabecular meshwork or the aqueous producing epithelium of the pars plicata of the ciliary body.

5.2.4.1
YAG-Laser Iridotomy

YAG-laser iridotomy is focused on the iris root peripheral to Fuchs' roll to create a shunt from the posterior to the anterior chamber bypassing the pupillary block. A small defect in the iris usually does not close because fibrin exudates of the wound edge are flushed by the aqueous flow. Occasionally thermic lasers focus on the brown iris stroma, causing shrinkage of this tissue later to facilitate YAG-laser iridotomy (see Sect. 5.3).

Laser iridoplasty focuses on the iris periphery, causing shrinkage of this tissue in an attempt to open the recently closed angle in plateau iris.

5.2.4.2
Mechanical Peripheral Iridotomy/Iridectomy

Mechanical peripheral iridotomy/iridectomy by scissors via a corneal or corneoscleral perforating incision is indicated if acute pupillary block angle closure glaucoma cannot be relieved by YAG-laser iridotomy. The failure to achieve an opening in the iris may be caused by corneal edema following endothelial decompensation and/or

Table 5.2.9. Indications for glaucoma surgery

I. *Angle closure* glaucomas
  1. Pupillary block: iridotomy/iridectomy
  2. Ciliary block
     Pars plana vitrectomy
     Restoration of anterior chamber (cataract extraction)
  3. Plateau iris

II. *Open angle* glaucomas
  1. Primary:
     Laser trabeculoplasty
     Filtrating surgery (with and without implants)
  2. Secondary:
     a) PEX: like II/1, but note:
        Blood aqueous barrier breakdown, zonular instability, poor mydriasis
        Corneal endothelial decompensation
     b) Rubeosis iridis: coagulation of retina by thermic laser and/or cryotherapy of ciliary body
     c) Others: remove obstructing material (blood, lens, silicone)
     d) Neoplasm: radiation, chemotherapy, enucleation

III. Congenital glaucomas
  1. Goniotomy, trabeculotomy if Schlemm's canal present
  2. See II.

Table 5.2.10. Terminology of mechanical glaucoma surgery

Iridectomy	von Graefe	1856
Filtrating surgery	Critchet	1858
Goniotomy	de Vincentis	1891
Iridencleisis	Holth	1906
Trephination	Elliot	1909
Trabeculotomy	Burian	1950
Sinusotomy	Krasnov	1962
Trabeculectomy	Cairns/Watson	1968
Deep sclerectomy	Fjodorov/Koslov	1989
Trabecular aspiration/ goniocurettage	Jacobi	1994/97
Viscocanalostomy	Stegmann	1999

Table 5.2.11. Glaucoma surgery – selection of implant types (filaments or channels)

Horsehair	Rollet/Moreau	1907
Silk fiber	Zorab	1912
Gold tube	Stefansson	1925
Silicone tube	Ellis	1960
Acryl tube with endplate	Molteno	1969
Molteno implant	Molteno	1973
Krupin implant	Krupin	1976
Baerveldt implant	Baerveldt	1990
Ahmed implant	Ahmed	1993
Ex-press		
Eye-pass	Brown	2002

Table 5.2.12. Terminology of non-mechanical glaucoma surgery (laser methods)

Laser trabeculopuncture	Hager	1970
Laser trabeculopuncture	Krasnov	1973
ALT	Wise/Witter	1979
XeCl excimer	Berlin	1988
Erbium-YAG	Fankhouser/Hill	1991
Selective laser trabeculoplasty	Latina	1998
Femtolaser	Toyran	2005

thickening of the iris stroma by ischemic necrosis especially in heavily pigmented iris. Peripheral mechanical iridectomy is also indicated in all filtering glaucoma surgery consisting of a through and through hole in the eye wall overlaying Schlemm's canal. The purpose of this peripheral iridectomy in these eyes is to prevent intra- and postoperative pupillary block (see Sect. 5.3).

5.2.4.3
Laser Trabeculoplasty

Laser trabeculoplasty consists of multiple 50-µm puncture thermic argon laser coagulation to the trabecular meshwork to improve the outflow by mechanisms poorly understood. The effect may be only temporary. Some prefer a "selective trabeculoplasty" (Holz and Lim, 2005).

5.2.4.4
Transscleral Thermic Diode Laser

Transscleral thermic diode laser directed to the pars plicata of the ciliary body destroys the non-pigmented epithelium producing the aqueous by absorption in the "oven" of the underlying pigmented ciliary epithelium. In contrast to the transscleral cryothermic or diathermic coagulation of the pars plicata, the overlying sclera is unaffected by these infrared lasers (see below).

5.2.4.5
Mechanical Goniotomy and Trabeculotomy

Mechanical goniotomy and trabeculotomy tend to dissect the trabecular meshwork in congenital glaucomas in a sector of 30–50° of the angle of circumference because of malformation of arrangements of the tissue in the chamber angle. Currently both the ab externo trabeculotomy and the ab interno approach goniotomy are relatively good methods with the available techniques. They involve vascularized tissue with marked liberation of growth factors from the seeping hemorrhage leading to unintended wound healing.

However, most attempts to treat adult POAGs by goniotomy or trabeculectomy are unsatisfactory (Fig. 5.2.13a–c). As the main obstacle to aqueous outflow in adult chronic open angle glaucomas is situated in the trabecular meshwork, it seems logical to try to establish a shunt between the anterior chamber and Schlemm's canal.

These procedures need to be improved. For the primary open angle glaucomas a currently *utopian* goal should include: (1) miniaturization, (2) avoidance of vascularized structures, and (3) preservation of the eye wall outside Schlemm's canal to maintain a closed eye system. Only then will *early* glaucoma surgery be a valid alternative option over medical therapy for established chronic open angle glaucomas lasting for years

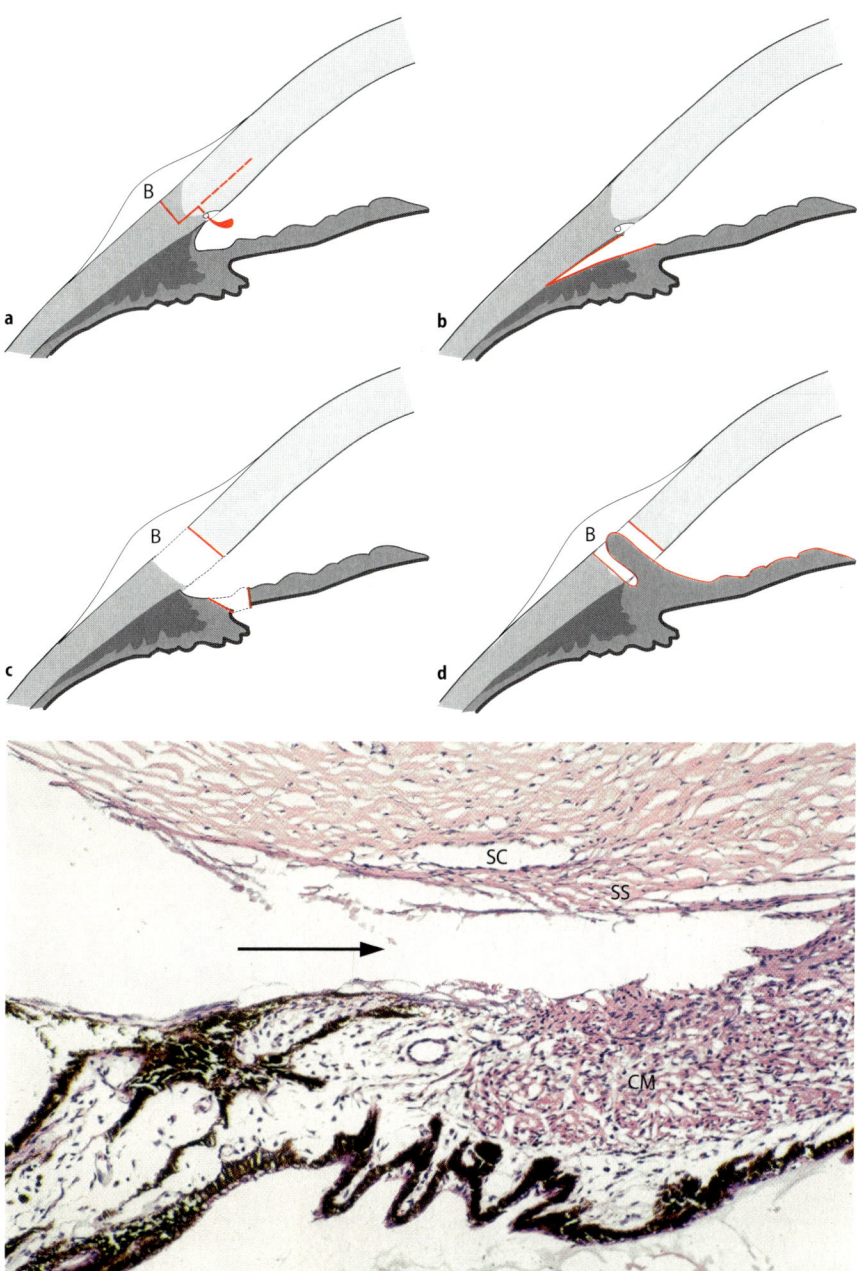

Fig. 5.2.12. Principles of glaucoma surgery. a Trabeculotomy and trabeculectomy covered by scleral flap with filtering flap (goniotomy without scleral flap): shunt from anterior chamber. b Cyclodialysis: separation of ciliary muscle from scleral spur. c Unprotected filtering after Elliot's principle with filtering bleb. d Iridencleisis iris root incarcerated into corneoscleral wound. In a, c and d, the peripheral iridectomy is indicated to prevent papillary block

Fig. 5.2.13. Histopathology after goniotomy (a). In congenital glaucoma showing incision of undifferentiated uveal tissue and separation of ciliary muscle from scleral spur (collection Maumenee-Green)

and decades. The potential of infrared femtolasers to achieve a shunt from the anterior chamber to Schlemm' canal (in this direction) deserves to be studied in detail (see below).

5.2.4.6
Procedures for Acute Secondary Open Angle Glaucomas

Urgent removal of material from the anterior chamber is required in the following entities: (1) coagulated blood clots with "*black ball hyphema*," (2) *macrophagocytic* open angle glaucomas (Table 5.2.4) with hypermature cataract phacolytic, following hemorrhage into the anterior chamber, hemolytic, after necrosis of melanin-containing tissue with liberation of granules, melanolytic, or siliconophagic glaucomas (Fig. 5.2.6). In view of the associated systemic complications of these acute open angle glaucomas, emergency microsurgical action is indicated not only to save the eye and optic nerve but also to prevent life-threatening complications. Like in all acute glaucomas, involvement of the parasympathetic system may lead to vomiting and ex-

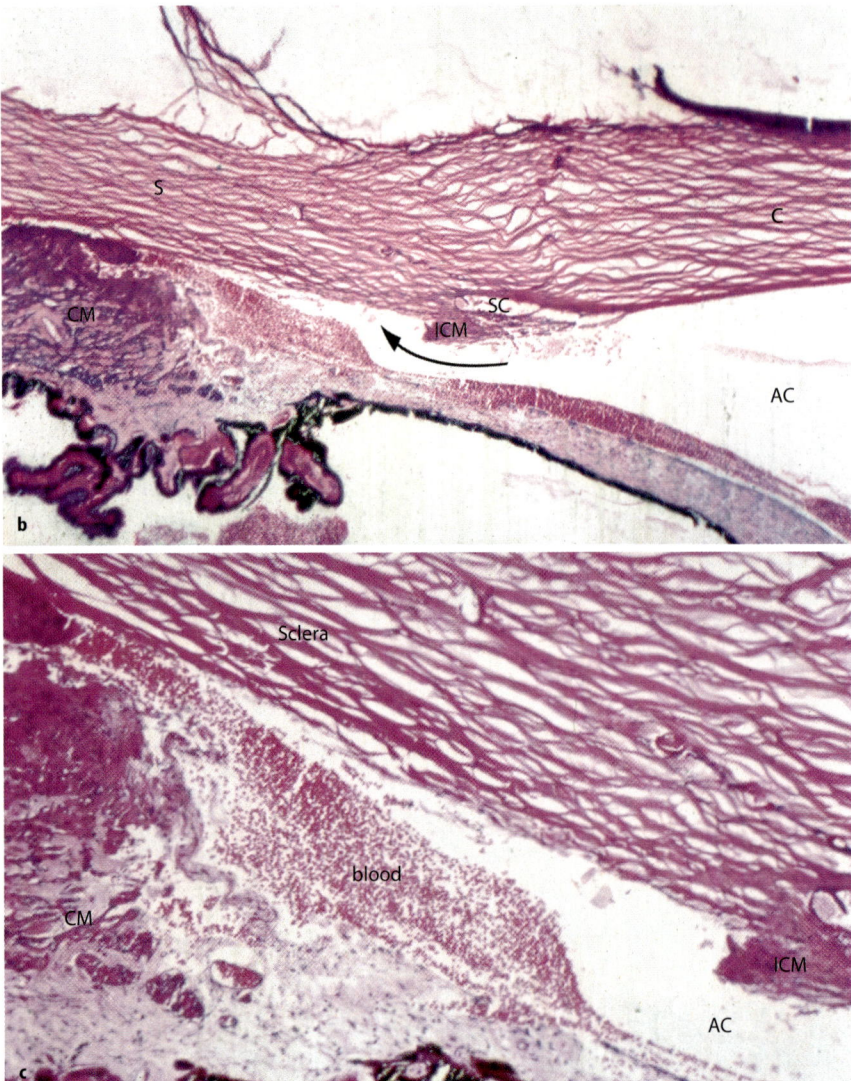

Fig. 5.2.13. b, c Attempted goniotomy in adult, leading to cyclodialysis with marked hemorrhage into anterior chamber. Insertion of ciliary muscle at scleral spur (*ICM*)

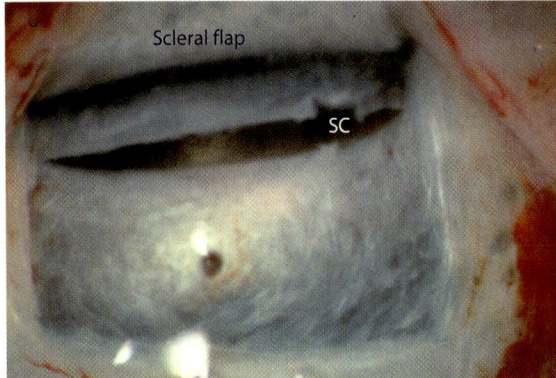

Fig. 5.2.14. Microanatomy beneath scleral flap. Opening of external wall of Schlemm's canal in "sinusotomy"

treme loss of fluid and exsiccosis. In other words: The urgent indication for microsurgical relief is both for life and vision.

Removal of the material may require larger incisions in black ball hyphema and in phacolytic glaucoma to remove the hard lens nucleus. Small transcorneal incisions for insertion of vitrectomy instruments are sufficient in hemolytic and siliconophagic glaucomas. In Radius-Maumenee syndrome, the secondary open angle glaucoma due to dilated episcleral veins (Fig. 5.2.8a–c). The surgical approach is the opening of the outer wall of Schlemm's canal, the so-called *sinosotomy* (Fig. 5.2.14). It represents the first step to other *variants* of *non-penetrating glaucoma* procedures (Table 5.2.10–12).

5.2.4.7
Filtrating Glaucoma Surgery

"Trabeculectomy" and its variants: All modifications have in common that they attempt to create a bypass canal between the anterior chamber and the subcon-

5.2.4 Indications and Contraindications for Microsurgery of Glaucomas

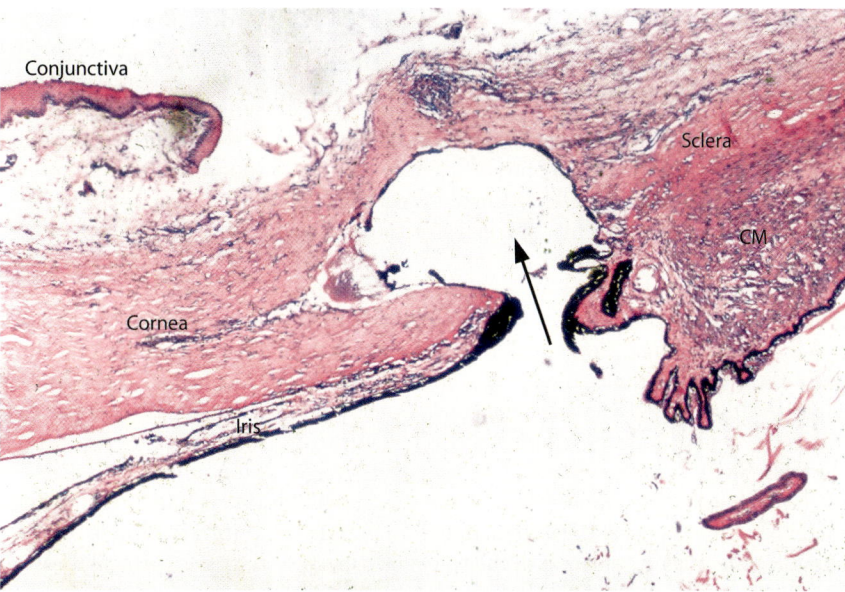

Fig. 5.2.15. Scarred filtering bleb after Elliot trephination (arrow): notice persistent broad anterior synechiae of the peripheral iris leading to secondary angle closure glaucoma (PAS stain)

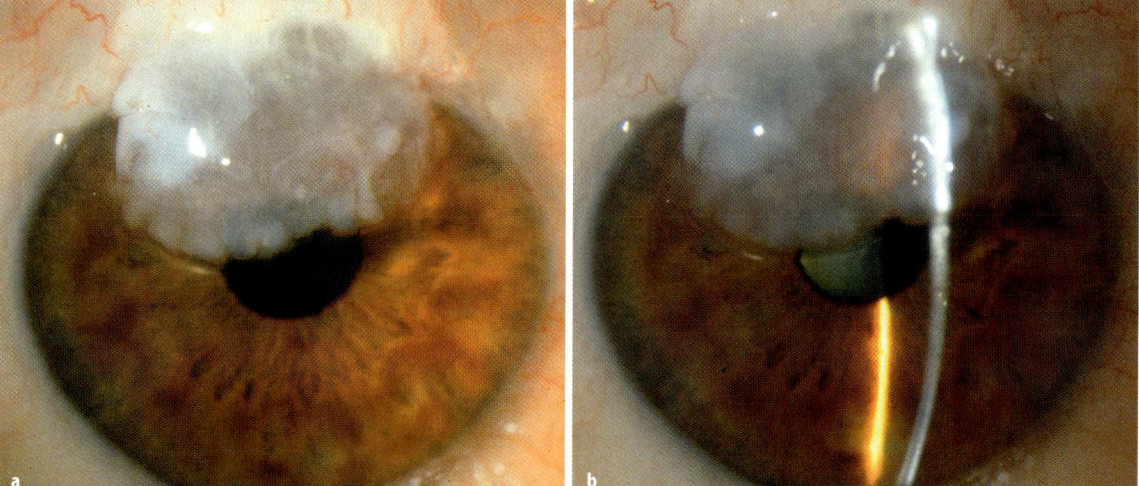

Fig. 5.2.16a, b. Luxuriant filtering bleb extending on the surface of the cornea anterior to Bowman's layer almost to the pupillary center. As Bowman's membrane is preserved *blunt* separation of the bleb and then reduction is achieved

junctival space in the region of the limbus (Table 5.2.10). They are usually performed after various periods of local medical therapy, which initiate *iatrogenic conjunctivitis*. Biopsies of subconjunctival hypervascular tissue and Tenon's capsule illustrate an increased number of lymphocytes indicating chronic inflammation with the risk of an increased tendency for scarring (Fig. 5.2.15). The intended episcleral pool of aqueous drainage is supposed to reach the aqueous veins, the lymphatic ring of Teichmann, the blood vessels and the general circulation. If an iatrogenic conjunctivitis is obvious, *preoperative treatment with local corticosteroids without preservatives might be considered*. Phacoemulsification alone can achieve a lowering of the intraocular pressure (IOP) for months or years (~ by clearing the trabecular meshwork?). The combination of trabeculectomy and phacoemuslification also is a valuable option.

The microsurgeon using a high magnification recognizes within the surgical limbus the following structures: peripheral edge of Bowman's layer, after creating the conjunctival flap; below a thick scleral flap the landmarks are the scleral spur, Schlemm's canal and Schwalbe's line. Although it is rare to obtain globes after successful or failed filtrating surgery for glaucomas, there is consensus that the initial scarring occurs not within the scleral canal but originates from the episcleral tissue and vessels (Table 5.2.13). To reduce the inflammatory response and excessive scarring, cytostatic medications such as mitomycin C and 5-fluorouracil are applied (Fig. 5.2.16).

5.2.4.8
Concept of a Transtrabecular Shunt Between the Anterior Chamber and Schlemm's Canal

According to McEwen, one opening alone in the trabecular meshwork of 20 µm would be sufficient to guarantee a normal aqueous outflow. Current methods of "rough" mechanical trabecular surgery probably scar to a considerable degree. They are probably successful only if a remnant of the outflow window with a minimum of 20 µm stays open. Wound healing is probably accelerated by growth factors within the blood leaking into the wound area after mechanical surgery (Table 5.2.10). The *currently utopian goal* to achieve the above shunt hypothetically could include the use of an ultrashort infrared femtolaser (10^{-15}) using doses in the terawatt range (10^{12} W). Ideally this infrared femtolaser would overcome the semi-opaque corneoscleral limbal zone transmission zone, starting ablation of the trabecular meshwork on the side of the anterior chamber and extending slowly to the level of Schlemm's canal. This would require preoperative determination of the exact depth of Schlemm's canal within the corneoscleral region measured by optical coherence tomography (OCT) or ultrasound biomicroscopy (UBM) (Fig. 5.2.17).

5.2.4.9
Transscleral Coagulation of the Ciliary Body

In contrast to the above mentioned procedures, transscleral coagulations aim to partially destroy the aqueous producing non-pigmented ciliary epithelium. Both cryo- and diathermic coagulation cannot avoid a coagulation of the adjacent sclera and ciliary muscle – more pronounced with diathermia. For this reason today cyclocoagulation is the preferred method. The transscleral infrared diode laser coagulation of the pars plicata has the principal advantage of avoiding necrotic

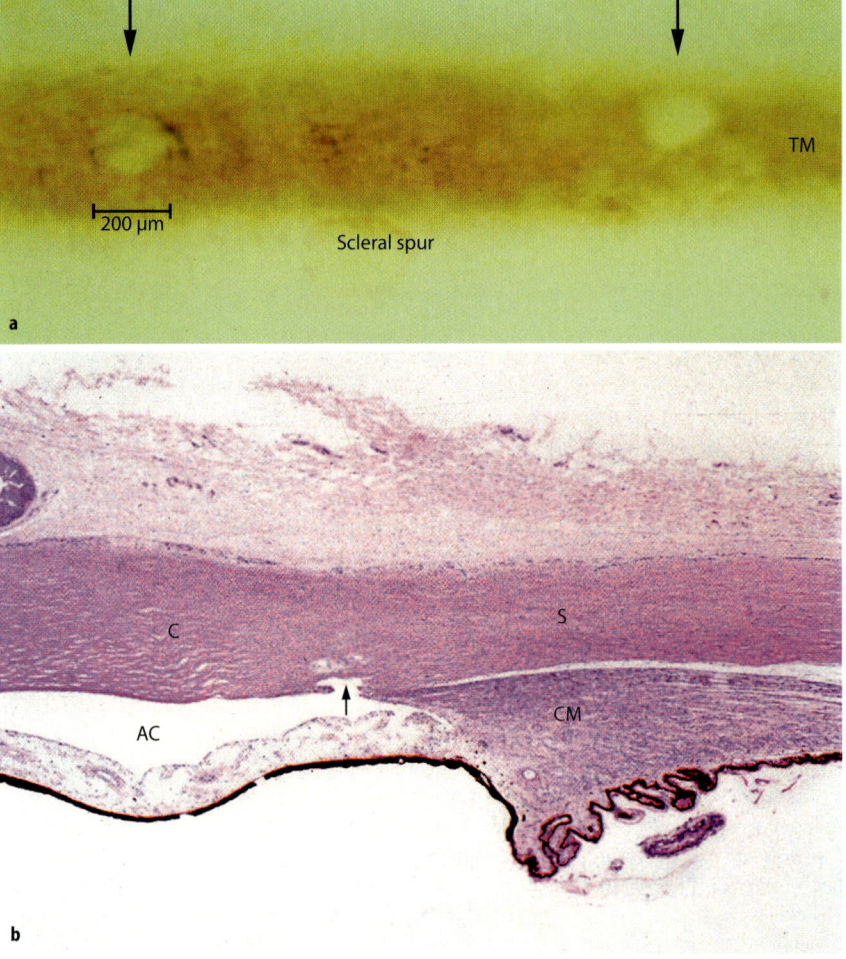

Fig. 5.2.17. Experimental erbium YAG-laser trabeculotomy from anterior chamber (*AC*) to Schlemm's canal (*SC*). **a** 200-µm perforation of trabecular meshwork (*arrows*). **b, c** Histology in donor eye (unpublished data from Jünemann)

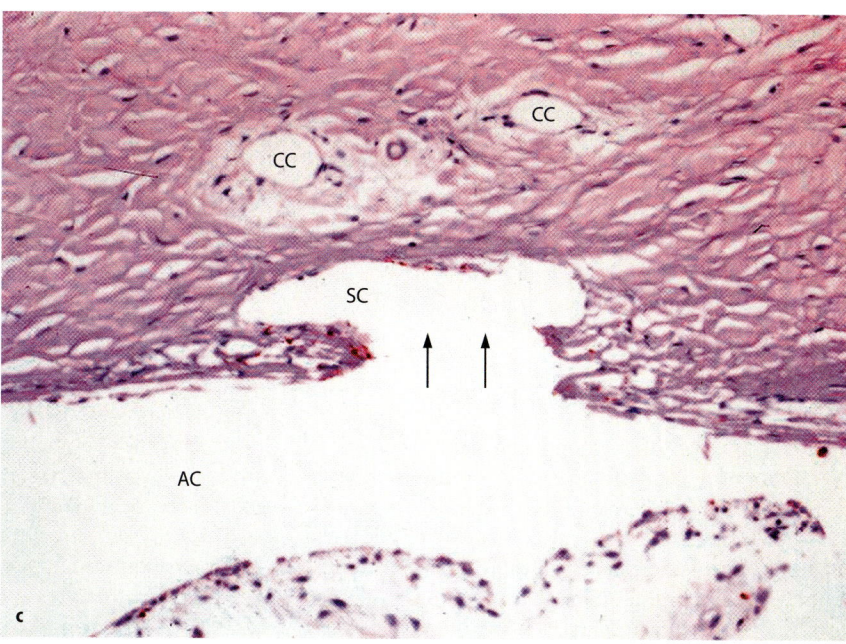

Fig. 5.2.17 (*Cont.*)

changes in the overlying sclera – as well as the risks associated with an opening of the eye (see Chapter 2, Sect. 2) – but as an exception scleral perforation may occur. Coagulation of the pigmented ciliary epithelium is associated with necrosis of the adjacent ciliary muscle (Fig. 5.4.32). Cyclodestructive procedures may pose extra risks in PEX (Zonula! BAB! See Chapter 6.3).

5.2.4.10
Contraindication to Filtering Procedures

Fresh angle closure glaucomas are best treated by YAG-laser iridotomy, if necessary mechanical peripheral iridectomy. Filtering procedures are accompanied by a risk of ciliary block angle closure glaucoma (malignant glaucoma, see below). The same is true for open but narrow angle glaucomas, especially with relative anterior microphthalmus (RAM, Auffarth and Völcker, 2000, 2006).

5.2.5
Complications with Excessive and Deficient Wound Healing

The most important considerations for avoiding complications are:

1. To clearly distinguish between *closed* angle glaucomas and *open* angle glaucomas
2. A narrow angle may still be open with the otherwise normal trabecular meshwork; it may be an imminent pupillary or ciliary block situation, if the anterior chamber is opened
3. A combination of both trabecular meshwork disease and imminent pupillary block is another possibility (Table 5.2.5)
4. A POAG with a very narrow angle represents only a particularly difficult type of open angle glaucoma (Table 5.2.1 and 5.2.5).

5.2.5.1
Acute Postoperative Decompensation of Intraocular Pressure

Complications of filtrating surgery are either an *insufficient* or *excessive* wound closure and healing. They are associated with acute postoperative decompensation either down or up:

Defects of wound healing from the conjunctival or corneo-conjunctival wound lead to persisting ocular *hypotony*, narrowing or flattening of the anterior chamber and detachment of the choroid (see Chapter 2). This situation requires posterior sclerotomy, reformation of the anterior chamber and revision of the conjunctival wound usually within a week – earlier if the lens touches the cornea.

Malignant postoperative ciliary block angle closure with loss of anterior chamber may follow filtrating surgery particularly in eyes with small anterior segments (RAM) showing all the signs of an acute glaucoma. This requires pars plana vitrectomy and/or removal of the lens and reestablishment of the anterior chamber.

Table 5.2.13. Growth factors in wound healing ("scar wars") (according to P. Khaw): Stimulation of migration, proliferation and collagen synthesis of human Tenon's capsule fibroblasts

Name	Abbreviation
Transforming growth factor beta 1 and beta 2	TGF β1 and β2
Epidermal growth factor	EGF
Basic fibroblast growth factor	bFGF
Insulin-like growth factor 1	IGF 1

5.2.5.2
Late Conjunctival Bleb Wound Dehiscence

Late conjunctival bleb wound dehiscence can be the precursor of a localized infection or *progressive endophthalmitis*. Debry et al. (2002) found in a series of 239 eyes, a bleb leak in 8% and a "blebitis" in 2% following trabeculectomy with mitomycin with a follow-up of 2.7 years. Inhibitors of growth factors to prevent scarring of the filtering bleb are insufficiently understood as are the rusulting "scar wars" (according to P. Khaw). The role of cytostatic substances like mitomycin C and/or 5-fluouracil is currently being intensively studied in many institutions around the world. Especially scarring in the tenon's tissue in relation to preexisting inflammatory infiltrate and growth factors from blood and sclera with conjunctival vessels needs to be considered in future studies of wound healing. *Large cystic blebs* may extend in front of Bowman's layer – they can be separated from the cornea by blunt instruments and then reduced in size (Fig. 5.2.16). The role of the corneal *endothelial proliferation* and *migration* from the inner opening of filtrating surgery and its extent in the episcleral region requires further study.

5.2.5.3
Failure of Goniotomy

As the procedure originates from the opposite side of the anterior chamber, simple rotation works with *twice the radius of Schlemm's canal*. Histopathologic studies show Schlemm's canal septated and following a variable course. This implies that it is difficult or impossible to maintain the same depth of incision into the structures of the chamber angle. The few globes available for histopathologic study after goniotomy and trabeculotomy often reveal evidence of an *atypical cyclodialysis* and not the intended shunt from the anterior chamber to Schlemm's canal over 120° (Fig. 5.2.13).

If Schlemm's canal is absent, both procedures cannot be performed "*lege artis*" of course. Correspondingly the results are very poor in these congenital complex anterior segment anomalies.

5.2.5.4
Failure of Filtering Surgery for Chronic Open Angle Glaucoma

Current methods of medical or microsurgical therapy are not satisfactory. Treatment of ocular hypertension is recommended if: (1) the pressure exceeds 30 mm Hg, because of the increased risk of CRVO (see Ch. 5.6) (2) there is definite reproducible threshold damage to the optic disc, defining "early glaucoma," or (3) there is definite reproducible change (delta) of the optic nerve head during follow-ups including in its interpretation the quantification of the disc area and its juxtapapillary zones (Jonas et al., 1999).

As current approaches by laser or filtering surgery are not yet optimal, treatment is started usually medically. After local therapy for months or years inevitably an *iatrogenic chronic conjunctivitis* develops with more or less pronounced hyperemia even if preservatives are not included in the eyedrops. This may be a cause of excessive scarring and closure of the filtering channel from episcleral wound healing.

5.2.5.5
Postoperative Peripheral Anterior Synechiae
5.2.5.5.1
Thermic Laser Trabeculoplasty

Thermic trabeculoplasty initiates thermal necrosis of approximately 40–50 μm spots around the trabecular meshwork. How this improves – often temporarily – the aqueous outflow in approximately two-thirds of treated patients is not exactly known. It is speculated that the trabecular endothelial cells adjacent to the thermal burn proliferate in the wound healing process and "*rejuvenate*" the trabecular meshwork. If the placement of the argon laser spot reaches the scleral spur or more posteriorly including the uveal tissue covering the ciliary band focal anterior hairlike synechiae often develop. This posterior application can induce secondary angle closure from confluent argon laser spots. If this occurs in more than one-half the circumference, secondary angle closure glaucoma is the most unpleasant complication.

5.2.5.5.2
Subsequent Filtering Procedures

Postoperatively the anterior chamber may be shallow or absent for a few days. If contact between lens and cornea is seen, immediate intervention to restore the anterior chamber is necessary. The same may be indicated if the anterior chamber does not deepen within a week. Failure to restore the anterior chamber in time may cause persistent anterior synechiae and even secondary angle closure glaucoma. This negates the goal of the procedure.

5.2.5.6
Consequences of Acute and Persistent Ocular Hypotony Following Filtrating Glaucoma Surgery

The hypotony may be the result of wound leak, excessive filtration without wound leak or, rarely, an unintentional atypical cyclodialysis. Regardless of the etiology the consequences are similar. Hyperemia of uveal vessels leads to a detachment of the choroid and ciliary body resulting in a visible *"choroidal" effusion*. This subacute-chronic process concerns the entire uvea and results mainly from obstruction of the outflow via the vortex veins. It displaces the origin of the zonular fibers anteriorly and induces a *subluxation* of the lens forward. In eyes with a small anterior segment (RAM) the lens may occlude the ring of the ciliary body and leads to a "malignant" ciliary block acute angle closure glaucoma. This requires immediate attention by a combination of posterior vitrectomy, reformation of the anterior chamber and extracapsular or even intracapsular cataract surgery.

Cystoid maculopathy may occur rather frequently after any opening of the eye, by trauma or microsurgically. This is usually reversible after the intraocular pressure is normalized (see Chapter 2, 4). High resolution OCT has improved our insight in this process.

Expulsive arterial hemorrhage originates from an acute rupture of a ciliary artery at the scleral entry into the choroid. Patients with arterial hypertension and high myopia may be at increased risk for this catastrophic event. Quick closure of the wound in the eye wall and posterior scerotomy 4 mm behind the limbus are attempted to save the eye.

5.2.5.7
Corneal Endothelial Proliferation and Migration After Filtrating Surgery

If the inner opening of the drainage channel reaches anteriorly of Schwalbe's line the contact inhibition between trabecular and corneoendothelium is not functioning: Therefore the corneal endothelium may proliferate through the canal into the episcleral tissue. This is difficult to prove in surgical specimens but may be a factor in the development of *cystic blebs*. Alternatively if the anterior chamber is so flat that the Fuchs' roll is in contact with the corneal endothelium, the barrier of Schwalbe's line again is not limiting the *vagaries of the corneal endothelium* leading to a persisting closure of the anterior chamber angle with ensuing secondary angle closure glaucoma.

References (see also p. 379)

Alvarado J, Murphy C, Polansky J, Juster R. Age-related changes in trabecular meshwork cellularity. Invest Ophthalmol Vis Sci 1981; 21: 714–727

Auffarth GU, Blum M, Faller U, Tetz MR, Völcker HE. Relative anterior microphthalmos: morphometric analysis and its implications for cataract surgery. Ophthalmology 2000; 107: 1555–60

Auffarth GU, Voelcker H-E. Cataract surgery in 79 patients with relative anterior microphthalmus (RAM). A review of anatomy, associated pathology and complications. Klin Monatsbl Augenheilk: 2006;216(6):369

CAT-1520102 Trabeculectomy Study Group, Khaw P, Grehn F, Hollo G, Overton B, Wilson R, Vogel R, Smith Z. A pahse III study of subconjunctival human anti-transforming growth factor beta (2) monoclonal antibody (CAT-152) to prevent scarring after first-time trabeculectomy. Ophthalmology 2007 Oct; 114(10):1822–1830

Debry PW, Perkins Trabekelwerk, Heatley G, Kaufmann P, Brumback LC. Incidence of late-onset bleb-related complications following trabeculectomy with mitomycin. Arch Ophthalmol 2002; 120:297–300

Grierson I, Howes RC, Wang Q. Age-related changes in the canal of Schlemm. Exp Eye Res 1984; 39: 505–512

He M, Foster PJ, Johnson GJ, Khaw PT. Angle-closure glaucoma in East Asia and European people. Different diseases? Eye 2006; 20:3–12

Holz HA, Lim MC. Glaucoma lasers: a Review of the Newer Techniques. Curr Opin Ophthalmol 2005; 16:89–93

Jonas JB, Budde WM, Panda-Jonas S. Ophthalmoscopic evaluation of the optic nerve head. Surv Ophthalmol 1999; 43:293–320

Jonas JB, Budde WM, Lang PJ. Parapapillary atrophy in the chronic open-angle glaucomas. Graefes Arch Clin Exp Ophthalmol 1999; 237: 793–9

Karlsberg, AMA Archiv Ophthalmology 1979: 86: 287: Wilmer 29294

Khaw PT, Occleston NL, Schultz G, Grierson I, Sherwood MB, Larkin G. Activation and suppression of fibroblast function. Eye 1994; 8(Pt 2): 188–195

Knorr HLJ, Jünemann A, Händel A, Strahwald H, Naumann GOH. Morphometrische und qualitative Veränderungen des Hornhautendothels beim Pseudoexfoliationssyndrom. Fortschr Ophthalmol 1991; 88: 786–789

Küchle M, Mardin C, Nguyen NX, Martus P, Naumann GOH. Quantification of Aqueous Melanin Granules in Primary Pigment Dispersion Syndrome. Am J Ophthalmol 1998; 126: 425–431

Küchle M, Nguyen NX, Mardin CY, Naumann G.O.H. Effect of neodymium:YAG laser iridotomy on number of aqueous melanin granules in primary pigment dispersion syndrome. Graefes Arch Clin Exp Ophthalmol. 2001 Jul;239(6):411–5

Kwong YY, Tham CC, Leung DY, Lam DS. Scleral perforation following diode laser transscleral cyclophotocoagulation. Eye 2006; 20: 1316–7

Mardin CY, Küchle M, Nguyen NX, Martus P, Naumann GOH. Quantification of Aqueous Melanin Granules, Intraocular Pressure and Glaucomatous Damage in Primary Pigment Dispersion Syndrome. Ophthalmology 2000; 107: 435–440

Quigley HA. New paradigms in the mechanisms and management of glaucoma. Eye, 2005; 19:1241–1248

Rummelt V, Naumann GOH. Cystic Epithelial Ingrowth after Goniotomy for Congenital Glaucoma. J Glaucoma 1997; 6: 353–356

Ruprecht KW, Naumann GOH. Unilateral secondary open-angle glaucoma with idiopathically dilated episcleral vessels. Klin Monatsbl Augenheilkd 1984; 184:23–27

Schlötzer-Schrehardt U, Naumann GOH. Trabecular meshwork in pseudoexfoliation syndrome with and without open-angle glaucoma. A morphometric, ultrastructural study. Invest Ophthalmol Vis Sci 1995; 36: 1750–1764

5.3 Iris

G.O.H. Naumann

Until the 1970s the iris was considered a special tissue incapable of wound healing. This is still true for small iridotomies that are flushed by aqueous, eliminating the fibrin scaffold which normally initiates wound healing. However, if the wound edges of the iris are *well adapted* by at least two sutures, healing of the iris tissue occurs in a similar fashion to in other tissues except that it takes much longer (see Hinzpeter et al. 1974).

The iris separates the anterior and posterior chamber and has the function of an optic diaphragm (Fig. 5.3.1). The pupil lies slightly inferior nasal to the center of the iris; its diameter varies from 1 to 8 mm. A dis-

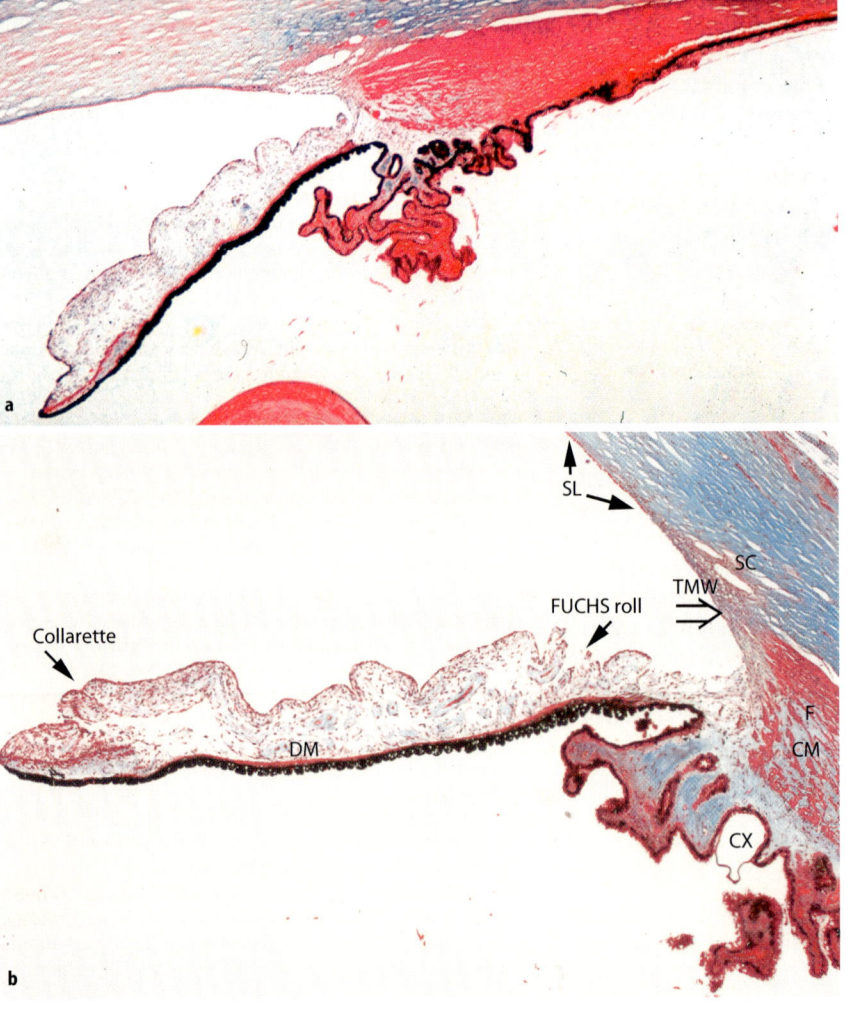

Fig. 5.3.1. Iris microanatomy: iris root and pupillary zone are significantly thinner than the rest of the iris. The iris root blends into the face of the ciliary body. **a** Child. **b** Adult: "collarette", Fuchs' roll (*FR*), Schwalbe's line (*SL*), Schlemm's canal (*SC*), scleral spur (*arrow*), ciliary muscles (*CM*), fibrosis within ciliary muscle (*F*). Separation of non-pigmented ciliary epithelium forming cystic space (*CX*). Anterior border layer and condensation of stroma. Note the loose arrangement of iris stroma sphincter pupillae (*SP*), dilator muscle (*DM*). Trabecular meshwork (*TMW*). Masson stain

crete asymmetry may occur in normal individuals; the average diameter decreases with age. The pupillary margin rests on the anterior lens capsule, causing the "*physiologic pupillary resistance*" leading to a pulsatile flow of aqueous into the anterior chamber. The iris capillaries are lined by *non-fenestrated* endothelial cells that are an important component of the blood-aqueous barrier (see Fig. 5.3.2). They contribute to the warming of the aqueous which has been cooled in the retrocorneal region contributing to the "paternoster phenomenon" of cells and melanin granules in the anterior chamber. They also furnish oxygen to the aqueous (Helbig et al., see Chapter 6.3).

5.3.1 Surgical Anatomy

The iris is cone shaped, and the pupillary margin is located more anteriorly than the root. This is more pronounced in hyperopic eyes with a shorter optical axis than in myopic eyes with a longer optical axis. Therefore in hyperopic eyes the anterior chamber is more shallow and the physiological pupillary resistance higher (Fig. 5.3.2).

The *anterior border layer of the iris* consists of a dense collection of fibroblasts and melanocytes within collagen fibers which extends from the collarette to Fuchs' roll. In this region the iris is significantly thicker than peripheral to Fuchs' roll and between the collarette and the pupillary margin. Pores within this layer allow free communication with the aqueous humor. Nests of uveal melanocytes appear as "freckles" and/or the relatively common iris nevi.

Dendritic melanocytes as remnants of the pupillary membrane are often seen on the anterior lens capsule. Using the slit lamp with high magnification ($\times 40$), one can recognize nuclei and uveal melanin granules. Melanin-containing macrophages appear on the slit lamp as round corpuscles (Table 5.3.1).

The *sphincter pupillae* muscle is approximately 1 mm wide and innervated by parasympathetic nerve fibers from the oculomotor nerves. The *dilator pupillae muscle* consists of the myoepithelial portion of the anterior iris epithelium, which is 4 µm thick and extends up around 50–60 µm in a radial direction. It is innervated by non-myelinated α-sympathetic fibers. Alpha-blocking agents for prostatic hypertrophy, e.g., tamsulosin, therefore as an unintended side effect produce a sluggish iris and a small pupillary diameter, making

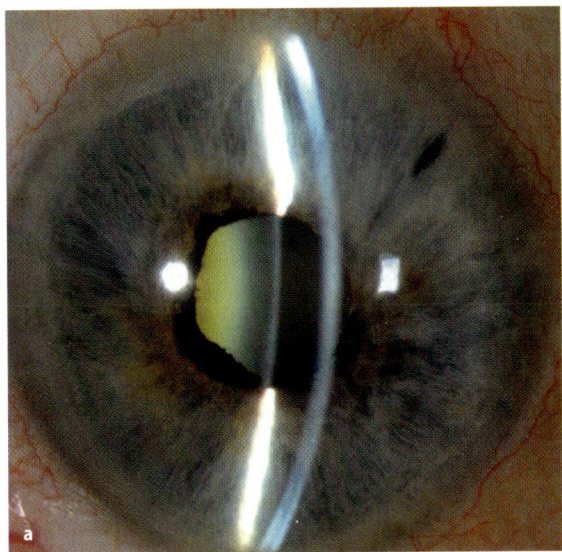

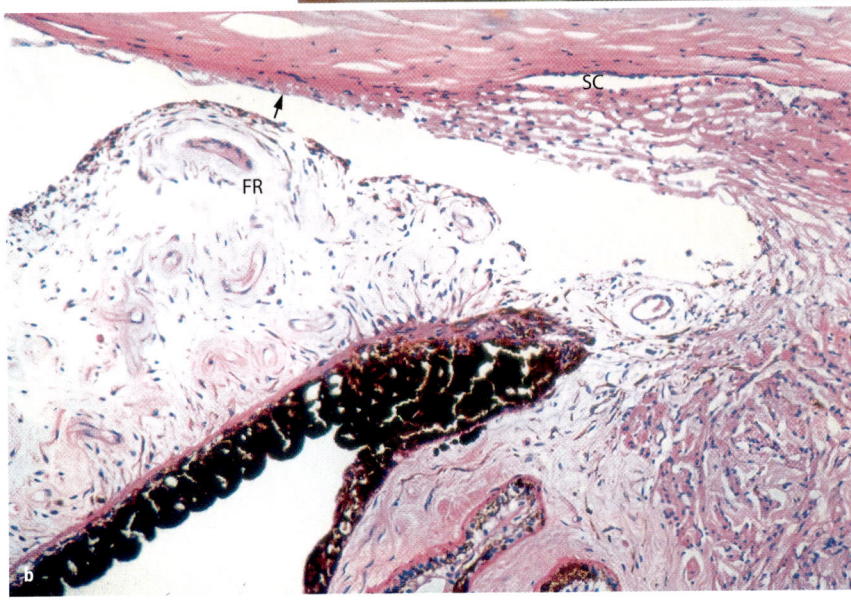

Fig. 5.3.2. Open, but very narrow chamber angle. **a** Nanophthalmus diameter 19 mm in 67 year old after iridotomy at 1 o'clock. **b** PAS stain: Schwalbe's line (*arrow*), Schlemm's canal (*SC*), Fuchs' roll (*FR*)

Table 5.3.1. Iris-pigment epithelium defects on transillumination

1.	Sectorial: uveitis:	Herpes simplex zoster pupillary block, angle closure glaucomas Essential iris-atrophy (ICE syndrome) Tumors Contusion Trauma direct
2.	Radial:	Melanin dispersion idiopathic Marfan syndrome Surgical trauma
3.	Pupillary region:	Pseudoexfoliation syndrome Aging
4.	Pinpoint:	Diabetic iridopathy Albinism variant
5.	Diffuse:	Viral keratouveitis Albinism, ocular and systemic

cataract surgery more demanding: intraoperative floppy iris syndrome (IFIS); see Chapter 5.5. The iris stroma contains myelinated and non-myelinated nerves originating from the nasociliary nerves via the long and short ciliary nerves of the trigeminus. They account for the pain sensitivity.

The pupillary portion of the iris pigment epithelium moves constantly against the anterior lens capsule. With age these cells lose some of their melanin granules, which are then distributed in the aqueous and phagocytized by the corneal and trabecular endothelium. The blood supply of the iris is characterized by many anastomoses. The incomplete major circle of the iris is present in the iris root, arriving from the anterior loops of the anterior ciliary artery branches. An incomplete minor arterial circle runs parallel to the collarette.

The iris root peripheral to Fuchs' roll is only 25–50% as thick as the central iris stroma. Its basal portions continue to the face of the ciliary body. Laser iridotomy should best be focused here preferably in the "stretched" iris associated with a pupil contracted by miotic drops such as pilocarpine.

5.3.1.1
Blood-Aqueous Barrier

In the iris the blood-aqueous barrier is based in the non-fenestrated endothelial lining of the capillaries surrounded by a thick collagenous sheath (see Fig. 2.1; and 2.6).

Congenital anomalies of the pupil are rare (Fig. 5.3.3). Congenital adhesions of the iris develop as part of the anterior cleavage syndrome (Fig 5.3.4).

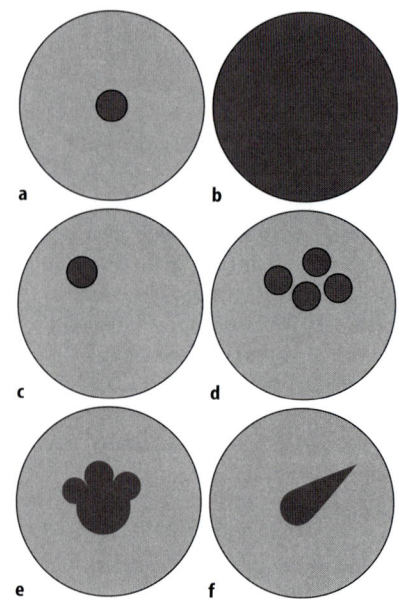

Fig. 5.3.3. Congenital anomalies and acquired deformation of the pupil. **a** Normal. **b** Aniridia. **c** Corectopia. **d** Multicoria. **e** Multiple posterior synechiae inhibit dilatation of the pupil. **f** Anterior synechiae from the iris to cornea after stab trauma

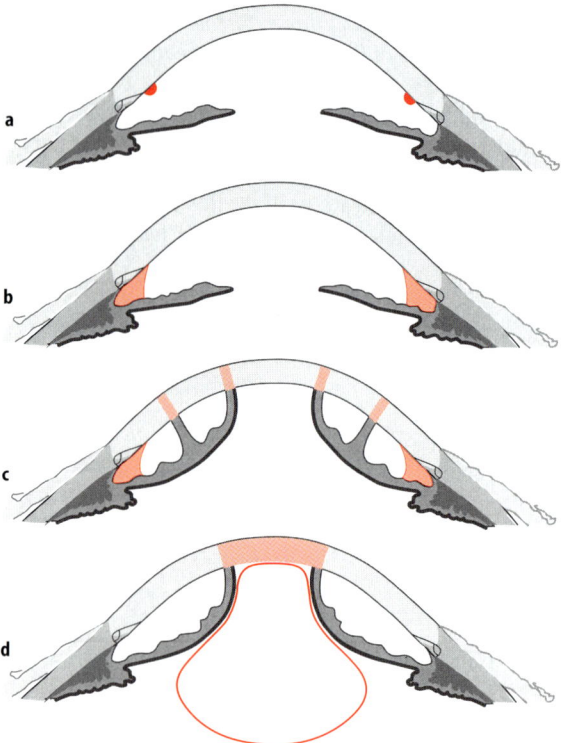

Fig. 5.3.4. Congenital anomalies of anterior uvea and cornea as a spectrum of the anterior chamber cleavage syndrome. **a** Prominent Schwalbe's rim. **b** Axenfeld anomaly. **c** Rieger's anomaly. **d** Peters' anomaly

5.3.1.2
"Biocytology" of Normal Pigmented Cells of the Iris

With high magnification we can distinguish between free melanin granules and hemosiderin-, or melanin-, containing cells: uveal melanocytes, melanophages, iris pigment epithelial cells and other pigmentation or melanin dispersion syndromes (Tables 5.3.2, 5.3.3, 5.3.5, 5.3.11, Figs. 5.3.5, 5.3.6).

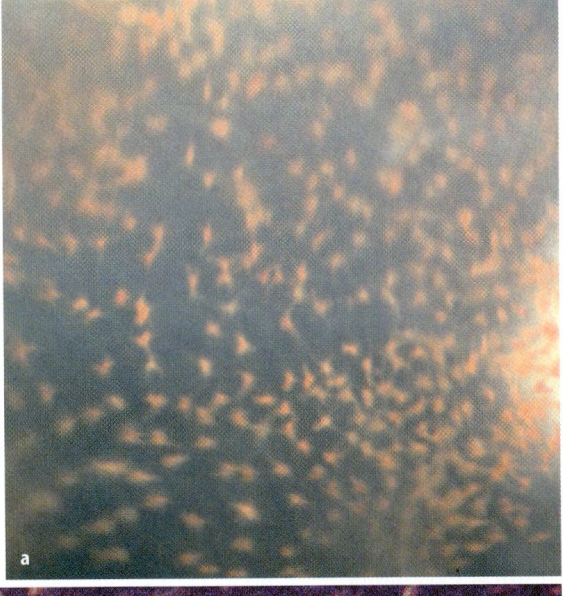

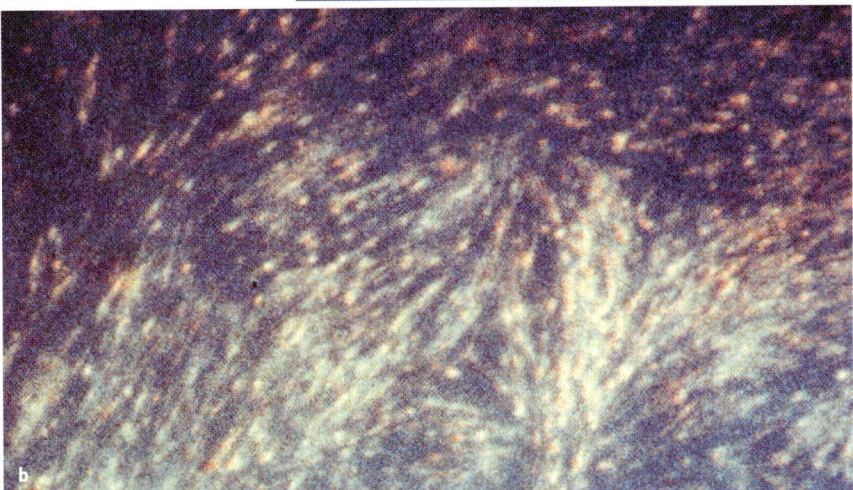

Fig. 5.3.5. Biocytology of uveal melanocytes: **a** *Dendritic* uveal melanocytes as remnants of pupillary membrane with ×40 magnification seen on the anterior lens surface. **b** Malignant slender *spindle* melanocytes on the anterior surface of the lens

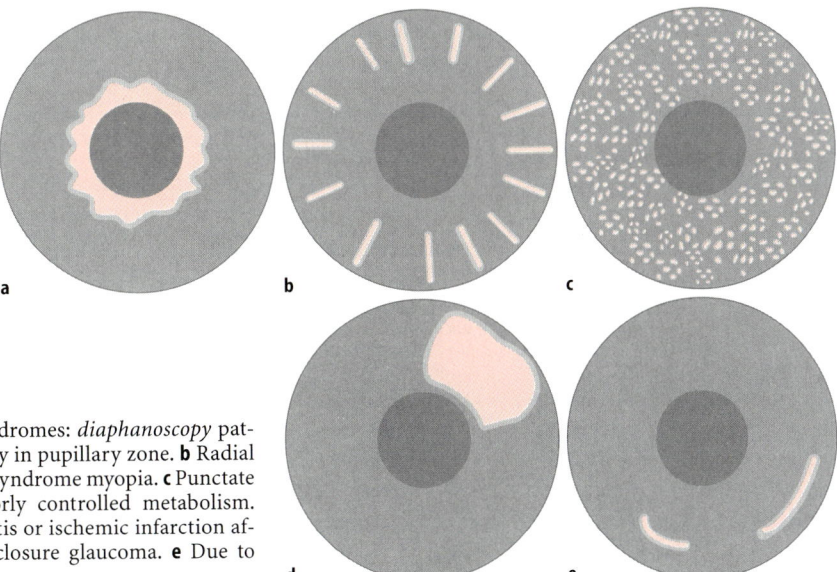

Fig. 5.3.6. Melanin dispersion syndromes: *diaphanoscopy* pattern (schematic). **a** PEX iridopathy in pupillary zone. **b** Radial in idiopathic melanin dispersion syndrome myopia. **c** Punctate in diabetic iridopathy with poorly controlled metabolism. **d** Sectorial necrosis from viral iritis or ischemic infarction after acute pupillary block angle closure glaucoma. **e** Due to blunt trauma

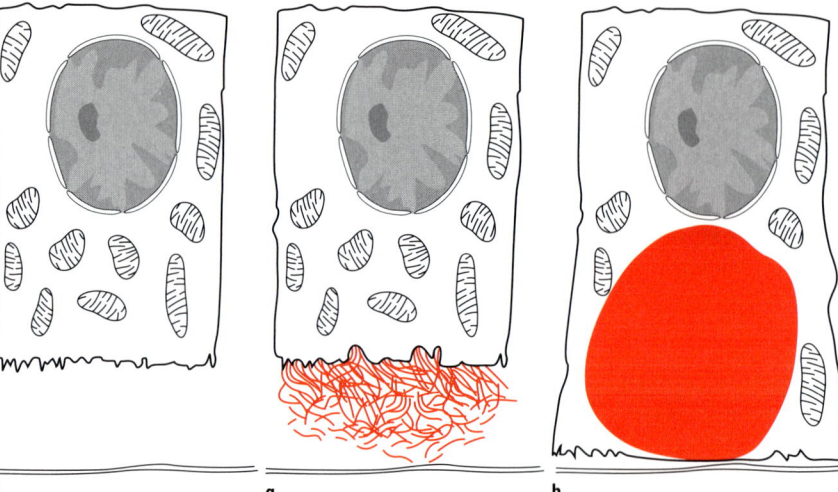

Fig. 5.3.6. Schematic *cellular* changes of iris-pigment epithelium: **f** normal; **g** *extra*cellular accumulation of PEX material ruptures cell membrane after pupillary traction; **h** *intra*cellular glycogen accumulation ruptures cell membrane and releases melanin granules

5.3.2 Surgical Pathology

5.3.2.1 "Biocytology" of Minimal Microsurgical Trauma

The uveal melanocytes of the stroma and the iris pigment epithelium are particularly vulnerable to microsurgical trauma by mechanical instruments, e.g., forceps and scissors, and/also by thermic argon or YAG-laser application. The collarette is exposed to very peripheral fundus-thermal-laser coagulation via three-mirror contact lens particularly if the pupil is dilating poorly. High magnification allows one to differentiate between the pigmented cell populations of the iris, particularly in patients who have a blue or gray iris (Table 5.3.2).

Any microsurgical trauma may lead to focal necrosis surrounded by a zone of depigmentation, visible melanophages and/or proliferation of the pigment epithelium often induce posterior synechiae. This is always associated with a circumscribed temporary breakdown of the blood-aqueous barrier which can be quantified by laser tyndallometry.

If the iris dilates poorly, e.g., in diabetic and pseudoexfoliation syndrome (PEX) iridopathy or with age, treatment of the peripheral fundus by thermic lasers may *accidentally burn* the edges of the collarette and lead to a peculiar superficial stroma necrosis (Fig. 5.3.5). Melanophages contain melanin from destroyed uveal melanocytes and/or pigment epithelium.

5.3.2.2 Melanin Dispersion from the Iris Pigment Epithelium

Liberation of melanin granules from the iris may be caused by: (1) blunt trauma, (2) penetrating trauma, (3) diffuse or sectorial necrosis, e.g., herpetic keratouveitis, (4) diabetic iridopathy, (5) PEX iridopathy involving the epithelium (see Fig. 5.3.6), (6) ischemic sector necrosis of the iris following angle closure glaucoma via pupillary or ciliary block, or (7) spontaneous or induced necrosis of uveal malignant melanomas (Table 5.3.2). Melanin is not the only intraocular pigment (Table 5.3.11).

5.3.2.3 Rubeosis Iridis Followed by Secondary Open and Angle Closure Glaucomas (Figs. 5.3.7, 5.3.8)

Hypoxic and ischemic processes of the retina induce capillary neovascularization of the anterior surface of the iris and angle leading to corneal endothelial proliferation and migration and open angle glaucoma. In later stages angle closure glaucomas develop by progressive contraction of the fibrovascular layer. The pseudoangle then is covered by migrating and proliferating corneal endothelium creating a basement membrane in continuity with Descemet's membrane (Fig. 5.3.7, Table 5.3.3). Laser coagulation of the ischemic retina may reduce the blood flow through the newly formed capillaries and decrease the breakdown in blood-aqueous barrier. However, the newly formed vessels will not regress after a capillary basement

Table 5.3.2. Iris-stroma necrosis: differential diagnosis

1. *Congenital:*	Rieger's anomaly
2. *Acquired:*	Ischemic infarct: angle closure glaucoma Anterior segment necrosis after encircling episcleral "retinal" implant Ischemic ophthalmopathy with carotid artery occlusion
	Thermic laser burns of iris colarette during laser coagulation of peripheral fundus Iridoschisis and ICE syndrome PEX iridopathy Xeroderma pigmentosum

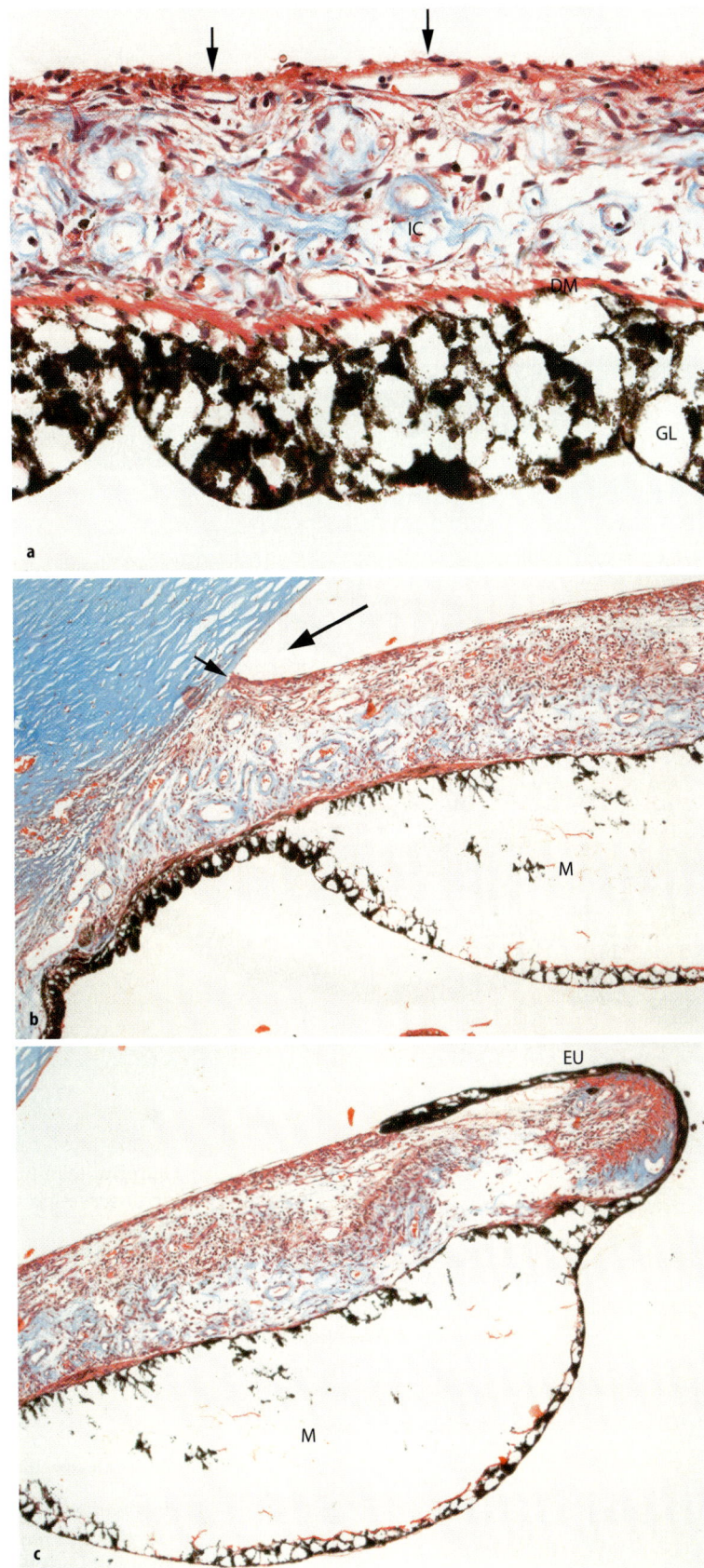

Fig. 5.3.7. Diabetic iridopathy: **a** Marked vacuolation of iris pigment epithelial layers by intracellular glycogen (*GL*) accumulation (lost in fixation) with massive rubeosis iridis: newly formed capillaries (*arrows*). Iris stroma vessels with collagen mantle (*IC*), dilator muscle (*DM*). **b** Massive splitting of iris pigment epithelial layer by glycogen accumulation in poorly controlled diabetes mellitus forming schisis-like space (*M*). **c** Ectropium uvea (*EU*), rubeosis iridis with anterior synechiae and corneal endothelial migration and proliferation forming pseudoangle (*broad arrow*), Schwalbe's line (*SL, small arrow*)

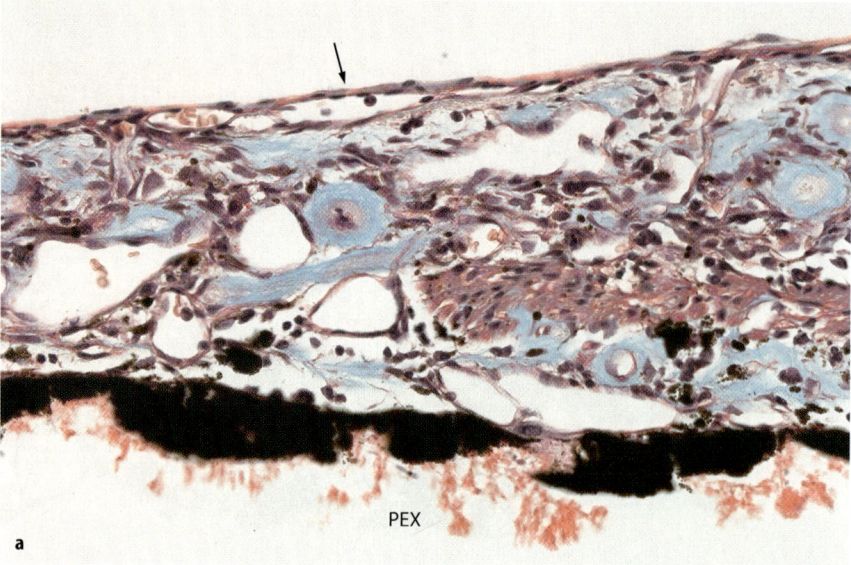

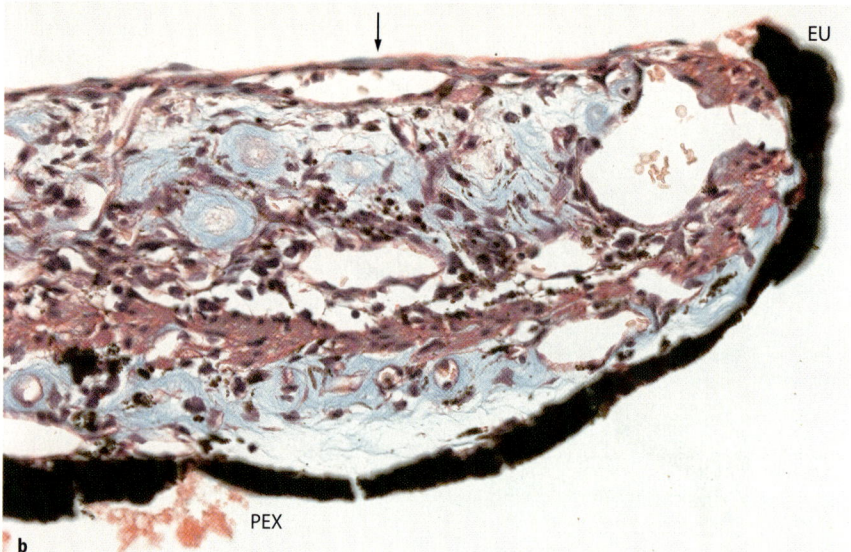

Fig. 5.3.8. Iridopathy of pseudoexfoliation syndrome: **a** Typical extracellular material (PEX) behind the iris pigment epithelium with rubeosis iridis leading to an ectropium uveae (*EU*) and secondary angle closure glaucoma following central retinal vein occlusion. **b** Pupillary zone with ectropium uveae

Table 5.3.3. "Biocytology" of anterior uvea, anterior lens capsule and cornea

1.	*Melanocytes:*	"Uveal dendritic" (persisting pupillary membrane) Uveal "fusiform" from diffuse malignant melanomas
2.	*Melanophages:*	Round spheroidal with melanin after necrosis of iris stroma: PEX, laser burns, viral iritis
3.	Iris pigment epithelium	
4.	Corneal endothelium (specular microscopy)	
5.	Lens epithelium	
6.	Keratocytes, trigeminal nerve axons (with Rostock module of HRT)	
7.	Erythrocytes (see Table 5.3.4)	

membrane is formed and cannot be removed by microsurgical manipulations – but they become less obvious in observation with the slit lamp (see Chapters 5.1 and 5.2).

Angle closure glaucoma due to iris-plateau syndrome is common in Asian eyes with a narrow anterior segment and crowding of ciliary processes behind the iris root. It may follow a chronic course by progressive closure of the angle.

5.3.2.4
Angle Closure Glaucomas Via Pupillary and Ciliary Block

In *pupillary block* acute angle closure glaucomas, the physiologic pupillary resistance is increased above a threshold by closer contact between the pupillary mar-

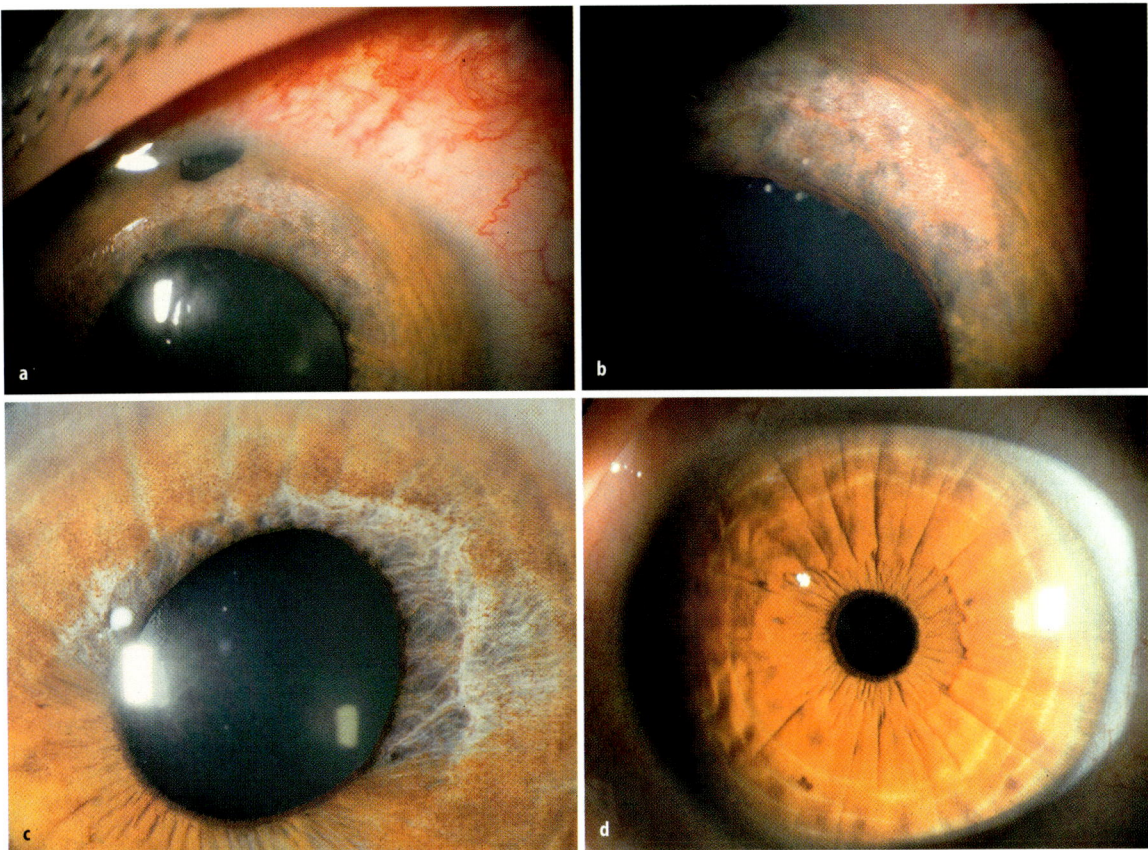

Fig. 5.3.9. Sectorial ischemic necrosis of iris following acute pupillary block angle closure glaucoma. **a, b** Acute phase after mechanical peripheral iridectomy; higher power shows melanophages in the iris stroma. **c, d** Scars after ischemic necrosis following pupillary block angle closure glaucoma from 9–10 and 12–4 o'clock with deformation of pupil in comparison to the not yet treated other eye with imminent pupillary block requiring prophylactic laser iridotomy

gin of the iris and anterior lens capsule following a decreased mobility of the pupillary margin and a larger lens in hyperopic eyes with age. PEX iridopathy, diabetic iridopathy and increased dimension of the anterior-posterior thickness of the lens with age are risk factors (Fig. 5.3.8). In contrast to ciliary block, the position of the lens is *not* altered in comparison to the other not yet involved eye, and the depth of the central anterior chamber is unchanged. During a fresh attack a shunt must be reestablished between the posterior and anterior chamber as soon as possible with a laser iridotomy. If the cornea is too opaque and/or the iris stroma is thickened by edema following adjacent ischemic iris necrosis – or in brown iris – laser iridotomy may be impossible: A surgical (mechanical) peripheral iridectomy via transcorneal or transcorneoscleral incision must be performed immediately. Sectorial ischemic necrosis develops if treatment is delayed (Fig. 5.3.9).

A *ciliary block* "misdirects" the aqueous into the vitreous and moves the lens forward. If cycloplegia and pars plana vitrectomy fail to relax strangulation of the lens by the ciliary muscle, the lens as obstacle to the aqueous flow from behind the lens to the posterior chamber must be removed by cataract extraction preceded by posterior sclerotomy (Fig. 5.3.9). In contrast to pupillary block, *the lens is moved forward* reducing the depth of the anterior chamber centrally – in comparison to the as yet uninvolved eye.

5.3.2.5
Iridodialysis

Blunt trauma may cause a tear in the iris at its thinnest portion peripheral to Fuchs' roll in front of the ciliary body. If located in the lid fissure, this may result in an optically disturbing diplopia and require closure by direct suturing under microscopic control (Figs. 5.3.10, 5.3.11). Before entering the eye using the McCannel technique – transcorneally or after transcorneoscleral opening of the eye – we must be aware of the associated potential zonula dialysis with sublocation of the lens and potential vitreous prolaps and loss (and the patient should be informed *pre*operatively).

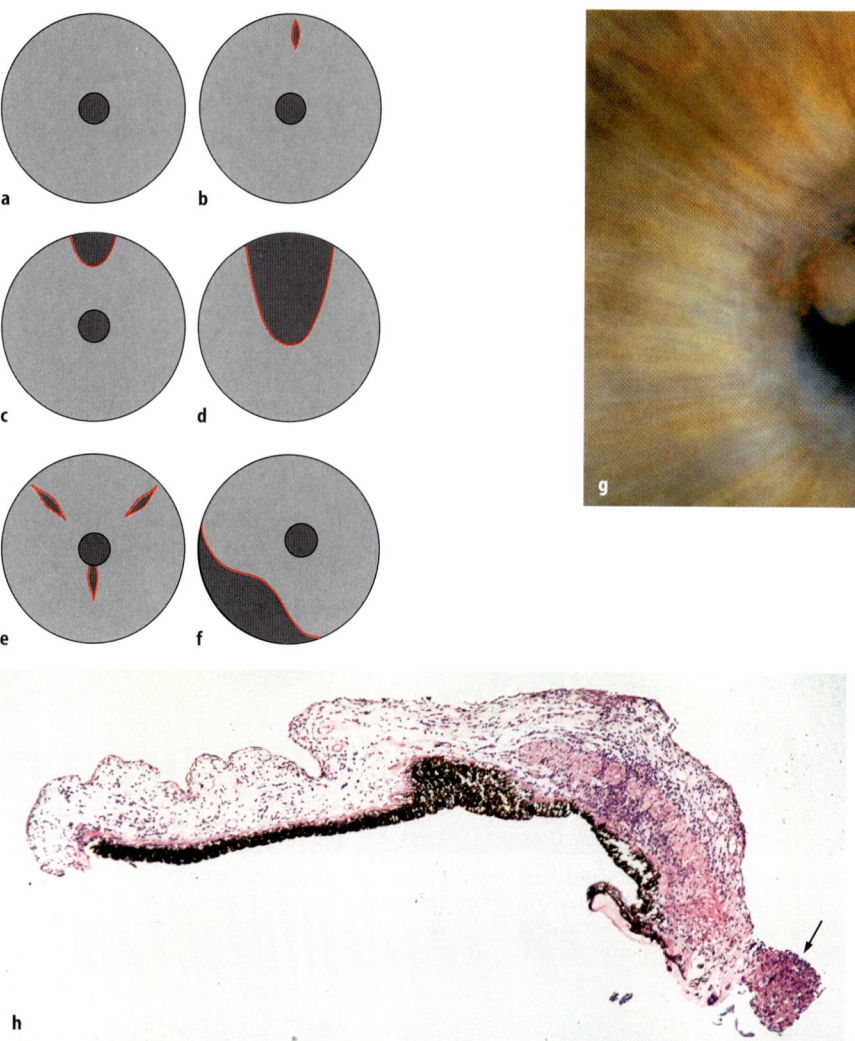

Fig. 5.3.10. Microsurgical procedures to iris (**a–e**). **a** Normal. **b** After laser iridotomy. **c** After mechanical peripheral iridectomy. **d** After sector iridectomy. **e** Peripheral iridotomies and sphincterotomy. **f** Iridodialysis after blunt trauma. **g** Two granulomas at pupillary margin in chronic anterior uveitis with posterior synechiae. Busacca nodules.

h Iris tissue from **g** obtained by sector iridectomy illustrating non-necrotizing granula (*arrow*) confirming diagnosis of sarcoidosis

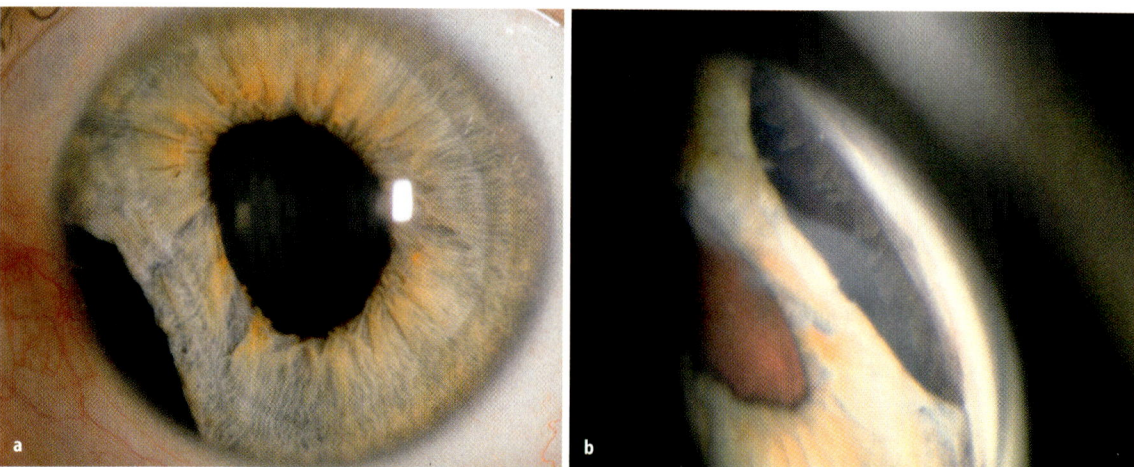

Fig. 5.3.11. Traumatic iridodialysis from 7–9 o'clock, contusion cataract and lens subluxation with bulging of iris from vitreous prolapse. **a, b** Preoperatively.

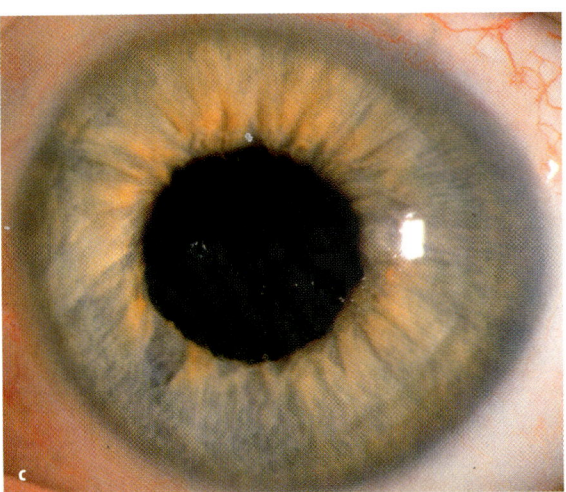

Fig. 5.3.11. c After phacoemulsification and anterior vitrectomy followed by iridopexy as part of the fixation of posterior chamber lens implant with transscleral sutures

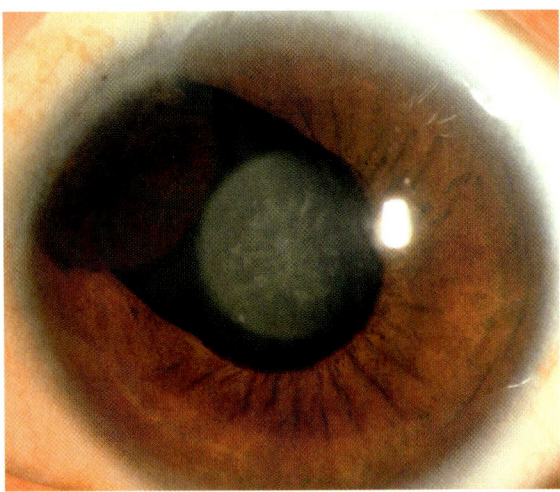

Fig. 5.3.12. Optical sector coloboma for central congenital cataract performed in 1939; occluded by retrocorneal uveal melanocytic proliferation and migration almost covering the optical opening by 1984

5.3.2.6
Tumors of the Iris

Cysts of the pigment epithelium of the pupillary margins (remnants of von Szily's ring sinus or following miotic therapy) or involving the retroiridal periphery usually do *not* require surgical intervention. If they enlarge, argon laser puncture of this single layer of epithelial cell layer wall liberates mucoid and the cyst collapses*. This can cause a temporary rise in intraocular pressure (Table 5.3.4).

Table 5.3.4. Spontaneous hyphema: causes

1. Congenital-hereditary diseases
   Persisting pupillary membrane
   Persistent hyperplastic primary vitreous (PHPV)
   Vitreoretinal dystrophies, e.g., juvenile retinoschisis
2. Rubeosis following retinopathy of prematurity (ROP), diabetes, central retinal vein occlusion (CRVO)
3. Uveitis: Fuchs' heterochromia complicata, Behçet disease viral
4. Tumors: malignant melanoma; iris metastasis (melanocytic nevus)
   Juvenile xanthogranuloma
   Hemangioma of iris
   Varix of iris
   Retinoblastoma
5. Clotting defects with hematologic disease
6. Following irido- or cyclodialysis from contusion of globe
7. Pseudoexfoliation syndrome (PEX)

Melanocytic freckles and nevi are very common and do *not* require any therapy.

Growing melanocytic lesions of the iris with suspected transition to a malignant melanoma: The course of therapy determines whether the process is still localized or if diffuse cellular dispersion into the anterior chamber is evident. This requires a careful *biocytology study* under high magnification at the slit lamp (Figs. 5.3.12, 5.3.13, Table 5.3.5). Only in the rare instances that the iris root is *not* involved is an *iridectomy* sufficient for a curative excision. Closure of the resulting defect in the iris requires *multiple* interrupted sutures to assure adaptation of the wound margins (Fig. 5.3.14). Single sutures will not induce wound healing. Wound healing of the iris occurs with delay only in those areas where the iris stroma is well adapted (Fig. 5.3.15 and below).

---

* Note: This approach is **contraindicated** in nonpigmented cystic epithelial ingrowth: here it converts the cyst into a diffuse epithelial ingrowth (see 5.4), which is usually resistant to any therapy. For cystic epithelial ingrowth of the iris root and chamber angle, *block excision* is the therapy of choice!

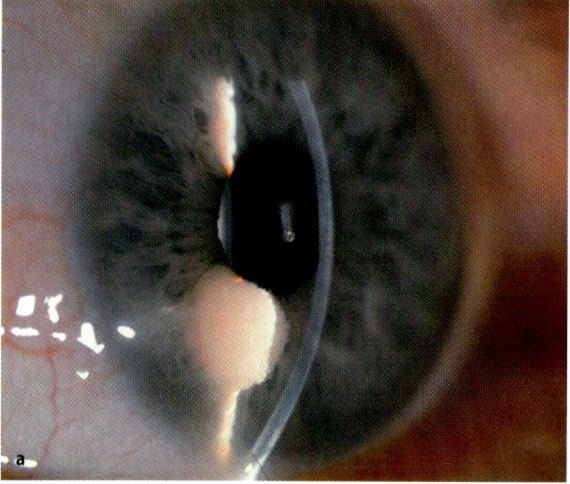
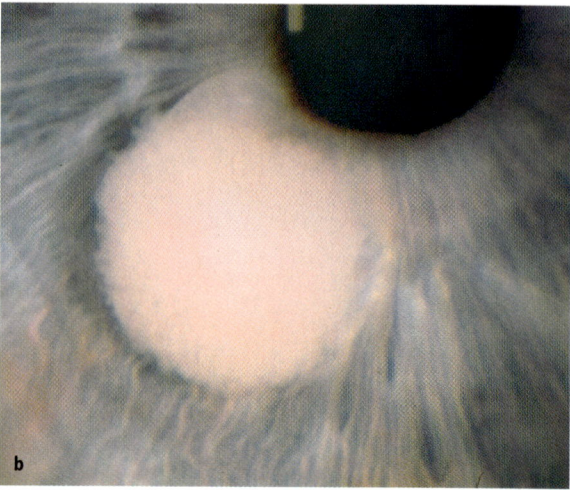
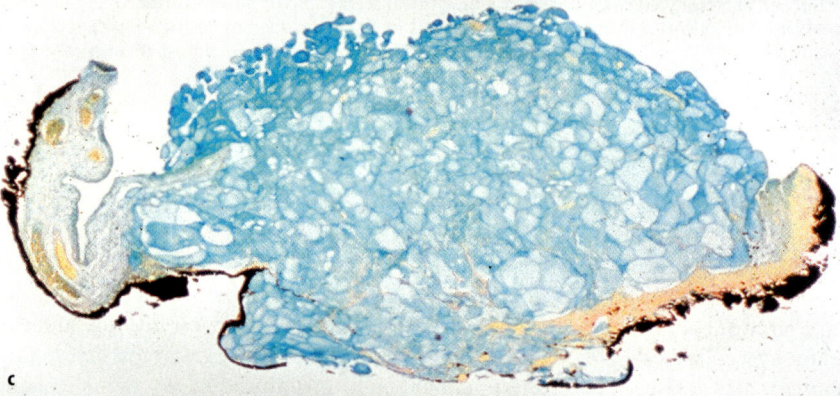
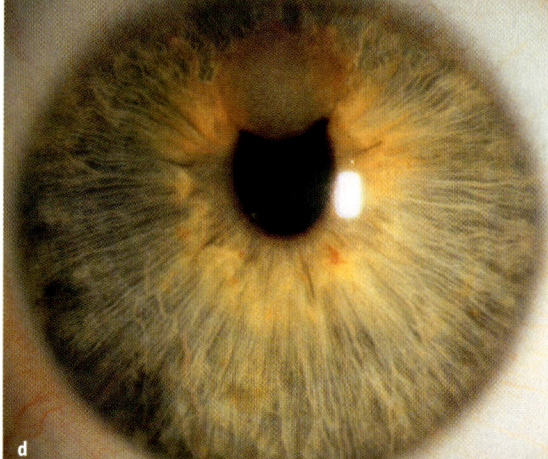

Fig. 5.3.13. *Localized iris tumors* not involving iris root sparing the chamber angle without signs of tumor cells shedding in the aqueous: suitable for curative iridectomy. **a–c** Xanthoma of the iris (Naumann and Ruprecht 1972). Colloidal iron stain for acid micropolysaccharides. **d** Leiomyoma of pupillary portion of the iris

Table 5.3.5. Heterochromia iridum – differential diagnosis of asymetric iris color (see Table 5.3.11)

A. *Congenital*
  1. Ocular melanocytosis
  2. Oculodermal melanocytosis (OTA and ITO)
  3. Waardenburg syndrome
  4. Hirschsprung's disease
  5. Iris bicolor
  6. Phakomatosis (Sturge-Weber-Krabbe)

B. *Acquired*
  1. Tumors
     – Diffuse iris melanoma
     – Diffuse iris nevus
     – Iris metastasis
     – Retinoblastoma
  2. Following hemorrhage: juvenile xanthogranuloma, trauma – hemosiderosis
  3. Metallosis, siderosis, chalcosis
     – Siderosis
     – Chalcosis
  4. Inflammations
     – Fuchs' heterochromic iridocyclitis
     – Chronic iridocyclitis
  5. Horner syndrome
  6. Pigment dispersion syndromes
     – Primary melanin-dispersion
     – Secondary (diabetes, trauma, myopia, pseudoexfoliation syndrome)

5.3.2 Surgical Pathology

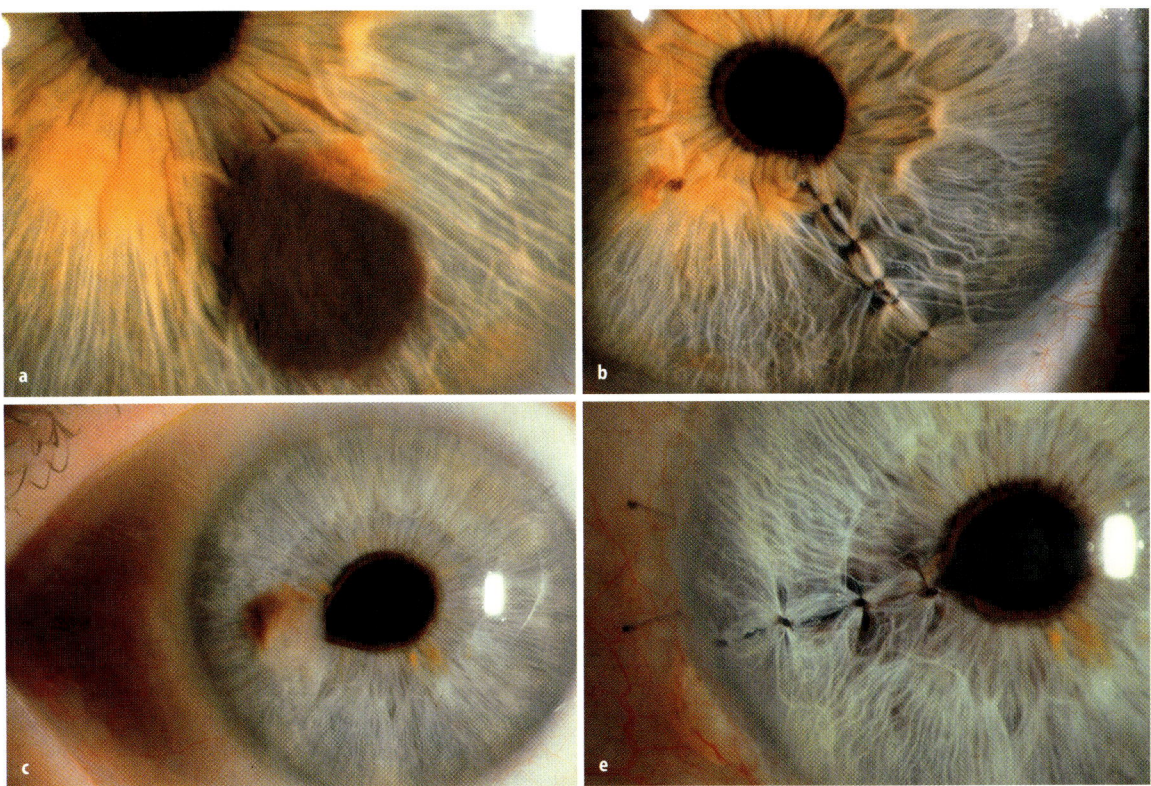

Fig. 5.3.14. Early melanomas of the iris (rare!) with *documented growth* sparing the chamber angle and sphincter pupillae. **a, b** Thirty-four-year-old male: **a** preoperatively; **b** after iridectomy sparing the sphincter pupillae and closing the iris defect with four interrupted 10-0 nylon sutures adapting the wound margins. Follow-up 16 years. **c** Preoperatively (52-year-old woman). **d** Curative excision. **e** Wound margins adapted by three interrupted 10-0 nylon sutures 1 year later

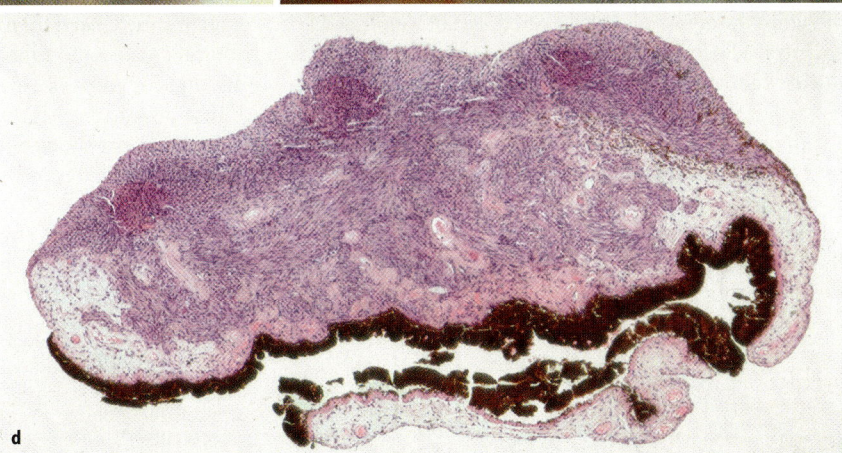

Table 5.3.6. Iris cysts: differential diagnosis

1. *Pigmented:*	Fixed at pupil or peripherally, floating into anterior chamber or vitreous
2. *Non-pigmented:*	a) Congenital: spontaneous or after amniocentesis
	b) Acquired: cystic ingrowth of corneal conjunctival epithelium or epidermis ("pearl cysts") floating in anterior chamber
	Parasitic

Table 5.3.7. Differential diagnosis: "Multiple iris nodules"

I. Melanocytic:
1. Diffuse malignant melanoma
2. Melanocytic nevi
3. Melanocytosis ocular or oculodermal
4. Brushfield spots
II. Neurofibromatosis I (Lisch nodules)
III. Granulomatous iritis
IV. ICE syndrome (Yanoff) and Rieger's anomaly
V. Metastasis
VI. Retinoblastoma

Table 5.3.8. Spectrum of laser effects on eye

I.	Cornea:	UV-excimer laser Femtolaser
II.	Trabecular meshwork:	Argon laser YAG laser
III.	Iris:	ALK *and* YAG
IV.	Lens:	YAG laser
V.	Retina starting at "oven" retinal pigment epithelium by thermic lasers (argon, krypton)	
VI.	Uveal tumors:	As adjunct

Table 5.3.9. Melanocytic processes of the iris

I.	Nevi
II.	Congenital melanocytosis a) Ocular b) Oculodermal (nevus of OTA) c) Oculofacial (nevus of ITO)
III.	Malignant melanoma: focal, diffuse
IV.	Pigmented epithelial cysts (see Table 5.3.6) and adenomas

Table 5.3.10. Non-pigmented tumors of iris

I.	Vascular:	Non-pigmented malignant melanoma Capillary hemangioma (rare), varix nodule
II.	Choristomas (congenital):	Non-pigmented epithelial cysts (see Table 5.3.6)
III.	Myogenic:	Leiomyoma Rhadomyosarcoma
IV.	Neurogenic:	Neurolemmoma (schwannoma) Neurofibroma
V.	Histiocytic:	Juvenile xanthogranuloma Xanthoma
VI.	Granulomatous inflammation, e.g., sarcoidosis	

Before considering local excision, two questions need to be clarified: (1) Is the process localized or are cells shedding into the aqueous? Diffuse shedding of tumor cells is a contraindication for local excision (Fig. 5.3.17). (2) Is the iris root and chamber angle involved? Then you *cannot* separate the process from the ciliary body.

All progressive melanocytic and other tumors localized to the iris root will therefore require *block excision* of the tumor including adjacent iris, pars plicata of the ciliary body, cornea and sclera (Fig. 5.3.16) – but only if the tumor is localized. The resulting defect in the eye wall needs to be closed by tectonic corneoscleral graft (see also Chapter 5.4).

5.3.2.7
Epithelial Ingrowth, Diffuse and Cystic

Epithelial ingrowth theoretically may follow surgical intervention or trauma with any opening of the anterior segment of the eye in spite of meticulous microsurgical techniques. Particularly puncture wounds of the peripheral cornea and limbus and their ensuing scars are difficult – or impossible – to detect with the slit lamp. Almost always the epithelial ingrowth covers the iris root and anterior face of the ciliary body and therefore requires *block excision* including adjacent iris, ciliary body, pars plicata of the ciliary body,* sclera and cornea – acting as a shell. A mechanical sector iridectomy or laser iridotomy is *contraindicated* in all non-pig-

---

* Removal of the pars plicata of the ciliary body up to 150° of the circumference by block excision does *not* lead to a cyclodialysis. This – to our own surprise – *never* occurred in over 200 patients successfully treated with block excision for tumors of the anterior uvea or epithelial ingrowths (see also "minimal eye" in Chapter 4, Sect. 4.7 and 5.4).

Fig. 5.3.15. Wound healing of the iris in the rabbit 3 weeks after iridotomy with several interrupted sutures adapting the wound margins illustrating stromal and iris-pigment epithelial wound healing. **a** Scheme of rabbit experiments showing the flat sections through healed scar (Hinzpeter et al. 1974).

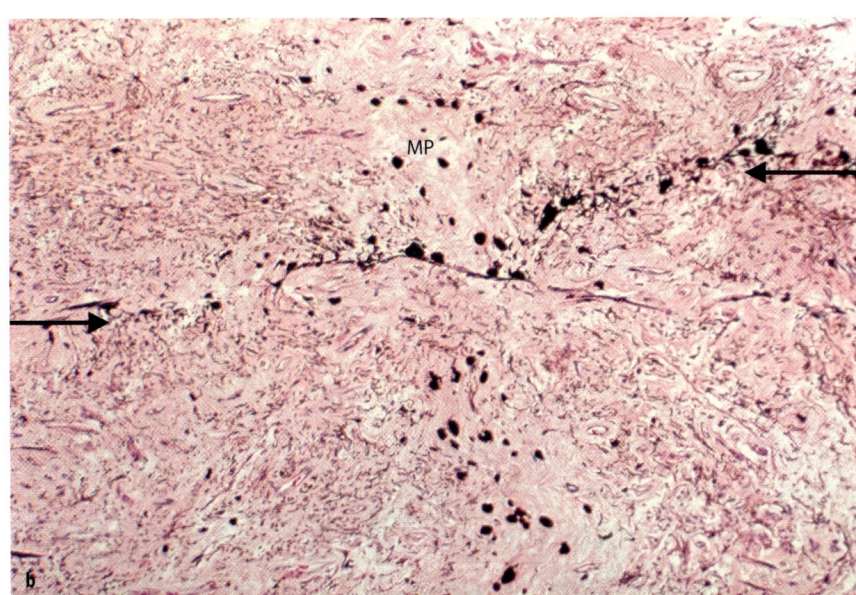

Fig. 5.3.15. b Histology: Closure of iridotomy (*arrows*) by fibro-vascular and pigment epithelial proliferation. Melanophages (*MP*) in area of iris-stroma necrosis

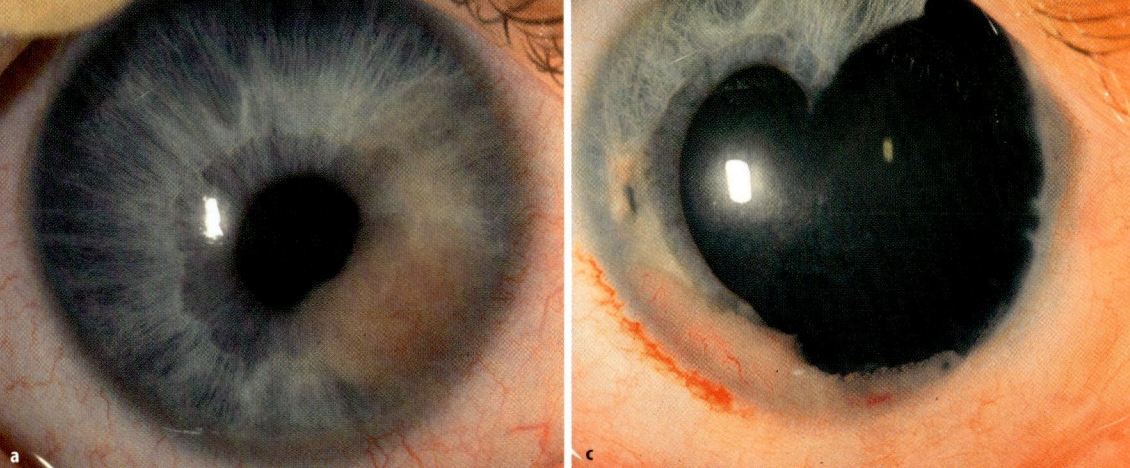

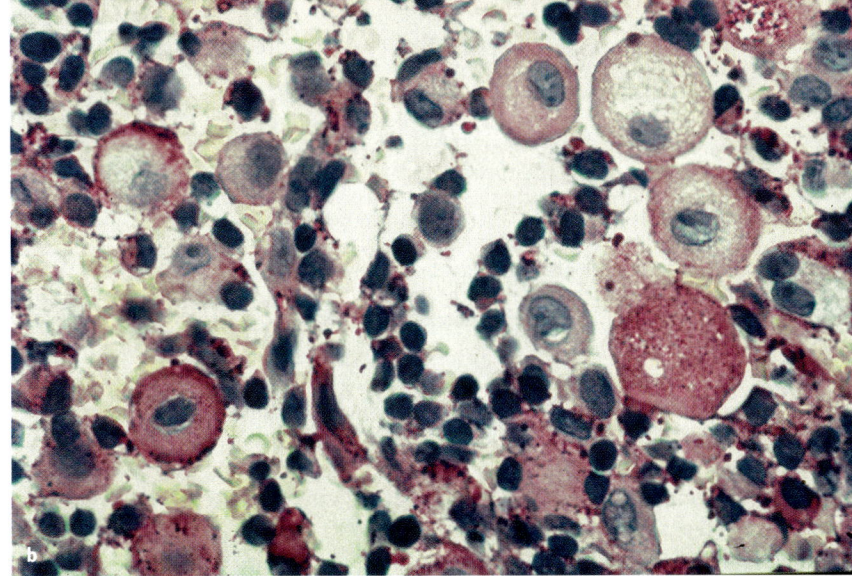

Fig. 5.3.16. Primary rhabdomyosarcoma of iris involving the iris root *and* chamber angle: iridectomy cannot be curative. **a** Preoperatively. **b** Histology of the iris biopsy with loosely arranged PAS-positive rhabdomyoblasts. **c** One year after sector iridectomy with massive recurrence in ciliary body and rest of the iris (Naumann et al., 1972). After radiotherapy and enucleation follow-up for 27 years without recurrence. PS: Involvement of the iris root *always* requires not only iridectomy but also excision of the adjacent pars plicata of the ciliary body as block excision (see Chapter 5.4, Fig. 5.4.13)

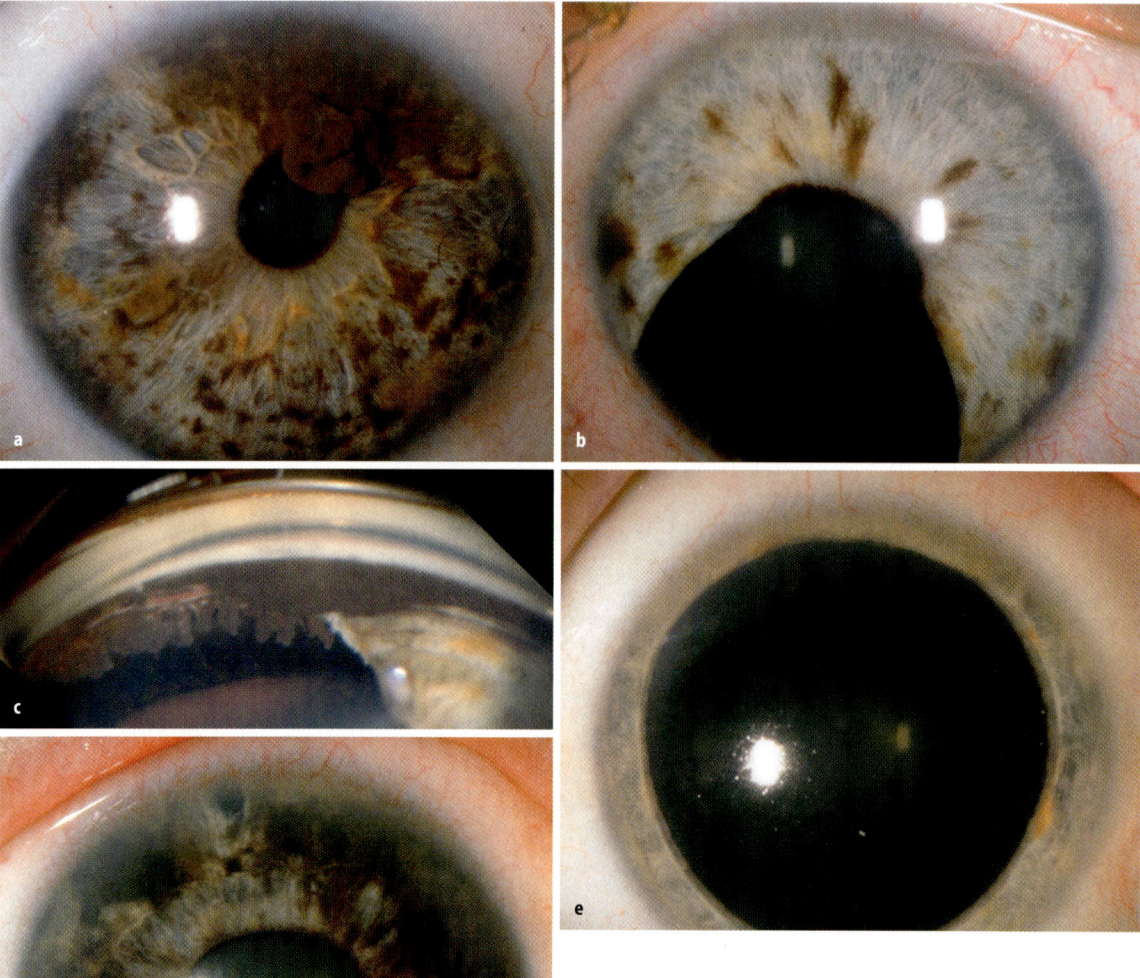

Fig. 5.3.17. Malignant melanomas of the iris root with diffuse shedding of the malignant melanocytes into the aqueous. Case 1: **a** Malignant melanoma of the iris from 11 to 2 o'clock between pupil and chamber angle with diffuse shedding of malignant melanocytes (53-year-old female patient). Case 2: **b** Recurrence of malignant melanoma after incomplete excision by sector iridectomy in 27-year-old male. **c** Ciliary body invasion. Case 3: **d, e** Diffuse malignant melanoma of the iris with invasion of the ciliary body (**d**) after laser iridotomy elsewhere. **e** Uninvolved other eye

mented epithelial cysts involving the iris root, because it *converts a cystic into a diffuse epithelial ingrowth*! As the epithelial tract connecting the surface epithelium with the intraocular portion of the epithelial ingrowth is non-pigmented it *cannot* usually be detected clinically – unless there is a (rare) fistula – in which case the adjacent sclera and cornea are potentially involved and it must be removed in full thickness. The resulting defect in the eye wall is then closed by a full thickness corneoscleral graft. Every cyst overlying the iris *root* will require this radical approach! (see Chapter 5.4).

Only tiny implantations-epithelial cysts located in the pupillary portion of the iris *not* involving the angle can be cured by simple iridectomy or sector iridectomy – and this in our exprience is rare (Figs. 5.3.18–5.3.20).

5.3.2.8
Non-invasive In Vivo Diagnostic Procedures for Processes of the Iris

These procedures include slit lamp including "biocytology" at ×40 magnification and gonioscopy, specular corneal endothelial microscopy (PEX), echography, ultrasound biomicroscopy (USB), and non contact optical coherence tomography (OCT). Laser tyndallometry measures blood-aqueous barrier breakdown and melanin dispersion.

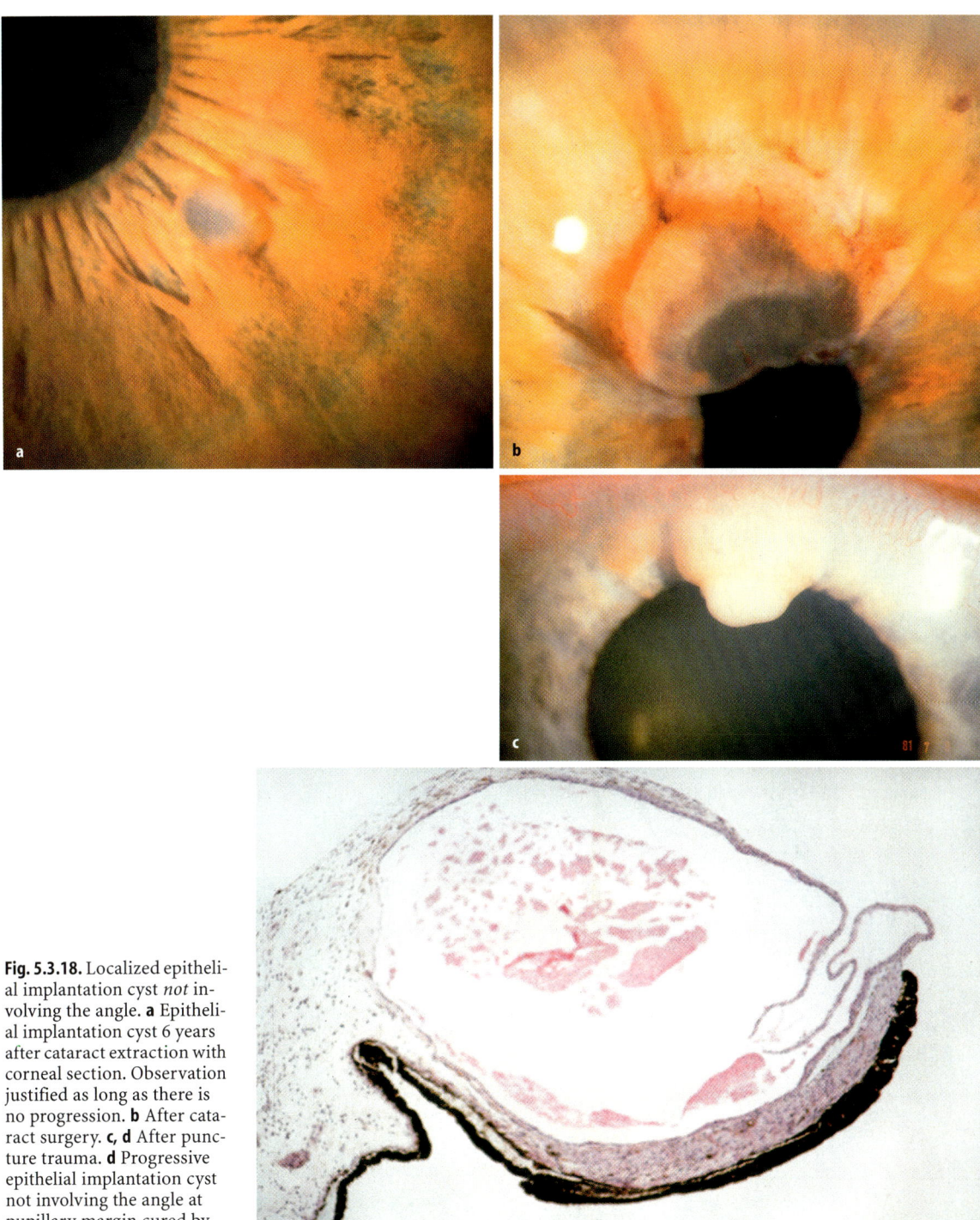

Fig. 5.3.18. Localized epithelial implantation cyst *not* involving the angle. **a** Epithelial implantation cyst 6 years after cataract extraction with corneal section. Observation justified as long as there is no progression. **b** After cataract surgery. **c, d** After puncture trauma. **d** Progressive epithelial implantation cyst not involving the angle at pupillary margin cured by sector iridectomy: removed cyst (PAS-positive)

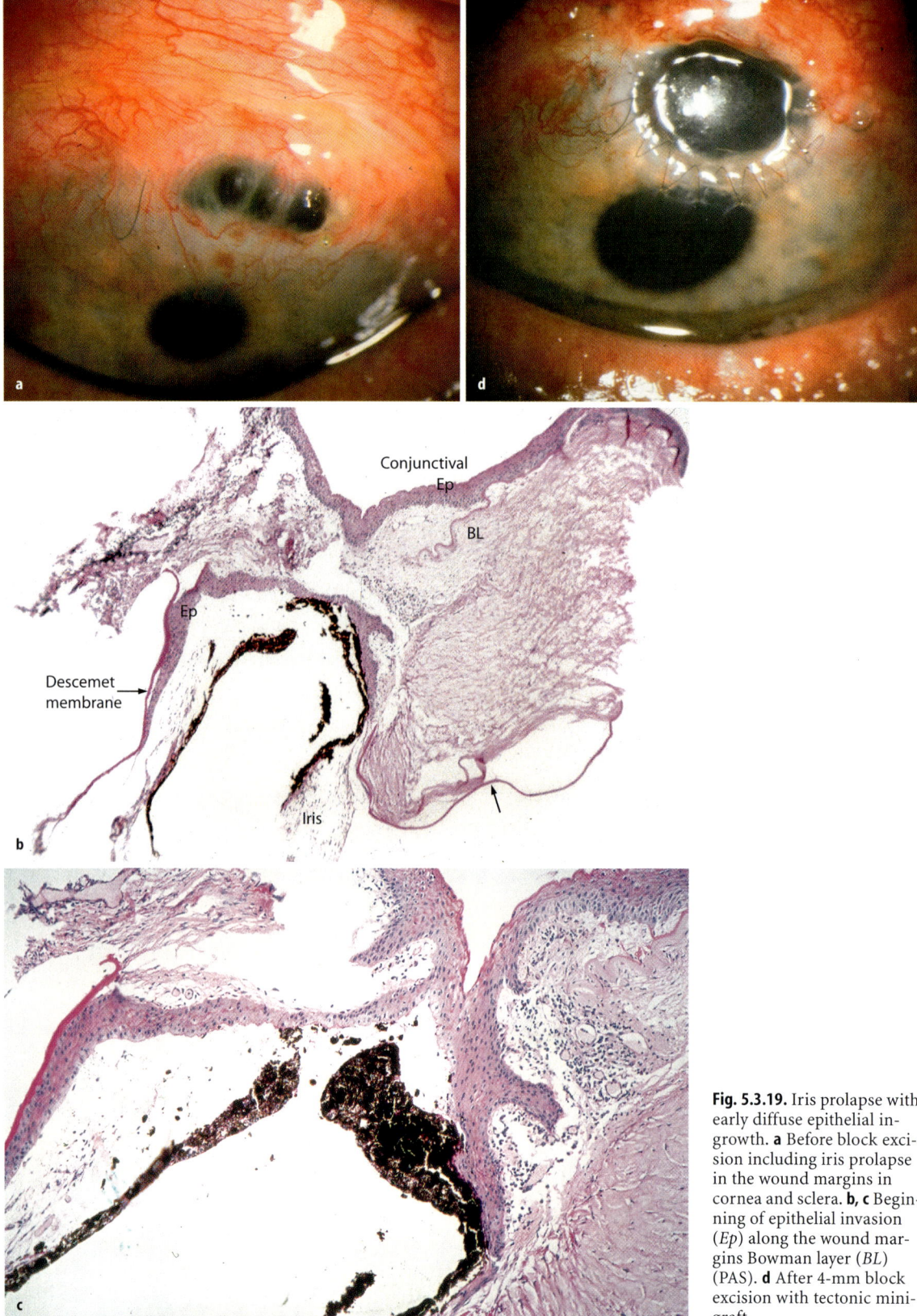

Fig. 5.3.19. Iris prolapse with early diffuse epithelial ingrowth. **a** Before block excision including iris prolapse in the wound margins in cornea and sclera. **b, c** Beginning of epithelial invasion (*Ep*) along the wound margins Bowman layer (*BL*) (PAS). **d** After 4-mm block excision with tectonic minigraft

Fig. 5.3.20. Diffuse epithelial ingrowth of variable thickness (*arrows*) of iris root, face of ciliary body and retrocorneal surface showing epithelial tract connecting with the surface epithelium. Diffuse ingrowth on iris root requires block excision including the adjacent sector of the pars plicata of ciliary body

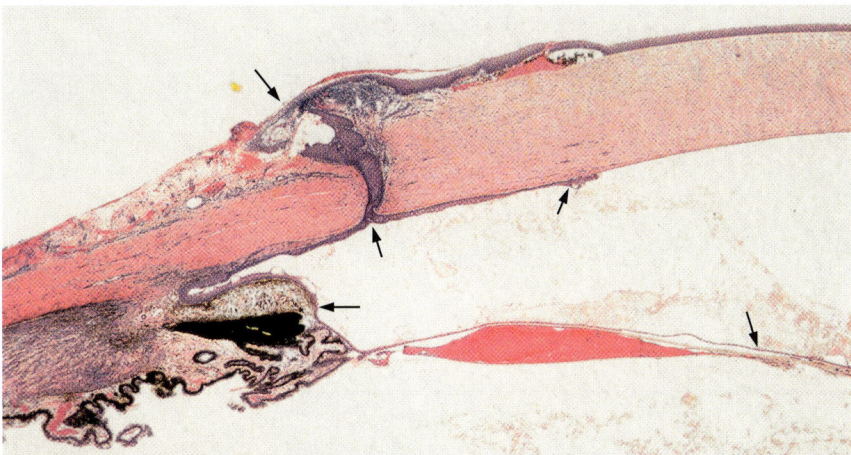

Fig. 5.3.21. Attempted YAG-laser iridotomy for angle closure glaucoma. **a** Posterior synechiae (*PS*), after necrosis of iris stroma and iris pigment epithelium (*PE*), defect in Descemet's membrane (*large arrow*), fragments shot and buried in iris stroma (*small arrow*), persisting angle closure.

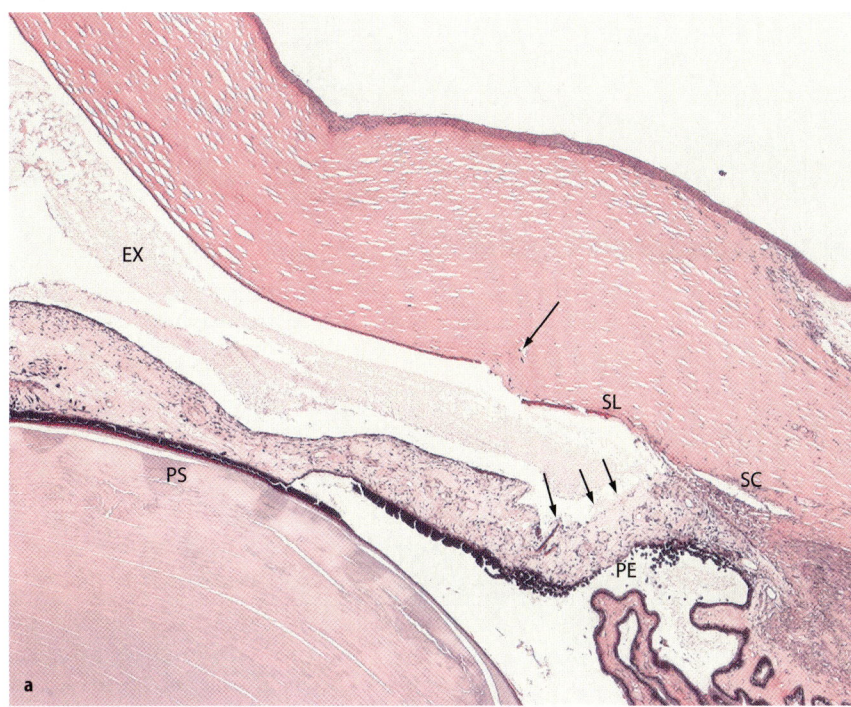

5.3.3 Indications for Surgical Procedures Involving the Iris

5.3.3.1 YAG-Laser Iridotomy and Iridoplasty

YAG-laser iridotomy for cure and prevention of manifest or imminent *pupillary block*: As the iris root peripheral to Fuchs' roll is the thinnest region of the iris stroma, every effort should be made to apply the laser here, because a through and through shunt from the posterior to anterior chamber can be achieved with little energy and few side effects (Figs. 5.3.10, 5.3.21).

Medical miosis pulls Fuchs' roll towards the pupil and exposes the iris root. The laser iridotomy should best be performed superiorly between 11 and 1 o'clock in order to avoid monocular diplopia from the iridotomy within the lid fissure (Fig. 5.3.10).

Non-penetrating argon-laser coagulation may facilitate perforating YAG iridotomy by burning and thinning a very dark-brown and thick-iris stroma as a preparatory first step.

In iris-plateau syndrome, argon *iridoplasty* also attempts to pull the Fuchs' roll away from Schwalbe's line to open a narrow or closed angle.

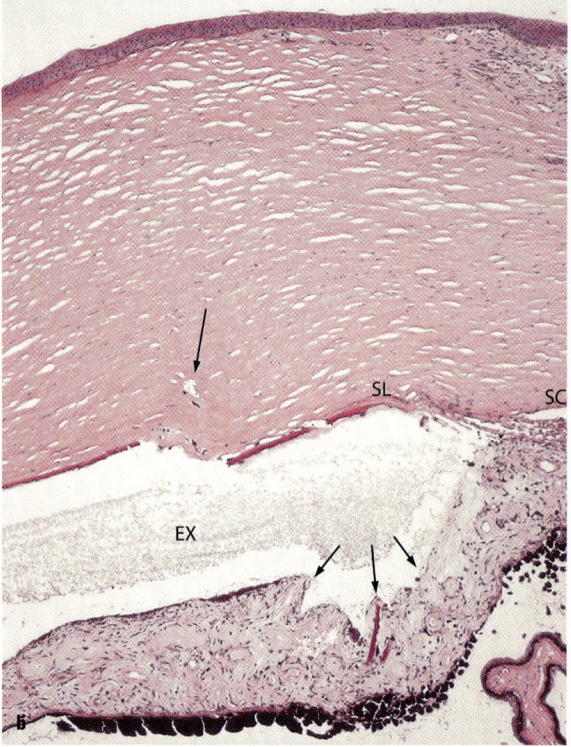
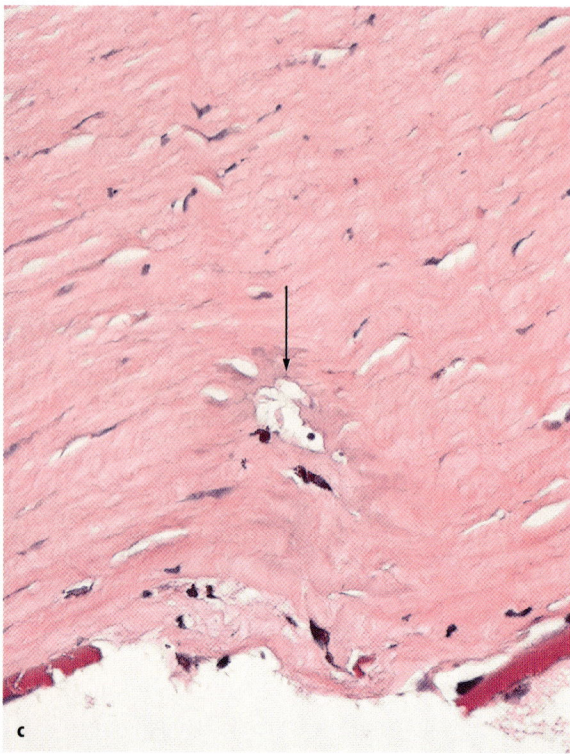
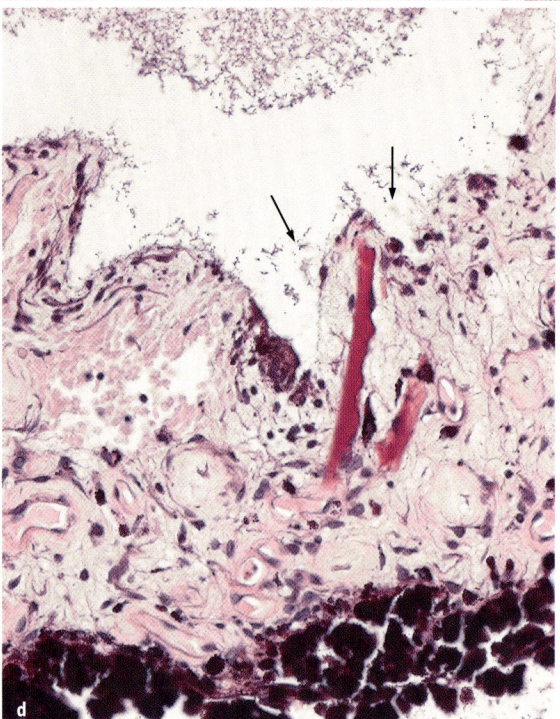

Fig. 5.3.21. b Higher power illustrates interruption of Descemet's membrane and melanophage cells in deep corneal stroma with vacuoles (from YAG laser). Exudate in anterior chamber (*EX*). Necrosis of iris stroma and iris pigment epithelium (*IPE*). **c** Higher power. **d** Descemet fragments buried in the iris stroma (PAS)

5.3.3.2
Mechanical Iridotomy and Iridectomy

Peripheral iridectomy must be performed by transcorneal or transcorneoscleral incisions if the cornea is too opaque and the iris stroma too thick to perforate it with lasers. Preferably these peripheral iridotomies should be performed superiorly between 11 and 1 o'clock to avoid monocular diplopia.

In adult extracapsular cataract extraction with lens implantation using today's technique, a peripheral iridectomy for prevention of pupillary block is usually not necessary. However, it is mandatory in intracapsular surgery and advisable for congenital cataracts – in view of the high permeability of infant blood-aqueous barriers.

5.3.3.3
Mechanical Mydriasis

Persisting posterior synechiae usually prevent medicamentous mydriasis and thus makes free access to the lens in cataract surgery impossible. Iris hooks and other devices achieve mechanical mydriasis and allow delicate maneuvers of the anterior lens capsule and inside the capsular bag. Mechanical mydriasis is also helpful in the triple procedure of simultaneous corneal transplantation and extracapsular cataract extraction with lens implantation in an open-sky technique (see Chapters 5.1, 5.5). This is particularly useful in eyes with pseudoexfoliation syndrome showing poor mydriasis and phacodonesis (see Chapters 5.1, 5.5, and 5.6, Sect. 5.6.3).

The *intraoperative floppy-iris syndrome* (IFIS) associated with generalized medication of α_1-blockers (tamsulosin for prostate hypertrophy) also requires mechanical mydriasis.

5.3.3.4
Sector Iridectomy

If mechanical mydriasis with iris hooks fails because of marked atrophy or fibrosis of the iris stroma, sector iridectomy may be less traumatic: starting with two small peripheral iridectomies at 11 and 1 o'clock, two radial incisions are performed into the pupillary area and then the iris tissue sector is removed using the slender and long iris scissors. To avoid recurrent pupillary block from the iris-sector wound margins attaching to the lens, we recommend one or two additional small peripheral iridotomies outside the sector iridotomy.

Optical sector iridectomy may be indicated as an alternative option for central corneal scars in microphthalmic eyes or in situations where corneal transplantation has a very poor prognosis, for instance, in Peters' anomaly (Fig. 5.3.18) – or in congenital cataracts in small eyes of very young infants (Fig. 5.3.10; Jünemann et al. 1996).

5.3.3.5
Closure of Iridodialysis

Closure of these defects is necessary only if the iridodialysis is causing monocular diplopia. Two approaches are possible: (1) McCannel recommended transcorneal sutures attaching the peripheral iris to the peripheral cornea always creating broad anterior synechiae, and (2) direct suturing under microscopic control after corneoscleral incisions minimizing the adhesions within the chamber angle. It is only rarely combined with cyclodialysis (see Chapter 5.4).

5.3.3.6
Localized Excision and Block Excisions of Iris Tumors and Epithelial Implantation Cysts

Localized excision is indicated only if there is *no* evidence of spreading of tumor cells into the aqueous. Removal of an iris tumor by "simple" *iridectomy* is proper in the rather *uncommon* situation that the iris root is *not* involved. Closure of the resulting defect requires *several* sutures in order to achieve wound healing in the well adapted iris stroma regions (Fig. 5.3.12, Fig. 5.3.22). If the tumor or epithelial ingrowth involves the iris root, it *always* involves the face of the pars plicata of the ciliary body and the insertion of the ciliary muscle to the scleral spur. Therefore an iridectomy cannot achieve a curative excision complete *block excision* requires removal of the adjacent pars plicata of the ciliary body as well as sclera and cornea. The defect is closed by a corneal or corneoscleral graft (see Chapter 5.4).

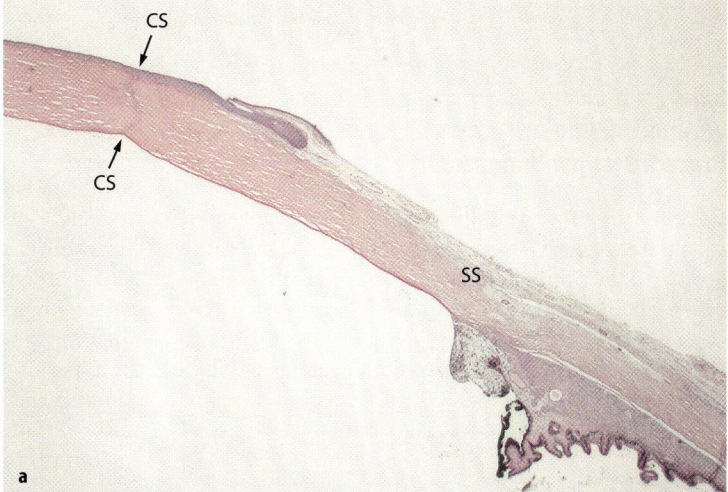

Fig. 5.3.22. a Diffuse malignant melanoma of iris. Scar of perforating wound of cornea (*CS*) as entrance for biopsy with recurrence in adjacent iris root and in the opposite angle. Endothelialization of the pseudoangle, pseudoexfoliation syndrome.
a Overview (PAS)

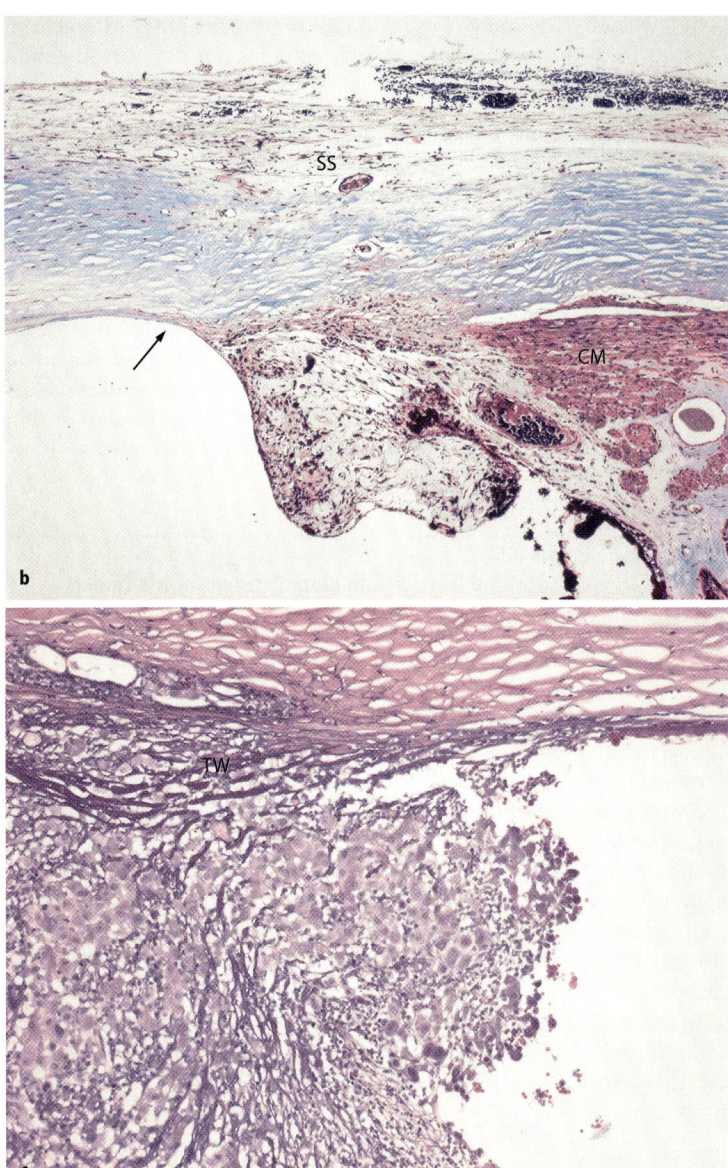

Fig. 5.3.22. b Iris root covering trabecular meshwork occluding angle endothelialization of pseudoangle (*arrow*), pseudoexfoliation syndrome, episcleral scar after trabeculectomy (*SS*), Ciliary muscle (*CM*) (MASSON). **c** Opposite angle shows massive recurrence with invasion of trabecular meshwork (*TW*), Schlemm's canal and collector channels and face of ciliary body

5.3.4
Wound Healing and Complications of Procedures Involving the Iris

Circumscribed defects in the iris stroma after mechanical or laser surgery – very fortunately for the microsurgeon and the patient! – usually do *not* heal spontaneously. The flow of aqueous from posterior to anterior chamber clears the wound edges from the fibrin scaffolding necessary for normal wound healing elsewhere in the eye or body (Fig. 5.3.23).

5.3.4.1
Iris Sutures

However, wound healing of adapted edges of iris wounds follows a similar pattern to wound healing elsewhere except that it takes a longer time (Fig. 5.3.12, Hinzpeter et al., 1974 a, b). A single 10-0 nylon suture usually does not induce the wound healing process because in the area of the suture the tissue is necrotic and the adjacent wound edges are retracted by the iris muscles and washed by the aqueous. In order to achieve sufficient adaptation, a *minimum of two interrupted iris sutures* is necessary.

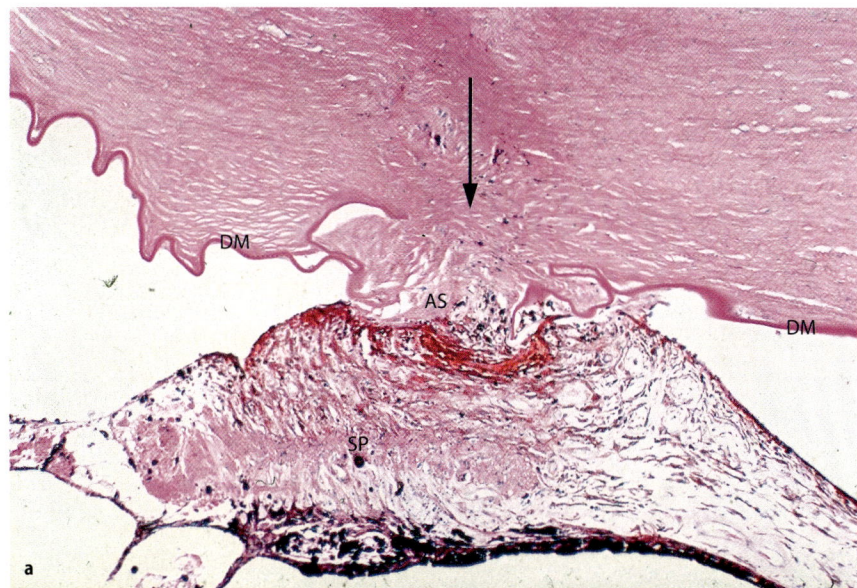

Fig. 5.3.23. Persisting anterior synechiae of iris to cornea (*AS*) after perforating injury. **a** Fibrotic partially vascularized corneal scar (*arrow*) connecting to pupillary iris 9 months after perforating injury, sphincter pupillae (*SP*). **b** Peripheral iris after failure to reestablish the anterior chamber and separating iris-root from trabecular meshwork. Schwalbe' line (*SL*), Descemet's membrane (*DM*) (PAS-stain)

Table 5.3.11. Ocular pigments

I. *Melanin*
   1. Free in anterior chamber and vitreous cavity from:
      a) Pigment epithelium
      b) Uveal melanocytes benign and malignant in necrotic tissue
   2. Intracellular
      a) Uveal melanocytes of iris and pigment epithelium
      b) Melanophages after liberation of melanin by necrosis of pigment epithelium and iris melanocytes
      c) Remnants of persisting pupillary membrane

II. *Hemosiderin/ferritin*
   a) Hudson-Stahli line and other iron lines of the cornea (Table 5.1.5)
   b) Hemosiderosis: in macrophages after i.o. hemorrhage
   c) Siderosis: intraocular iron foreign body

III. *Lipofuscin*
   a) In scars of corneal stroma
   b) In the RPE
   c) In macrophages overlying choroidal tumors

IV. *Metallosis*: hepatolenticular dystrophy Wilson: Kayser-Fleischer ring (multiple myeloma, rare) Argyrosis: exogenous and endogenous

V. *External pigments*: gold, medications, local and systemic

VI. *Xanthophyll* in retinal ganglion cells

5.3.4.2
Laser Iridotomy and Hemorrhage from Iris

Laser iridotomy usually results in a very small defect that remains patent (Tesumoto et al. 1992) (Figs. 5.3.10, 5.3.21). Occasionally proliferations of the pigment epithelium may close these small openings. These secondary occlusions can simply be reopened by low dose argon-laser applications.

Hemorrhages from involved iris vessels may result from laser and mechanical manipulations. They are

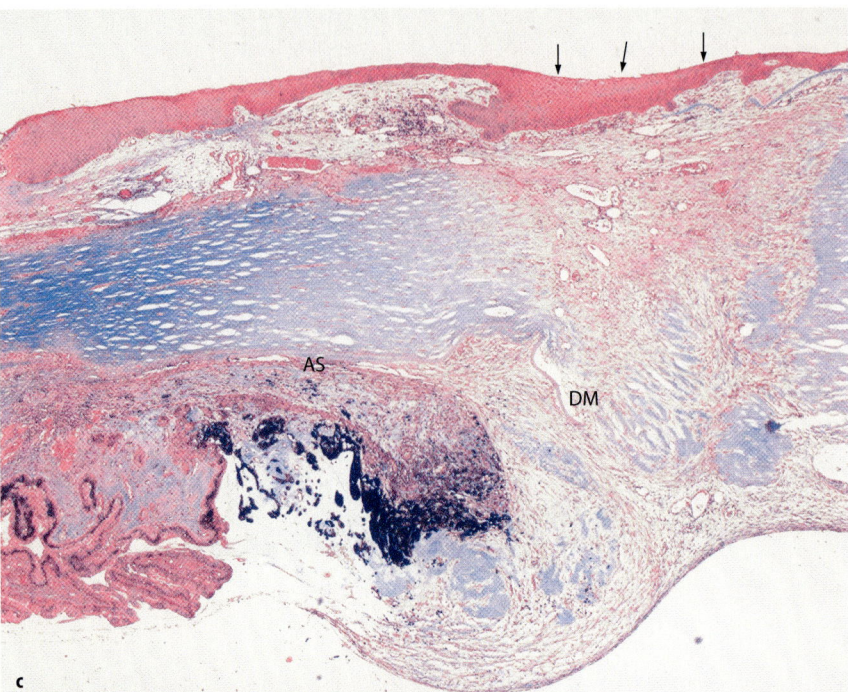

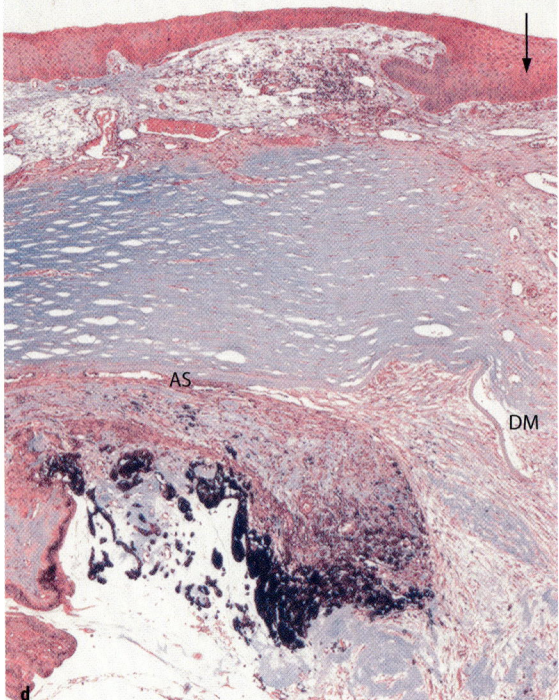

Fig. 5.3.23. c, d Crushed iris stroma and pigment epithelium remnants attached to extensive limbal scar, (MASSON-stain). Descemet's membrane (*DM*)

rare in both instances. Such hemorrhages usually stop spontaneously as soon as the intraocular pressure rises. The nature of ocular pigments varies widely (Table 5.3.11).

Spontaneous hemorrhages from the iris without direct microsurgical trauma may occur after opening the anterior chamber in eyes with rubeosis iridis, with PEX iridopathy and with heterochromia complicata (Fuchs) and should alert the surgeon to these entities.

Laser iridotomy in very narrow or flat anterior chambers may be accompanied by a defect in the adjacent Descemet's membrane and corneal endothelium. This induces transitory circumscribed edema of the corneal stroma. Fragments of the broken Descemet's membrane may be dislocated by the laser application into the iris stroma (Fig. 5.3.20). Traces of microsurgical manipulations of the iris – e.g., by forceps or during trephination in perforating keratoplasty (PRP), remain visible indefinitely because the iris does not possess any repair mechanisms. This is more obvious in brown irides.

References (see also page 379)

Braun UC, Rummelt V, Naumann GOH. Diffuse maligne Melanome der Uvea. Eine klinisch-histopathologische Studie über 39 Patienten. Klin Monatsbl Augenheilkd 1998; 213: 1–10

Hinzpeter EN, Demeler U, Naumann G. Iriswundheilung nach zweifacher Naht einer experimentellen Iridotomie I. Lichtmikroskopische Betrachtungen am Kaninchen Albrecht v Graefes Arch Ophthmol 1974; 191: 215–229

Hinzpeter EN, Ortbauer R, Naumann G. Healing of a sutured iridotomy in man Ophthalmologica 1974; 169: 390–396

Jünemann A, Gusek GC, Naumann GOH Optische Sektoriridektomie: Eine Alternative zur perforierenden Keratoplastik bei Petersscher Anomalie Klin Monatsbl Augenheilkd 1996; 209: 117–124

Jünemann A, Holbach L, Naumann GOH. Leiomyom der Iris Klin Monatsbl Augenheilkd 1992; 201: 322–324

Küchle M, Naumann GOH. Varixknoten der Iris mit Spontan-Regression Klin Monatsbl Augenheilkd 1992; 200: 233–236

Mühlenweg I, Naumann GOH. Sekundäres Pigmentdispersions-Syndrom nach medikamentöser Dauer-Mydriasis über 24 Jahren Klin Monatsbl Augenheilkd 1981; 178: 24–25

Naumann G, Font RL, Zimmerman LE. Primary Rhabdomyosarcoma of the Iris. Am J Ophthalmol 1972; 74:110–118

Naumann G, Ruprecht KW. Xanthom der Iris Ophthalmologica 1972; 164: 293–305

Taban M, Behrens A, Newcomb RL, Nobe MY, Saedi G, Sweet PM, McDonnell PJ. Acute endophthalmitis following cataract surgery. Arch Ophthalmol 2005; 123: 613–620

Tetsumoto K, Küchle M, Naumann GOH. Late Histopathological Findings of Neodymium: YAG Laser Iridotomies in Humans. Arch Ophthalmol 1992; 110: 1119–1123

5.4 Ciliary Body

G.O.H. Naumann

The ciliary body serves the essential functions of: (1) *equilibrium of the intraocular pressure* by secretion of aqueous from the ciliary epithelium and influencing the outflow by contraction of the ciliary muscle to the scleral spur and therefore indirectly the trabecular meshwork; also by the secretion of hyaluronic acid from the ciliary epithelium of the pars plana. (2) *Accommodation* by the activity of the ciliary muscle which is transmitted to the lens via the zonula fibers originating from the pars plicata and pars plana of the ciliary body. Contraction of the ciliary muscle also regulates the "foveal stretch," the orientation of the photoreceptor outer segments by pulling at the Bruch's membrane. (3) All intraocular tissues are firmly *anchored* at the scleral spur anteriorly and the juxtapapillary Elschnig's spur posteriorly (Fig. 5.4.1).

Several concerns have made direct surgery of the ciliary body, particularly the pars plicata, an untouchable taboo zone until recently (ca 5.4.1). Except for the removal of malignant tumors, direct contact or cutting of the ciliary body was considered *contraindicated*. Only cyclodestruction or access for pars plana vitrectomy had been routine. We shall illustrate how these risks can be controlled, if some nuances are observed.

Table 5.4.1. Concerns with direct surgery of the ciliary body

1. Intraocular hemorrhage
2. Hypotony – atrophy of the globe
3. Lens: Decentration-subluxation
   Nuclear cataract
4. Retinal detachment
5. Remnants – recurrence

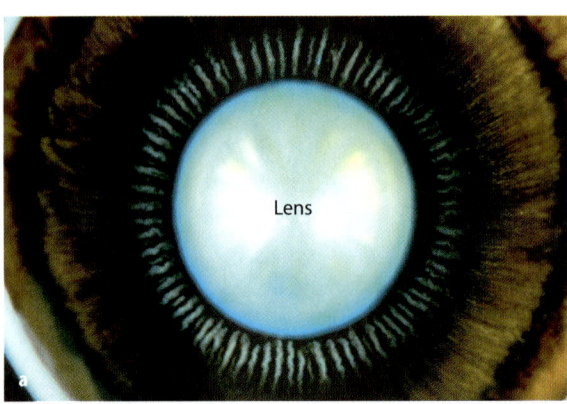
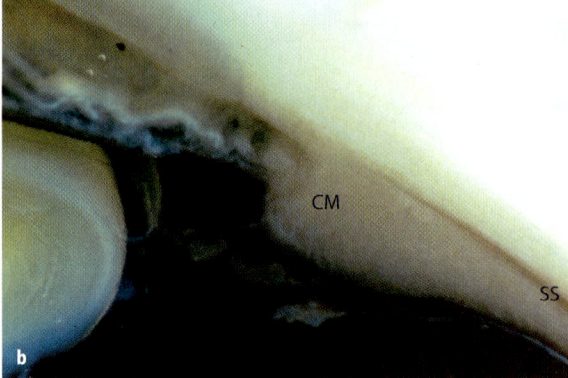
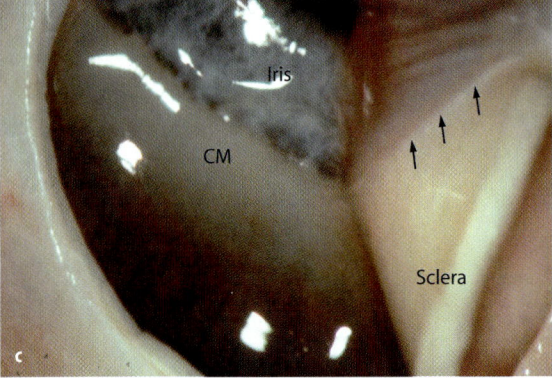

Fig. 5.4.1. Normal ciliary body. **a** View from vitreous showing ciliary processes and pars plana up to the ora. **b** Cross section: ciliary muscle and sclera in loose contact allowing contraction for accommodation. Supraciliary space (*SS*). **c** Only the ciliary muscle (*CM*) is fixed with a fine line to the scleral spur (*arrow*): donor eye with preparation of corneoscleral graft to cover defect after block excision

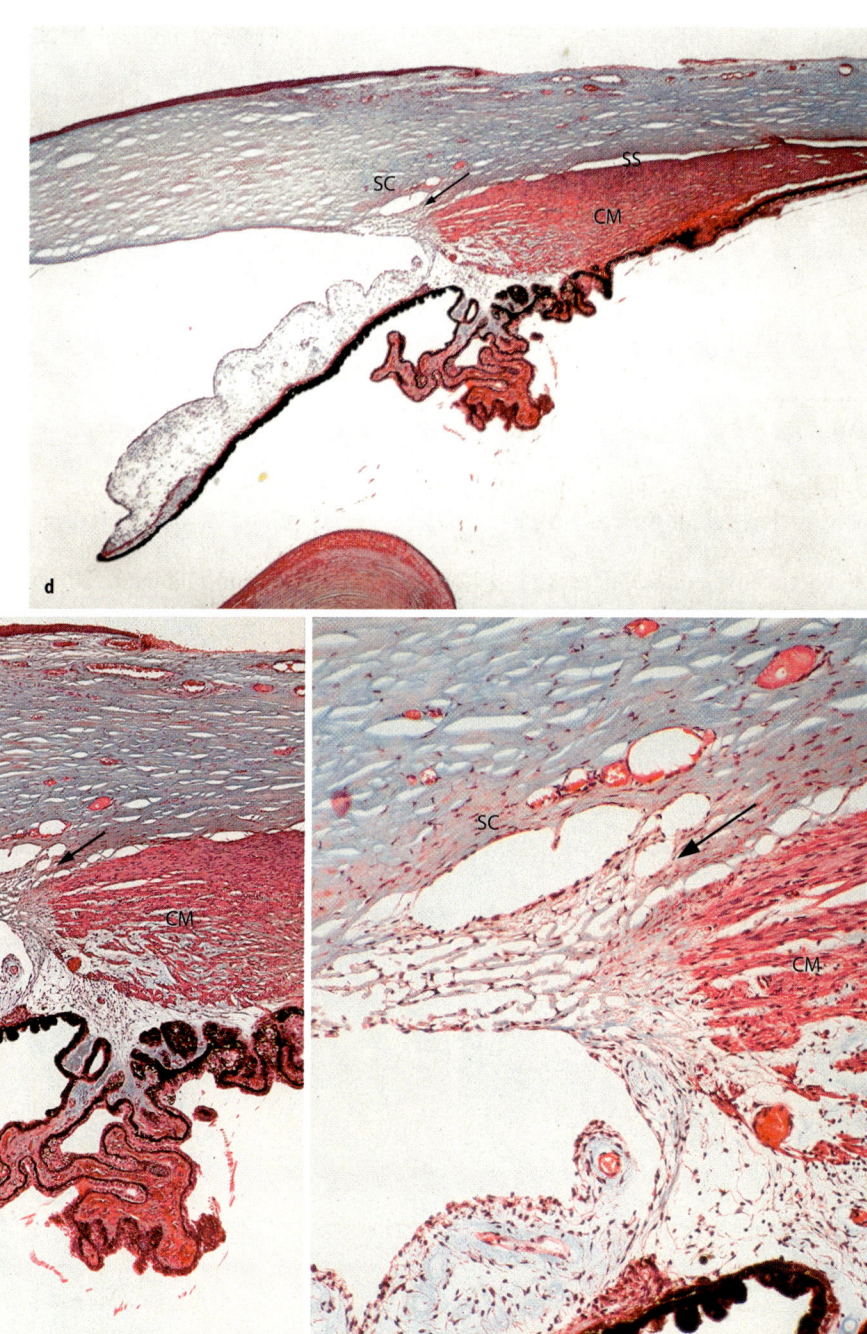

Fig. 5.4.1. d–f Histopathology demonstrating ciliary muscle insertion to scleral spur. Schlemm's canal (*SC*) and collector channels partially filled with blood. Supraciliary space extending up to scleral spur (*arrow*)

From our own experience of over 200 patients with block excision of expanding *tumors of the anterior uvea* including the angle and for *epithelial ingrowth*, we know that the pars plicata of the ciliary body can be excised up to 150° (5 h of the circumference) *without* inducing a persisting hypotony. Also, treatment of *traumatic cyclodialysis causing persisting ocular hypotony* can be cured by direct cyclopexy under microscopic control.

5.4.1
Surgical Anatomy

The ciliary body extends between the scleral spur visible by gonioscopy to the ora serrata recognizable by funduscopy and indentation or by diaphanoscopy. The ciliary muscle extends between the scleral spur and the peripheral end of Bruch's membrane as "tensor choroideae" which is responsible also for the "foveal tilt of the photoreceptors" during accommodation (Enoch et al. 1975). The circular portion of the ciliary muscle contains more mitochondria than that close to the sclera. Between the ciliary muscle and sclera there is the *potential supraciliary space* allowing almost free movement of the ciliary muscle – against the sclera. The non-pigmented ciliary epithelium frequently shows aging changes (Fig. 5.4.2). Also part of the ciliary muscle is progressively replaced by collagenous tissue distributed in between the muscle fibers (Fig. 5.4.3).

The *vitreous base* is attached to the posterior 1–2 mm of the pars plana and extends towards the peripheral sensory retina adjacent to the ora serrata. The zonula apparatus originates from the pars plicata and the pars plana, fusing with the vitreous base, extending towards the anterior and posterior lens capsule, and reaching up to the ring-shaped Wieger's hyalocapsular ligament (see Chapters 5.5, 5.6).

The *blood supply* of the ciliary body originates from the long posterior ciliary arteries and anterior ciliary arteries forming a network of anastomosing vessels in connection with the major circle of the iris (Fig. 5.4.4). The ciliary processes contain many capillaries with a large diameter lined by *fenestrated* endothelium – even minor mechanical trauma may lead to marked hemorrhage. This was until recently one reason the ciliary body was considered a "taboo zone." Venous outflow occurs posteriorly through the vortex vein and to a lesser degree via the anterior ciliary veins.

The *ciliary body* has a dense network of parasympathic sympathetic and sensory nerves. The sensory innervation originates from the nasociliary nerves of the first branch of the trigeminus.

Blood-Aqueous Barrier. In the pars plicata of the ciliary body this is formed by the zonulae occludentes of the non-pigmented ciliary epithelium. There is a physiologic defect in the transition between the face of the ciliary body and iris root which may contribute to spontaneous hemorrhages following opening of the anterior chamber in Fuchs' complicated heterochromia and PEX iridopathy (see Chapter 2, Fig. 2.3; Chapter 6.3).

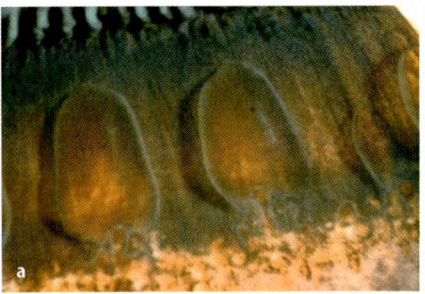 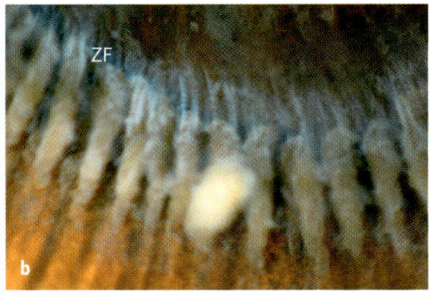

Fig. 5.4.2. Aging changes of ciliary epithelium: **a** "Pars plana cysts": de facto separation of the non- from the pigmented ciliary epithelium. **b** Pseudoepitheliomatous hyperplasia of the non-pigmented ciliary epithelium (Fuchs' adenoma) in 25% of autopsy eyes here in eye with pseudoexfoliation syndrome and interrupted zonular fibers (*ZF*)

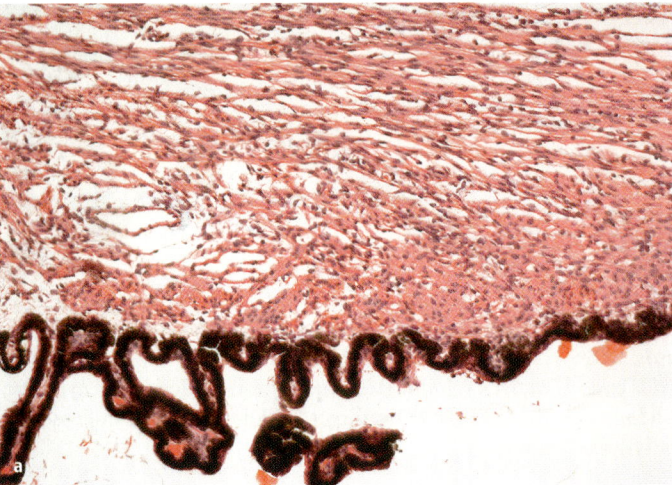

Fig. 5.4.3. Aging of the ciliary muscle: collagenous fibrous tissues (blue with Masson stain) increase progressively from birth to over 95 years: **a** 3 months

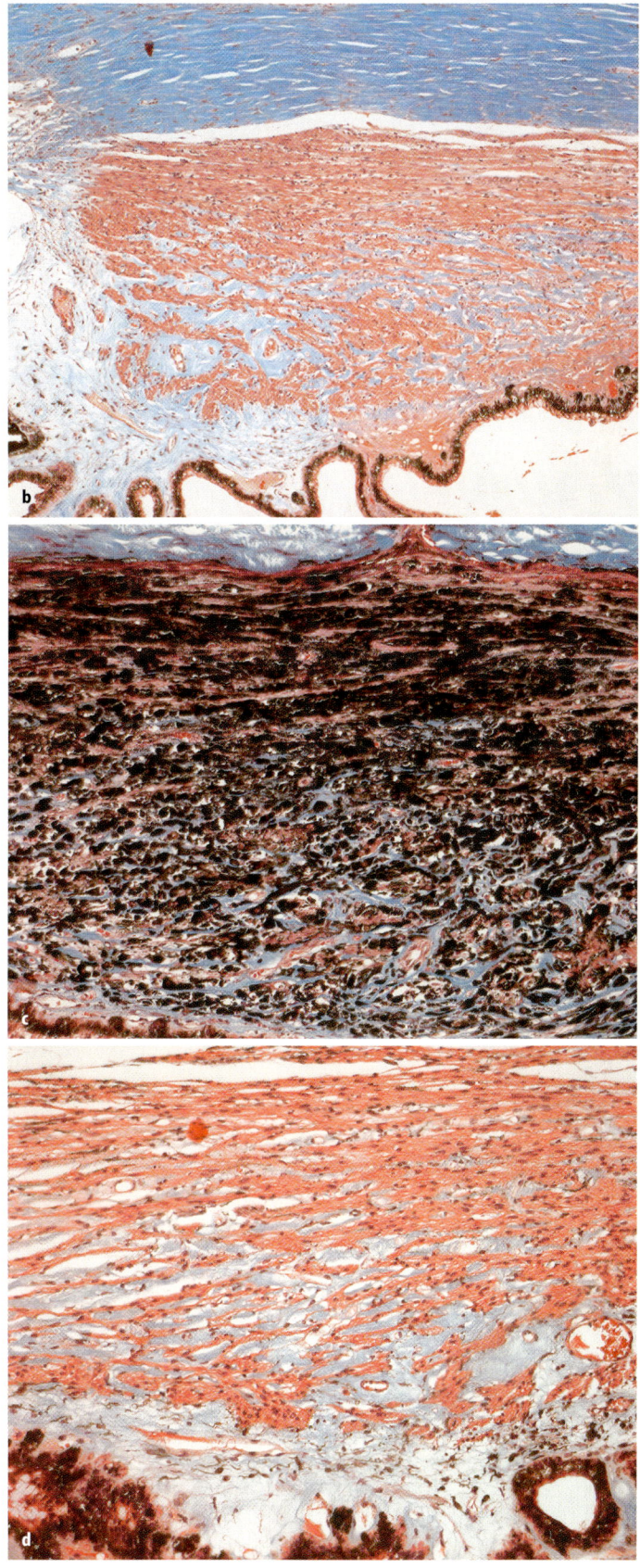

Fig. 5.4.3. b 46 years; **c** 56 years in an African person; **d** 60 years

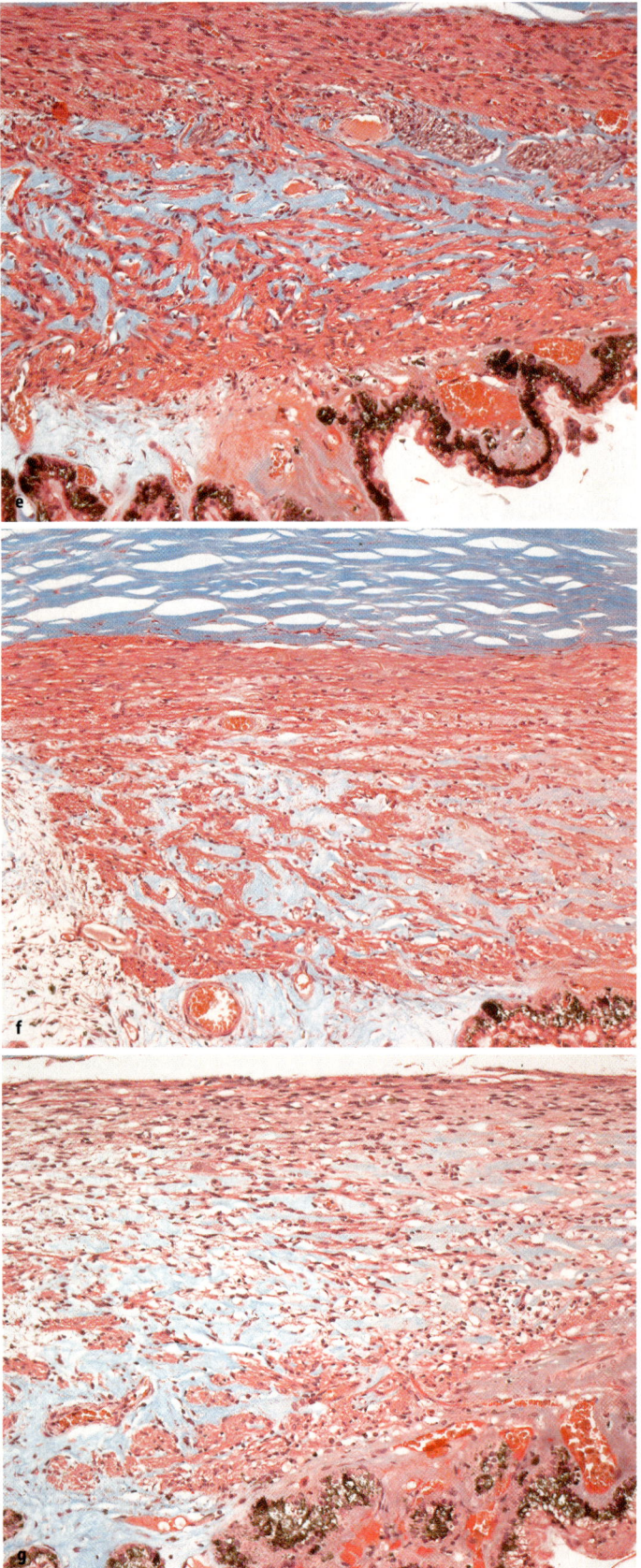

Fig. 5.4.3. e 71 years; **f** 73 years; **g** 77 years

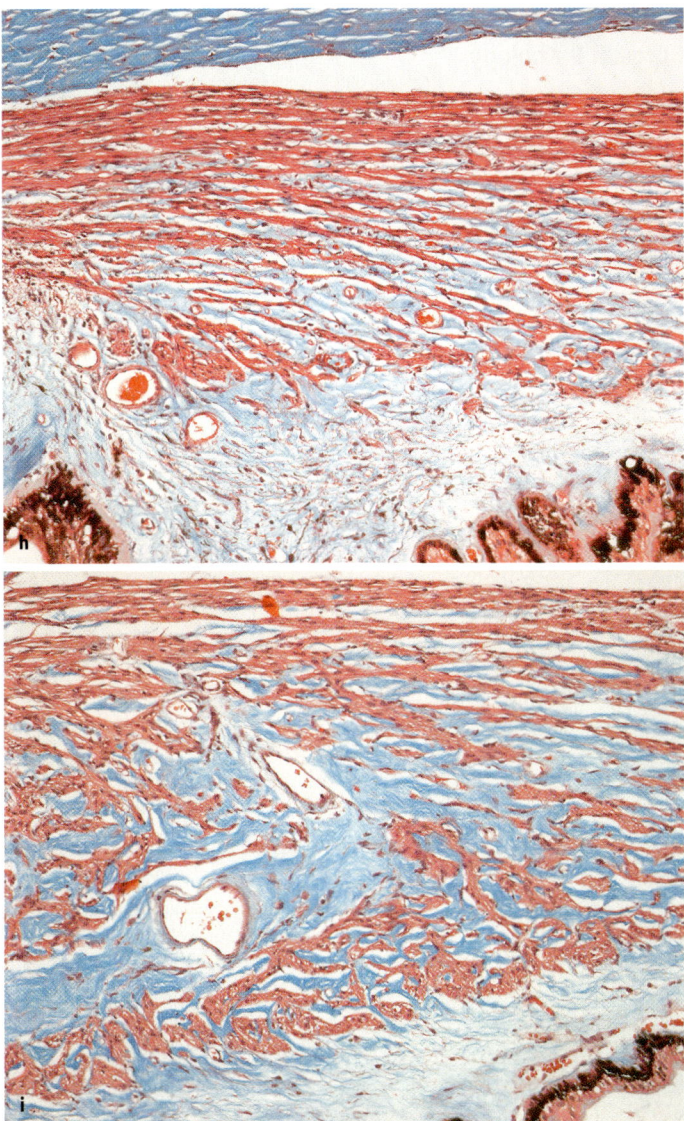

Fig. 5.4.3. h 87 years; **i** 95 years

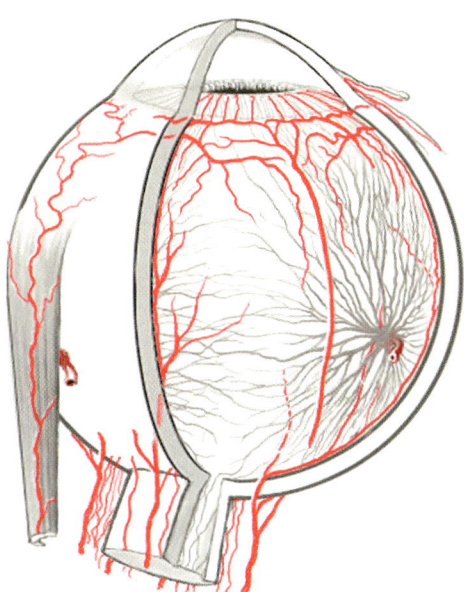

Fig. 5.4.4. Blood supply of the pars plicata of the ciliary body by anastomosing branches from the long posterior ciliary artery and the anterior ciliary arteria via the four straight extraocular muscles

5.4.2
Surgical Pathology

5.4.2.1
Presbyopia

In children the ciliary muscle, on light microscopy, does not show obvious connective tissue between the muscle fibers. Beyond 60 years of age more than half of the cross-section of muscle fibers is replaced by collagenous fibrous tissue, suggesting a limited function of the muscle fibers in between the acquired connective tissue scaffold (Fig. 5.4.3).

5.4.2.2
Cataract Surgery

All intra- and extracapsular cataract surgery cannot avoid traction on the lens capsule. This traction is transmitted via the zonular apparatus to the pars plicata and pars plana of the ciliary body and via the vitreous base also to the peripheral sensory retina. Most attempts at recovering accommodation after extracapsular cataract surgery and lens implantation rely on the residual action of the ciliary muscle. In view of the aging changes, skepticism regarding the function of the ciliary muscle in recovering pseudo-accommodation in the aged is justified and indicated.

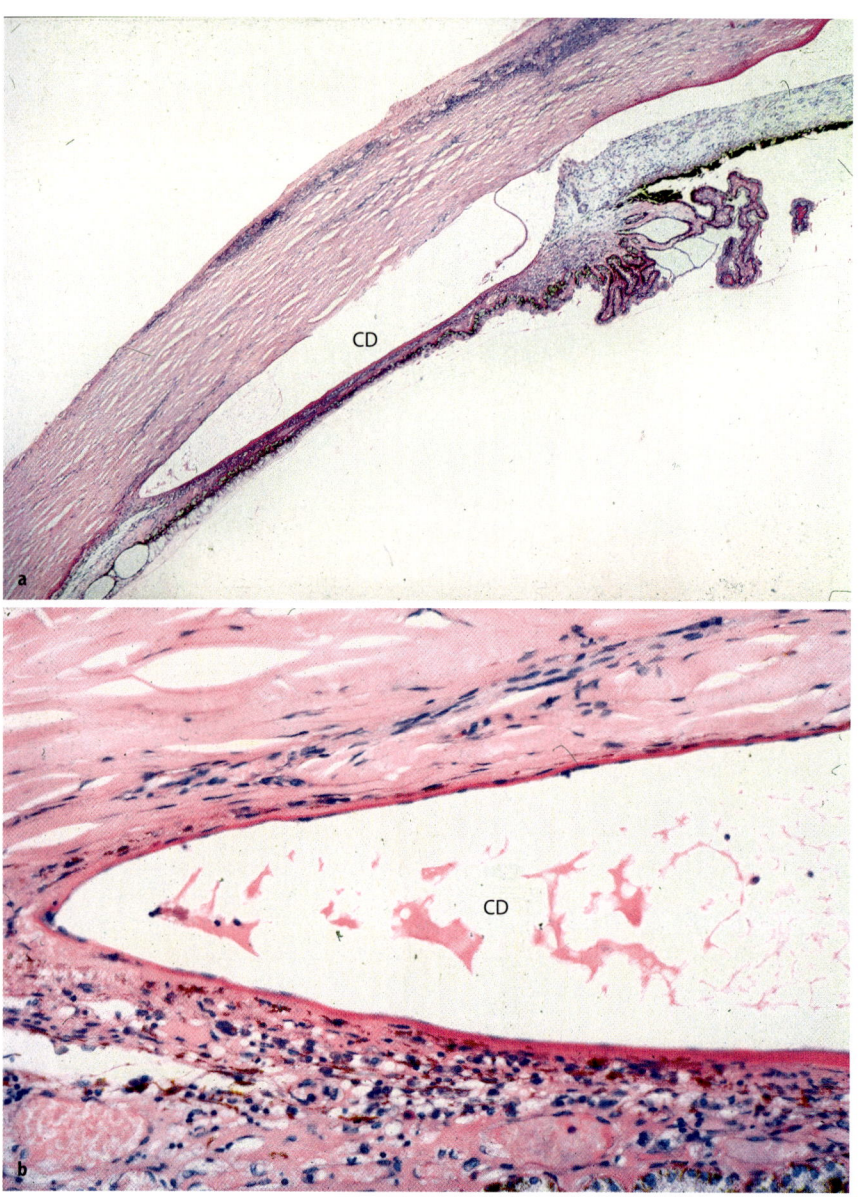

Fig. 5.4.5. Traumatic cyclodialysis (*CD*) showing separation of ciliary body from sclera with focal anterior synechiae of iris root, untreated. **a** The cleft reaches almost to the region of the ora serrata. **b** Sclera and ciliary muscle covered by corneal endothelium producing basement membrane material (PAS stain) (from Völcker and Enke 1983, with permission)

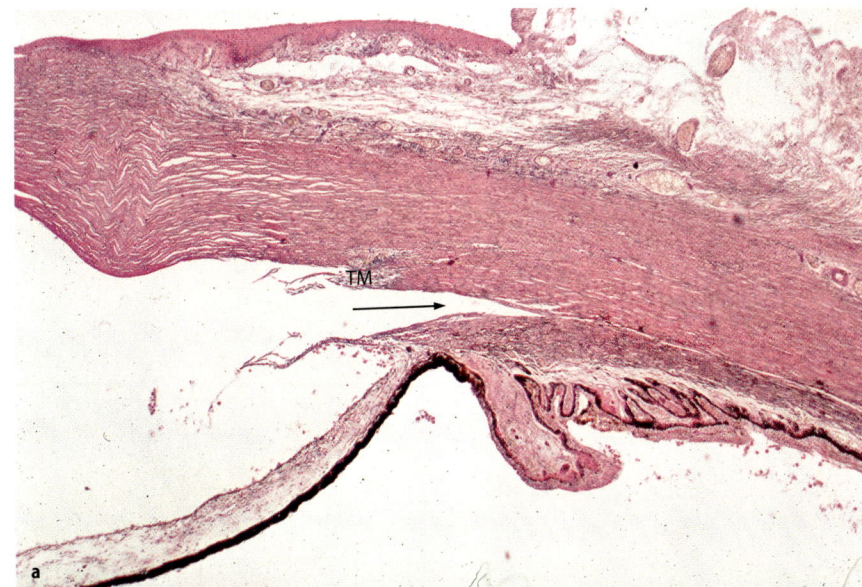

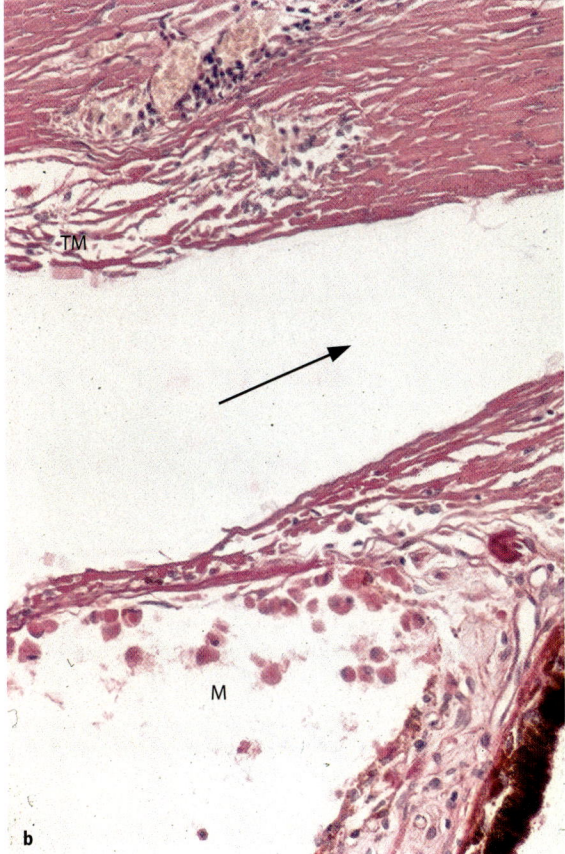

Fig. 5.4.6. Surgically intended cyclodialysis showing cleft above scarred ciliary muscle (*arrow*) in eye with phacolytic open angle glaucoma.
a Overview. **b** Higher power showing macrophages (*M*) and scarred trabecular meshwork (*TM*)

5.4.2.3
Contusion Deformity

Blunt trauma to the eye may create a tear between the longitudinal and circular portion of the ciliary muscle combined with a retroplacement of the iris insertion and an abnormally wide open angle. These contusion effects are not limited to the ciliary muscle but also affect the trabecular meshwork, probably followed by disturbance of the contact inhibition between corneal and trabecular endothelial cells. The endothelial cells of the cornea proliferate and migrate posteriorly covering the surface of the trabecular meshwork and producing a basement membrane which may further increase outflow resistance and contribute to a *secondary open angle glaucoma* (see Chapter 5.2).

5.4.2.4
Traumatic Cyclodialysis

More intensive contusion may separate a sector of the insertion of the ciliary muscle completely from the scleral spur, producing a *cyclodialysis* opening the supraciliary space. The cyclodialysis increases the uveoscleral outflow and may induce persisting ocular hypotony (Fig. 5.4.5). If *ocular hypotony* persists longer than 6 weeks and the cyclodialysis extends for more than 60° (or 2 clock hours) of the circumference, spontaneous recovery of pressure is unlikely.

Surgically intended cyclodialysis today is rarely performed (Fig. 5.4.6). Direct cyclopexy is discussed below (Figs. 5.4.7, 5.4.8, Table 5.4.2).

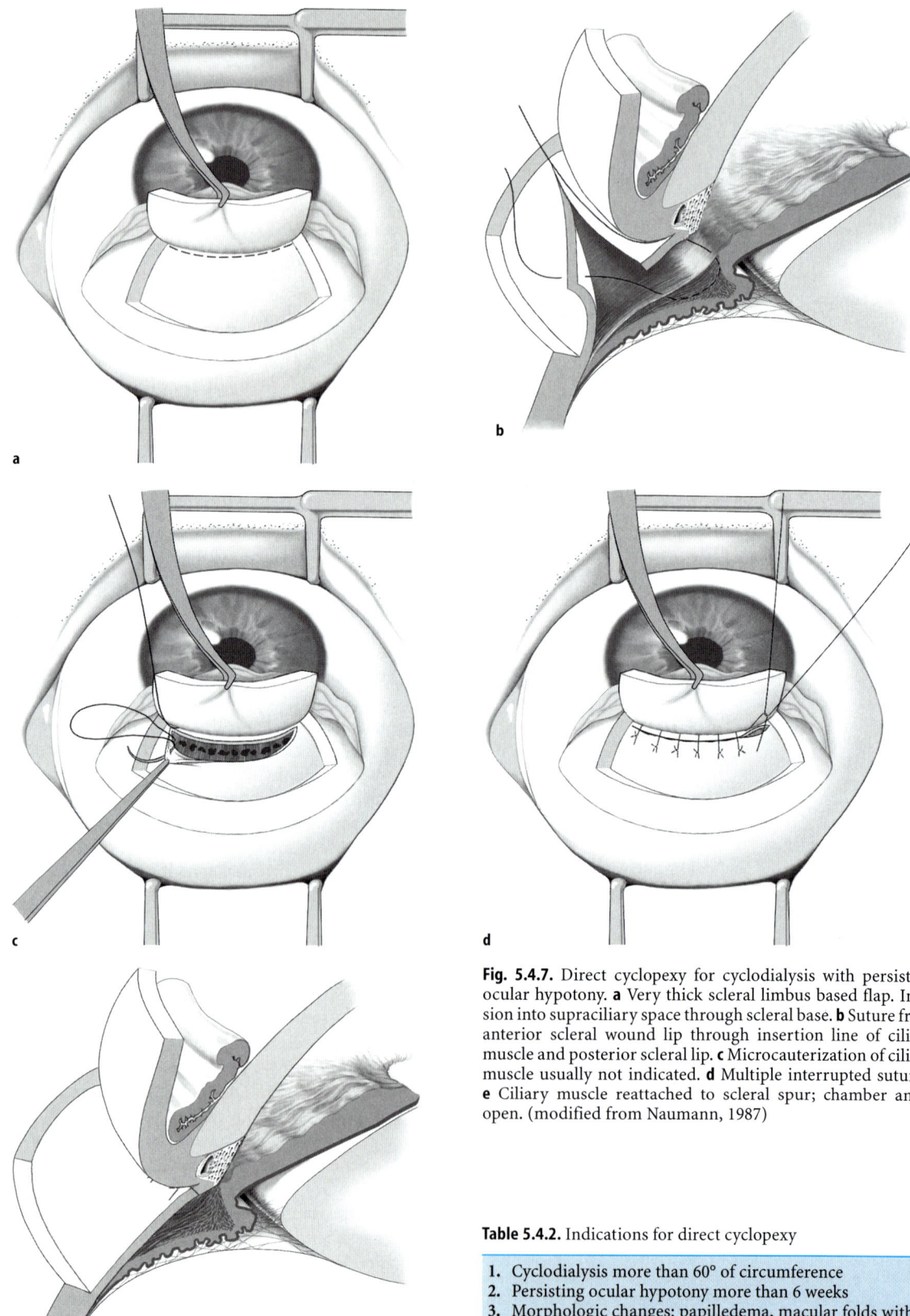

Fig. 5.4.7. Direct cyclopexy for cyclodialysis with persisting ocular hypotony. **a** Very thick scleral limbus based flap. Incision into supraciliary space through scleral base. **b** Suture from anterior scleral wound lip through insertion line of ciliary muscle and posterior scleral lip. **c** Microcauterization of ciliary muscle usually not indicated. **d** Multiple interrupted sutures. **e** Ciliary muscle reattached to scleral spur; chamber angle open. (modified from Naumann, 1987)

Table 5.4.2. Indications for direct cyclopexy

1. Cyclodialysis more than 60° of circumference
2. Persisting ocular hypotony more than 6 weeks
3. Morphologic changes: papilledema, macular folds with cystoid maculopathy
4. Functional defects

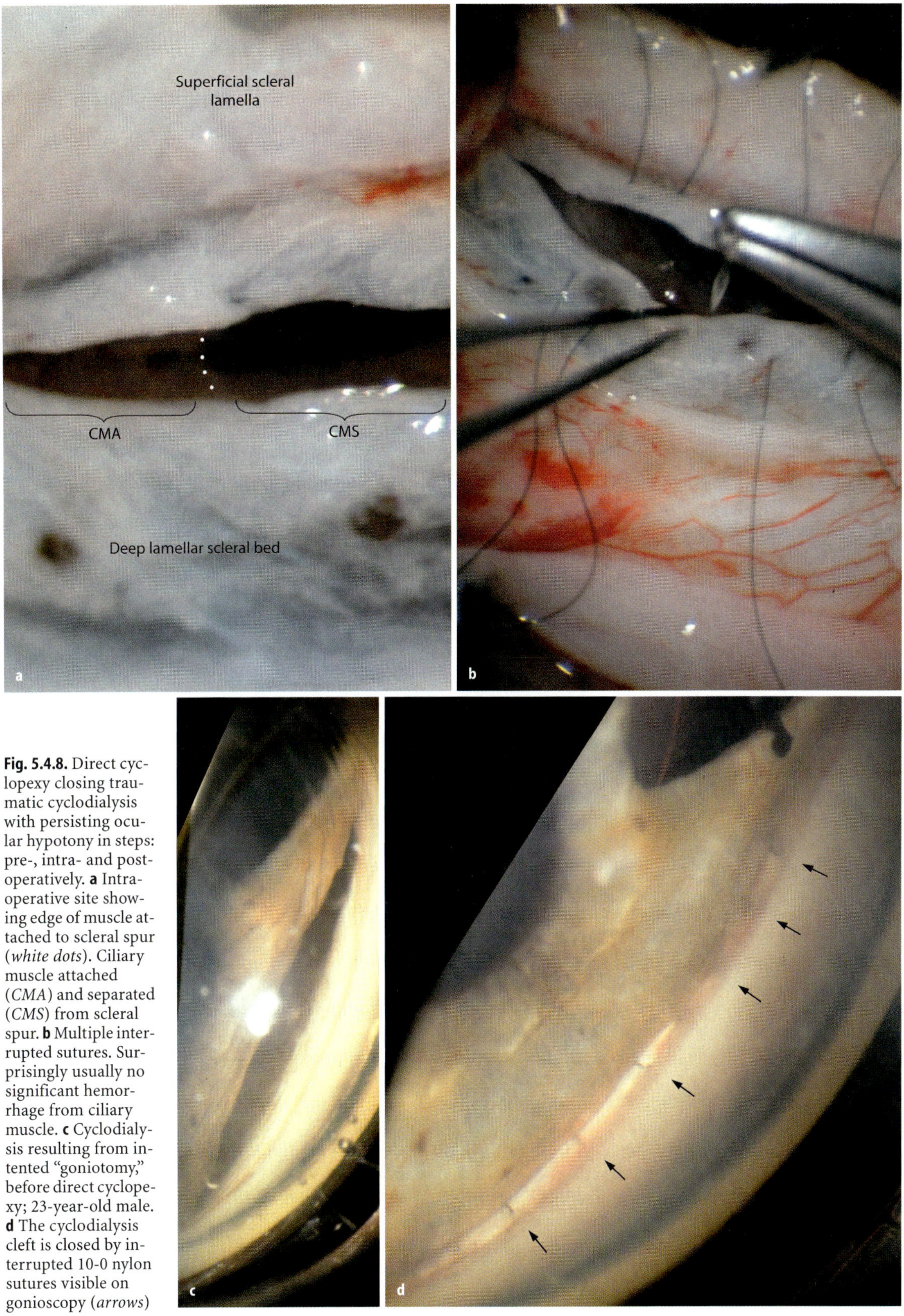

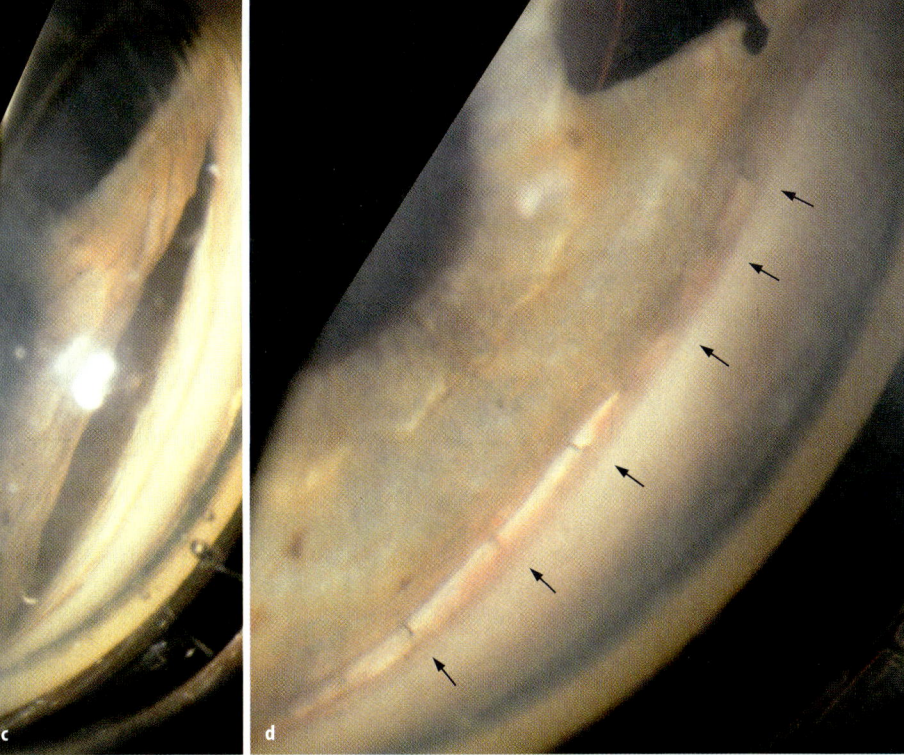

Fig. 5.4.8. Direct cyclopexy closing traumatic cyclodialysis with persisting ocular hypotony in steps: pre-, intra- and postoperatively. **a** Intraoperative site showing edge of muscle attached to scleral spur (*white dots*). Ciliary muscle attached (*CMA*) and separated (*CMS*) from scleral spur. **b** Multiple interrupted sutures. Surprisingly usually no significant hemorrhage from ciliary muscle. **c** Cyclodialysis resulting from intented "goniotomy," before direct cyclopexy; 23-year-old male. **d** The cyclodialysis cleft is closed by interrupted 10-0 nylon sutures visible on gonioscopy (*arrows*)

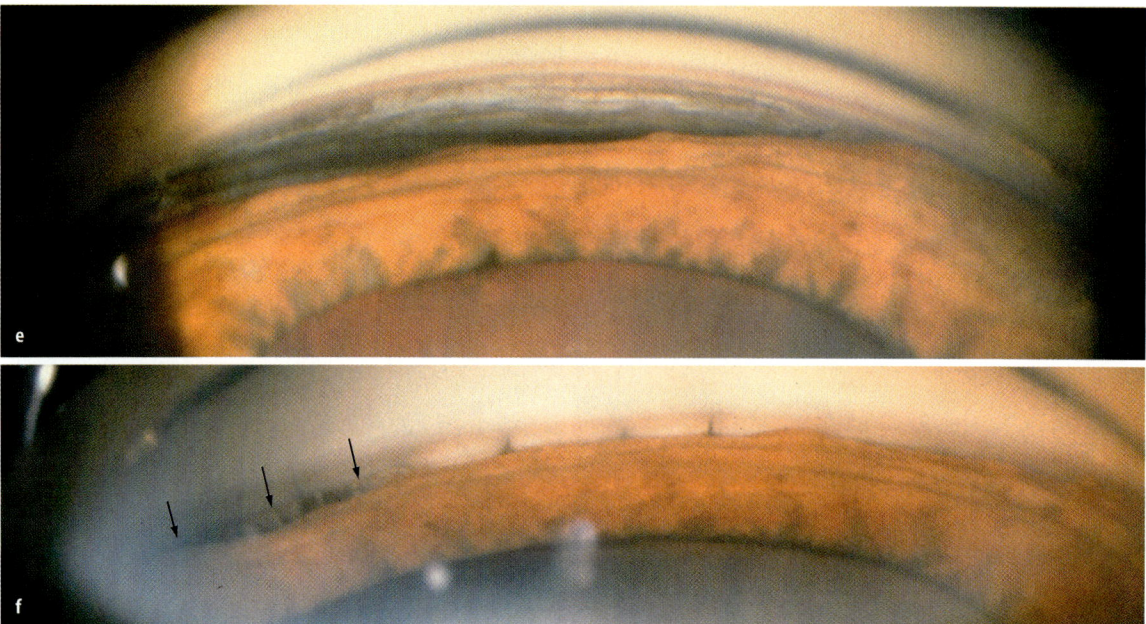

Fig. 5.4.8. e Another traumatic cyclodialysis: preoperatively; **f** postoperatively with closure of the deep cleft except residual cleft of less than 1 h (*arrows*) – i.o. pressure compensated

5.4.2.5
Pseudoadenomatous Hyperplasia ("Fuchs' Adenoma")

This is present in 25% of autopsy eyes (Hillemann and Naumann 1972; Fig. 5.4.2). The process is rarely larger than 1 mm in diameter. As an exception large processes may cause a focal narrowing of the chamber angle by pushing the iris root forward. Clinically they can be detected by ultrasound biomicroscopy and OCT. Usually this process requires no microsurgical intervention.

5.4.2.6
Tumors of the Ciliary Body

Malignant melanomas of the anterior uvea are most frequently observed (Table 5.4.3). Ninety percent of them show histopathologically invasion of the inner layers of the sclera and chamber angle in serial section – most pronounced between the scleral spur and Schwalbe's line into Schlemm's canal and its collector channels (Fig. 5.4.7). The extent of the scleral invasion cannot be judged clinically if the tumor is not pigmented. Shedding of tumor cells into the aqueous and the adjacent structures occurs frequently and must be ruled out by biocytology (see Chapter 5.3). Only then can a curative local excision be achieved.

Local removal and preservation of the eye can be achieved by block excision involving the adjacent anterior uvea together with the *adjacent full-thickness sclera* and cornea (Tables 5.4.4–5.4.8). The ensuing defect in the eye wall needs to be closed by corneal or corneoscleral graft (see below).

Table 5.4.3. Tumors of the ciliary body: differential diagnosis

A. *Neuroepithelial*
 I. Glioneuroma
 II. Embryonal forms
  Medulloepithelioma (diktyoma)
   Benign
   Malignant
  Teratoid medulloepithelioma
   Benign
   Malignant
 III. Adult forms
  Adenoma
  Adenocarcinoma
 IV. Pseudoadenomatous hyperplasia (Fuchs' adenoma)

B. *Pigmented ciliary epithelium*
 I. Adenomas
 II. "Ringschwiele," subretinal and reactive hyperplasia in cyclitic membrane

C. Stroma of ciliary body:
 Leiomyoma
 Neurofibroma
 Schwannoma
 Rhabdomyosarcoma

Benign Tumors. Progressive tumors of the ciliary body with a benign histology account for more than approximately 25% of our 135 patients with progressive tumors of the anterior uvea treated by block excision (Tables 5.4.5–5.4.7).

Table 5.4.4. Block excision of processes of the anterior uvea in 210 patients (Universities of Hamburg, Tübingen, Erlangen)

University	Tumors	Epithelial ingrowth
Hamburg (1971–1975)	12	4
Tübingen (1975–1980)	19	12
Erlangen (1980–2003)	104	59
Total	**135**	**75**

Table 5.4.5. Block excisions of tumors of the anterior uvea (including iris, ciliary body, peripheral cornea and sclera): rationale

1. Tumors of chamber angle and iris root *always* involve ciliary body
2. Tumors must be *localized*: no seeding of tumor cells in aqueous and vitreous (biocytology)
3. Angle of not more than 150° involved
4. Full thickness removal of adjacent sclera, cornea and other tissues. Invasion of inner sclera and outflow system cannot be detected clinically if not pigmented
5. >25% of expanding tumors of ciliary body and iris root are benign and radioresistant

Table 5.4.6. Block excisions of epithelial ingrowth: reasons

1. Cysts of angle and iris root always involve face of ciliary body
2. Location of non-pigmented epithelial strands in cornea, limbus and sclera cannot be recognized clinically (unless fistula)
3. Variable thickness of epithelial lining (1–20 layers) prevents indirect total destruction by laser or toxic solutions
4. Direct manipulation of one to two cell layers would disrupt cyst and convert to diffuse epithelial ingrowth
5. Iridectomy alone converts from cystic to diffuse ingrowth
6. Diameter of epithelial cyst can be reduced by aspiration (through parts of limbus later removed)
7. Adjacent iris, pars plicata of ciliary body – full thickness cornea and sclera forming a "shell" for block excision allowing complete curative removal

Table 5.4.7. Block excision of expanding ciliary body tumors involving chamber angle: histopathologic diagnosis: 26 "benign"! (Erlangen 1980–2003, n=104) (evaluated by Arne Viestenz, MD, 2004)

Malignant	
Malignant melanoma	74 (12% extrascleral)
Adenocarcinoma ciliary epithelium	3 (2×NPE, 1×PE)
Medulloepithelioma	1
Benign	
Melanocytoma/nevi	11 (2% extrascleral)
Melanocytic nevi	5
Adenoma ciliary epithelium	6
Leiomyoma	2
Schwannoma	2

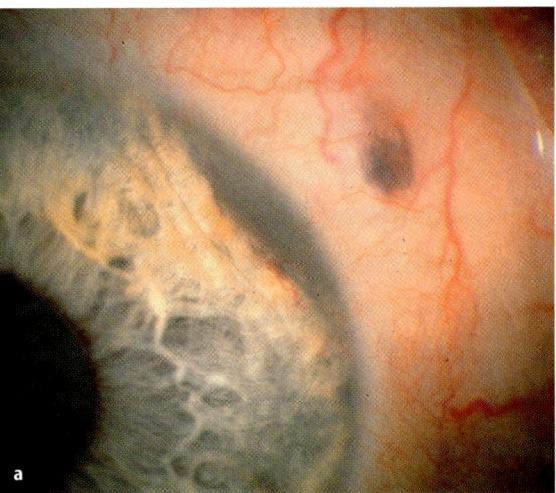

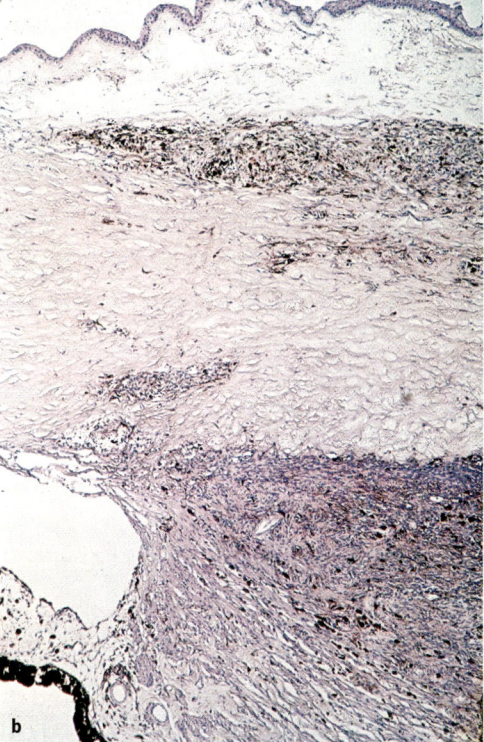

Fig. 5.4.9. Malignant melanomas of the ciliary body and iris root: invasion of sclera, Schlemm's canal and outflow channels. **a** Episcleral extension from malignant melanoma of ciliary body and iris root. **b** Histology showing invasion of Schlemm's canal, outflow channels up to the episcleral conjunctival tissue

Table 5.4.8. Block excision of epithelial ingrowth (Erlangen 1980–2003; n=59) (evaluated by Arne Viestenz, MD, 2004, personal communication)

Cause:		*Histopathology:*	
Penetrating trauma	22	Cystic	54
Cataract surgery	15	Diffuse	4
Perforating keratoplasty	5	Both	1
Amniocentesis	2		
Others/unknown	15		

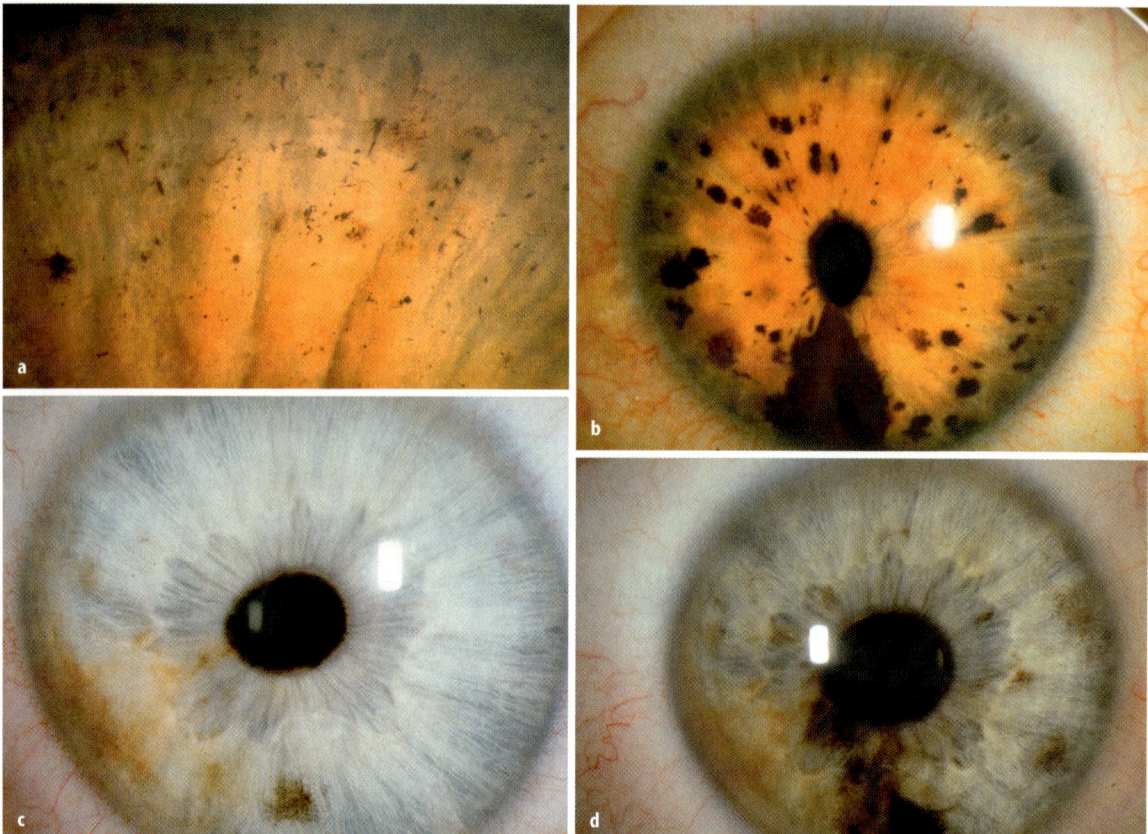

Fig. 5.4.10. Diffuse shedding of malignant melanocytes into aqueous and adjacent structures in different patients showing unilateral ocular hypertension or glaucoma. **a** Malignant melanocytes on the surface of the iris recognized by biocytology. **b** Progressive diffuse malignant melanoma with seeding into the surface of the iris. **c** Diffuse malignant melanoma of iris in 35-year-old male. **d** Same eye 33 months later

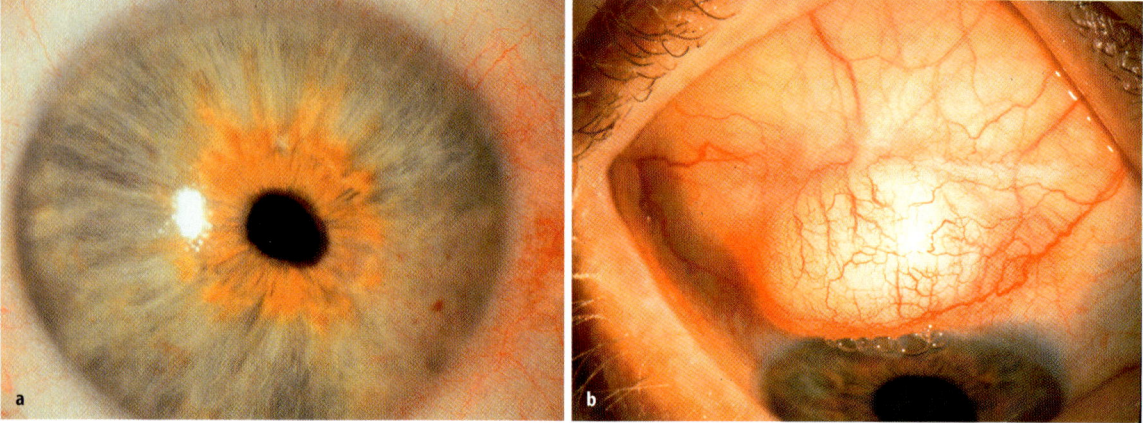

Fig. 5.4.11. Diffuse non-pigmented malignant melanoma of the iris (ring melanoma) masquerading as "glaucoma." **a** Preoperatively. **b** After filtering procedure "cystic" bleb

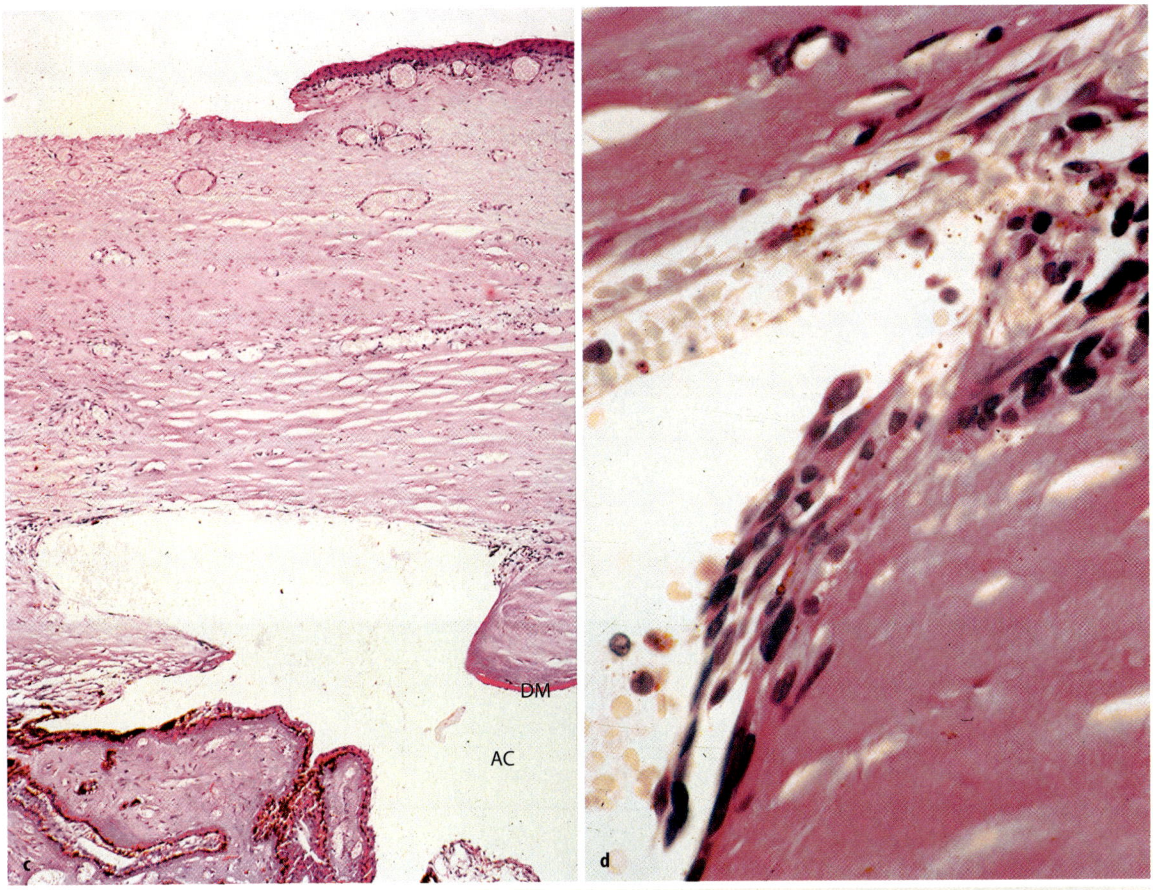

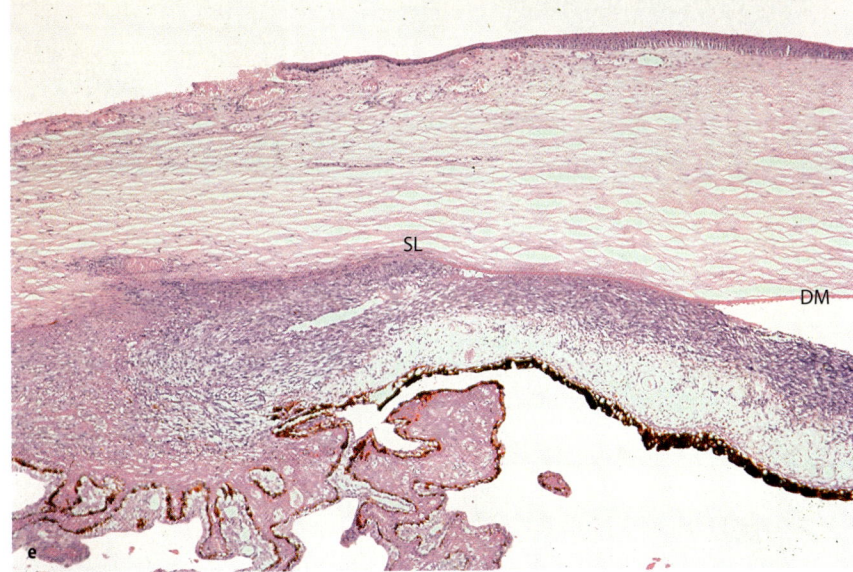

Fig. 5.4.11. c, d Filtering channel lined by malignant melanocytes: anterior chamber (*AC*), Descemet membrane (*DM*). **e, f** Ring melanoma invading ciliary body and outflow channels in opposite chamber angles (PAS)

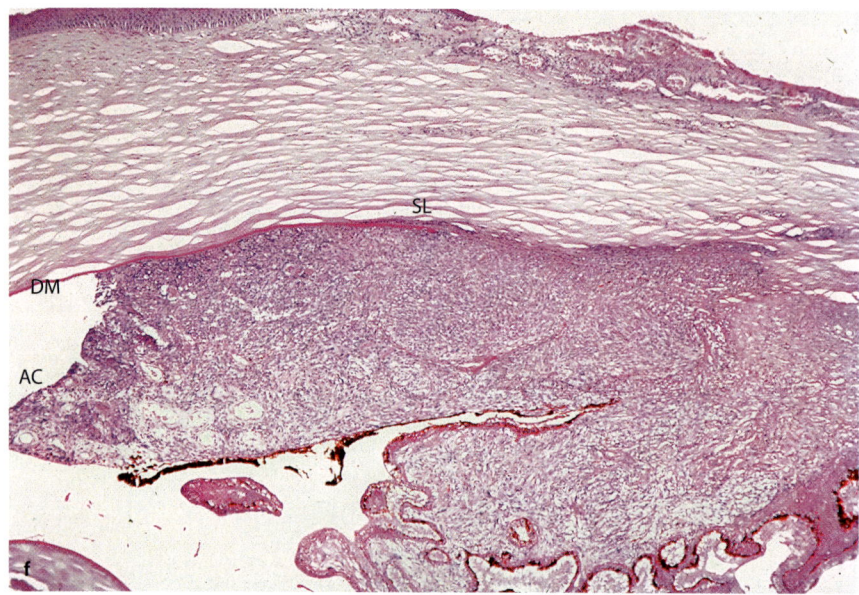

Fig. 5.4.11 (*Cont.*)

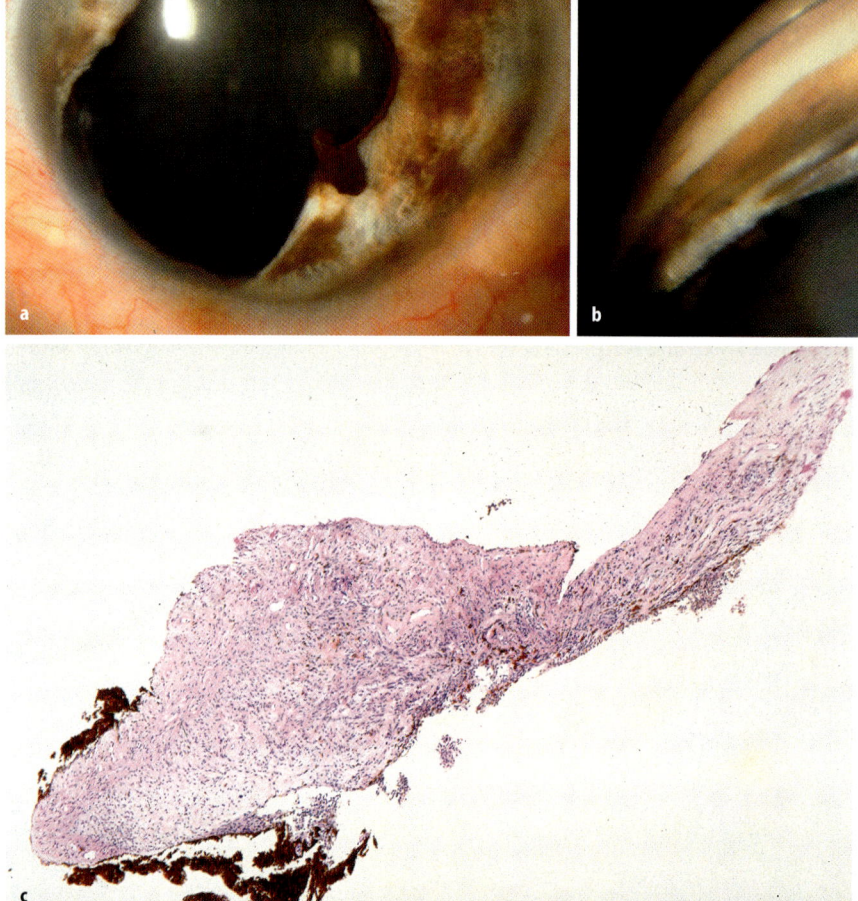

Fig. 5.4.12. Recurrence and subconjunctival extension of malignant melanoma of the anterior uvea 14 years after sector iridectomy via corneal scleral incision. Starting at age 33 years this patient was observed for 10 years because of an iris tumor. Then secondary glaucoma (32 mm Hg) and a pigmented tumor of the iris roof was described. Histologically the tumor was considered a "nevus of the iris." Twelve years later he developed diffuse malignant melanoma of the anterior uvea, pressure of 40 mm Hg and advanced cupping. He refused enucleation, which was performed later, 14 years after the sector iridectomy for the initial biopsy. **a** Diffuse malignant melanoma of iris and ciliary body with extrascleral extension. **b** Gonioscopy showing invasion of the ciliary body. **c** Histopathology of sector iridectomy specimen, 14 years before enucleation

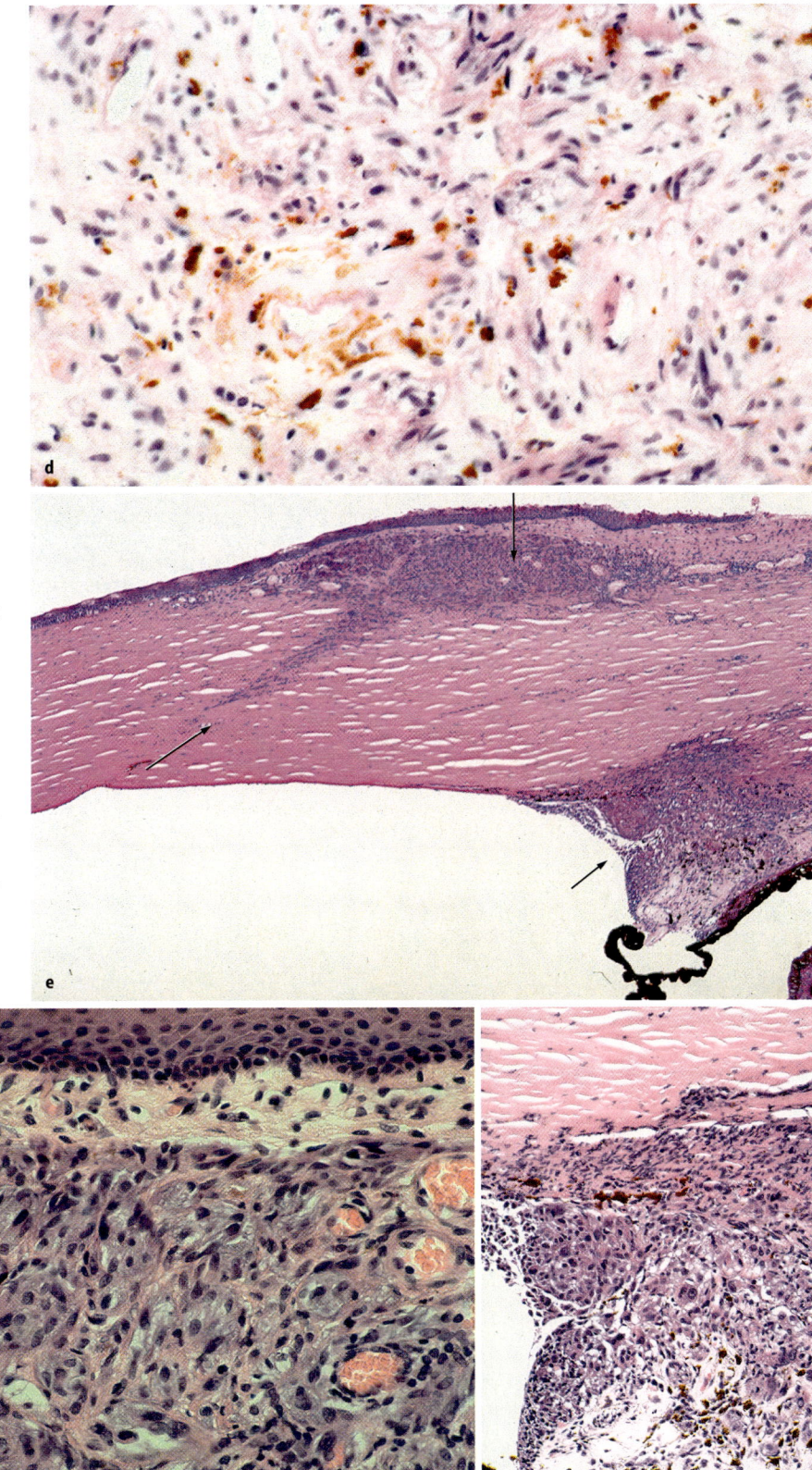

Fig. 5.4.12. d Higher power from **c**. Relatively benign looking melanocytes.
e–g Recurrence of malignant melanoma in the iris root and ciliary body within the intracorneal scar and with extrascleral extension (*arrows*) (PAS stain), also higher power. This case illustrates the need to perform "biopsy" of the iris only through the *avascular corneal access* to allow earlier recognition of recurrence. (Case reported to Joint Meeting of Verhoeff Society and European Ophthalmic Pathology Society, Philadelphia, 1986)

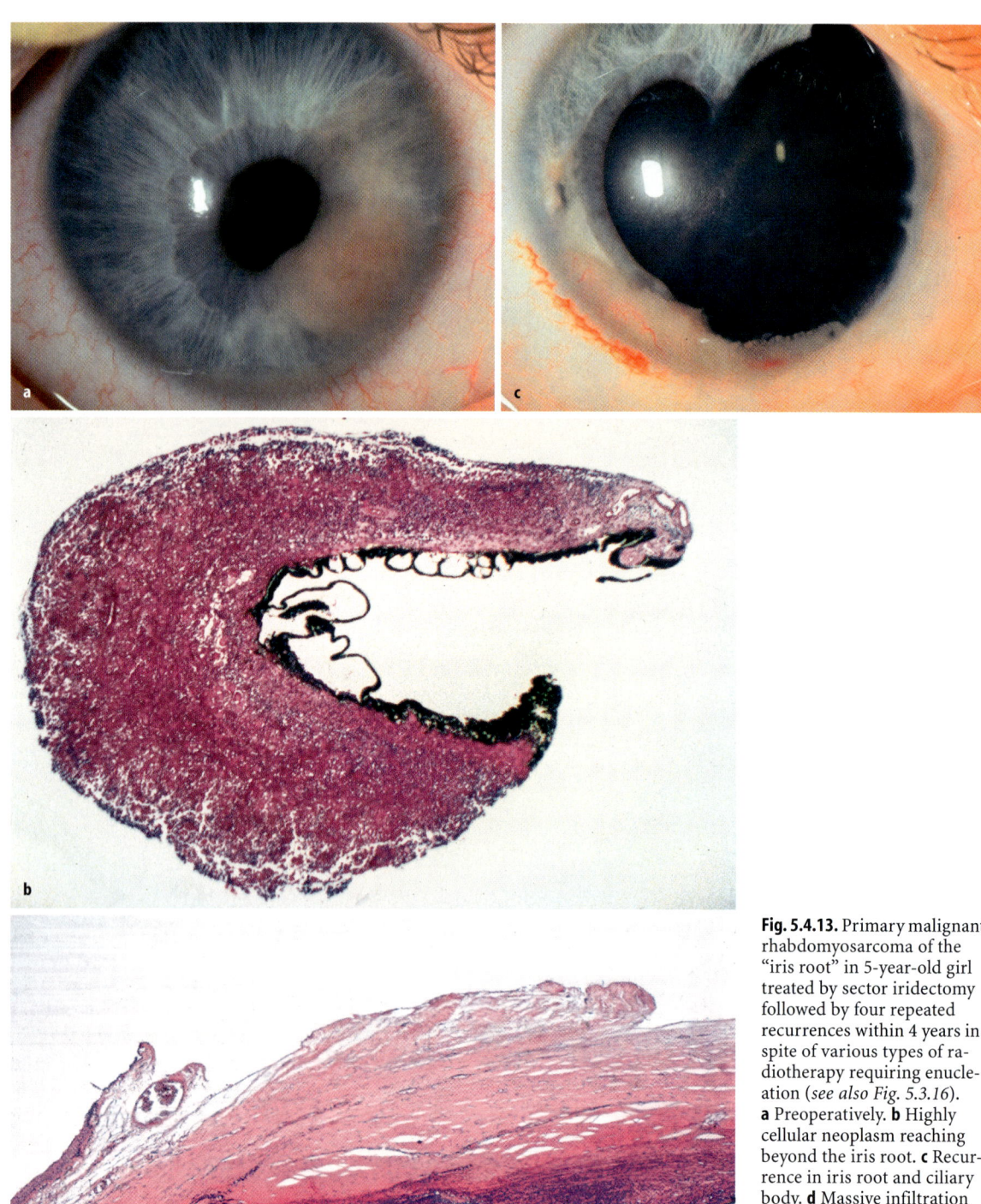

Fig. 5.4.13. Primary malignant rhabdomyosarcoma of the "iris root" in 5-year-old girl treated by sector iridectomy followed by four repeated recurrences within 4 years in spite of various types of radiotherapy requiring enucleation (*see also Fig. 5.3.16*). **a** Preoperatively. **b** Highly cellular neoplasm reaching beyond the iris root. **c** Recurrence in iris root and ciliary body. **d** Massive infiltration of the ciliary body. Processes of the iris root cannot be removed completely with a sector iridectomy, they require block excision including the adjacent pars plicata of the ciliary body. After 36-year-old follow-up patient is in good health. (Reported by Naumann et al. 1972)

5.4.2.7
Epithelial Ingrowth Involving the Anterior Chamber Angle

Any epithelial ingrowth both of the diffuse and cystic type involving the anterior chamber angle covers not only the surface of the iris root and the back of the cornea but – by necessity – also the *"face of the ciliary body,"* or in other words: the insertion of the ciliary muscle to the scleral spur. As direct manipulation and separation of the delicate corneal, conjunctival or epidermal epithelial layers – often only one to two cell layers – is impossible, the adjacent tissues must be "used as a shell," resulting in block excision together with cornea, sclera, and pars plicata of the ciliary body and iris (Fig. 5.4.8). Partial excision attempted by sector iridectomy or laser application will convert the cystic into a diffuse type of epithelial ingrowth – both approaches are contraindicated (Tables 5.4.6, 5.4.8).

5.4.2.8
Zonular Apparatus in Pseudoexfoliation Syndrome and Homocystinuria

Both in pseudoexfoliation syndrome and homocystinuria basement membrane material and microfibrillar intercellular matrix is interposed between the origin of the zonular fibers and the non-pigmented ciliary epithelium. This causes weakening of the anchoring of the zonules at their origin in the ciliary body leading to phacodonesis or spontaneous dislocation or even luxation of the lens (see Chapter 5.5).

5.4.2.9
Non-invasive In Vivo Diagnostic Procedures

Echography, ultrasound biomicroscopy, optical coherence tomography (OCT), diaphanoscopy in addition to gonioscopy and funduscopy with indentation of the ora serrata are used. Laser tyndallometry measures the involvement of the blood-aqueous barrier.

5.4.3
Indications for Procedures Involving the Ciliary Body

The ciliary body itself until recently was considered a "taboo zone" for direct intraocular microsurgery because of concerns about hemorrhage, vitreous loss, lens subluxation and their complications. We shall show that these concerns can be controlled.

5.4.3.1
Posterior Sclerotomy

Penetrating incisions of the sclera 4 mm behind the limbus open the supraciliary space and allow drainage of fluid from the choroidal detachment particularly with postoperative or post-traumatic defects in the anterior segment causing *acute or persisting ocular hypotony*. The anterior ciliary arteries are avoided by entering in the sectors between the rectus muscles. Choroidal detachments develop after *all* perforating injuries that do not seal spontaneously. If wound closure is delayed, reforming the anterior chamber may be possible only after the fluid of the choroidal detachment is released by posterior sclerotomy.

5.4.3.2
Pars Plana Vitrectomy

This approach, pioneered by Machemer (1972), has revolutionized not only vitreal surgery but has also set an example for minimally invasive microsurgery in other organs of the body. It starts with posterior sclerotomies and traverses both the sclera *and* the pars plana of the ciliary body.* It is indicated: (1) in acute ciliary block angle closure glaucomas with abnormal accumulation of aqueous in the vitreous behind the lens and (2) to treat a multitude of vitreoretinal pathologies via multiple ports combining infusion, cutting, suction and illumination – and implantation of gas and silicone (see Chapter 5.6).

5.4.3.3
Direct Cyclopexy for Treating Persisting Ocular Hypotony Resulting from Traumatic or Iatrogenic Cyclodialysis

Cyclodialysis for up to 2 h (60°) may close and heal spontaneously or after thermal argon laser coagulation. Closure of larger clefts by direct thermic lasers usually is not successful – nor is intravitreal gas injection, with or without capsular tension rings placed in the sulcus ciliaris. Direct cyclopexy describes the reattachment of the anterior attachment line of the ciliary muscle to the scleral spur by suturing under direct microsurgical control (Fig. 5.4.7, 5.4.8 and Table 5.4.2). This procedure is only indicated: (1) if there is *functional impairment*, (2) morphologic consequences of ocular hypotony like *macular star* with cystoid maculopathy, choroidal edema and *papilloedema ex vacuo* persist, (3) the cyclodialysis

---

* Historically a similar entry into the globe was suggested by Celsus (Chapter 1) to achieve couching of the cataractous lens (see Chapter 1).

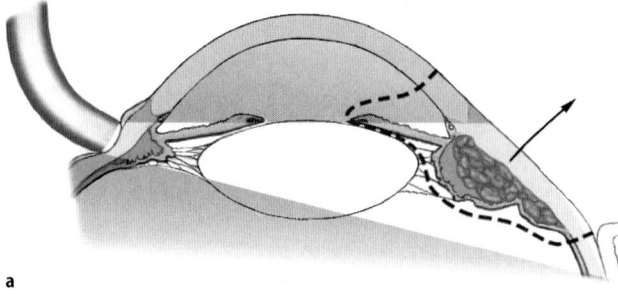

Fig. 5.4.14. Block excision of tumors of the anterior uvea: ciliary body with adjacent iris and/or choroid and full thickness cornea and sclera, followed by corneoscleral graft. Sketches of surgical steps. **a** Transillumination outlining the borders of the tumor by scleral sutures. **c** Removal of the tumor with adjacent tissue of ciliary body, iris, full thickness sclera and cornea en block usually with sector iridectomy and anterior vitrectomy

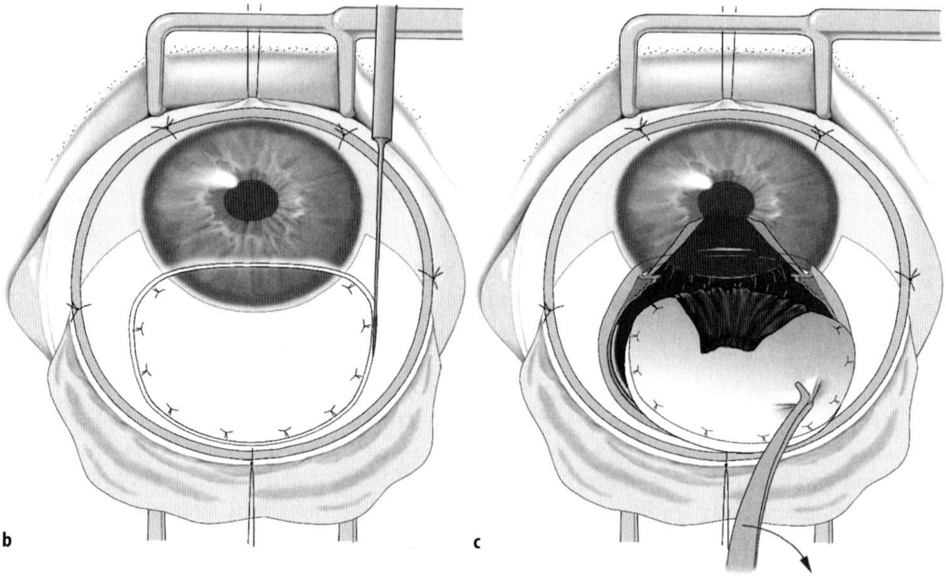

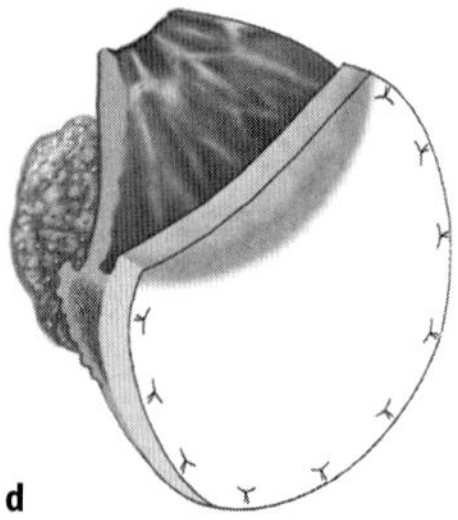

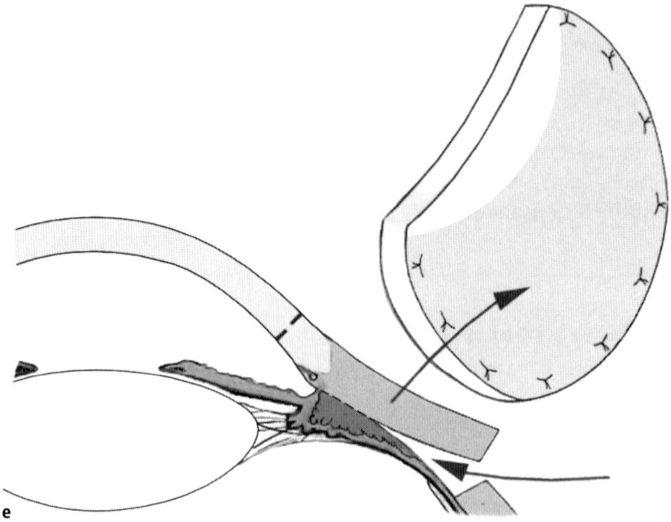

Fig. 5.4.14. d Excised tumor and shell. **e** Corneoscleral graft from donor eye corresponding to the defect of the wall resulting from the block excision. **f** Corneoscleral graft in place (modified from Naumann, 1987)

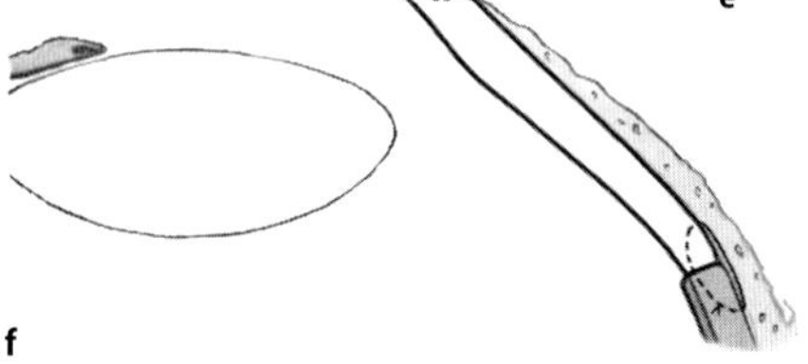

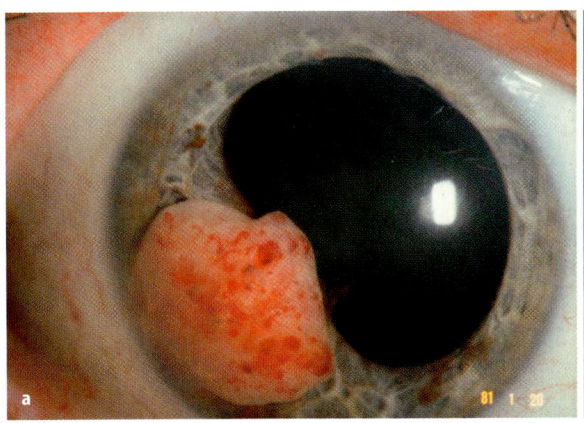
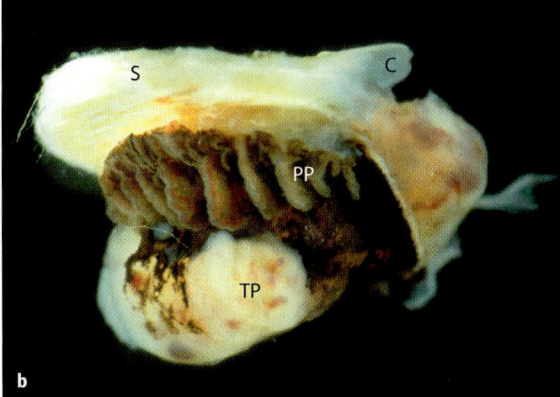
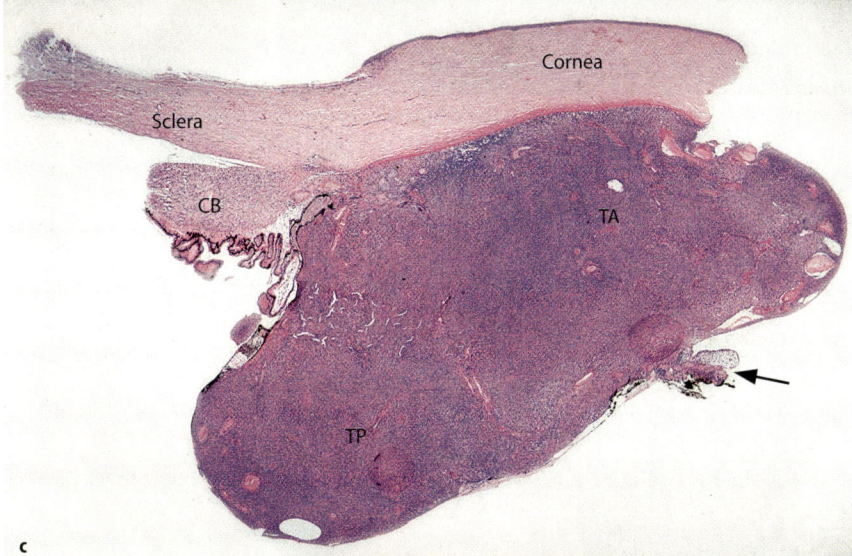

Fig. 5.4.15. Highly vascularized malignant melanoma of the iris extending into the ciliary body in a 47-year-old male. **a** Preoperatively. **b** Block excision of 7,5 mm. **c** Histopathology of block consisting of the tumor and adjacent full-thickness sclera and cornea. Iris (*thick arrow*). **d** After follow-up of 13 years partially vascularized tectonic corneoscleral graft. Iron staining of corneal epithelium of host (*arrow*) – not to be confused with recurrence! Extent of graft (*dots*). Tumor anterior (*TA*) and posterior to iris (*TP*). Pars plicata (*PP*) of ciliary body (*CB*)

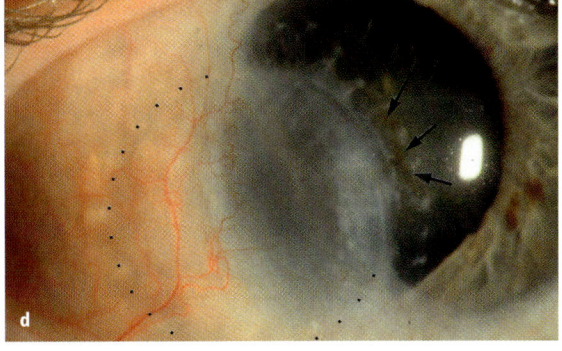

extends for more than 60° (2 clock hours), and (4) no spontaneous improvement has occurred within 6 weeks. Our technique avoids anterior synechiae resulting in persisting closure angle glaucoma (Table 5.4.3) (Naumann and Völcker 1981; Küchle and Naumann 1991).

Transitory acute pressure spikes in the first days after direct cyclopexy should be treated medically. In more than 60 consecutive patients no persisting secondary glaucomas developed.

5.4.3.4
"Block Excision" of Tumors and Epithelial Ingrowth of Anterior Uvea

Block excision is defined as in toto removal of the process involving the anterior uvea and angle structures together with the adjacent iris, pars plicata of the ciliary body, full thickness sclera and cornea up to 150° of the circumference.

The defect in the eye wall then is closed by a corresponding corneoscleral tectonic graft (Tables 5.4.4–5.4.8; Naumann and Rummelt 1996; Rummelt et al. 1994) (Fig. 5.4.15–22).

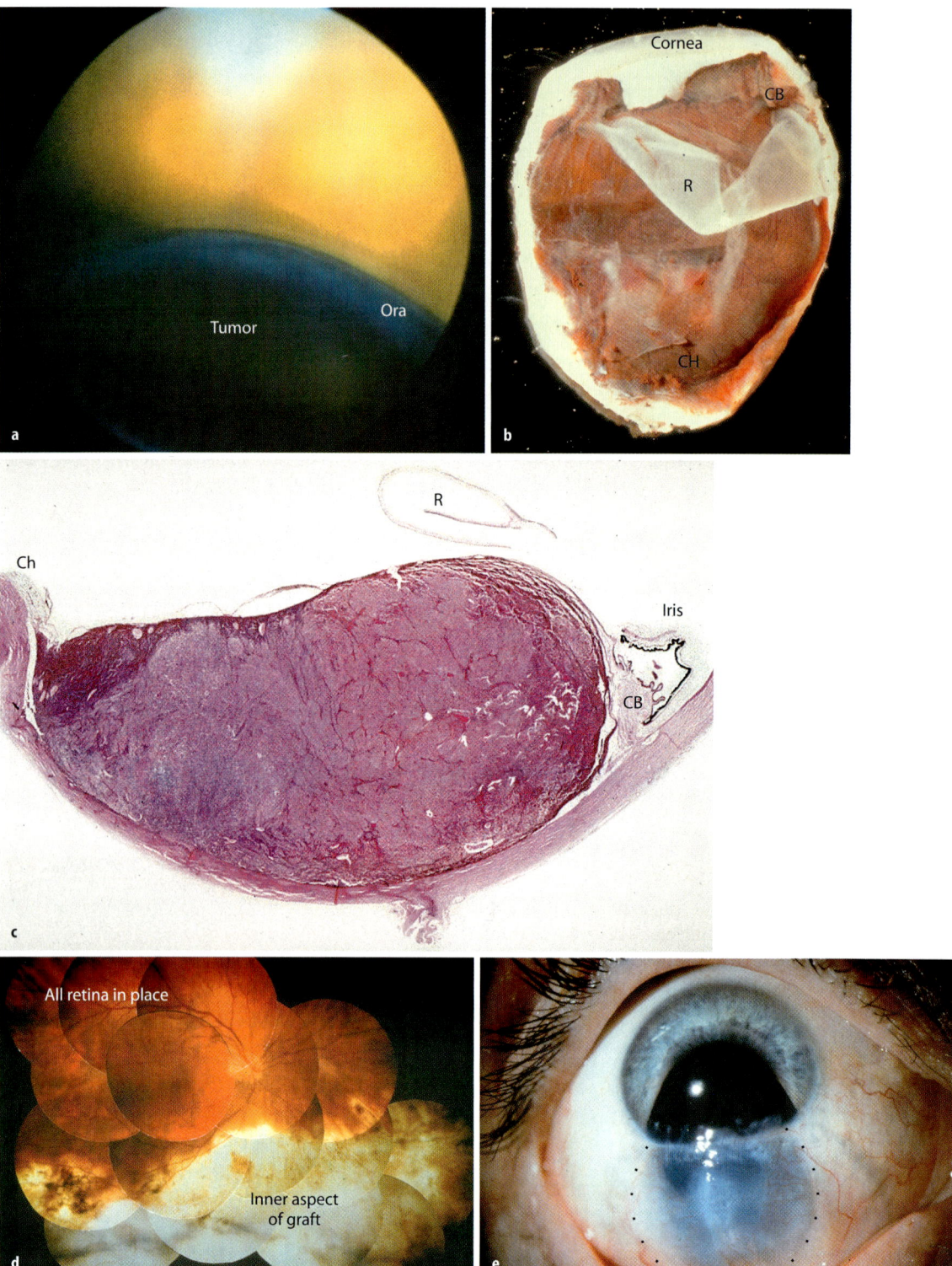

Fig. 5.4.16. Large malignant melanoma of the anterior uvea extending to the level of the inferior temporal retinal vessel arcade located inferiorly in 55 years old male. **a** Preoperatively with infrared photography. **b** Excised tumor with adjacent full thickness sclera and cornea and retina (preceded by retinopexy 2 weeks earlier): 18 × 18 × 9 mm. Retina (*R*) over tumor detached. Ciliary Body (*CB*). **c** Histopathology. **d** Extensive chorioretinal scarring following broad cryoretinopexy. **e** Sixteen years postoperatively, external aspect with visual acuity of 0.2 – 0.3. Extent of graft (*dots*)

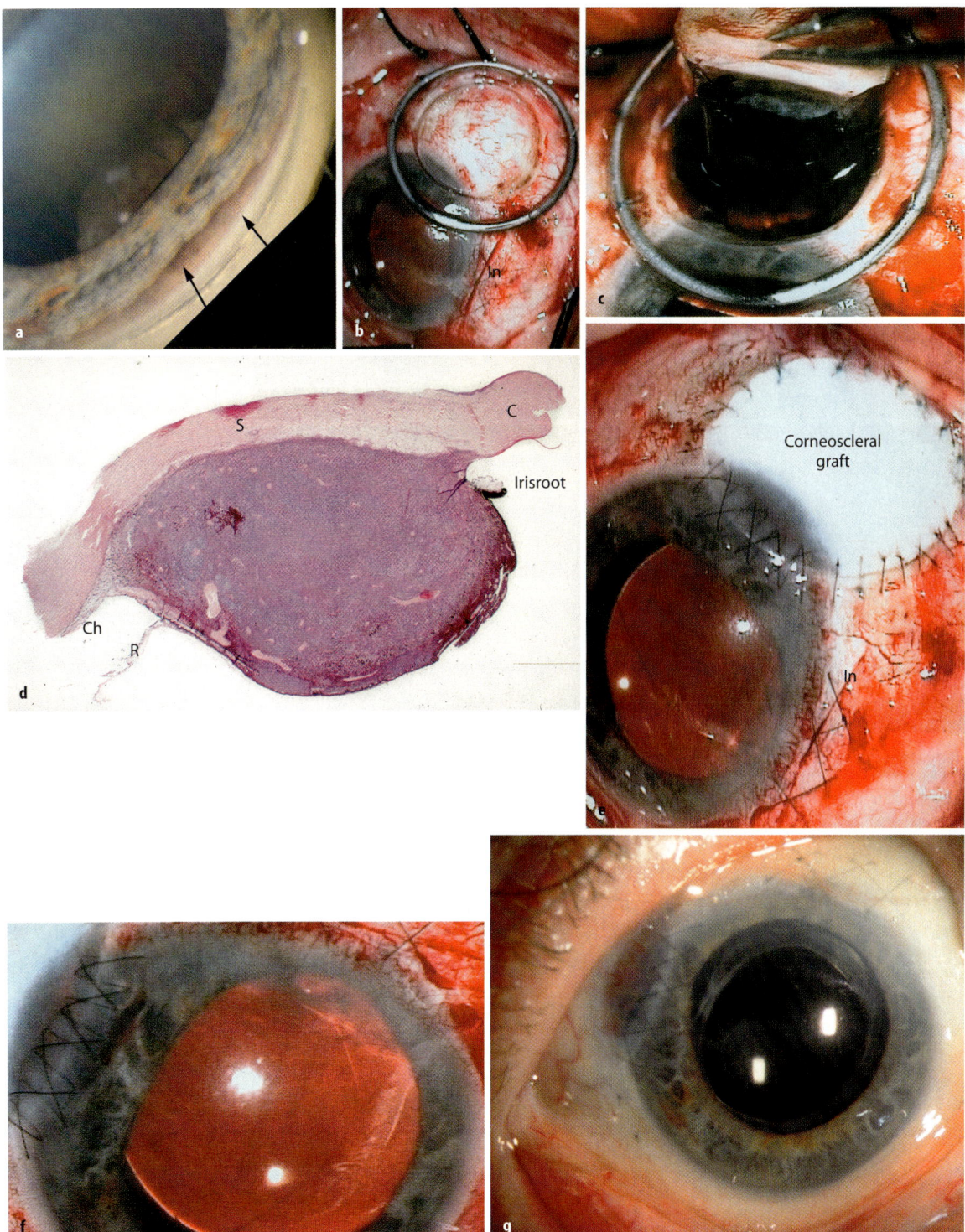

Fig. 5.4.17. Malignant melanoma of the anterior uvea with extension into the iris root, 74-year-old male: microsurgical steps. **a** Preoperative gonioscopy: tumor in iris root (*arrow*). **b** Flieringa ring after phacoemulsification and implantation of rigid PMMA lens. **c** Block excision 9 mm in diameter. **d** Excised tumor with adjacent structure and peripheral iris. **e** With tectonic corneoscleral graft scleral cataract incision (*In*), Sclera (*S*), Cornea (*C*), Choroid (*Ch*), Retina (*R*). **f** One year later corneoscleral graft, clear optic media, peripheral iris coloboma. **g** Fifteen months postoperatively: good function

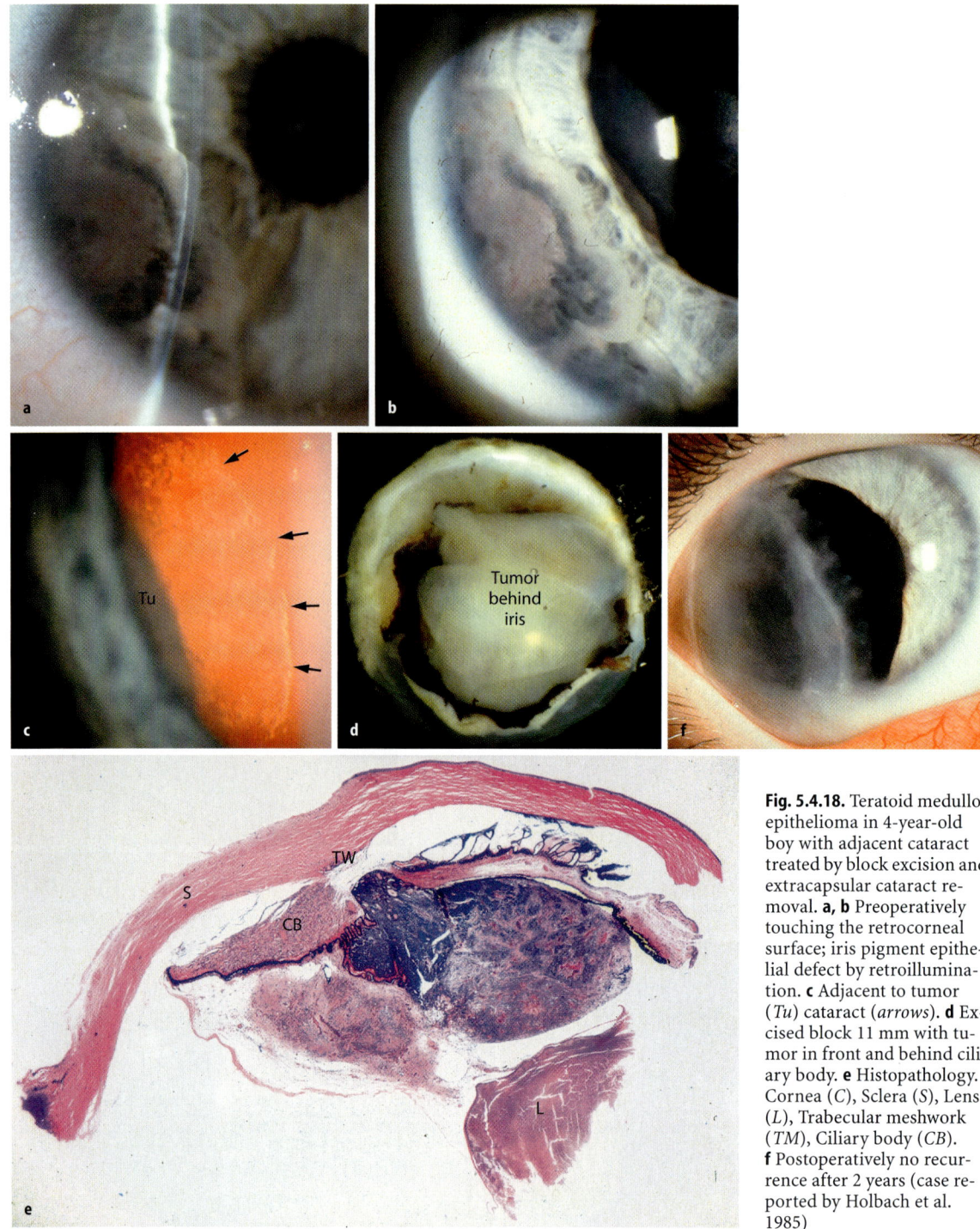

Fig. 5.4.18. Teratoid medulloepithelioma in 4-year-old boy with adjacent cataract treated by block excision and extracapsular cataract removal. **a, b** Preoperatively touching the retrocorneal surface; iris pigment epithelial defect by retroillumination. **c** Adjacent to tumor (*Tu*) cataract (*arrows*). **d** Excised block 11 mm with tumor in front and behind ciliary body. **e** Histopathology. Cornea (*C*), Sclera (*S*), Lens (*L*), Trabecular meshwork (*TM*), Ciliary body (*CB*). **f** Postoperatively no recurrence after 2 years (case reported by Holbach et al. 1985)

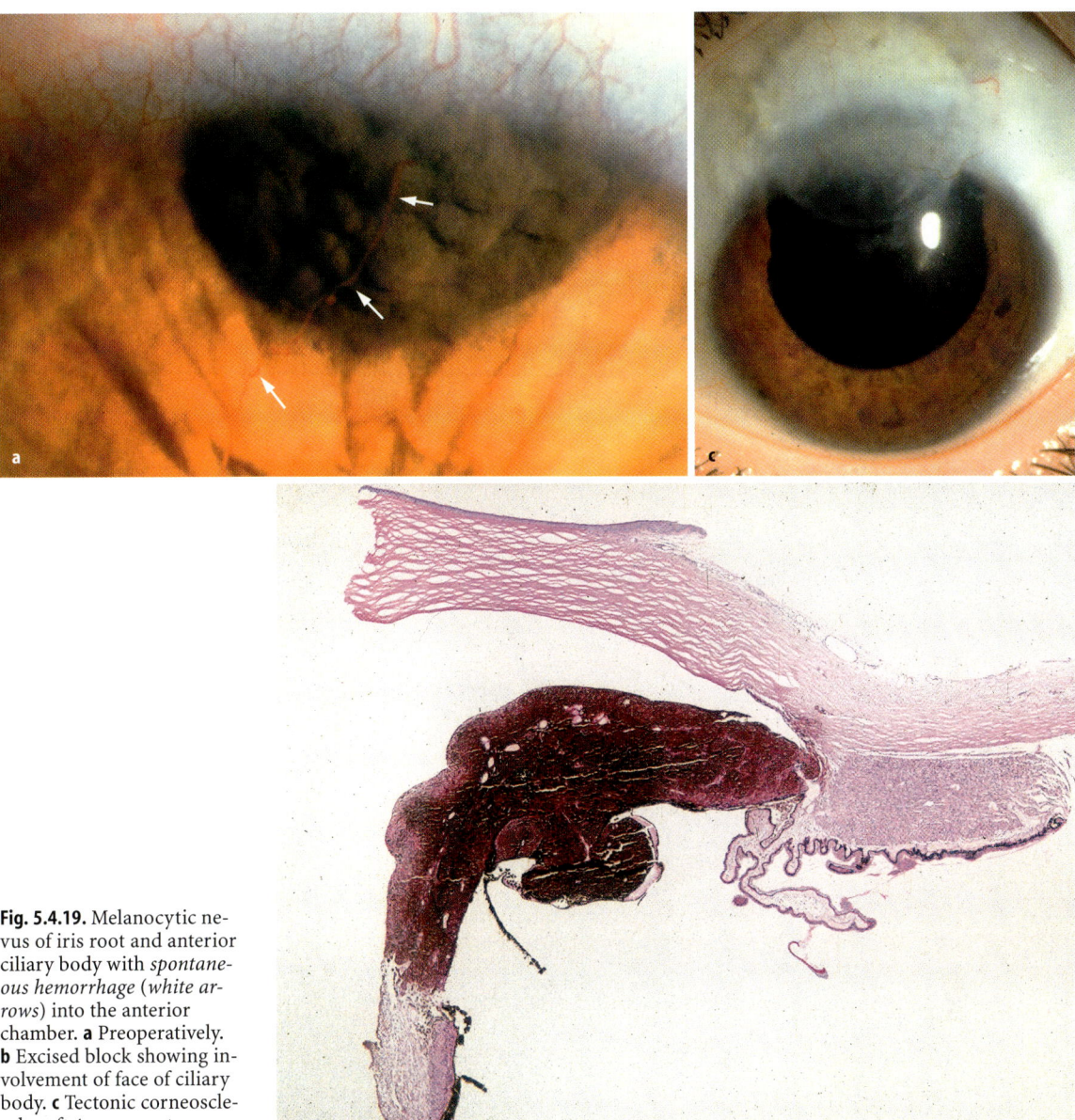

Fig. 5.4.19. Melanocytic nevus of iris root and anterior ciliary body with *spontaneous hemorrhage* (*white arrows*) into the anterior chamber. **a** Preoperatively. **b** Excised block showing involvement of face of ciliary body. **c** Tectonic corneoscleral graft 4 years postoperatively, full vision

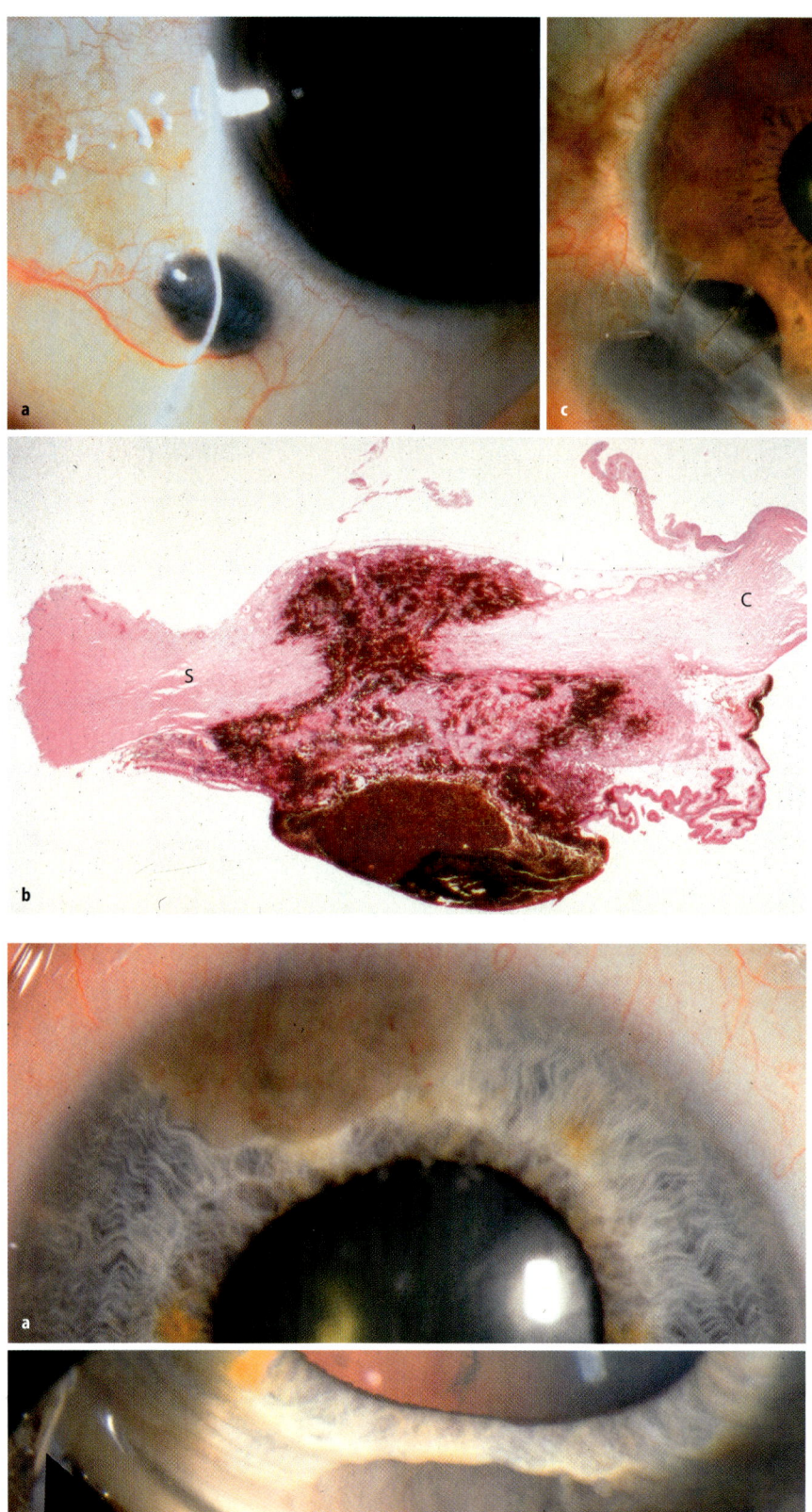

Fig. 5.4.20. Episcleral extension of partially necrotic melanocytoma of the ciliary body. **a** Preoperatively: no significant episcleral hyperemia. **b** Histopathology showing partially necrotic *benign* melanocytes. **c** 6.5 mm tectonic corneal graft 2 years postoperatively

Fig. 5.4.21. Adenoma of the non-pigmented ciliary epithelium extending into the anterior chamber in 62-year-old female patient. **a–c** Preoperatively including gonioscopy and ultrasound biomicroscopy

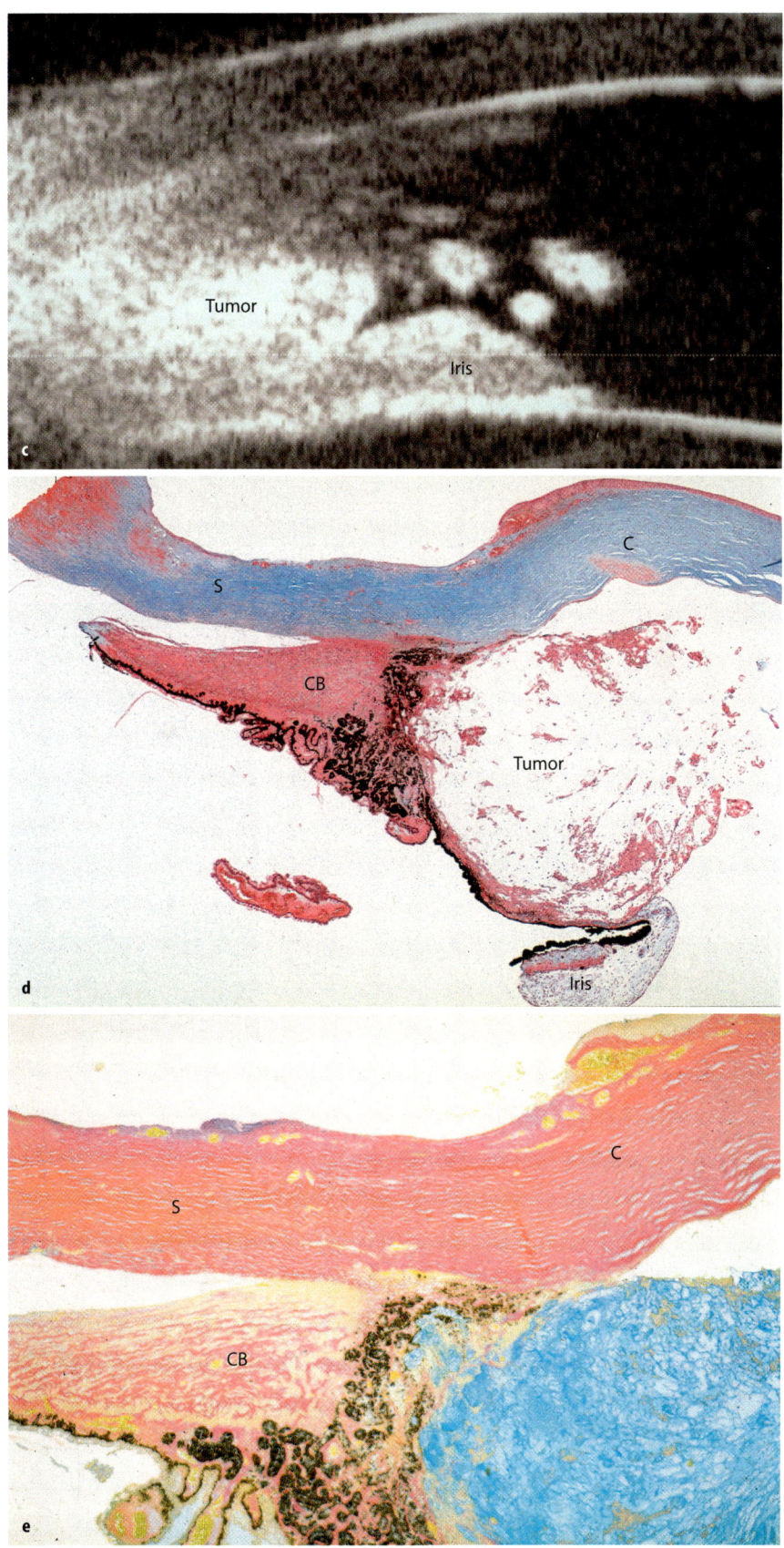

Fig. 5.4.21. d After phacoemulsification implantation of rigid PMMA-lens. Nine-millimeter block including tumor, iris, pars plicata of ciliary body (*CB*) and full thickness sclera and cornea. Ciliary body (*CB*). **e** Stained for acid mucopolysaccharides

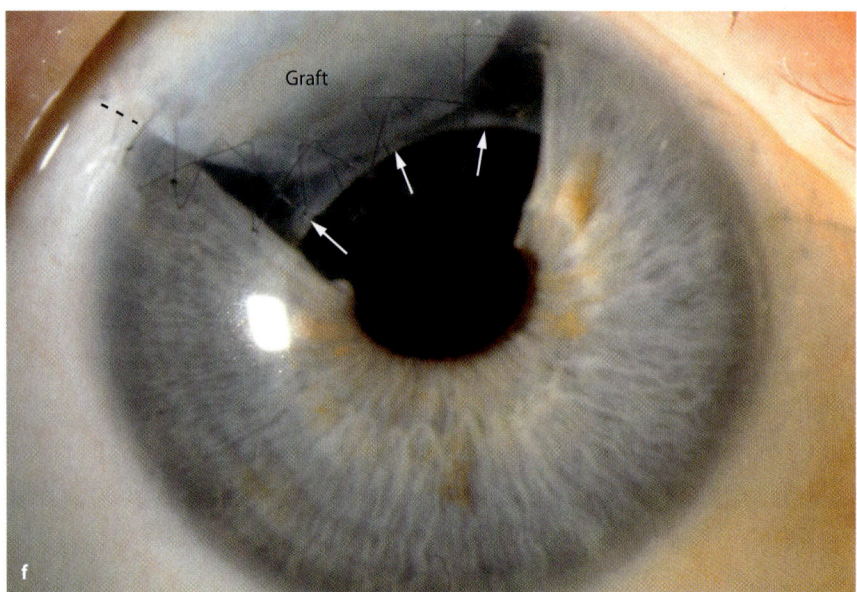

Fig. 5.4.21. f Corneoscleral graft 15 months later with good visual acuity edge of anterior lens capsule covering endocapsular PMMA-lens (*arrows*) (case reported by Cursiefen et al. 1999)

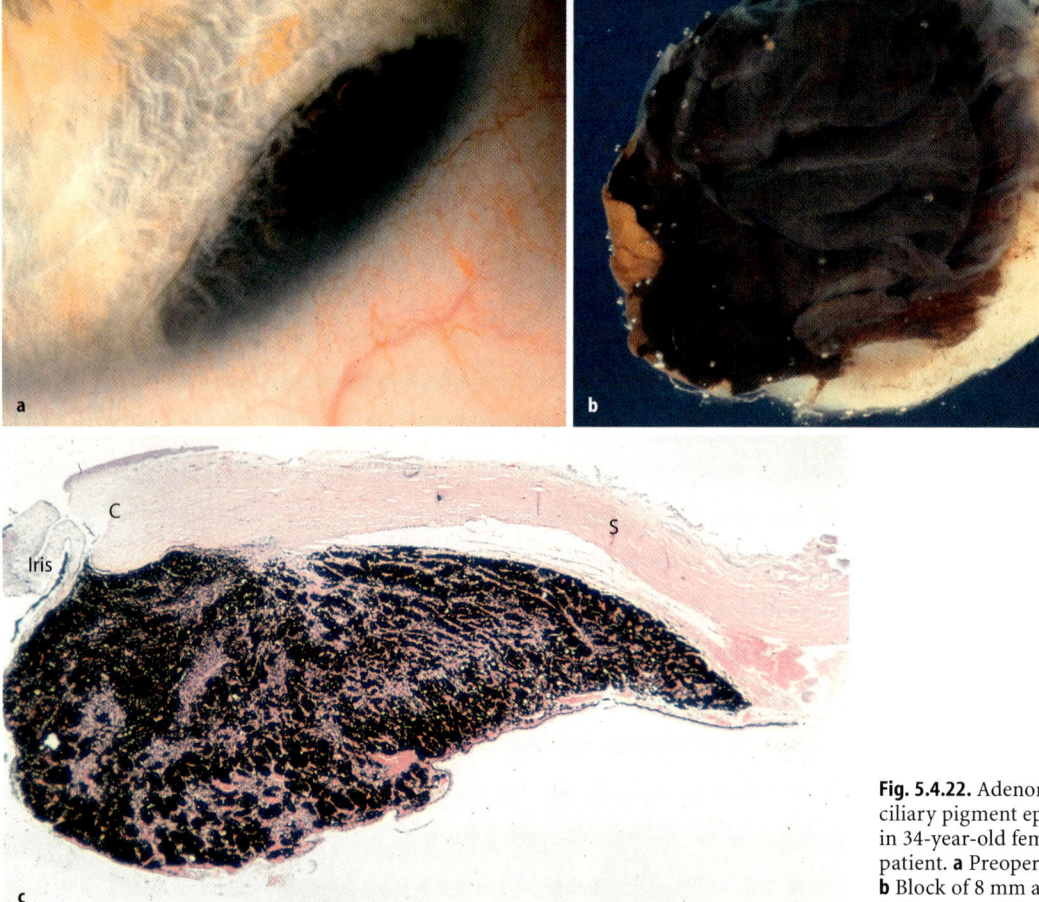

Fig. 5.4.22. Adenoma of the ciliary pigment epithelium in 34-year-old female patient. **a** Preoperatively. **b** Block of 8 mm and sector-iridectomy. **c** Histology

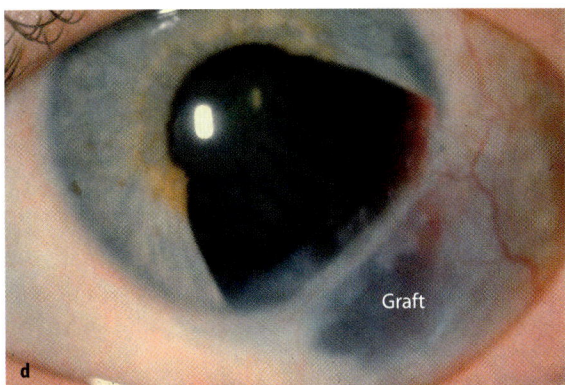

Fig. 5.4.22. d Postoperatively (case reported by Naumann et al. 1976)

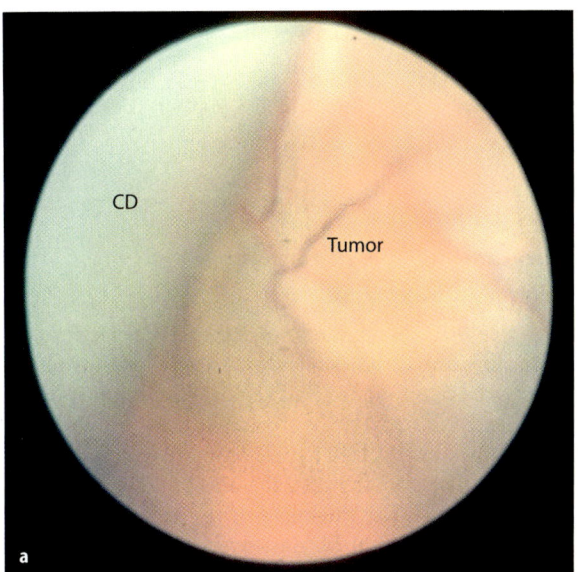
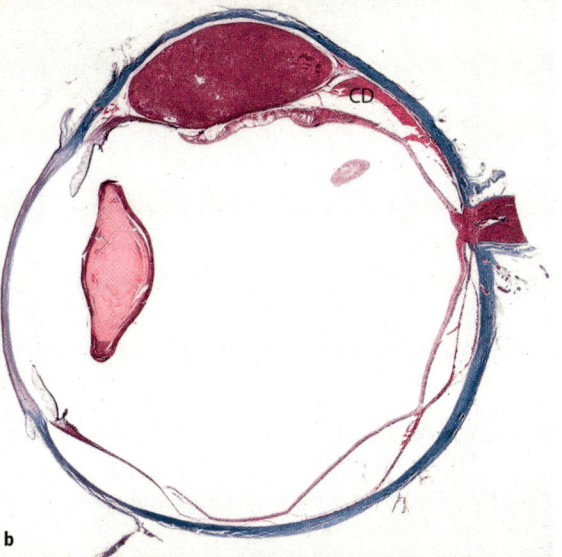
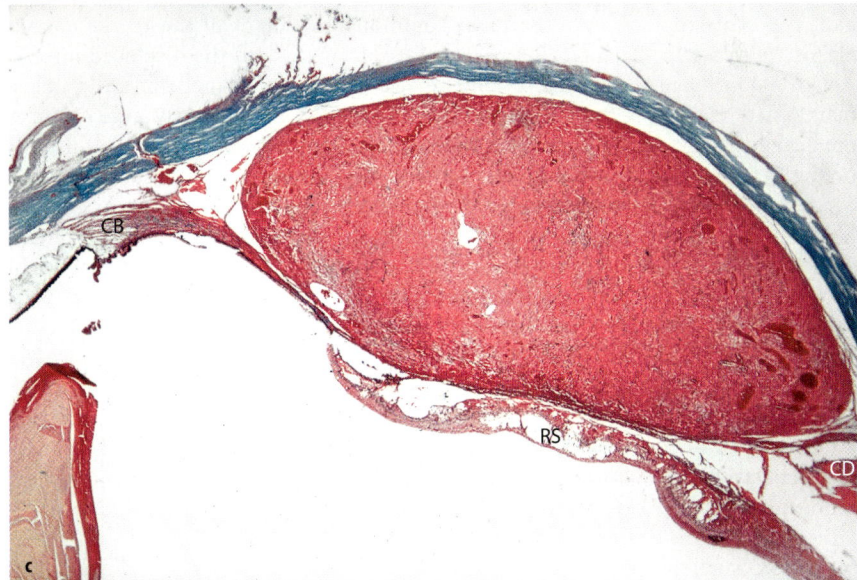

Fig. 5.4.23. Leiomyoma of ciliary body and choroid with collateral and distant retinal detachment in 17-year-old boy treated by enucleation. **a** Preoperatively showing extensive collateral detachment (*CD*). **b, c** Histology showing collateral detachment, ciliary body (*CB*) and retinoschisis (*RS*) overlying the tumor. Choroid and retina in cross-section of globe opposite to tumor arteficially detached

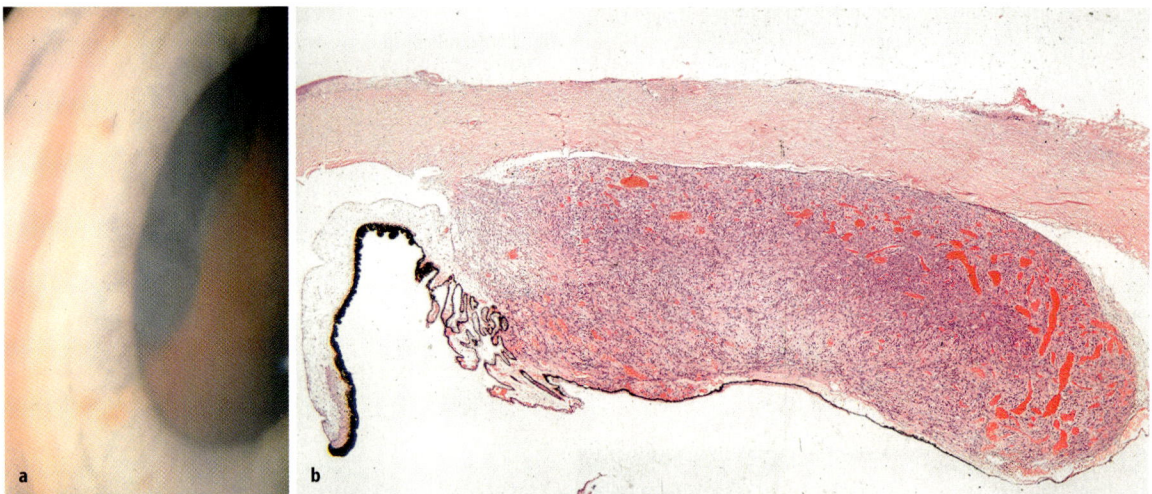

Fig. 5.4.24. Leiomyoma of the ciliary body and choroid treated by 10-mm block excision in 43-year-old man. **a** Preoperatively. **b** Block excision preceded by transcorneal extracapsular cataract extraction with PMMA rigid lens implant. Postoperatively, visual acuity 1.0 (case report by Schlötzer-Schrehardt et al. 2002)

5.4.3.4.1
Block Excision of Localized Tumors of the Anterior Uvea

The anterior uvea is only justified if there is *no* evidence of seeding of tumor cells into the aqueous and/or vitreous cavity. *Biocytology* – that is slit lamp examination by × 40 magnification – allows recognition of individual tumor cells against a background of blue-gray iris tissue on the lens surface and/or fundus red (see Chapter 5.3). Against the backdrop of a brown iris this is often difficult or impossible to recognize (Fig. 5.4.11). Of 104 consecutive expanding tumors of the ciliary body, 26 were histopathologically benign. Among the malignant types melanomas were the most common (Table 5.4.7; Fig. 5.4.15 – 22; 5.4.24).

Normal intraocular pressure postoperatively can be maintained if not more than 150° (or 5 clock hours) of the circumference of the pars plicata is excised. Surprisingly the block excision – contrary to our original concerns – does *not* usually create a cyclodialysis and is not associated with persisting ocular hypotony if 210° of the pars plicata is preserved. It is not well understood why the unavoidable opening of the supraciliary space associated with block excision does *not* induce a persisting ocular hypotony (Tables 5.4.1, 5.4.2).

Reasons for this radical approach for tumors of the anterior uvea are: (1) uveal malignant melanomas have a tendency to invade the sclera, (2) the extent of the scleral invasion cannot be judged clinically if the tumor is non-pigmented, (3) every involvement of the iris root indicates invasion of the ciliary body and cannot be separated from the pars plicata of the ciliary body. Therefore an iridectomy cannot achieve a curative excision in processes of the iris root (Table 5.4.5).

5.4.3.4.2
Block Excision of Epithelial Ingrowth

(1) Both the diffuse and cystic variants show marked *variable thickness* of the lining epithelial layer from 20 to – often only 1 or 2 cell layers. This delicate structure cannot be manipulated and separated mechanically or uniformly destroyed by alcohol injection and other toxic substances. (2) Reliable complete removal is only possible by removing also the adjacent tissue "acting as a shell." (3) The thickness of the epithelial layer is variable and cannot be destroyed with uniform certainty by lasers or coagulation. (4) The location and extent of the tracks connecting the surface epithelium and the displaced intraocular elements cannot be determined clinically, unless there is an obvious external fistula. (5) Large cystic epithelial ingrowth can be reduced in diameter if part of the fluid within the cyst is drained (via an access later removed) and the diameter of the cyst compressed by injection of Healon into the anterior chamber outside the cyst. This permits a smaller diameter of the block excision without risking incomplete removal (Table 5.4.6; Naumann and Völcker 1975; Naumann and Rummelt 1990, 1992a, b, 1997; Rummelt et al. 1993, Fig. 5.4.26 – 31).

Important: Attempts to treat cystic epithelial ingroth with laser-puncture or sector-iridectomy shall convert the process to the diffuse type – originating from remaining epithelium in the angle at the face of the ciliary body (Groh et al. 2002; Viestenz et al. 2003).

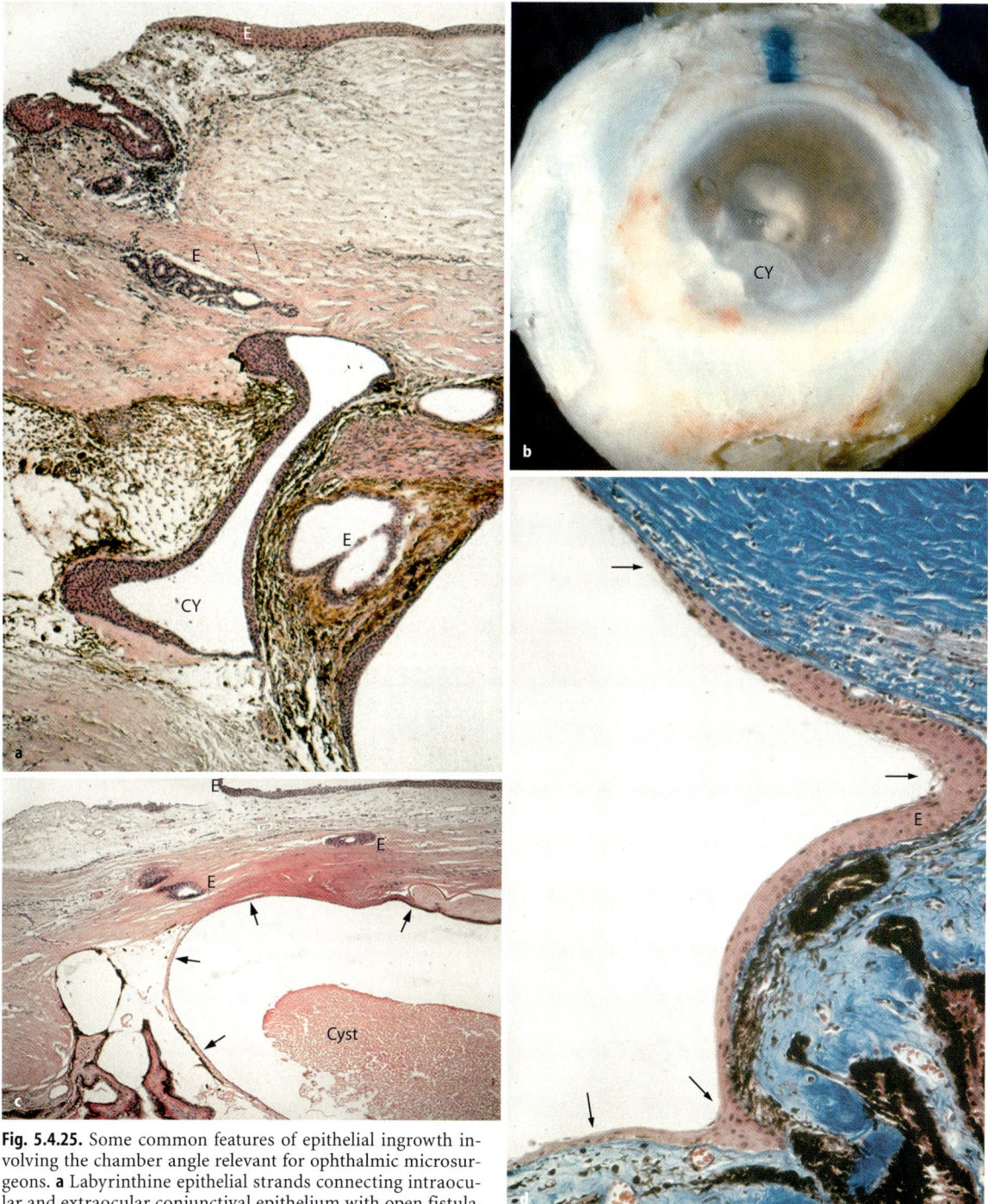

Fig. 5.4.25. Some common features of epithelial ingrowth involving the chamber angle relevant for ophthalmic microsurgeons. **a** Labyrinthine epithelial strands connecting intraocular and extraocular conjunctival epithelium with open fistula. **b, c** Globe with cystic ingrowth (*CY*) and cross-section of nonpigmented epithelial strands connecting intra- and extraocular epithelium (*E*). **d** Involvement of the chamber angle *always* involves the face of the ciliary body in diffuse and cystic epithelial ingrowth (*arrow*)

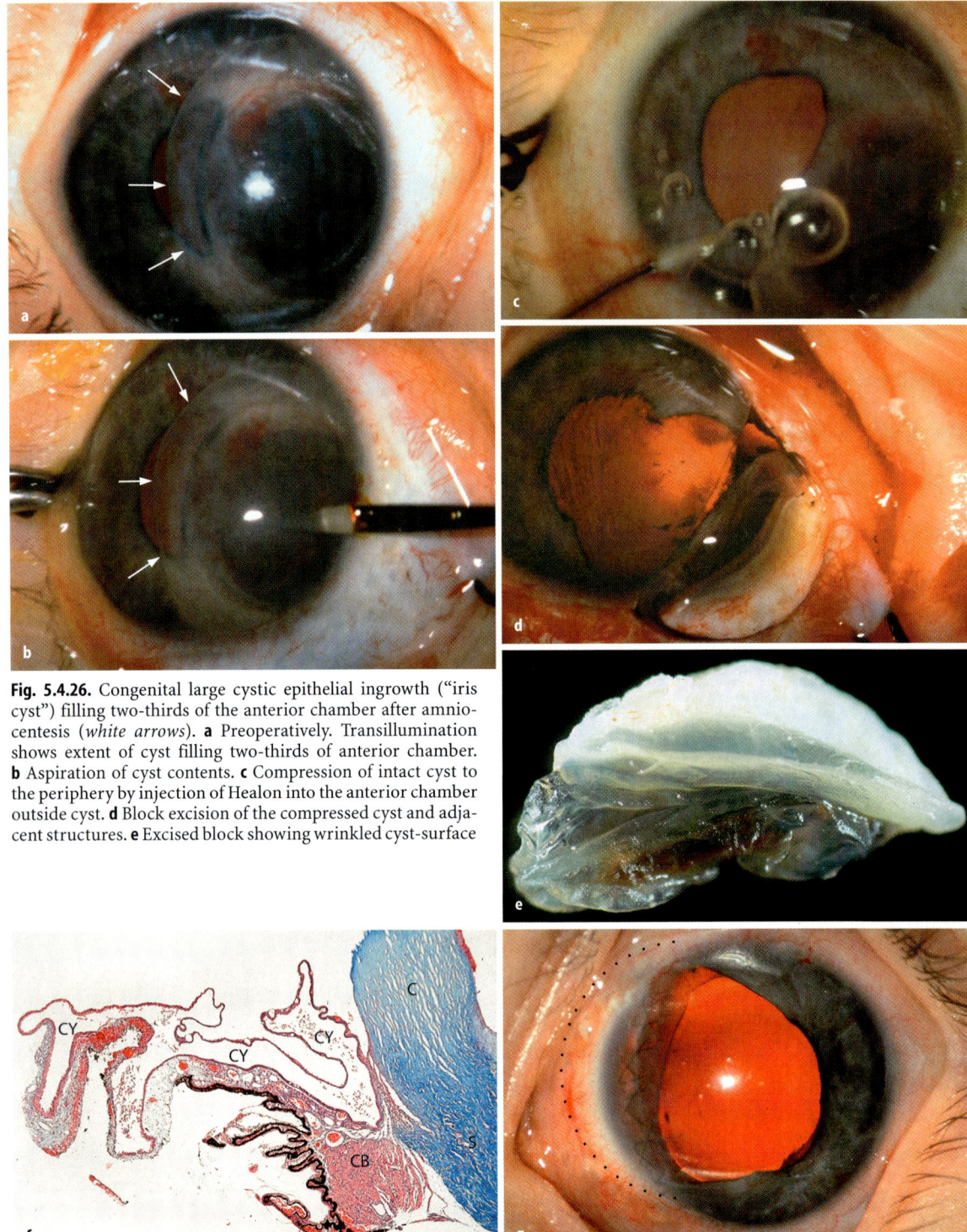

Fig. 5.4.26. Congenital large cystic epithelial ingrowth ("iris cyst") filling two-thirds of the anterior chamber after amniocentesis (*white arrows*). **a** Preoperatively. Transillumination shows extent of cyst filling two-thirds of anterior chamber. **b** Aspiration of cyst contents. **c** Compression of intact cyst to the periphery by injection of Healon into the anterior chamber outside cyst. **d** Block excision of the compressed cyst and adjacent structures. **e** Excised block showing wrinkled cyst-surface **f** Histology showing intimate contact of epithelial lining of the cyst (*CY*) to face of ciliary body (Masson stain). **g** One year postoperatively. Extent of graft (*dots*)

5.4.3 Indications for Procedures Involving the Ciliary Body

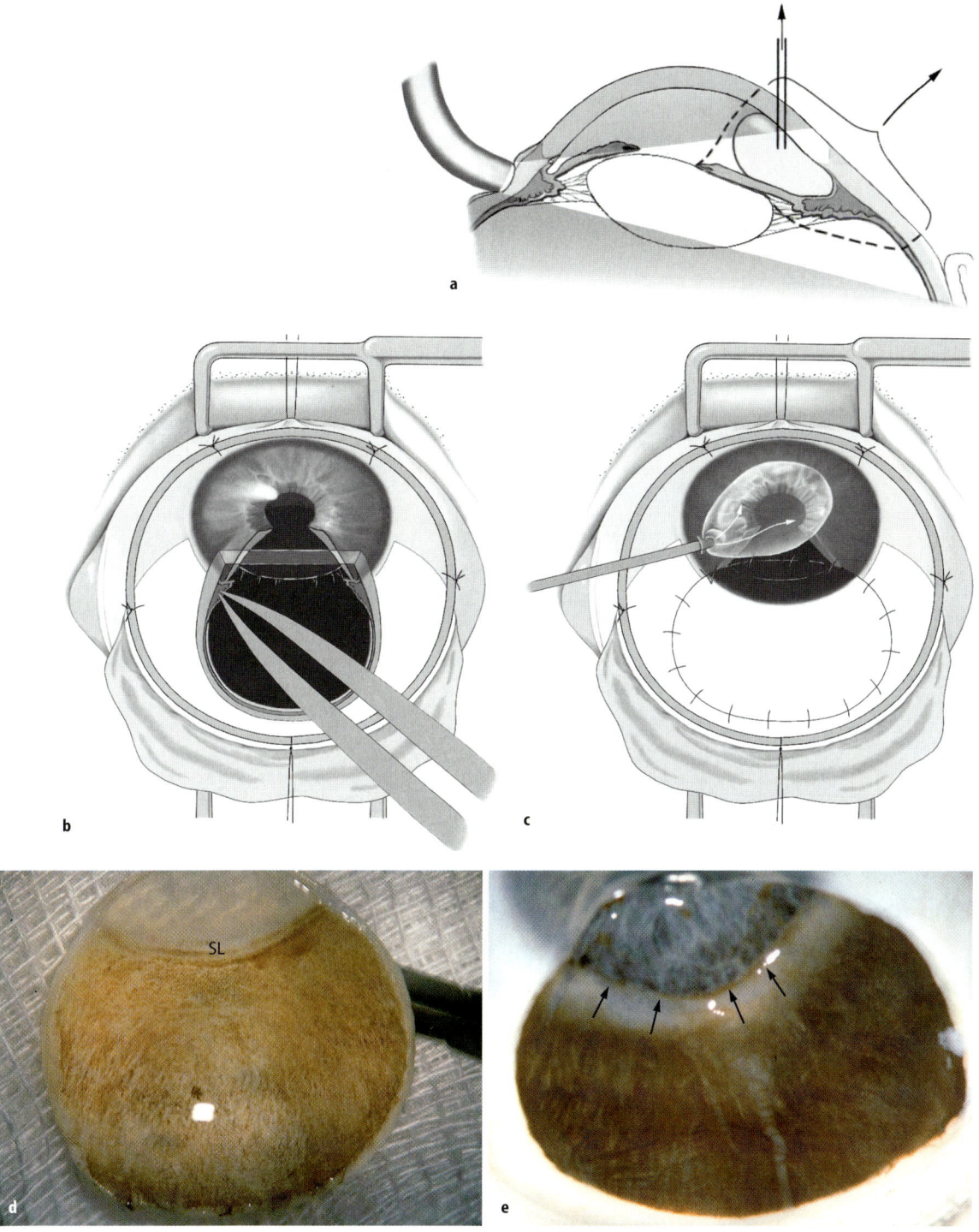

Fig. 5.4.27. Surgical steps of block excision of epithelial ingrowth in sketches. **a** Transillumination and aspiration of cystic contents later followed by injection of Healon into the anterior chamber compressing the cyst to reduce diameter of excision. **b** Block excision of cyst with adjacent tissue of iris, ciliary body, sclera and cornea acting as a shell in one block. Microcautery of ciliary vessels. **c** Corneoscleral transplant covering the defect in the globe and restoration of the anterior chamber (modified after Naumann, 1987). **d** Corneoscleral graft obtained from donor eye showing scleral spur and Schwalbe's line (*SL*) separating sclera and cornea and **e** exposed anterior uvea illustrating the fine gray band of ciliary muscle insertion in one line (*arrows*) separated from scleral spur

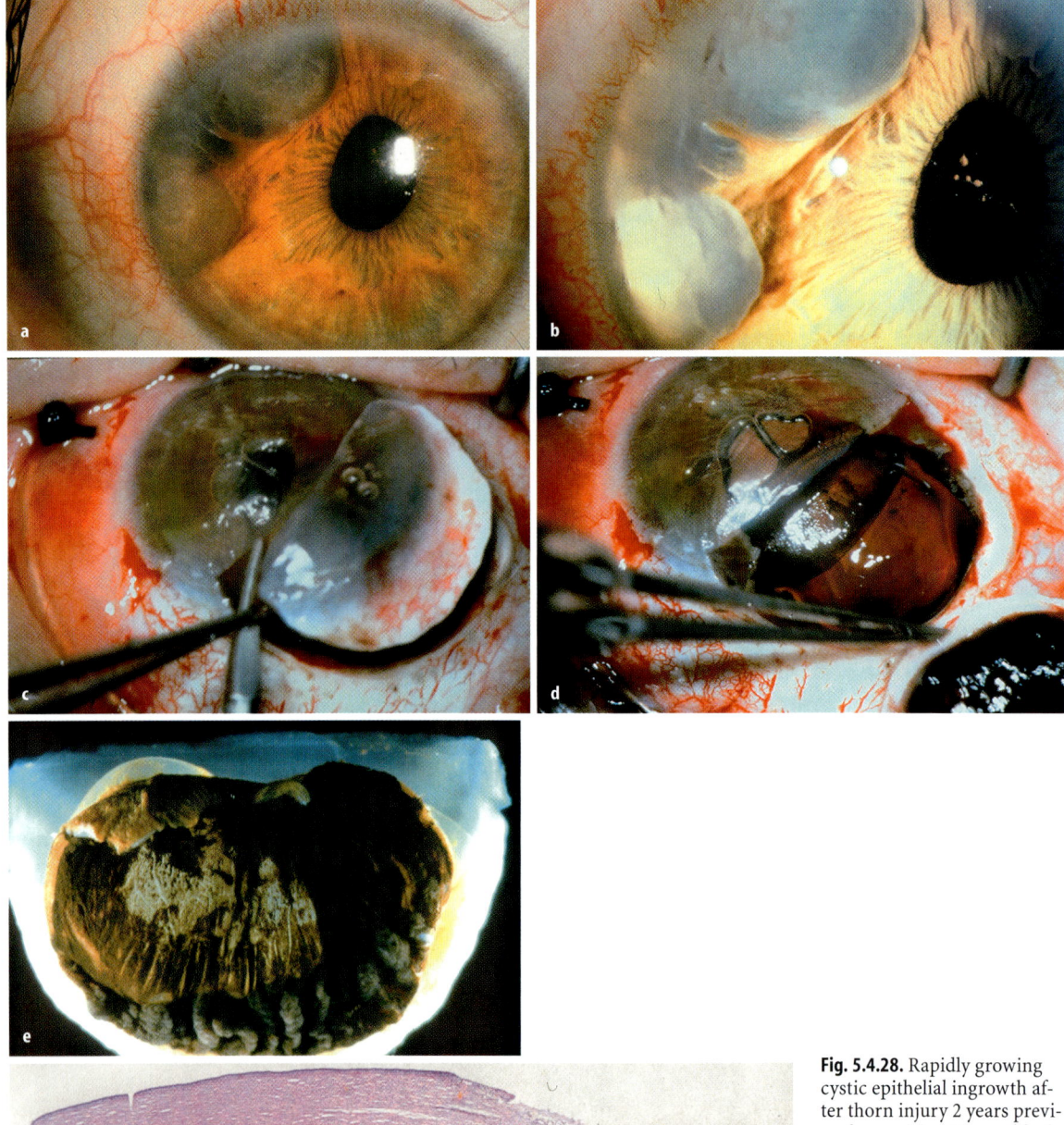

Fig. 5.4.28. Rapidly growing cystic epithelial ingrowth after thorn injury 2 years previously requiring 10-mm block excision. **a, b** Preoperatively showing extent of the cyst from 8 to 12 o'clock. Transillumination illustrating extent of cyst posteriorly. Outlining excision with "open trephine." **c** Block excision after posterior sclerotomy with von Graefe knife and scissors. **d** Defect in global wall exposing lens equator and still intact anterior face of vitreous. **e** Excised block, inner aspect, pars plicata (*PPL*). **f–h** Histology: large cyst lined by very thin layer of epithelium (*arrows*) shown in front of ciliary muscle (*CM*) and processes

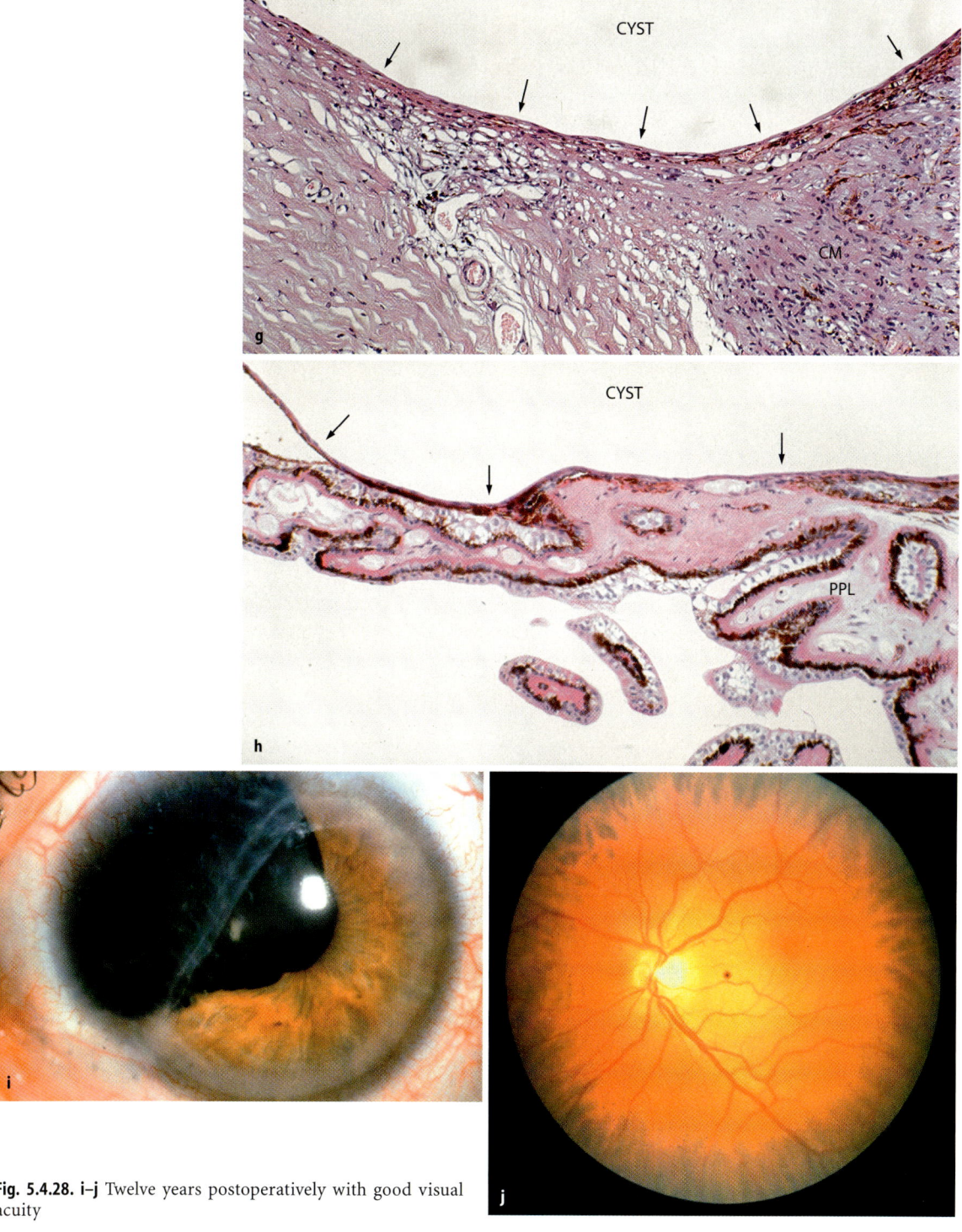

Fig. 5.4.28. i–j Twelve years postoperatively with good visual acuity

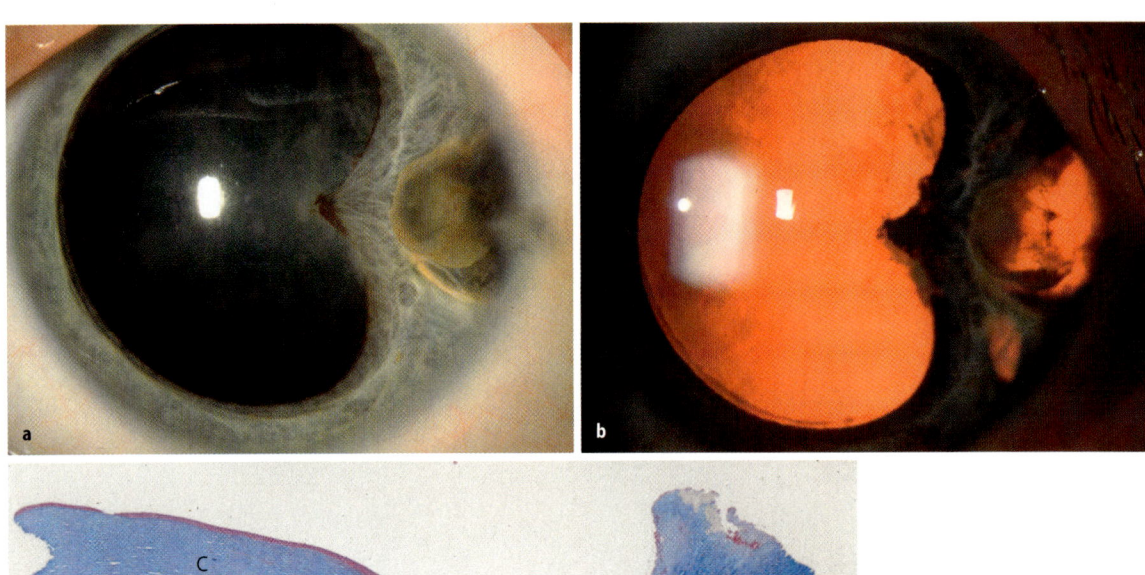
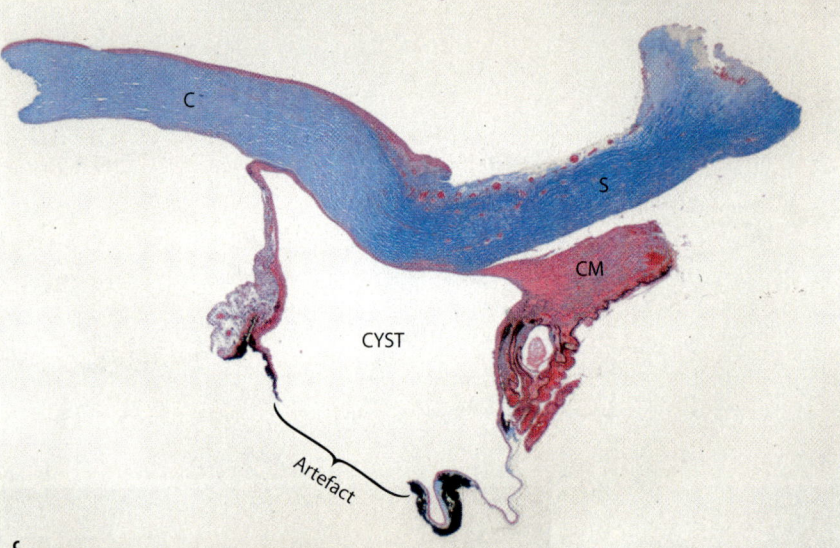

Fig. 5.4.29. Cystic epithelial ingrowth with *impression cataract* extending to posterior pole of lens in one-eyed 26-year-old patient requiring simultaneous extracapsular cataract extraction, implantation of rigid PMMA lens implant and block excision 7 mm in diameter. **a, b** Preoperatively including retroillumination showing posterior subcapsular cataract.
c Excised tissue-block with cyst intact. Thin cystoid wall ruptured *after* removal (Masson stain)

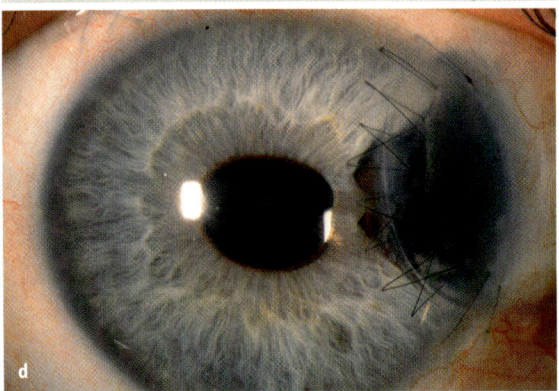

◁
d After block excision simultaneously with implantation of rigid PMMA lens after extracapsular cataract extraction. Visual acuity 1.0

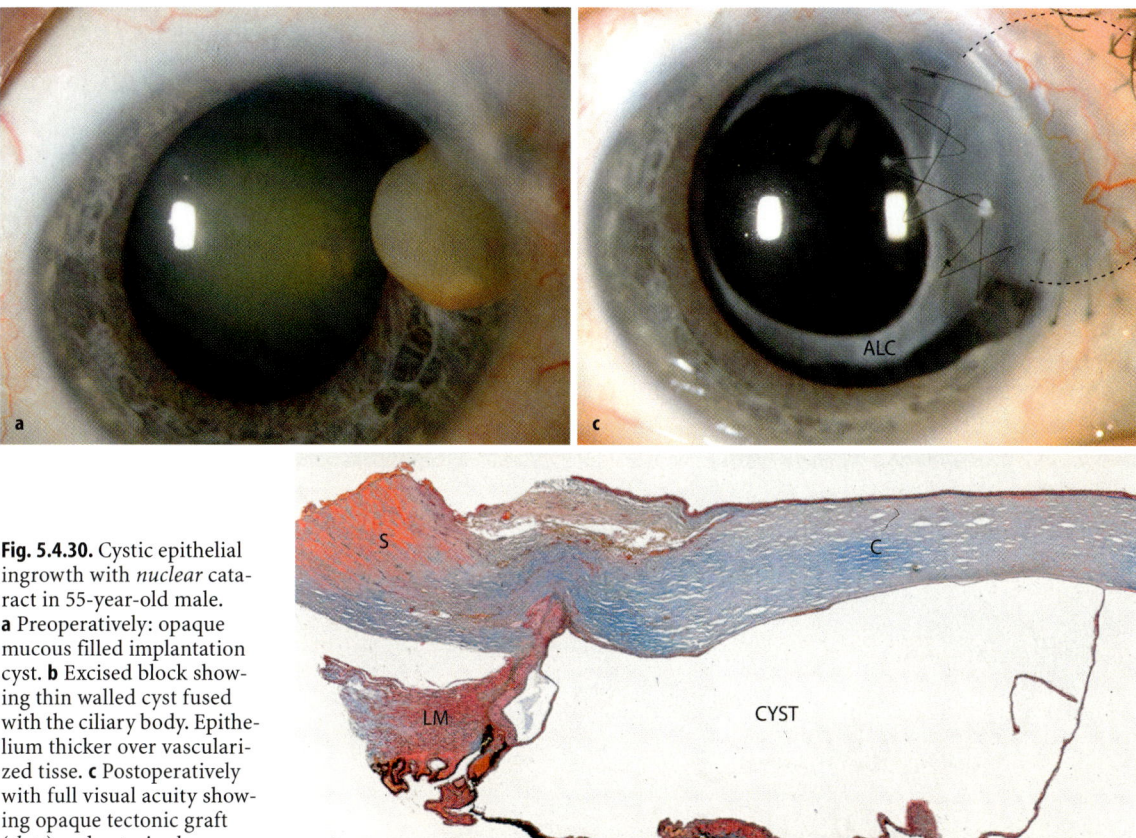

Fig. 5.4.30. Cystic epithelial ingrowth with *nuclear* cataract in 55-year-old male. **a** Preoperatively: opaque mucous filled implantation cyst. **b** Excised block showing thin walled cyst fused with the ciliary body. Epithelium thicker over vascularized tisse. **c** Postoperatively with full visual acuity showing opaque tectonic graft (*dots*) and anterior lens capsule (*ALC*) covering lens implant

Our own experience of block excision of cystic and diffuse epithelial ingrowth of the anterior chamber with 59 consecutive patients in Erlangen is summarized as follows: diameter of block excision 8.0 ± 1.5 mm (5.5–12 mm), in all anterior vitrectomies. Eleven (17%) combined simultaneous surgeries concerning the lens: 8 × phakoemulsification and implantation of posterior chamber intraocular lens, 2 × intracapsular cataract extraction and one lens implant explantation (Table 5.4.8).

Complications. Fourteen intraoperative vitreous hemorrhages, 14 postoperative vitreous hemorrhages (11 spontaneous resorptions), 10 bullous keratopathies (× 6 preexisting), two retinal detachments, one atrophia bulbi. There was no recurrence in this series.

Histopathologic Classification ($n=59$). Fifty-three cystic, one cystic and diffuse, five diffuse, one each for mucogenic and foreign body granuloma.

Causes of visual acuity less than 20:200 ($n=16$ out of 53): ten reversible corneal decompensations, one irreversible preexisting secondary glaucoma, one atrophy of the globe. Visual acuity always better than preoperatively.

Block excision both after removal of tumors and epithelial ingrowth results in huge defects in the eye wall that need to be closed by corneal or corneoscleral tectonic grafts. These grafts do *not* enjoy immune privilege and almost all develop an irreversible immunologic graft reaction with consecutive vascularization and scarring.

If this affects the optical axis an ipsilateral autologous rotational graft may be indicated (see Chapter 5.1). The eye tolerates removal of up to 150° of the pars plicata of the ciliary body (see "minimal eye" in Sect. 7, Chapter 4).

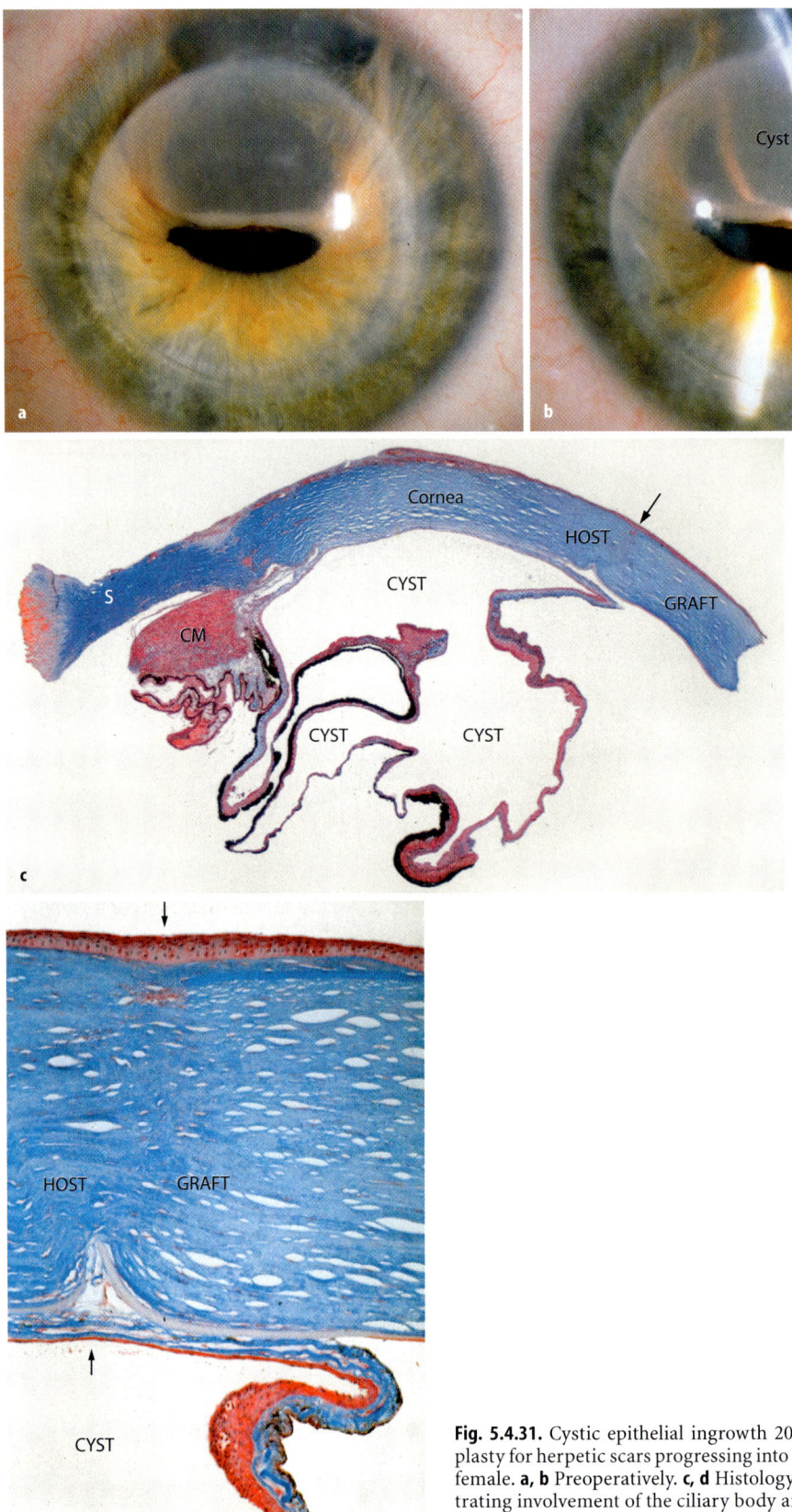

Fig. 5.4.31. Cystic epithelial ingrowth 20 years after perforating keratoplasty for herpetic scars progressing into the pupillary area in 30-year-old female. **a, b** Preoperatively. **c, d** Histology of 7.5-mm block excision illustrating involvement of the ciliary body and variable thickness of the epithelial lining and thinning of the retrocorneal portion, scar of host – graft junction (*arrow*)

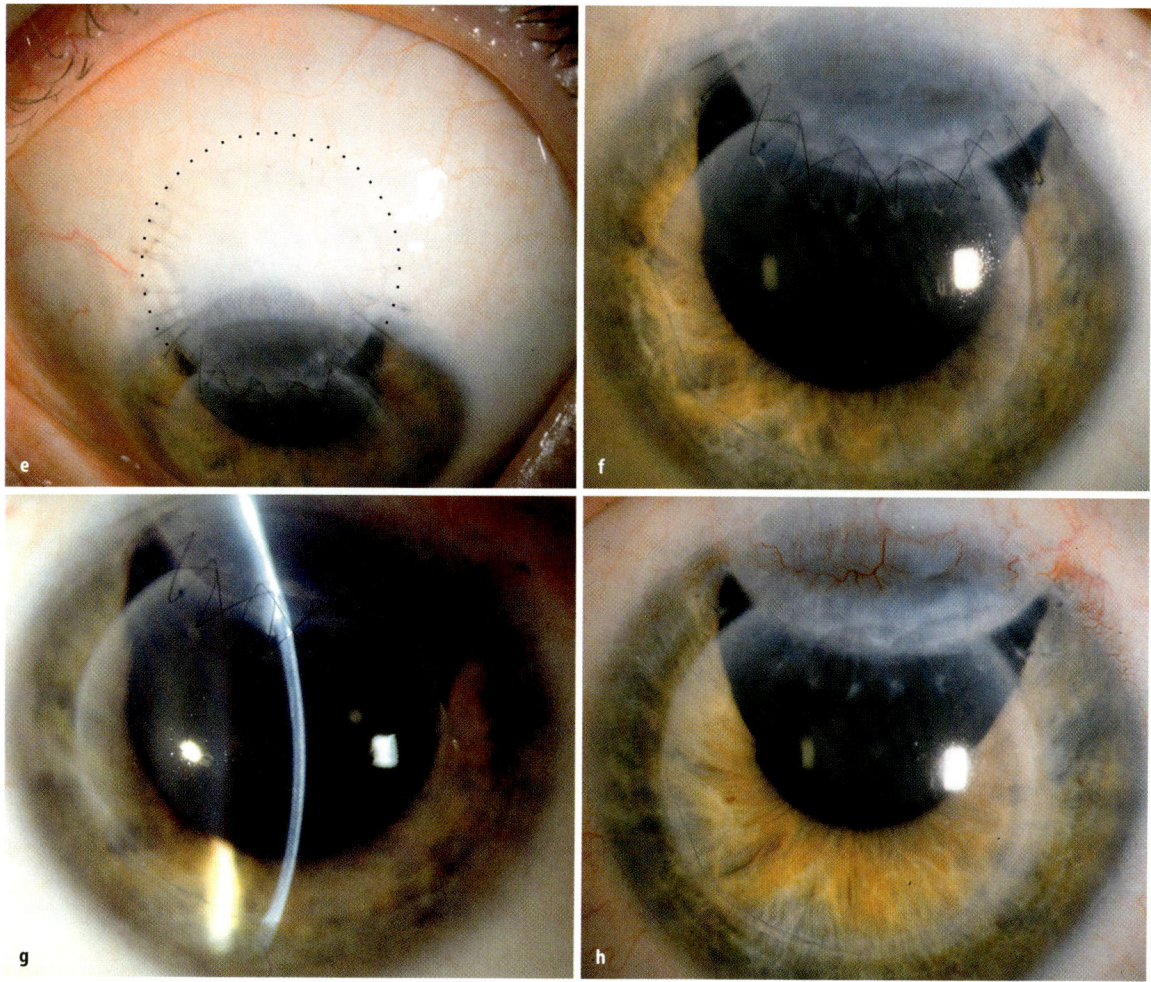

Fig. 5.4.31. e–g Postoperative appearance after block excision of intact cyst compressed by Healon, with adjacent iris, ciliary body, sclera, cornea and part of the original graft. **h** Two years later, visual acuity 0.5. Tectonic graft vascularized; original graft still clear

5.4.3.5
Cyclodestruction

Cyclodestruction may be indicated as the "ultima ratio" in secondary angle closure glaucoma with rubeosis iridis.

Transscleral coagulation of the pars plicata of the ciliary body is performed by transscleral *diode laser* coagulation and *cryo-* or *diathermic* applications. Diathermy always causes severe scleral necrosis, cryothermy to a somewhat lesser degree. All affect not only the "oven" pigmented ciliary epithelium *but also destroy the exposed ciliary muscle* (Fig. 5.4.32).

Antiglaucomatous Pars Plicata Excision

For far advanced intractable secondary angle-closure glaucoma with partial athalamia, aphakia after perforating injury excision of a sector of the Pars plicata may save the eye as an ultima ratio (see Naumann, 1987). It can make restoration of the anterior chamber possible.

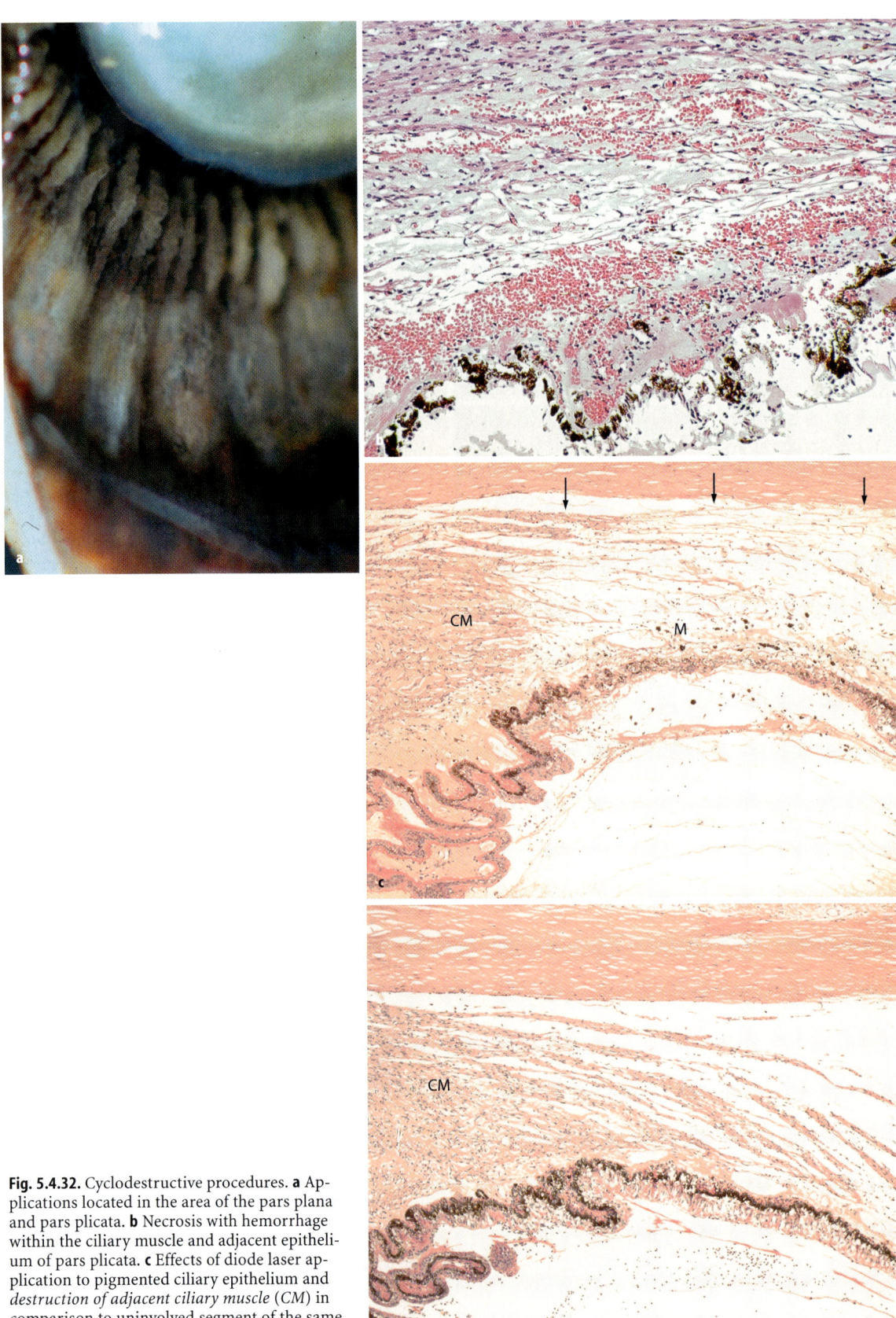

Fig. 5.4.32. Cyclodestructive procedures. **a** Applications located in the area of the pars plana and pars plicata. **b** Necrosis with hemorrhage within the ciliary muscle and adjacent epithelium of pars plicata. **c** Effects of diode laser application to pigmented ciliary epithelium and *destruction of adjacent ciliary muscle* (*CM*) in comparison to uninvolved segment of the same eye (**d**) melanophages (*M*)

5.4.4
Wound Healing and Complications After Procedures Involving the Ciliary Body

5.4.4.1
Intraoperative Hemorrhage

Intraoperative hemorrhage develops if the ciliary processes are touched mechanically and if the excision includes the pars plicata of the ciliary body with its supplies from the major anterior circle of the iris and ciliary body. Surprisingly, in "direct cyclopexy" intra- or postoperative hemorrhage is *not* usually marked. During block excisions particularly with malignant melanomas, the ciliary body vessels have a large caliber and may cause a marked and sometimes persisting vitreous hemorrhage – in spite of direct microcautery – requiring later vitrectomy in a second procedure. In contrast, benign tumors and epithelial ingrowth of the anterior uvea do not usually present serious bleeding problems during block excisions – apparently their blood supply is lower.

The pigmented and non-pigmented ciliary epithelium participate in the formation of *cyclitic membranes by fibrovascular proliferations in the vitreous*. Other repair mechanisms are not evident in the pars plicata and ciliary body.

5.4.4.2
Local Recurrence and Metastasis of Tumors

Recurrence of tumors occurs rarely only if seeding of tumor cells into the aqueous is overlooked. The frequency of metastasis of malignant melanomas compares favorably with enucleation (Naumann and Rummelt 1996).

Traction to the pars plicata of the ciliary processes develops from cyclitic membranes, and scar formation around the lens may lead to a *"cilioschisis"* leading to persisting ocular hypotony due to a reduction in aqueous secretion.

Tectonic corneoscleral grafts after block excisions do not enjoy the immunologic privileges of a corneal graft placed in the center of an avascular cornea. Early or later they all develop in the graft corneal endothelial decompensation, bullous keratopathy, ingrowth of newly formed vessels and scarring (see Sect. 5.1). Migration and proliferation of corneal endothelium of the patient's cornea to the retrocorneal surface of the scarred graft may lead after decades to a reduced corneal endothelial count of the host and decompensation of the patient's own central cornea.

5.4.4.3
Prevention of Retinal Detachment

If the tumors of the ciliary body extend into the choroid beyond the ora serrata, extensive preoperative *prophylactic retinopexy* by cryo- or laser coagulation is indicated to prevent retinal detachment. Additionally pars plana vitrectomy with membrane peeling must be evaluated to avoid macular pucker (see Sect. 5.6). Retinal detachment is relatively rare considering the extent of the block excision:

In our series of 144 consecutive block excisions (87 for tumors, 57 for intraocular epithelial indentation cysts), the diameter ranged between 5.5 and 20 mm. In 39 patients the tumor extended posterior to the ora serrata. Retinal detachment occurred in 10 (6.9%) of 144 patients (2 of 57, or 3.5%, with cysts; 8 of 87, 9.2%, with tumors) 3–12 months after block excision. After scleral buckling procedures and primary pars plana vitrectomy with temporary ocular endotamponade, the retina has remained attached in all patients after a mean follow-up of 31 months. Large diameters and posterior location were risk factors. The detachment usually developed from retinal tears *opposite* the site of the block excision (Jonas et al. 1999).

5.4.4.4
Corneal Endothelium Proliferation and Migration in Traumatic Postcontusional Cyclodialysis

Völcker and Enke (1983) pointed out that an untreated cyclodialysis cleft after years can be covered by proliferating/migrating corneal endothelial cells both on the scleral and ciliary muscle surface. How this influences the intraocular pressure is poorly understood.

5.4.4.5
Ocular Hypotony After Block Excision for Tumors or Epithelial Ingrowth

In 210 consecutive patients persisting ocular hypotony and atrophy of the globe occured if more than 150° of the pars plicata was excised. In the Departments of Ophthalmology in Hamburg, Tübingen and Erlangen, we treated 135 patients for tumors of the anterior uvea and 75 mainly for cystic (but a few for diffuse) epithelial ingrowth. Larger excisions – which we do not recommend – are complicated by proliferative retinopathy, retinal detachment and cyclitic membrane.

5.4.4.6
Relative Ocular Hypertension After Block Excision

Immediately postoperatively within the first week high intraocular pressure spikes due to residua of Healon or hemorrhage within the anterior chamber can develop and are usually compensated in a few days.

5.4.4.7
Lens Decentration/Subluxation and Cataract Formation After Block Excision

Depending on the extent of removal of the ciliary body, the lens or pseudophakos can be slightly decentered or subluxated – usually not preventing recovery of satisfactory vision. After 2 years many patients with a clear lens develop a nuclear or progressive sectorial cataract formation. Therefore today we recommend a *lens exchange with endocapsular implantation of a rigid polymethylmethacrylate (PMMA)* lens implant in the same session immediately before completion of the block excision. This simultaneous procedure stabilizes the anterior segment and spares the patient a second procedure. Extracapsular cataract surgery is otherwise technically more difficult because of the sectorial zonula defect.

References

Cursiefen C, Schlötzer-Schrehardt U, Holbach LM, Naumann GOH. Adenoma of the nonpigmented ciliary epithelium mimicking a malignant melanoma of the iris. Arch Ophthalmol 1999; 117: 113–116

Enoch JM. Retinal receptor orientation. Am J Optom Physiol Optics 1975; 52:375

Groh MJM, Nguyen NX, Küchle M, Naumann GOH. Umwandlung der zystischen in eine diffuse Epithelinvasion durch Laser Zysteneröffnung. Bericht über 4 Patienten. Klin Monatsbl Augenheilkd 2002; 219: 37–39

Hillemann J, Naumann G. [Benign epithelioma (Fuchs) of the ciliary body] Ophthalmologica. 1972;164(4):321–5 (in German)

Holbach L, Völcker HE, Naumann GOH. Malignes teratoides Medulloepitheliom des Ziliarkörpers und saures Gliafaserprotein – Klinische, histochemische und immunhistochemische Befunde. Klin Monatsbl Augenheilkd 1985; 187: 282–286

Jonas JB, Groh MJM, Rummelt V, Naumann GOH. Rhegmatogenous retinal detachment after block excision of epithelial implantation cysts and tumors of the anterior uvea. Ophthalmology 1999; 106: 1942–1946

Küchle M, Holbach L, Schlötzer-Schrehardt U, Naumann GOH. Schwannoma of the ciliary body treated by block excision. Br J Ophthalmol 1994; 78: 397–400

Küchle M, Naumann GOH. Direct Cyclopexy for Traumatic Cyclodialysis with Persisting Hypotony Report in 29 Consecutive Patients Ophthalmology 1995; 102: 322–333

Küchle M, Naumann GOH. Mucogenic Secondary Open-Angle Glaucoma in Diffuse Epithelial Ingrowth Treated by Block-Excision. Am J Ophthalmol 1991; 111: 230–234

Machemer R (1972) Vitrectomy. A pars plana approach. Grune & Stratton, New York, pp 1–136

Naumann G. Über pigmentierte Naevi der Aderhaut und des Ciliarkörpers (eine klinische und histopathologische Untersuchungsreihe). Adv Ophthalmol 1970; 23: 187–282

Naumann GOH. Surgery of the Ciliary Body, chapter 3 in: Koch DD, Spaeth GL (eds.) Vol II "Cornea Glaucoma Lens" in: "Atlas of Ophthalmic Surgery" (3 Vol), Heilmann K, Paton D. (eds), Stuttgart, Thieme Verlag, 3.1–3.40, 1987

Naumann G, Green WR. Spontaneous nonpigmented iris cysts. Arch Ophth 1967; 78: 496–500

Naumann G, Font RL, Zimmerman LE. Primary Rhabdomyosarcoma of the Iris. Am J Ophthalmol 1972; 74: 110–118

Naumann G. Blockexcision intraokularer Prozesse I. Tumoren der vorderen Uvea. Klin Monatsbl Augenheilkd 1975; 166: 436–448

Naumann GOH, Völcker HE, Lerche W. Adenom des pigmentierten Ziliarepithels. Albrecht v. Graefes Arch Klin exp Ophthalmol 1976; 198: 245

Naumann G, Völcker HE. Blockexcision intraokularer Prozesse II. Epitheleinwachsung in den vorderen Augenabschnitten. Klin Monatsbl Augenheilkd 1975; 166: 448–457

Naumann GOH, Völcker HE. Direkte Zyklopexie zur Behandlung des persistierenden Hypotonie-Syndroms infolge traumatischer Zyklodialyse. Klin Monatsbl Augenheilkd 1981; 179: 266–270

Naumann GOH, Rummelt V. Block Excision of Tumors of the Anterior Uvea. Report on 68 Consecutive Patients. Ophthalmology 1996; 103: 2017–2028

Naumann GOH, Rummelt V. Block-excision of cystic and diffuse epithelial ingrowth of the anterior chamber. Report on 32 consecutive patients. Arch Ophthalmol 1992; 110: 223–227; Arch Ophthalmol 1992; 10: 214–218 (see also Chinese and Spanish editions)

Naumann GOH, Rummelt V. Congenital nonpigmented epithelial iris cyst removed by block-excision. Graefes Arch Clin Exp Ophthalmol. 1990; 228: 392–397

Rummelt V, Naumann GOH, Folberg E, Weingeist T. Surgical management of melanocytoma of the ciliary body with extrascleral extension. Report on 4 patients. Am J Ophthalmol 1994; 117: 169–176

Rummelt V, Naumann GOH. Block excision of congenital and infantile nonpigmented epithelial iris cysts – Report on 8 infants. Ger J Ophthalmol 1992; 1: 361–366

Rummelt V, Naumann GOH. Blockexzision mit tektonischer Korneoskleralplastik wegen zystischer und/oder diffuser Epithelinvasion des vorderen Augensegments (Bericht über 51 konsekutive Patienten, 1980–1996). Klin Monatsbl Augenheilkd 1997; 211: 312–323

Rummelt V, Rummelt C, Naumann GOH. Congenital Nonpigmented Epithelial Iris Cyst after Amniocentesis Ophthalmology. 1993; 100: 776–781

Schlötzer-Schrehardt U, Jünemann A, Naumann GOH. Mitochondria-rich epithelioid leiomyoma of the ciliary body. Arch Ophthalmol 2002; 120: 77–82

Viestenz A, Küchle M, Naumann GOH. Blockexzision der Epithelinvasion nach Kataraktoperation – Bericht über 15 Patienten. Klin Monatsbl Augenheilkunde 2003; 220: 465–470

Völcker HE, Enke P. Diffuse endothelialization of a cyclodialysis cleft: a light and electron microscopic study. Klin Monatsbl Augenheilkd 1983 Sep;183(3):195–200 (in German)

Zagórski Z, Shrestha HG, Lang GK, Naumann GOH. Sekundärglaukome durch intraokulare Epithelinvasion. Klin Monatsbl Augenheilkd 1988; 192: 16–20

Lens and Zonular Fibers

U. Schlötzer-Schrehardt, G.O.H. Naumann

Cataract extraction is the most common surgical procedure in medicine. Knowledge of the structure of the lens and its suspensory apparatus and their changes with age may help the cataract surgeon to manage successfully this very common disease and avoid potential intra- and postoperative complications.

Today extracapsular cataract extraction with nuclear expression or by phacoemulsification is the therapy of choice. Until approximately the 1970s intracapsular cataract extraction was preferred. In view of the difficulties of fixation of intraocular lens implants and the vitreous complications leading to traction on the retina causing more frequent detachment or cystoid maculopathy, intracapsular cataract extraction is today considered obsolete. It is now only applied in special situations of dislocated lenses with particularly hard cataracts. Since Ridley's pioneering work in 1949, lens implants have been developed and a broad range of choices concerning the *site* for *fixation*, *material* of the pseudophakos and method of implantation have been developed. The main disadvantage of extracapsular cataract extraction is the development of secondary cataract, which is inherent in the approach to leave the lens capsule inside the eye together with adherent lens epithelial cells that postoperatively *always* proliferate.

5.5.1 Key Features of the Lens

The lens of the eye is a transparent, biconvex, elliptical organ located between the iris and the vitreous (Fig. 5.5.1). It is held in position by the zonular fibers and by its close apposition to the vitreous on its posterior and equatorial aspects. It is a highly organized structure of specialized surface ectoderm-derived cells, which constitute an important component of the optical system of the eye. The function of the lens is to focus images on the retina by altering the refractive index of light entering the eye. While it has less refractive power (15–20 diopters) than the cornea (42 diopters), the lens has the advantage of the ability to change its shape, under the influence of the ciliary muscle, and thus alter its refractive power. In addition, it acts as a spectral filter absorbing the more energetic wavelengths of the spectrum (300–400 nm) that have the potential to damage the retina and particularly the macula. The transparency of the lens is based on the shape, arrangement, internal structure, and biochemistry of the lens cells or lens fibers and on the lack of any innervation or blood supply after regression of the tunica vasculosa lentis in fetal development. It receives its nourishment from the aqueous and vitreous humors.

The lens is remarkable for being an "inside-out" structure. During embryonic development, the lens,

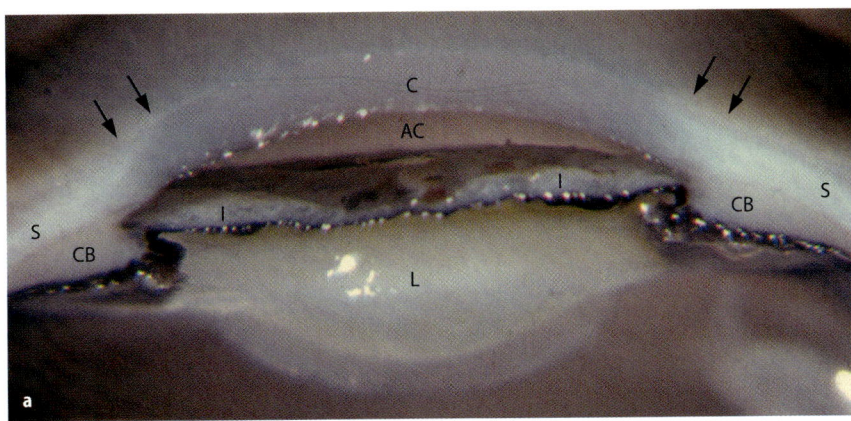

Fig. 5.5.1. Anatomy of the lens. **a** Macroscopic view by parasagittal section of the globe: Lens (*L*), Ciliary body (*CB*), Cornea (*C*), Sclera (*S*), Limbus (*arrows*), Anterior chamber (*AC*) Iris (*I*)

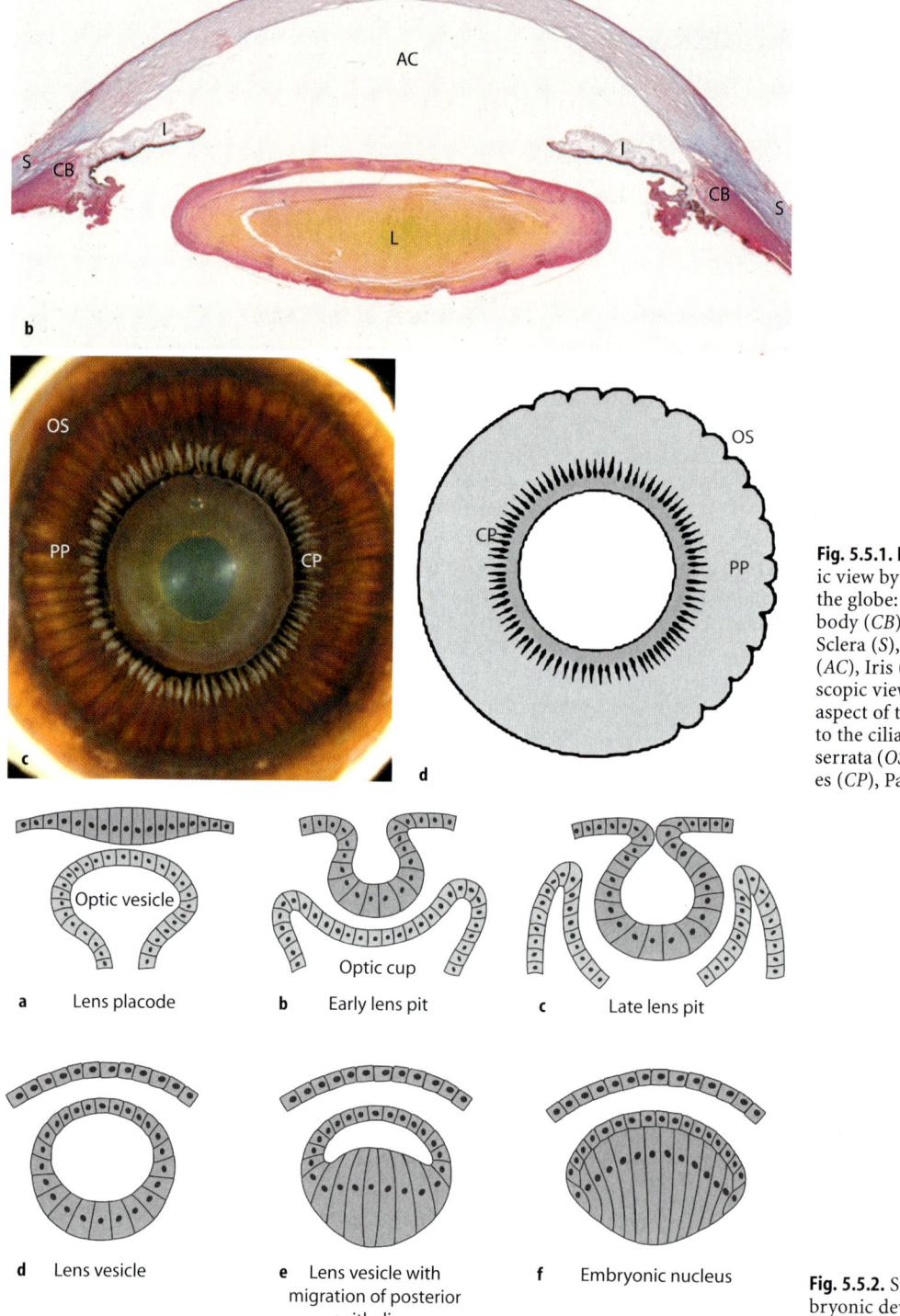

Fig. 5.5.1. b Light microscopic view by sagittal section of the globe: Lens (*L*), Ciliary body (*CB*), Cornea (*C*), Sclera (*S*), Anterior chamber (*AC*), Iris (*I*). **c, d** Macroscopic view of the posterior aspect of the lens in relation to the ciliary body and ora serrata (*OS*), Ciliary processes (*CP*), Pars Plana (*PP*)

Fig. 5.5.2. Stages in the embryonic development of the lens

which originates from the surface ectoderm, invaginates toward the optic cup and then separates and migrates posteriorly (Fig. 5.5.2). Thus the basement membrane, i.e., the lens capsule, is peripheral, and the cells are enclosed within. This encapsulation process "isolates" the lens anatomically from the rest of the eye from the 3rd gestational week on (Marshall et al. 1982). The lens is also unique among internal organs in that it

Table 5.5.1. Phakogenic intraocular disease

1. Phakogenic uveitis
2. "Endophthalmitis phakoanaphylactica": ocular hypotony
3. Acute glaucomas (see Chapter 5.2)
   a) Phakolytic open angle glaucoma
   b) Angle closure glaucoma via:
      Pupillary block
      Ciliary block

contains cells solely of a single epithelial type, in various stages of differentiation, and retains within it all the cells formed during its lifetime. The oldest cells are contained within the central nucleus of the lens, and throughout life new cells are added superficially to the cortex in concentric layers. Thus, the lens demonstrates cells at varying stages of senescence permitting an excellent opportunity to study age-related structural and metabolic alterations.

The lens tissue consists of about 35% protein, a protein content about twice as high as that of other tissues. The lens crystallins account for nearly all the protein. The crystallins were once thought to be unique to the lens, but, in fact, are widely distributed throughout other body tissues as well. Nevertheless, any disruption of the lens capsule will provoke under certain circumstances an immunologic response with antibody formation and macrophage mobilization against lens proteins ("phacogenic uveitis," "phacoanaphylactic endophthalmitis," phacolytic secondary open-angle glaucoma") (Halbert and Manski 1965; Marak 1992) (Table 5.5.1).

Because of its avascularity, primary inflammatory diseases of the lens do not exist. Also, even though the lens epithelium constantly undergoes physiologic replication, primary neoplasms of the human lens have not been recognized.

5.5.2
Basic Aspects of Intraocular Anatomy for Microsurgery of the Lens

Microsurgery of the lens is influenced by the individual anatomy of the anterior segment of the eye and systemic factors such as the arterial blood pressure. In the view of the high frequency of cataract surgery, all nuances are of particular practical significance. In children and young adults with cataracts, the lens tissue is soft, but the vitreoretinal adhesions are strong. Extracapsular surgical aspirations of the lens cortex and nucleus are usually facile. Intracapsular cataract surgery should be avoided. In contrast, the surgeon dealing with age-related cataract is confronted with an increasingly fragile capsule and zonular apparatus, a liquefied vitreous body, and a hardened nucleus.

5.5.2.1
Position of the Lens and the Lens-Iris Diaphragm

The position of the lens is determined by the stability of the zonular apparatus proper and by the location of the zonular insertion into both the nonpigmented ciliary epithelium and the lens capsule. Zonular instability can be pronounced in pseudoexfoliation (PEX) syndrome (see Chapter 6.3). The position of the ciliary body moves towards the lens in acute hypotony with the paracentesis effect associated with any opening of the aqueous space – in the course of "vis a tergo" (Chapters 2, 3, 4) – and in extreme expulsive hemorrhages. In the latter cases, the hemorrhage extends into the supraciliary space separating the ciliary muscle from the sclera. Patients with uncontrolled arterial hypertension are at particular risk to show a rapid anterior movement of the lens-iris diaphragm if the anterior chamber is opened (see Chapter 4). Quick restoration of the anterior chamber establishing a "positive pressure" can be achieved with microincision techniques using an access through the clear cornea stabilizing the position of the lens in the anterior segment. As long as the "open eye" situation persists, any outer pressure to the globe (e.g., lid specula, fluid injected into the orbit) leads to a forward movement of the lens-iris diaphragm.

In contrast, loss of aqueous from the liquefied vitreous may result in a posterior movement of the lens, particularly in highly myopic eyes. Zonular dialysis by contusion trauma or due to metabolic diseases (see Table 5.5.4) causes lens subluxation or dislocation and is prone to vitreous loss as soon as the eye is opened.

5.5.2.2
Characteristics of the Lens Capsule

The anterior capsule is significantly thicker than the posterior capsule and increases in thickness with age. In children, the anterior lens capsule is more elastic, more difficult to perforate during capsulorrhexis, and prone to accidental tears of the equatorial region due to a more central anterior insertion of the zonules in a smaller lens. Although the posterior lens capsule is only about 8 μm thick (corresponding to the maximal diameter of an erythrocyte), its resistance to mechanical microsurgical manipulations is astounding, as long as the instruments have a smooth surface. The slightest mechanical irregularity of a polishing cannula may lead to capsular rupture and consecutive vitreous loss.

5.5.2.3
Hyalocapsular Ligament (Wieger's Ligament)

In children, this vitreolenticular connection is so firm that any attempt at intracapsular lens extraction causes extensive removal of vitreous and retinal complications.

Senile cataracts can be removed intracapsularly, facilitated by α-chymotrypsin digestion of the zonules, while leaving the vitreous face intact during surgery. However, the vitreous face may become defective in the postoperative phase filling the anterior chamber with vitreous. In view of this vitreolenticular connection via Wieger's ligament and the posterior origin of the zonular fibers close to the vitreous base, *all microsurgery of the lens indirectly involves the peripheral retina*, because any lens microsurgery exerts traction on the lens capsule and zonules.

5.5.2.4
Features of Lens Epithelial and Fiber Cells

Congenital cataracts may be restricted to the lens nucleus or the cortical layers; the cataractous and clear tissues are soft and can be relatively easily aspirated. In rubella cataract, living virus particles can be recovered from the lens tissue and should be considered infectious (rubella vaccination of surgical nurses participating in this situation is advisable). In senile cataracts, both the opaque and the clear tissues are more firm and can only be aspirated after phacoemulsification.

Usually, the subcapsular lens epithelium is at least partially preserved in most variants of cataract and remains firmly attached to the lens capsule. Current methods of extracapsular surgery do not achieve complete removal of all lens epithelial cells, which always proliferate in an "attempt at wound healing" leading to formation of secondary cataract. Whereas its peripheral portions may contribute to fixation of the haptic, its extension into the optical axis obscures vision and requires a posterior YAG-laser capsulotomy.

5.5.2.5
Iatrogenic Mydriasis

Wide dilatation of the pupil is a prerequisite for "atraumatic" manipulation of the anterior lens capsule and endocapsular cataractous tissue. Even with proper doses and timing of mydriatic drugs, the pupil may not dilate sufficiently in the presence of iris synechiae, after long-standing iatrogenic miosis, and in certain systemic diseases such as diabetes mellitus (diabetic iridopathy) and PEX syndrome (PEX-associated iridopathy, see Chapter 6), which both are associated with secondary melanin dispersion due to rupture of the iris pigment epithelium. Postoperatively, the formation of posterior synechiae is difficult to avoid due to iris tissue damage and a compromised blood-aqueous barrier.

5.5.2.6
Pseudophakic Lens Implants

Regardless of the variability of lens implants and techniques, the goal of the cataract surgeon should be to avoid any collateral damage to adjacent tissues including the iris, ciliary body, cornea, and chamber angle, and to assure good axial centration. In situations of traumatic or other acquired zonular instability, the surgeons as well as the patients have to be aware of the risks before the surgery. This is frequently neglected in patients suffering from PEX syndrome.

5.5.3
Surgical Anatomy of the Lens

5.5.3.1
Gross Anatomy

The equatorial diameter of the adult lens measures 9–10 mm and its axial width about 4.5 mm (Table 5.5.2) (Tripathi and Tripathi 1983). The lens equator is typically adjacent to the midpoint of the ciliary body with a space of 0.3–0.5 mm between the ciliary processes and the lens equator, which is necessary for accommodation (Fig. 5.5.1). It shows a number of indentations corresponding to the attachment of the zonular fibers. The anterior pole of the lens is about 3 mm from the posterior surface of the cornea, depending on the size of the eye and depth of the anterior chamber. The radius of curvature of the less convex anterior surface averages 10 mm (range 8–14 mm). The more convex posterior surface has an average radius of 6 mm (range 4.5–7.5 mm). It lies in a fossa lined by the hyaloid face – also called a "mem-

Table 5.5.2. Lens measurements throughout life

	At birth	80 years
Equatorial diameter	5.0–6.5 mm	9.0–10.0 mm
Axial diameter	3.5–4.0 mm	4.75–5.0 mm
Weight	65 mg	270 mg
Anterior curvature	14.0 mm	8.0 mm

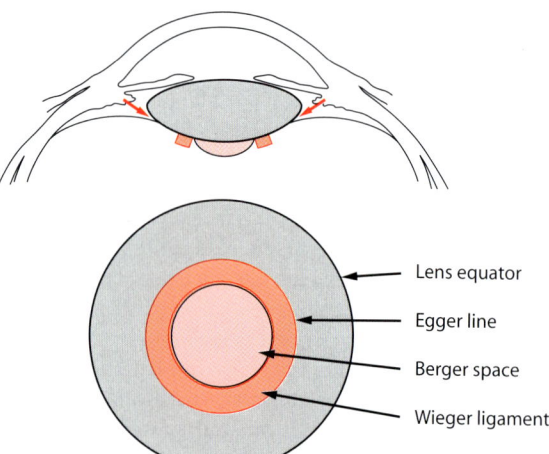

Fig. 5.5.3. Relationship between the lens and the anterior vitreous face. **a** Schematic drawing.

brane" – of the vitreous. This retrolenticular space, filled with aqueous humor, was described by Berger in 1882 (Fig. 5.5.3). The circular hyalocapsular ligament of Wieger surrounds the space of Berger and firmly connects the vitreous with the lens; it is inseparable in infants but can be gently loosened in adults over 40 years of age.

Remnants of the embryonic hyaloid vasculature (tunica vasculosa lentis) can commonly be observed at or slightly nasally to the posterior pole of the lens. These include the remnants of the primary vitreous ("Mittendorf dot") and the "white arcuate line of Vogt"; both only rarely impair vision.

Because of its location, the lens, with the exception of the equator, can be easily examined by biomicroscopy allowing differentiation of various zones of discontinuities corresponding to the embryonic, fetal, infantile, and adult nucleus surrounded by the cortex (Hockwin 1989).

Histologically, the lens consists of three major components: the lens capsule, the lens epithelium, and the lens cells or fibers making up the bulk of the lens substance.

5.5.3.2
Lens Capsule

The lens capsule, which is the basement membrane of the lens epithelium and the thickest basement membrane in the body, completely envelops the lens. It is produced anteriorly by the lens epithelium and posteriorly by the elongating fiber cells and serves to contain the epithelial cells and lens fibers as a structural unit and as a metabolic barrier allowing the passage of small molecules both into and out of the lens (Fig. 5.5.4). Due to its elastic properties, the lens capsule also plays a major role in molding the shape of the lens during the process of accommodation. For this purpose, it receives the insertion of the zonular fibers anteriorly and posteriorly at the lens periphery as well as at the lens equator.

The capsule is of variable thickness, being much thicker on the anterior than on the posterior surface, and being thickest both pre- and postequatorially within the attachment of the zonules and thinner at the

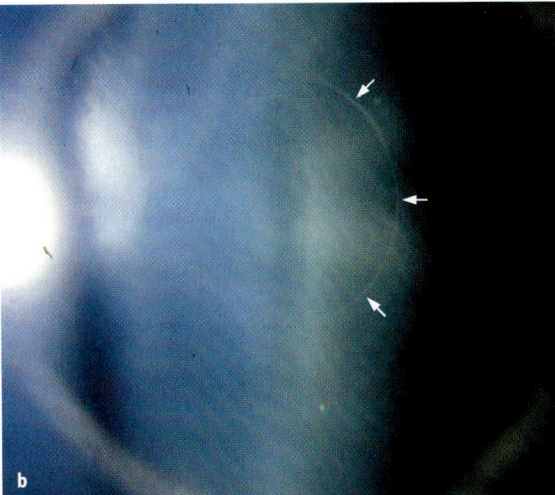

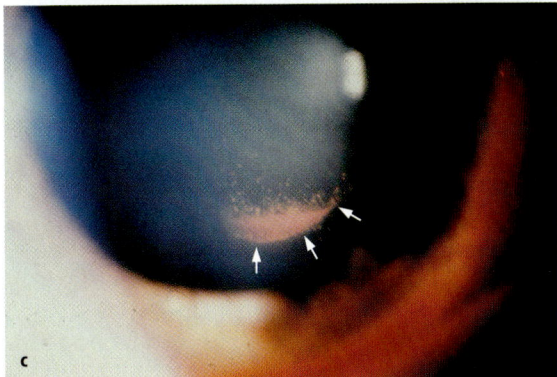

Fig. 5.5.3. b Clinical appearance of Wieger's ligament (*arrows*) (courtesy of Dr. A. Bergua, Erlangen). **c** Hemorrhage into vitreous and Berger's space (*arrow*) following blunt trauma to the eye

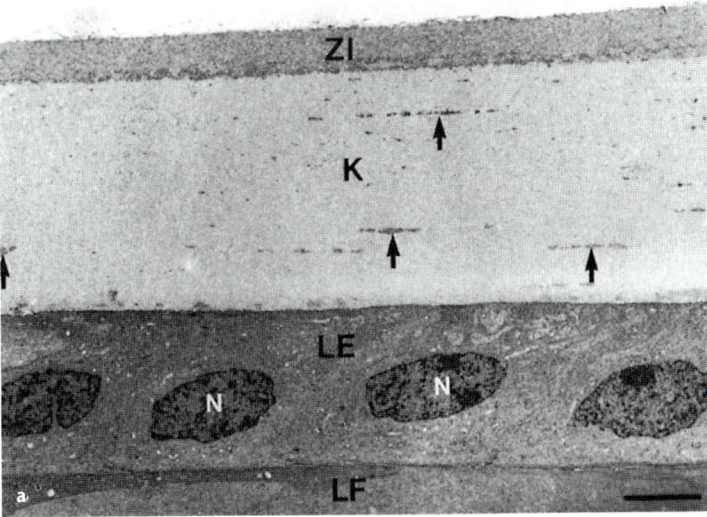

Fig. 5.5.4. Ultrastructure of the lens epithelium and the lens capsule. **a** Preequatorial lens epithelium (*LE*), lens capsule (*K*) with zonular lamella (*Zl*) and intracapsular microfibrillar inclusions (*arrows*) (*LF* lens fibers, *N* nuclei, *scale bar* 5 µm).

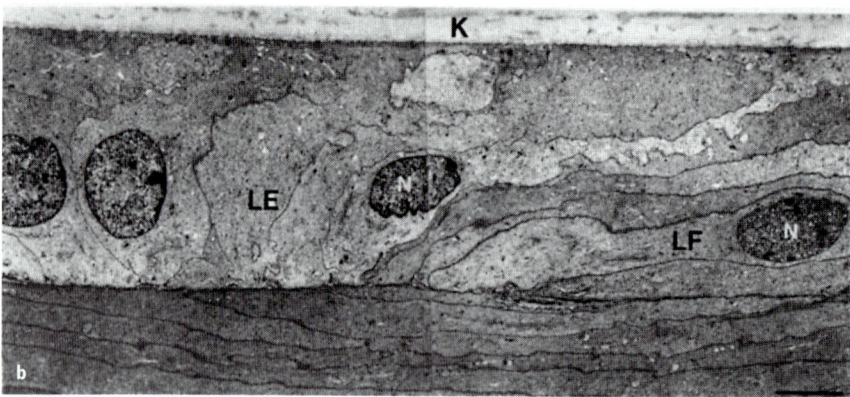

Fig. 5.5.4. b Differentiation of equatorial lens epithelial cells (*LE*) into fiber cells (*LF*) (*K* lens/capsule, *N* nuclei) (*scale bar* 5 µm)

Table 5.5.3. Lens capsule thickness throughout life (µm)

Age (years)	Anterior pole	Anterior mid-periphery	Equator	Posterior pole	Posterior periphery
2–5	8	12	7	3.5	12
35	12	16	7	4	9
70	16	20	7	4	9

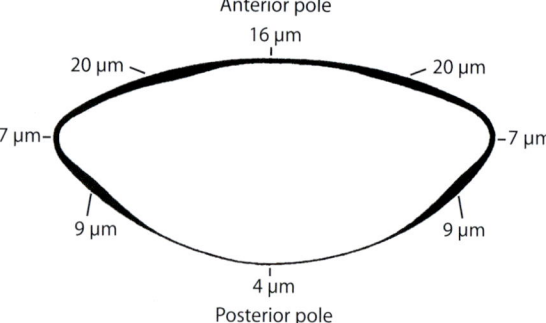

Fig. 5.5.5. Schematic view of the lens capsule showing the relative thickness of various portions (unpublished data, 2007)

anterior and posterior poles (Table 5.5.3, Fig. 5.5.5). Whereas the posterior capsule is thickest in an area about 1 mm from the equator, the anterior capsule is thickest in a midperipheral concentric area about 3 mm from the anterior pole; more peripherally, the capsule thins considerably. This, in addition to the zonular insertion, may be part of the reason why a capsulorrhexis placed too far peripherally extends into the equatorial region due to capsular tears. In a recent study, the anterior zonular insertion was actually related to a local preequatorial thinning of about 7 µm, which remained unchanged with age (Barraquer et al. 2006). The lens capsule continues to grow throughout life (Table 5.5.3). The capsule is normally under tension, so when cut or ruptured, its edges curl up due to its intrinsic elasticity. This property of elastic recoil is useful during Nd:YAG laser capsulotomy of the posterior capsule following secondary cataract formation, by causing an expansion of the opening made by the laser pulse.

Ultrastructurally, the capsule is not homogeneous but displays a lamellar substructure and a parallel alignment of scattered microfilaments (Fig. 5.5.4). In the anterior and equatorial capsule, electron dense inclusions (linear densities) consisting of small bundles of elastic microfibrils occur, which increase in number during aging (Seland 1992). They are not found in the posterior capsule. These microfibrillar bundles have been suggested to represent deep zonular insertions; however, no connection with the zonules has been demonstrated. The most superficial layer of inserting zonular fibers is termed the zonular lamella, which is 1.0–1.7 µm in thickness. It is restricted to a narrow zone around the equator, related to the insertion of the zonules. The capsule consists of typical basement membrane constituents, such as collagen type IV, laminin, entactin, fibronectin, and heparin sulfate proteoglycan, which is responsible for its prominent PAS-positive staining properties in histologic sections (Mohan and Spiro 1986). The capsule is freely permeable to water, ions, and small molecules, and offers a barrier to larger protein molecules.

5.5.3.3
Lens Epithelium

The lens epithelium is a single layer of cuboidal cells on the anterior surface of the lens beneath the anterior capsule, extending to the equator (Figs. 5.5.4a, 5.5.6). It consists of about 500,000 cells with a density of 4,000–6,000 cells/mm² increasing from the center towards the periphery (Karim et al. 1987). Interestingly, women have a higher average epithelial cell density (5,780 cells/mm²) than men (5,009 cells/mm²) (Guggenmoos-Holzmann et al. 1989). The presence of lens epithelium beneath the posterior capsule is observed as so-called Wedl bladder cells only in pathologic situations (cataract), reflecting posterior migration of epithelial cells from the equatorial region.

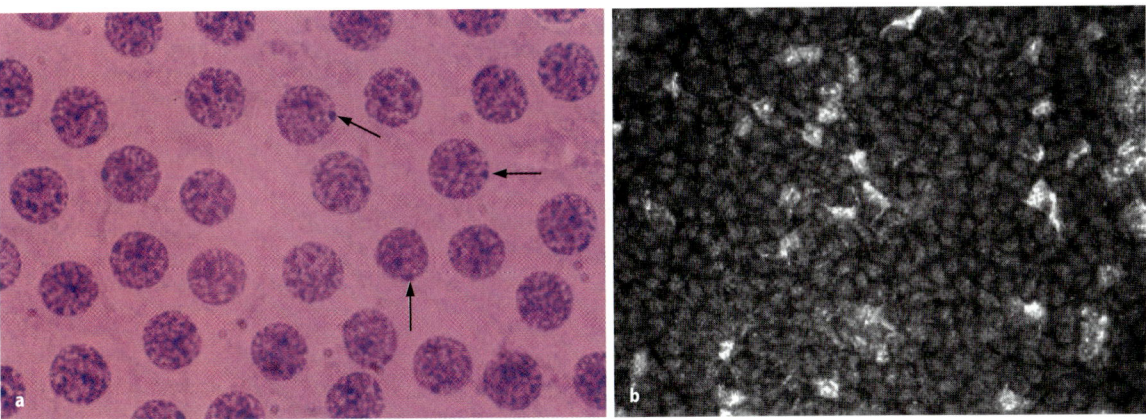

Fig. 5.5.6. Surface view of lens epithelium. **a** Histological flat preparation of lens epithelium of a female patient; the *arrows* mark Barr bodies (from Konofsky et al. 1987). **b** Clinical imaging of lens epithelium with the confocal laser scanning ophthalmoscope (courtesy of M. Pollhammer, Erlangen)

The epithelial cells are polygonal or hexagonal in surface view, and 11–17 μm wide and 5–8 μm high. Their basal surface adheres to the anterior capsule, whereas their apical surface smoothly adjoins the most superficial lens fibers. The cells have large indented nuclei and a regular array of organelles, including ribosomes, polysomes, smooth and rough endoplasmic reticulum, mitochondria, Golgi bodies, lysosomes, and glycogen particles. Cytoskeletal elements, including microfilaments (containing actin), intermediate filaments (containing vimentin), and microtubules (containing tubulin), form a network which provides structural support and distribution of mechanical stress. Hemidesmosomes attach the basal aspects of the cells to the lens capsule. The highly undulating, interdigitating lateral membranes of adjacent cells are attached to each other by desmosomes, tight junctions, and gap junctions providing adhesion and transfer of mechanical stress, restricted permeability of macromolecules through the extracellular space, and direct communication between cells, respectively (Marshall et al. 1982).

The proliferative capacity of epithelial cells varies according to their location. In the central zone, cells are normally mitotically inactive, but they can proliferate in response to damage. Mitotic activity is greatest in the preequatorial lens epithelium (about 20 divisions per day), known as the germinative or proliferative zone (von Sallmann et al. 1962). The cells in this zone constitute the stem cell population of the lens and are responsible for the continuous formation of lens fibers throughout life. During this process, the epithelial cells move from the midperiphery to the equatorial region, become more cylindrical in shape with their cell axis rotating through 180° following cell division (Fig. 5.5.4b). The transition between epithelial cells and lens fibers is accompanied by a pronounced elongation of the basal and apical portions of the cells, which extend backwards along the inner surface of the capsule and

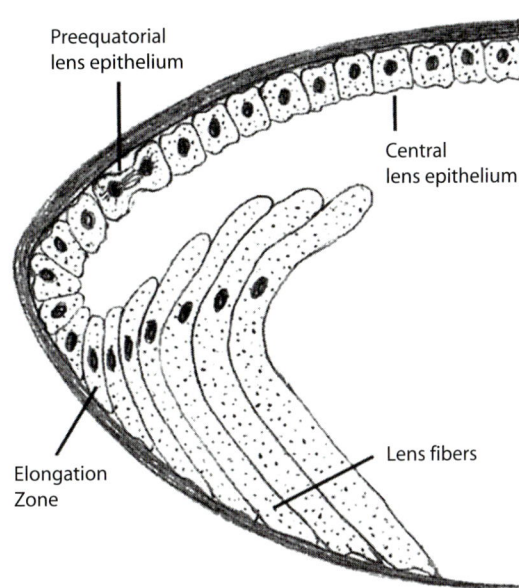

Fig. 5.5.7. Schematic view of the (pre)equatorial lens epithelium differentiating into lens fibers

forward under the epithelium, respectively (Fig. 5.5.7). The cell nuclei migrate *anteriorly* as the cells are pushed deeper into the lens body, hence creating the *nuclear bow* that curves forward in a crescent shape from the epithelial region toward the lens cortex. With increasing differentiation, the cell nuclei become pyknotic and finally disappear, and the cell organelles are lost. Because of the constant formation of new fiber cells, the following generations of lens fibers are displaced more and more into the nucleus associated with a condensation of the lens tissue with an increased protein content (Kuwabara 1975).

Whereas the lens fibers peel off easily during cataract extraction, the anterior epithelial cells remain adherent to the anterior and equatorial capsule during stripping and aspiration, because the capsule representing the epithelial basement membrane is part of the cell itself and not only a neighboring structure.

5.5.3.4
Lens Fibers

The lens substance is composed of about 2,500 densely packed fiber cells with very little extracellular space in between (Fig. 5.5.8). The adult lens substance consists of the nucleus and the cortex, two regions that are often histologically indistinct. Although the size of these two regions is age dependent, studies of lenses with an average age of 61 years indicate that the nucleus accounts for approximately 84% of the mass of the lens and the cortex for the remaining 16%. The nucleus is further subdivided into embryonic, fetal, infantile, and adult

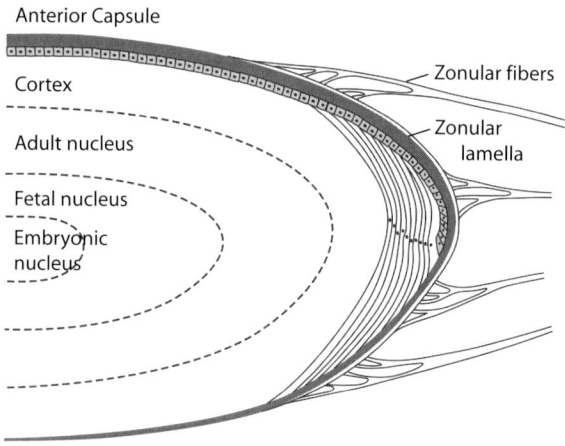

Fig. 5.5.9. Schematic representation of the adult lens showing the nuclear and cortical zones and the attachment of zonular fibers at the lens capsule

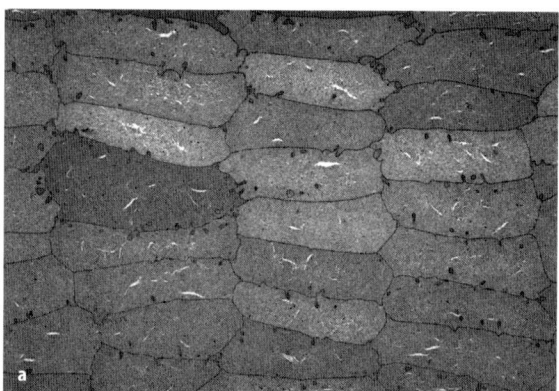

Fig. 5.5.8. Ultrastructure of lens fibers. **a** Transmission electron micrograph of cortical lens fibers in cross section. **b** Clinical imaging of cortical lens fibers in longitudinal section with the confocal laser scanning ophthalmoscope (courtesy of M. Pollhammer, Erlangen)

nucleus (Fig. 5.5.9). The embryonic nucleus contains the original primary lens fibers that are formed in the lens vesicle; the rest of the nuclei are composed of secondary fibers, which are added concentrically at the different stages of growth until sexual maturation. The cortex is composed of all the secondary fibers continuously formed after sexual maturation.

The lens fibers are band-shaped cells, which are hexagonal in cross section, 10–12 µm in width, 1.5–2 µm in thickness, and up to 12 mm long (Tripathi and Tripathi 1983). Lens fibers from concentric growth shells are aligned so that radial columns extend from the center of the lens to the periphery (Fig. 5.5.8). The tips of the fibers meet at the poles to form sutures, which become increasingly complex with lens growth. The sutural arrangement may be reflected in certain forms of cataract.

Superficially located fibers still contain most of the organelles present in epithelial cells. As the fibers are internalized and elongate further, the cell nucleus is displaced anteriorly, which results in the formation of the lens bow. Mature lens fibers have lost their nuclei and organelles and show a dense, amorphous granular cytoplasm due to high concentrations of structural proteins, i.e., the lens crystallins, and cytoskeletal elements (Kuwabara 1975). Lens fibers contain the highest protein content of any cell in the body, with about 35% of its wet weight being protein. Retention of cell nuclei occurs in certain pathologic conditions, most notably in rubella cataract. The cell membranes of adjacent fibers are connected by gap junctions to provide metabolic coupling and are firmly interlocked by ball-and-socket joints arranged regularly along the length of the fibers to resist zonular stress during accommodation. In the deeper layers of the cortex and in the nucleus, the ball-and-socket structures are further supplemented by a complex series of tongue-and-groove interdigitations (Kuszak et al. 1988; Stirling and Griffiths 1991).

The transparency of the lens is mainly based on the regular spatial arrangement of the organelle-free fibers and the highly organized substructural distribution of their structural proteins forming a "biological crystal" and causing only minimal light scattering (Benedek 1983).

5.5.3.5
Suspensory Apparatus

The suspensory ligament of the lens consists of the zonular fibers and the hyalocapsular ligament of Wieger, holding the lens in a position posterior to the iris in the patellar fossa of the vitreous.

5.5.3.5.1
Zonular Fibers

The ciliary zonules (zonules of Zinn) consist of a complex three-dimensional system of fiber *bundles*, the total number of which varies between 220 and 350, passing from the ciliary body to the lens. They hold the lens in position and enable the ciliary muscle to act on it during accommodation. The definite site of synthesis of the zonules is not known; however, they are probably synthesized and maintained by the nonpigmented ciliary epithelial cells of the pars plana. The vast majority of the zonules arise from the posterior end of the pars plana up to 1.5 mm from the ora serrata, where they blend with the basement membrane of the nonpigmented ciliary epithelium without entering their cytoplasm (Raviola 1971; Rohen 1979). The fibers pass forward over the pars plana, spread into the zonular plexus, which passes through the ciliary valleys between the ciliary processes. Tension fibers leave the main strands and anchor to the basement membrane within the depths of the valleys and are thought to play an important role in the accommodation process by stabilizing the zonules. Towards the anterior margin of the pars plicata, each plexus divides into a zonular fork consisting of three fiber groups running to the anterior, equatorial, and posterior lens capsule, respectively (Rohen 1979). These main fibers transmit the force of the ciliary muscle upon the lens during accommodation by relaxing the tension of the zonules. The space between the anterior and posterior zonules and the lens equator is known as the canal of Hannover. Contraction of the ciliary muscle relaxes tension on the zonules, allowing the lens to become more spherical and increasing its refractive power.

Each fiber bundle, 5–30 µm in diameter, is composed of *microfibrils* 10–12 nm in diameter and tubular in cross section, with a beaded substructure and a microperiodicity of 12–14 nm or 40–55 nm following lateral aggregation. The beaded structure, evident by rotary shadowing electron microscopy, may be an expression of the elastic properties of the fibrils (Wallace et al. 1991). The microfibrillar subunits are composed of the glycoprotein fibrillin-1, a major component of elastic fibers and elastic microfibrils. Marfan's syndrome, which is associated with lens dislocation, has been shown to be due to mutations in the fibrillin-1 gene on chromosome 15q21.1 (Lee et al. 1991). Rupture of the elastic zonules requires 100 g in children and 60 g in adults. The zonules are susceptible to digestion by α(chymo)trypsin, a property utilized in intracapsular lens extraction (Barraquer 1961).

The preequatorial insertion of the zonules occurs at approximately 1.5–2 mm from the equator in a zone about 0.5 mm in width. The zonular bundles split up into smaller brush-like processes, which fan out and finally blend with the superficial lens capsule to form the *zonular lamella* on the capsular surface (1.0–1.7 µm thick) (Fig. 5.5.4a). The zonular lamella may contribute to zonular adhesive mechanisms due to the presence of adhesive glycoproteins, such as fibronectin and vitronectin. Smaller fibrils penetrate the capsular surface to a depth of 0.5–1.5 µm, but have not been observed to penetrate the entire capsule. The equatorial fibers are sparse and poorly developed and also fan out in a brush-like manner to insert into the capsule at right angles. The posterior zonules insert over a zone of 0.4–0.5 mm wide about 1.25–1.5 mm from the equatorial margin.

The zonules have a high stretching capability before they rupture. The mean mechanical zonular stretch tolerance has been reported to vary from 3.2 to 3.8 mm (Assia et al. 1991; Saber et al. 1998). Patients with PEX showed a significantly decreased stretching capability (2.6 mm) before rupturing (Assia et al. 1991).

During extracapsular cataract extraction, as traction is applied on the zonules, the zonules may tear partially. About 5% of these dehiscences may be detected at the time of surgery (Guzek et al. 1987). Due to particularly weak zonules and poor mydriasis in pseudoexfoliation (PEX) syndrome, cataract surgery in PEX eyes has been recognized as an increased risk and is considered a particular challenge. Intraoperative and postoperative surgical complications, such as zonular ruptures, vitreous loss, blood-aqueous barrier breakdown, anterior capsule fibrosis/contraction, secondary cataract, and decentration or dislocation of the intraocular lens implant (IOL), have been reported to be significantly more common and more serious than in eyes without PEX (Skuta et al. 1987; Naumann et al. 1989; Küchle et al. 1997; Hayashi et al. 1998). Zonular fragility has been associated with a three- to tenfold increased risk of zonular rupture and an approximately fivefold increased risk of vitreous loss. In a prospective study of 1,000 extracapsular cataract extractions the only significant risk factors for zonular ruptures and vitreous loss were the presence of PEX and small pupil size (Guzek et al. 1987). As PEX eyes often respond poorly to mydriatics due to the iris dilator muscle atrophy, mechanical dilatation of small pupils is frequently required intraoperatively. Today, the common use of phacoemulsification with anterior capsulorrhexis has provided significantly better results compared with the conventional extracapsular cataract extraction technique including nuclear expression (Hyams et al. 2005). However, improvements in intraoperative results may merely reflect a shift of complications to the postoperative period, as reflected by a growing number of case reports on *late* IOL dislocation due to progressive zonular weakening (Jehan et al. 2001). Continued destabilization of the zonules appears to result from anterior capsule fibrosis and contraction exerting additional centripetal stress on the compromised zonules.

The thickness and volume of the capsular bag are greatly reduced after IOL implantation. The thickness of a normal lens in a 70-year-old is approximately 4.5 mm and the thickness of an IOL is typically 1 mm. The volume of the crystalline lens is 250–300 mm³ and the volume of an IOL implant is only 30–40 mm³ (Assia and Apple 1992a, b). In the axis of the haptics, the capsular bag will stretch, and in the axis opposite the haptics, the zonules will be maximally relaxed. These observations indicate that physiologic accommodation is effectively impossible with any thin IOL. For an IOL to allow physiologic accommodation, a precondition would be to fill the entire capsular bag and retain the physiologic position and stretch of the zonules (Assia and Apple 1992a, b). In view of the progressive fibrosis of the ciliary muscle with age, any expectations of a "pseudophakic accommodation" deserve some skepticism (see Chapter 5.4).

5.5.3.5.2
Wieger's Ligament

Posteriorally, the lens is attached to the vitreous by Wieger's ligament or the hyalocapsular ligament. This structure is not a true ligament, but a circular area of adhesion between the anterior vitreous face and the posterior lens capsule, about 8–9 mm in diameter, located approximately 2 mm posterior to the lens equator (Fig. 5.5.3). The peripheral ring-like line of attachment is also called Egger's line, and the central retrolenticular space, filled with aqueous humor, is called Berger's space. Wieger's ligament is readily visible by slit-lamp examination and corresponds to the most anterior aspect of Cloquet's canal, the remnant of the primary vitreous (Fig. 5.5.10). In traumatic lens subluxation, Berger's space and Egger's line may be outlined by hemorrhage (Fig. 5.5.3.c). This adhesion is strong in infants and children, but weak in older persons.

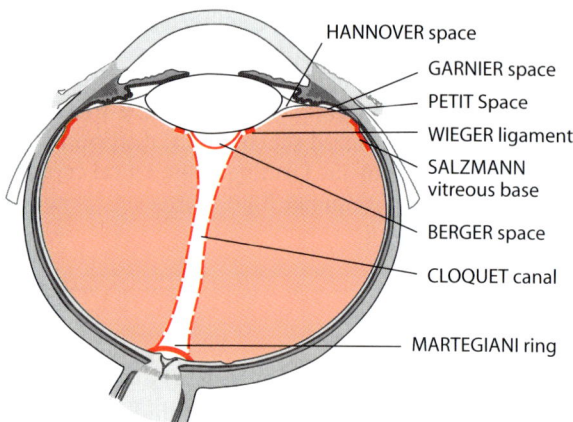

Fig. 5.5.10. Schematic representation of the vitreous body and its relationship to neighboring tissues

5.5.4
Aging Changes

5.5.4.1
Gross Anatomy

The lens continues to grow (0.023 mm per year) and alters its shape throughout life, becoming more flattened with age (Bron et al. 2000; Tripathi and Tripathi 1983) (Table 5.5.2). During an average life span, the *surface area* of the lens increases from 80 mm² at birth to 180 mm² by the seventh decade. The *equatorial diameter* of the lens increases from approximately 5 mm in the newborn to 9–10 mm in the second decade with little change thereafter. Its *axial thickness*, which is 3.5–4.0 mm at birth, increases throughout life reaching 4.75–5.0 mm in old age. *Lens weight* increases by approximately 1.4 mg/year to reach about 260 mg by the age of 90 years (65 mg at birth). The lenses of men are heavier than those of women of the same age, the mean difference being 7.9±2.5 mg. The thickness of the nucleus decreases with age, as the result of compaction, whereas the *cortical thickness* increases as more fibers are added at the periphery. The *radius of curvature* of the anterior surface decreases from 14 mm at the age of 10 years to 8 mm by the age of 80 years. There is very *little* change in the radius of curvature of the posterior surface, which remains approximately 6 mm. This ongoing growth changes the topographic relationships between lens, ciliary body and cornea and leads to flattening of the anterior chamber.

The amplitude of accommodation decreases throughout life from 13–14D at the age of 10 years to 6–8D at 40 years and almost 0D by the age of 60 years. This decline in accommodative power is attributable to a number of factors, including a decrease in capsular elasticity, an increase in stiffness of the lens substance (nuclear sclerosis), a decrease in the radius of curvature of the anterior lens surface, and an associated atrophy and fibrosis of the ciliary muscle. Consequently, the lens fails to change shape sufficiently during accommodation (presbyopia).

5.5.4.2
Lens Capsule, Epithelium, Fibers, and Zonules

As the lens ages, many morphological changes occur to the epithelial cells, lens fibers, and capsule. The lens capsule thickens throughout life (about 0.2 μm per year) resulting in an about twofold increase in anterior capsule thickness with age (Fig. 5.5.11), whereas there is little change at the posterior pole and the equator. The capsule at the posterior periphery appears to decrease slightly in thickness with age (Tripathi and Tripathi 1983; Barraquer et al. 2006) (Table 5.5.3).

Aging of the human anterior lens capsule is associated with a progressive loss of mechanical strength (0.5% per year) and elasticity (1% per year). The young capsule is strong, tough, and highly extensible, whereas the older, thicker capsule is less extensible and much more brittle (Krag et al. 1997). Mechanical strength of the posterior lens capsule also markedly decreases with age, and extensibility of the posterior capsule decreases by a factor of two during the life span (Krag et al. 2003).

Age-related changes in the composition of the lens capsule might be responsible for these altered mechanical properties. Ultrastructural changes include the loss of its lamellar substructure and an increase in the number of linear densities in the anterior and equatorial portions (Fig. 5.5.11). However, the median suction pressure (200 mm Hg), tolerated by the posterior lens capsule before disruption during cataract surgery, did not significantly decrease with age (Saber et al. 1998). Changes in capsular elasticity may be related to the age-related loss in accommodation.

The *cell density* of the lens epithelium *declines* with age (7.8 cells/mm^2/year), due to a decrease in its proliferative capacity, which is compensated by cellular flattening and enlargement (Konofsky et al. 1987; Guggenmoos-Holzmann et al. 1989). Ultrastructurally, the epithelial cells develop degenerative signs, such as inclusion of electron-dense bodies and vacuoles.

Lens fibers show remarkable biochemical and structural alterations of plasma membrane and cytoskeletal proteins as the lens ages (Vrensen 1995; Vrensen et al. 1990). The term "nuclear sclerosis" describes the compaction and increasing rigidity of the nuclear fibers with age (Fig. 5.5.12). It results from changes in structure and composition of the lens fiber membranes (age-related increase in the cholesterol-to-phospholipid ratio) and the degradation of cytoskeletal proteins. Advanced sclerosis is a major obstacle to phacosonication of the nucleus. If it is too sclerotic, the nucleus must be removed in toto.

With age, the zonular fibers are finer and more sparse, especially the equatorial ones, and rupture more easily due to a decline in their elasticity. The zonular stretch tolerance has been reported to decrease significantly with age by approximately 0.1 mm per year (Assia et al. 1991; Saber et al. 1998). This is of benefit in intracapsular cataract extraction procedures.

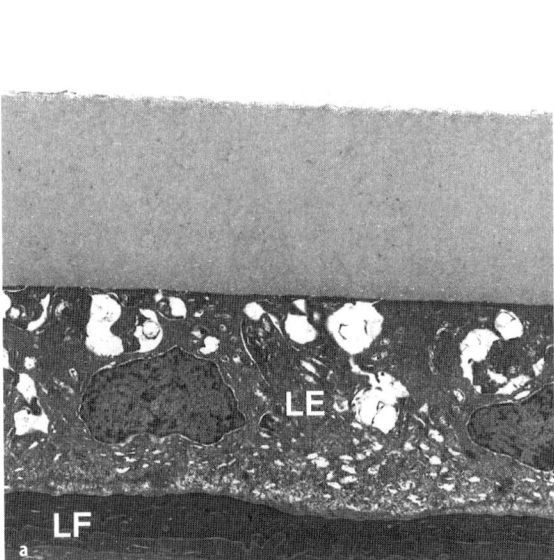
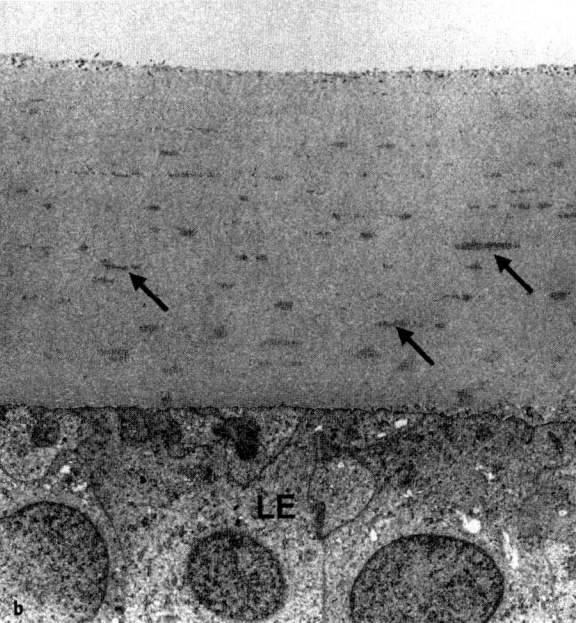

Fig. 5.5.11. Aging changes of the lens capsule. **a** Lens capsule of a 17-year-old individual. **b** Lens capsule of an 86-year-old individual showing increased thickness and microfibrillar inclusions (*arrows*) (*LE* lens epithelium, *LF* lens fibers)

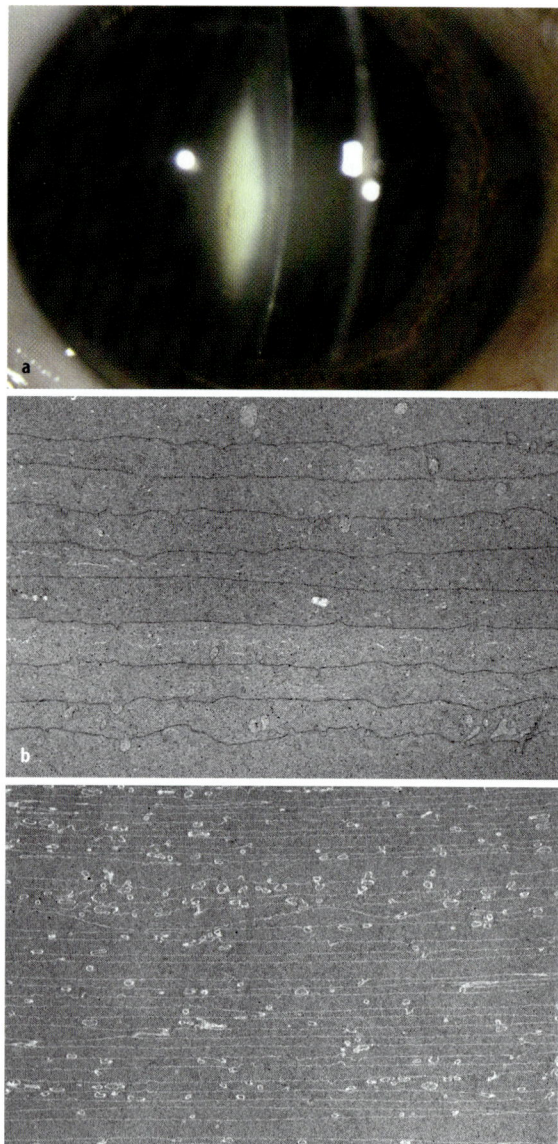

Fig. 5.5.12. Aging changes of the lens fibers. **a** Age-related nuclear cataract caused by nuclear sclerosis. **b** Electron micrograph of nuclear lens fibers of a 17-year-old individual. **c** Electron micrograph of nuclear lens fibers of a 86-year-old individual

Moreover, the site of the anterior zonular insertion becomes displaced more centrally with age (Sakabe et al. 1998). Thus, the width of the zonule-free area of the anterior capsule reduces from about 7.5 mm in young adults (age 20) to 6.5 mm in the eighth decade, so that the insertion may intrude into the region selected for capsulorrhexis during surgery (Farnsworth and Shyne 1979; Stark and Streeten 1984; Sakabe et al. 1998). To create the capsulorrhexis within the zonule-free zone, it is recommended to stay within the central 6.8-mm area of the anterior capsule, which is the average diame-

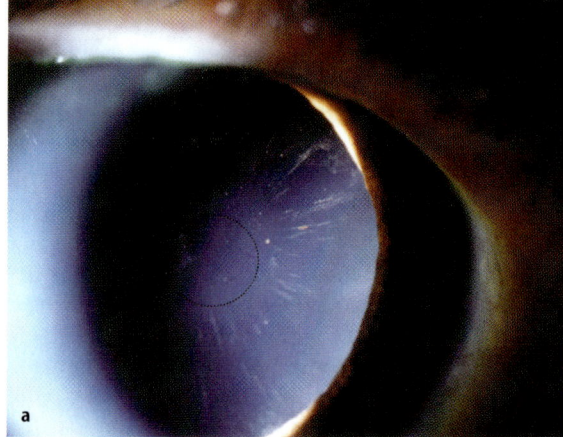
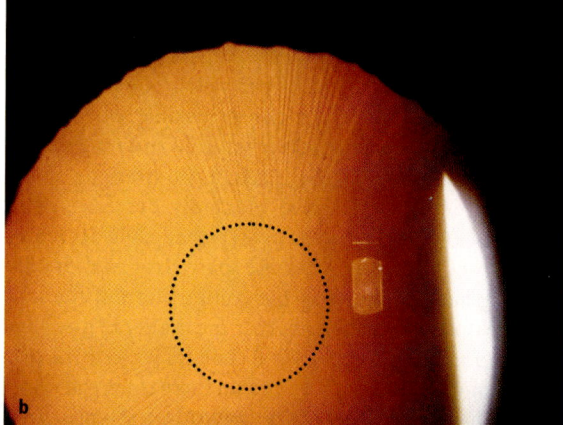

Fig. 5.5.13. Long anterior zonules. **a, b** Centrally displaced insertion of anterior zonules on the anterior lens capsule in a 66-year-old patient (from Moroi et al. 2003)

ter of the zonule-free zone (Sakabe et al. 1998). The origin of the zonule from the pars plana is also thought to move anteriorly with age (Farnsworth and Shyne 1979).

It has to be considered that a small percentage of cataract patients may disclose an unusual centrally displaced anterior zonule insertion, a phenomenon which has been described as "long anterior zonule syndrome" (Moroi et al. 2003) (Fig. 5.5.13).

5.5.4.3
Biochemical Changes

As the lens ages, it *changes in color* from colorless to pale yellow to darker yellow in adulthood, and brown or even black in old age (brunescence of the lens). These changes in coloration, which are limited to the nucleus, are thought to result from biochemical production and accumulation of yellow-pigmented fluorescent protein derivatives and advanced glycation end products. They result in an *increased absorption of both ultraviolet and visible light, particularly the blue part* of the spectrum, and an age-related shift in the spectral transmission of the lens. In addition, there is an age-related increase in light scattering of the nucleus due to the accumulation of insoluble high molecular weight aggregates of crystallins and nonenzymatically glycated proteins (Berman 1994; Bron et al. 2000). The increased capacity of the lens to absorb light, in combination with the increased scattering properties of the lens, results in a decrease in transparency. This increase in the amount of absorbed light is accompanied by an age-related loss in antioxidant levels (e.g., catalase, superoxide dismutase, ascorbate, glutathione, glutathione peroxidase), which, therefore, increases the amount of photo-oxidative stress and damage to the lens (Hockwin 1993; Ohrloff and Hockwin 1983; Dawczynski and Strobel 2006).

5.5.5
Surgical Pathology of the Lens

Lens abnormalities may be divided into three categories: (1) abnormalities of lens size and shape, which are largely developmental, (2) lens dislocations, and (3) abnormalities of lens transparency, or cataract, which may be congenital or acquired.

5.5.5.1
Anomalies of Size and Shape

5.5.5.1.1
Aphakia

Aphakia may be primary or secondary due to regression or resorption of a previously formed lens. Primary aphakia, i.e., the lack of any lens anlage, is a rare condition associated with gross malformations of the globe, such as microphthalmos, microcornea, and nystagmus. It is proposed that a primary defect in surface ectoderm or in the formation of the optic cup is responsible. Secondary aphakia is distinguished from primary aphakia by the presence of some remnants of lens tissue or capsule. It may be associated with developmental abnormalities, such as microcornea, or it may occur as a result of partial or complete absorption of the lens in congenital cataract from rubella.

5.5.5.1.2
Duplication of the Lens (Biphakia)

A metaplastic change in surface ectoderm may prevent the invagination of the lens placode and thereby the formation of a single vesicle, which may lead to a duplication of the lens. This extremely rare condition is usually associated with corneal metaplasia and coloboma of the iris and choroid.

5.5.5.1.3
Microspherophakia

Microspherophakia is a rare bilateral condition, in which a defect in the development of lens zonules leads to the formation of small, spherical lenses. The condition may be familial and occur as an isolated defect or it may be associated with other defects, e.g., in the Weill-Marchesani syndrome, hyperlysinemia, Alport syndrome, and trisomy 13. The condition may result in lenticular myopia and lens dislocation, which occurs usually downward. As a result, pupil block and angle closure glaucoma are common complications.

5.5.5.1.4
Lens Coloboma

In lens coloboma, a rare congenital indentation of the lens periphery occurs as a result of localized defects of the zonules (Apple 1979) (Fig. 5.5.14). The lenses are frequently microspherophakic. The condition is usually unilateral, rarely isolated, and may be associated with colobomas of the iris, ciliary body, and choroid.

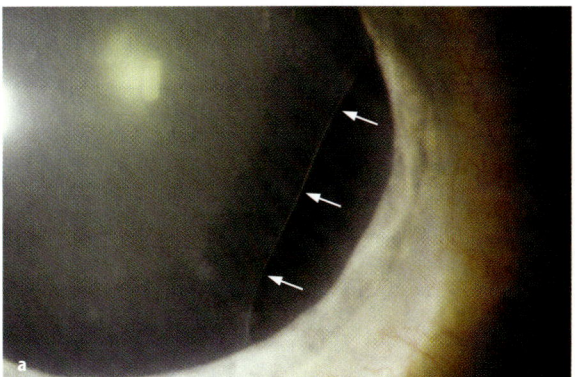 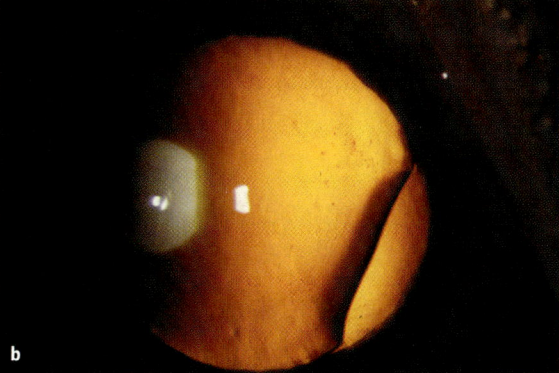

Fig. 5.5.14. Lens coloboma. **a, b** Indentation of the lens equator (*arrows*) in a 59-year-old patient (courtesy of A. Bergua, Erlangen)

5.5.5.1.5
Lenticonus and Lentiglobus

In both lenticonus and lentiglobus, an abnormality of the central lens curvature occurs, associated with thinning of the lens capsule and deficiency of epithelial cells in the affected region (Fig. 5.5.15). It may be caused by traction of a persisting hyaloid artery on the posterior lens surface or the presence of a weak, underdeveloped lens capsule (Gibbs et al. 1993; Lang and Naumann 1983). The resultant protrusion of the lens surface may be more conical, as in lenticonus, or spherical, as in lentiglobus. The protrusion may be anterior or, more commonly, posterior and measures 2–7 mm in diameter. The abnormality may occur sporadically or may be inherited as an autosomal recessive trait or in association with other abnormalities, such as Alport syndrome or oculocerebral syndrome of Lowe.

Histopathologically, the lens capsule is considerably thinned in the affected area. For instance, the thickness of the anterior lens capsule in *Alport syndrome* is reduced to 4 µm and shows an abnormal ultrastructure with numerous cleft-like dehiscences facilitating capsular rupture (Streeten et al. 1987) (Fig. 5.5.15b). The central epithelial cells appear degenerative in these regions.

Both lenticonus and lentiglobus may cause lenticular myopia with irregular astigmatism and an oil droplet reflex on retinoscopy. The conditions are commonly associated with progressive circumscribed opacification of the posterior pole fibers. Spontaneous rupture of the extended lens capsule may frequently occur, particularly at the edge of the ectasia.

5.5.5.1.6
Persistent Hyperplastic Primary Vitreous

Persistent hyperplastic primary vitreous (PHPV) is a common developmental anomaly of unknown cause, in which the embryonic hyaloid artery and primary vitreous fail to regress normally (Fig. 5.5.16) resulting in an abnormal lenticular development and secondary changes of the retina and the globe (microphthalmia). The condition is almost invariably unilateral and is

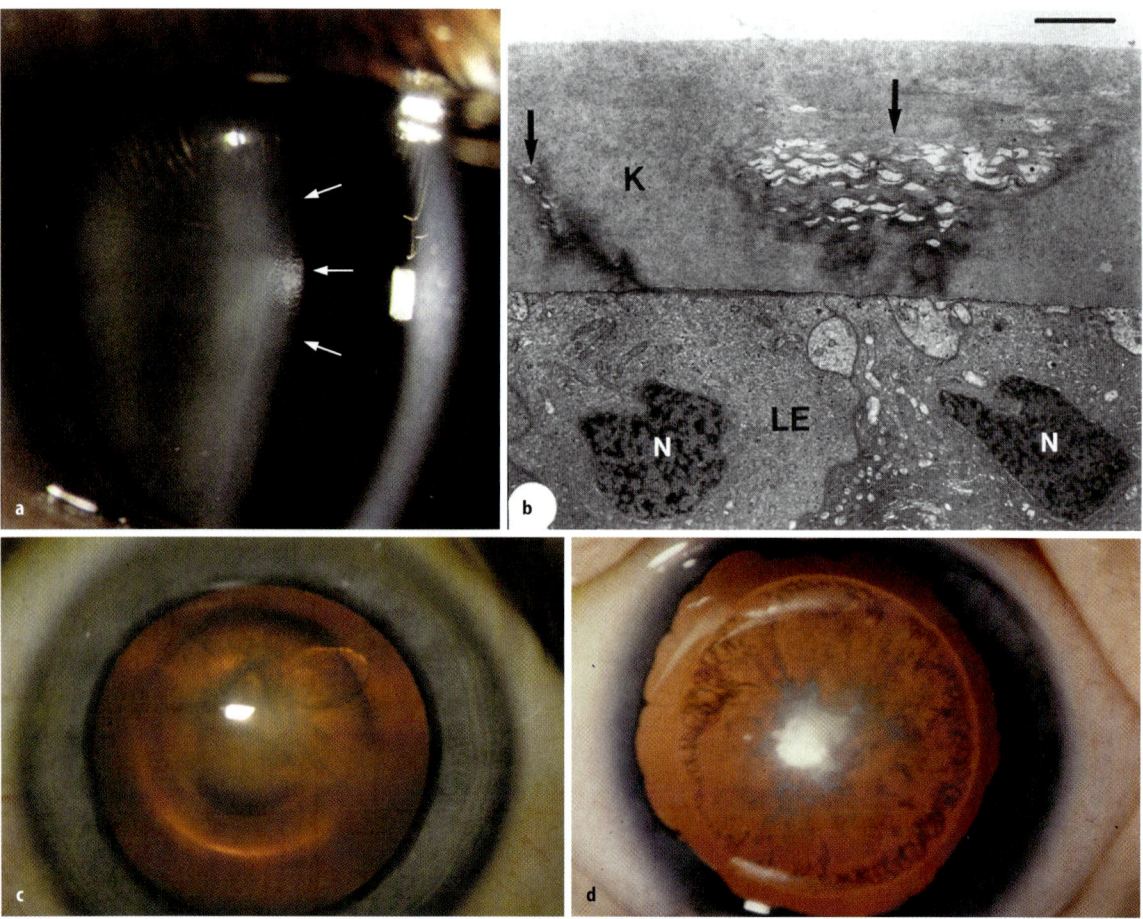

Fig. 5.5.15. Lenticonus anterior and posterior. **a, b** Lenticonus anterior in Alport's syndrome; fragile structure of the thinned lens capsule with intracapsular dehiscences (*arrows*) (*K* lens capsule, *LE* lens epithelium, *N* nuclei). **c, d** Lenticonus posterior

characterized by the presence of a vascularized membrane behind the lens. Eyes with PHPV frequently develop cataract, which may range from a tiny opacity to posterior polar cataract over a widespread vascularized plaque up to a total hypermature white cataract (Fig. 5.5.17), and atrophy of the globe or glaucoma. In addition, the pupil often does not dilate well. The ciliary processes are connected to the retrolental plaque. Surgical removal of the vascular membrane and associated cataract in order to preserve the eye is advisable, but surgery for PHPV is complicated by a higher rate of retinal detachment and most children will develop amblyopia. Without modern imaging methods the entity was often confused with retinoblastoma (see Goldberg, 1997; see also 5.6).

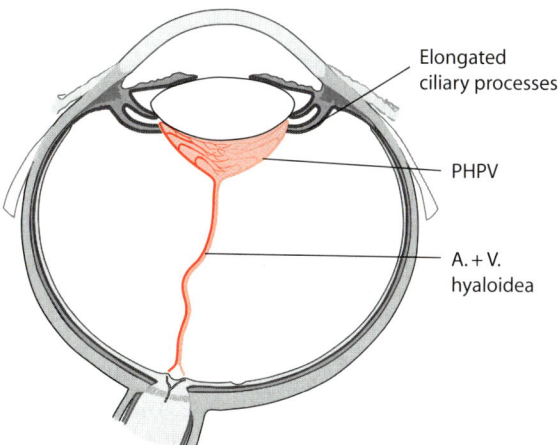

Fig. 5.5.16. Schematic representation of persistent hyperplastic primary vitreous

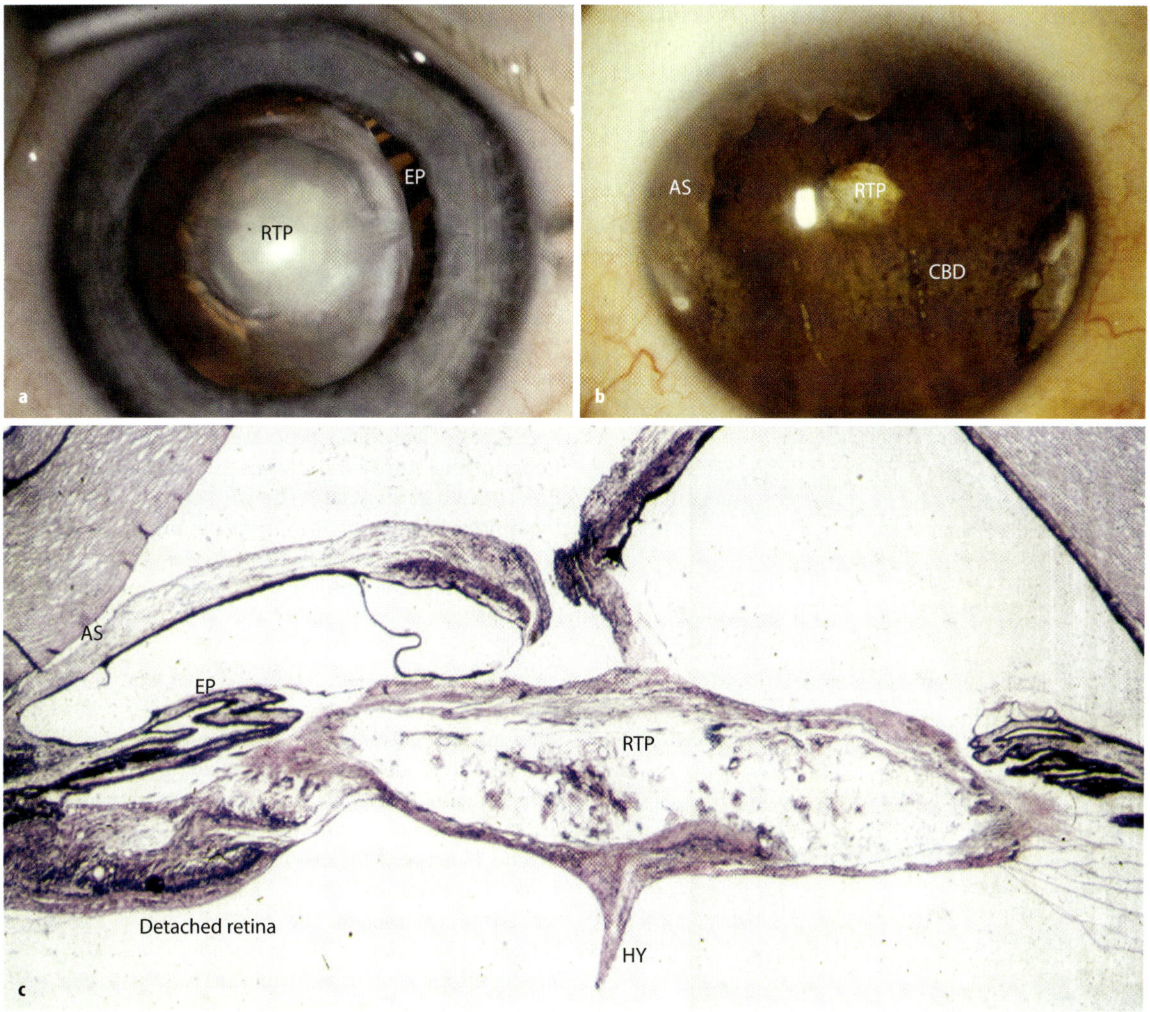

Fig. 5.5.17. Spontaneous course of persistent hyperplastic primary vitreous. **a** Early posterior polar cataract and retrolental vascularized tissue-plaque (*RTP*) with elongated ciliary processes (*EP*). **b** Untreated PHPV in an adult with atrophy of the globe: Corneal band-degeneration (*CBD*); anterior synechiae (*AS*), retrolental tissue plaque (*RTP*). **c** Histopathology showing the presence of an iris bombata with formation of anterior and posterior synechiae, stretched ciliary processes, and a resorbed lens substance and retrolental plaque of adipose tissue (pseudophakia lipomatosa) (*EP* elongated ciliary processes, *HY* hyaloid vessel)

5.5.5.2
Lens Dislocations (Ectopia Lentis)

Any defect of the zonules (developmental abnormalities or degenerative alterations) can lead to partial (subluxation) or complete (luxation) displacement of the lens from its normal position. Ectopia lentis can occur as an isolated entity, congenital or spontaneous in adult age, in association with a number of systemic connective tissue diseases, or secondary to trauma, intraocular tumors, uveitis, PEX syndrome, hypermature cataracts, and other causes (Table 5.5.4; Nelson and Maumenee 1982). Traumatic ectopia is by far the most common cause of lens displacement. The majority of isolated zonular defects is congenital and developmental and usually leads to a bilateral and symmetric dislocation of the lens and/or anomaly in shape. When a lens is dislocated, the metabolic relationships with other structures are compromised, leading to opacifications in later stages. Posterior displacement of the lens may cause lens-induced uveitis.

5.5.5.2.1
Isolated Dislocation

A congenital, isolated dislocation of the lens (ectopia lentis simplex), frequently occurring upward and temporally, can result from maldevelopment of the zonules due to a genetic defect in the fibrillin-1 gene on chromosome 15 (Kainulainen et al. 1994). This is sometimes associated with a coloboma-like defect of the lens border in the affected region. Ectopia lentis, mostly downward, can also occur spontaneously in older age due to a general degeneration of the zonules (Malbran et al. 1989). Rarely, a simultaneously dislocated lens and pupil can be observed (ectopia lentis et pupillae), which is associated with other abnormalities of the iris (Cruysberg and Pinckers 1995).

5.5.5.2.2
Systemic Diseases and Lens Dislocation

A usually bilateral, progressive dislocation of the lens may be also associated with a number of systemic conditions. The four most important systemic lens displacement syndromes are Marfan's syndrome, homocystinuria, Weill-Marchesani's syndrome, and PEX syndrome.

Marfan's Syndrome

This autosomally dominant inherited syndrome is characterized by ocular, cardiovascular, and skeletal anomalies with variable expressivity (Maumenee 1981; Nemet et al. 2006). Due to a segmental zonular defect, the lens is usually displaced upward and temporally in 60–80% of the patients (Fig. 5.5.18a). The cause of this disease is a genetic defect in the gene for fibrillin-1 on chromosome 15 (Lee et al. 1991). Histopathologically, the rarefied zonules may be focally fragmented or totally lacking (Cross and Jensen 1973). In addition, the anterior chamber angle may have an "undifferentiated" appearance: The ciliary processes are elongated and the fibers of the ciliary muscle reach as far as Schwalbe's line (Burian et al. 1960). The iris shows sector-shaped hypopigmentation of the posterior pigment epithelium. The dilator muscle is sometimes focally absent; hence, pharmacologic dilatation of the pupil is often incomplete.

Homocystinuria

This autosomal-recessive disorder commonly affects blond individuals. It is characterized by a risk toward generalized systemic vascular thromboses and associated symptoms resembling those of Marfan's syndrome. However, lens dislocation typically occurs inferonasal in more than 90% of patients due to a progressive degeneration of the entire zonular apparatus (Fig. 5.5.18b) (Hagee 1984). Histopathologically, a pathognomonic layer of amorphous PAS-positive material, consisting of fragmented zonular fibrils, may be identified near the origin of the zonular fibers on the surface of the nonpigmented ciliary epithelium of the pars plicata (Cross and Jensen 1973). The zonular fibers separate from the ciliary epithelium and retract to their

Table 5.5.4. Major causes of ectopia lentis

I. *Congenital and hereditary lens dislocation*
1. Isolated
1.1. Simple ectopia lentis
1.2. Ectopia lentis et pupillae
2. Ocular disease
2.1. Congenital glaucoma
2.2. Aniridia (hemiphakia)
2.3. Megalocornea
3. Systemic disease
3.1. Marfan's syndrome
3.2. Homocystinuria
3.3. Weill-Marchesani syndrome
3.4. Rare conditions (Ehlers-Danlos syndrome, hyperlysinemia, sulfite oxidase deficiency, Refsum disease, Crouzon syndrome, osteogenesis imperfecta, Sturge-Weber syndrome, Beals' syndrome)
II. *Acquired causes*
1. Trauma (blunt and penetrating)
2. Uveitis
3. Hypermature cataract
4. Intraocular tumors
5. High myopia/buphthalmus
6. Uveal staphyloma
7. Ciliolenticular block
III. *Unknown etiology*
1. Pseudoexfoliation syndrome

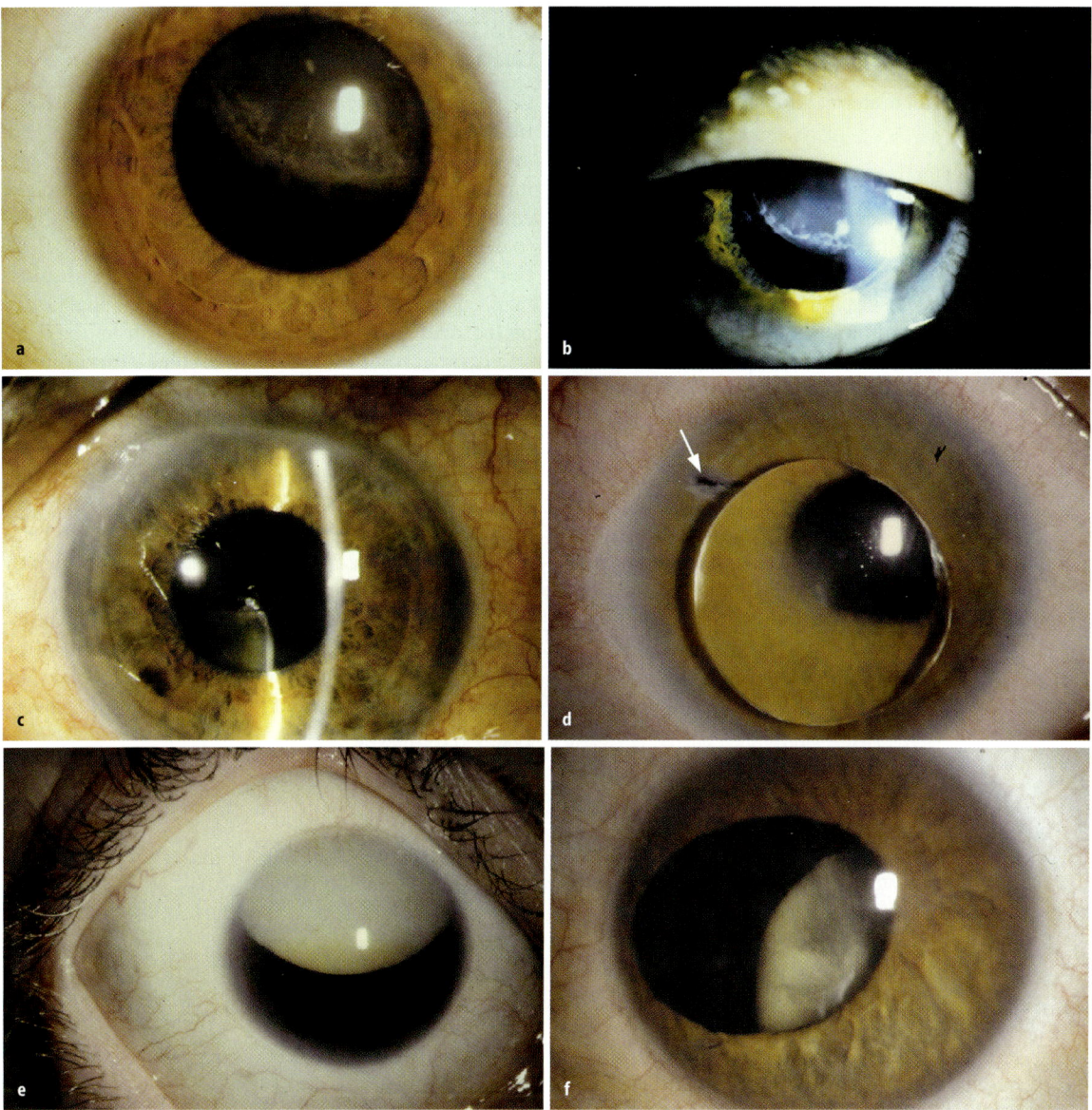

Fig. 5.5.18. Ectopia lentis. a Marfan's syndrome. b Homocystinuria. c Pseudoexfoliation syndrome. d Lens luxation into the anterior chamber with YAG-iridotomy (*arrow*) (courtesy of A. Bergua, Erlangen). e Aniridia with hemiphakia and hypermature cataract with sunken heminucleus. f Traumatic subluxation (courtesy of A. Bergua, Erlangen)

insertion at the anterior lens capsule – visible as a rim of shrunken undulated zonular fibers in the periphery of the lens. The cause of this disease is a lack of the enzyme cystathionine-β-synthetase (Mudd et al. 1964). Therefore, a lack of cysteine for the formation of the cysteine-rich zonular fibers may be causally involved in zonular alterations.

Marchesani's Syndrome

This autosomal-recessive disorder is associated with small body size, brachycephaly, brachydactyly, and microspheric lenses, which usually subluxate inferiorly or anteriorly in most patients due to a progressive degeneration of the zonular fibers. The ocular findings of this syndrome are practically identical to those of homocystinuria (Jensen et al. 1974).

Pseudoexfoliation Syndrome

Due to a pronounced weakness of the zonular fibers, eyes with PEX syndrome have a higher risk of phacodonesis and lens subluxation, which can occur in about 5% of patients either spontaneously or after minor trauma (Fig. 5.5.18c) (Bartholomew 1970; Freissler et al. 1995). This zonular instability results from a mechanically loosened anchorage of the zonular fibers into the basement membranes of ciliary epithelium and lens epithelium by locally produced intercalating PEX fibers (Schlötzer-Schrehardt and Naumann 1994).

Aniridia with Hemiphakia

Aniridia is a rare bilateral congenital autosomal dominant hereditary condition characterized by the absence of the iris and numerous defects of corneal, lens, optic nerve, and retinal tissues. It is caused by a mutation in the *PAX6* gene on chromosome 11 and is associated with cataract and ectopia lentis in up to 60% of patients (Fig. 5.5.18e). In *sporadic* cases a Wilms' tumor of the kidney should be excluded (Miller syndrome).

5.5.5.2.3
Traumatic Luxation

Blunt or perforating trauma is the most frequent cause of lens displacements (Völcker 1984) (Fig. 5.5.18f). Traumatic (sub)luxations are not progressive, but often associated with secondary cataracts, particularly contusion rosettes (Asano et al. 1995). The lens may be dislocated into the vitreous or the anterior chamber.

5.5.5.3
Cataracts

Lenticular opacification still remains the most common cause of visual reduction and the leading cause of avoidable blindness worldwide (Sommer 1977; Thylefors 1999; Resnikoff et al. 2004). The classification of cataracts can be based on the time of development (congenital, infantile, juvenile, senile), on the localization of opacifications (polar, capsular, subcapsular, cortical, equatorial, nuclear), on the pattern of opacification (coronary, zonular, cuneiform, etc.), or on the etiology (primary, secondary). The detailed description of the various cataract types is beyond the scope of this chapter, which focuses on general mechanisms of cataract formation instead. Table 5.5.5 summarizes the major clinical forms. Examples for congenital and secondary cataracts are presented in Figs. 5.5.19–5.5.21. Age-related or senile cataract is the most prevalent type of cataract and cataract extraction is the most frequently performed surgical procedure. Significant advances in the surgical methods for cataract extraction, from intracapsular to extracapsular and phacoemulsification techniques, have allowed the development of rapid, small-incision surgery and markedly reduced recovery time.

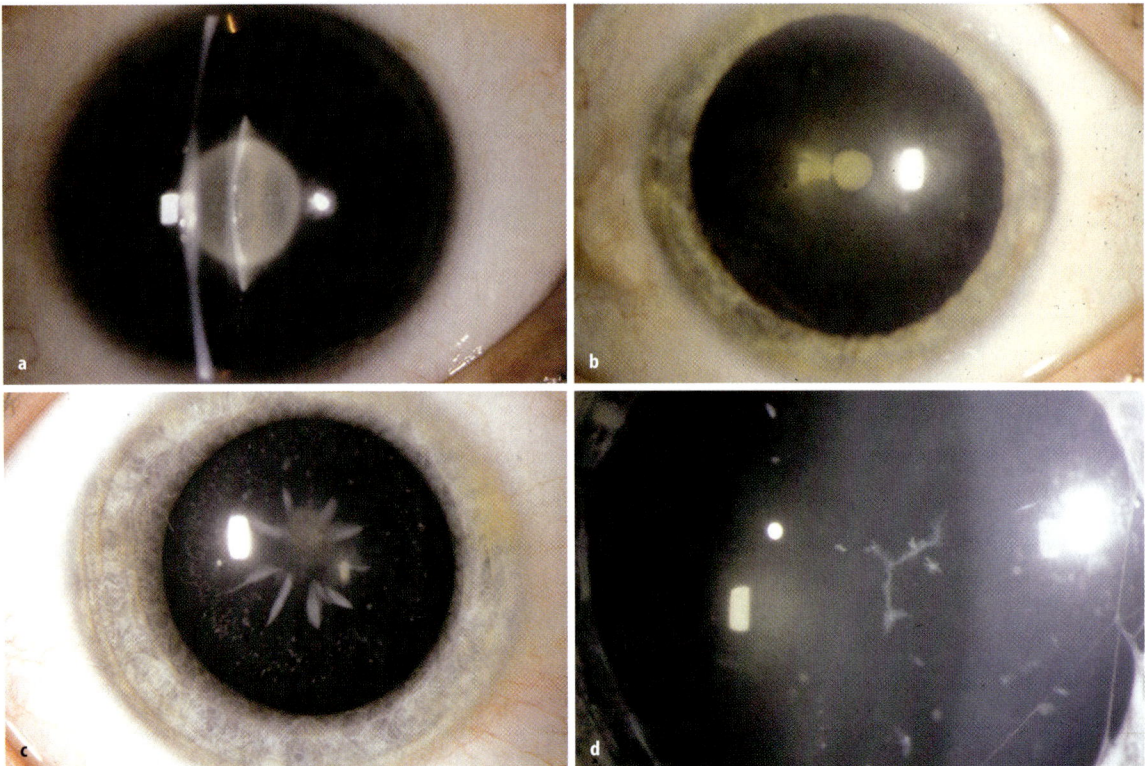

Fig. 5.5.19. Congenital cataracts. **a** Nuclear cataract (cataracta pulverulenta). **b** Cataracta polaris posterior. **c** Cataracta floriformis. **d** Cataracta suturalis ("anterior axial embryonal nuclear cataract": common, no relevant optical consequences)

Table 5.5.5. Cataract types

Cataract type	Special features
1. Congenital cataracts	
Total congenital cataract	Degenerated and liquefied lens fibers at birth; milk-like appearance of the lens, or partial or complete resorption of the lens substance
Nuclear cataract	Solid, granular, or powder-like central opacity of the embryonic lens nucleus
Zonular cataract	Discrete shell-like zones of opacity due to a transient disturbance in lens fiber differentiation; radially coursing opacities in the equatorial region ("riders")
Crystalline cataracts	Deposition of crystalline substances, e.g., tyrosine, cystine or calcium sulfate
Anterior polar cataract	Focal anterior subcapsular opacification of 1–2 mm diameter; often secondary to persistence of the embryonic pupillary membrane or a perforating injury during intrauterine life; pseudofibrous metaplasia of the central anterior lens epithelium
Posterior polar cataract	Focal posterior subcapsular opacification; often secondary to disturbances in regression of the tunica vasculosa lentis of the primary vitreous; degeneration of the posterior subcapsular cortex and bladder cell formation
Lenticonus anterior and posterior	Localized defect or deformation in the anterior or posterior lens capsule allowing a conical protrusion of the lens surface, which produces an "oil droplet" appearance on retinoscopy
Rubella cataract	Caused by rubella virus infection during gestation; mostly nuclear or total opacification; persistence of pyknotic nuclei within lens fibers
Persistent hyperplastic primary vitreous (PHPV)	Posterior polar cataract, associated with microphthalmos and extended ciliary processes
Cataracts with congenital syndromes	e.g., Down's syndrome (trisomy 21), Alport's syndrome, Lowe's syndrome, trisomy 13, 15
2. Age-related cataracts	
Subcapsular cataract	
– Anterior subcapsular cataract	Proliferation and fibrous pseudometaplasia of the lens epithelium, formation of a connective tissue plaque underneath the anterior capsule
– Posterior subcapsular cataract	Posterior migration of the lens epithelium producing a focal opacification beneath the posterior capsule; formation of Wedl bladder cells
Cortical cataract	
– Cortical cataract	Progressive opacification of the lens cortex occurring as scattered punctate opacities, vacuoles, water clefts, and spoke-like white opacities due to degenerative alterations of lens fibers
– Mature cataract	Opacification of the entire cortex
– Hypermature cataract	Leakage of the liquefied cortex through the lens capsule
– Morgagnian cataract	Descent of the nucleus within the liquefied cortex
Nuclear cataract	Progressive sclerosis and brunescence of the lens nucleus due to accumulation of macromolecular protein aggregates within lens fibers
3. Etiology of cataracts	
Cataracts caused by *ocular* diseases ("Cataracta complicata")	Typically posterior subcapsular cataract; anterior subcapsular cataract may develop in anterior uveitis
– Chronic uveitis	
– Adjacent tumors and cysts	
– Retinal dystrophies	
– Angle-closure glaucomas	
Cataracts associated with systemic disorders	
– Diabetes mellitus	Osmotic stress due to lenticular accumulation of sorbitol leading to increased water uptake and to initially reversible, later irreversible opacities
– Galactosemia	Osmotic stress due to accumulation of galactitol in the lens
– Hypocalcemia	Small white cortical opacities
– Wilson's disease	Characteristic stellate or sunflower opacities in anterior lens capsule
– Myotonic dystrophy	Multicolored lens opacities ("Christmas tree" cataract)
– Dermatologic disorders	Polar or subcapsular cataract
– Pseudoexfoliation syndrome	Nuclear cataract
Cataracts caused by *exogenous* factors	
– Trauma (blunt or penetrating)	Opacities in the anterior or posterior subcapsular region with delayed onset; mature cataract after traumatic rupture of the capsule
– Metallosis (siderosis, chalcosis)	Accumulation of iron ions in anterior lens epithelium and anterior subcapsular cataract; accumulation of copper ions in lens capsule and "sunflower cataract" formation
– Radiation (UV, X-ray, β, infrared)	Opacities in the anterior or posterior subcapsular regions with a latency period of months or years
– Electrical shock	Anterior or posterior subcapsular opacifications, often with a fern-like or starburst appearance
– Medication (corticosteroids topical/systemic, cytostatics/immunosuppressives, antiglaucoma drugs)	Anterior and especially posterior subcapsular opacifications

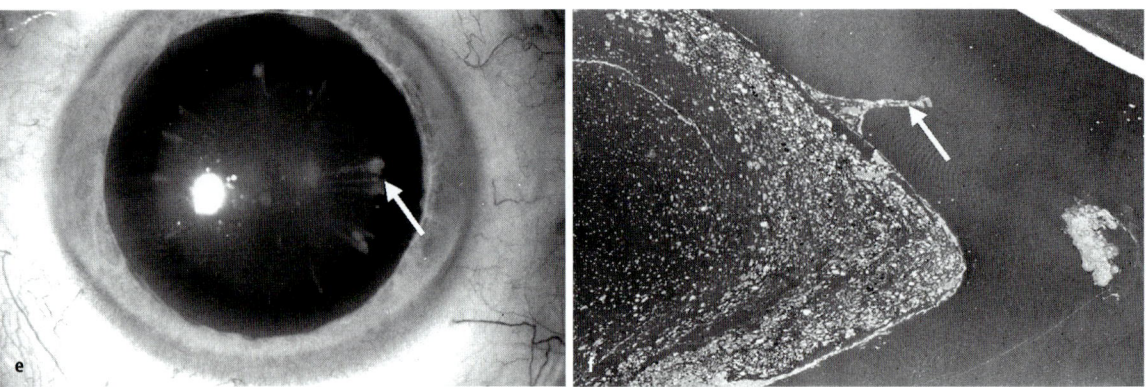

Fig. 5.5.19. e, f Cataracta zonularis with a shell-like zone of opacification and "riders" (*arrows*) in the equatorial region

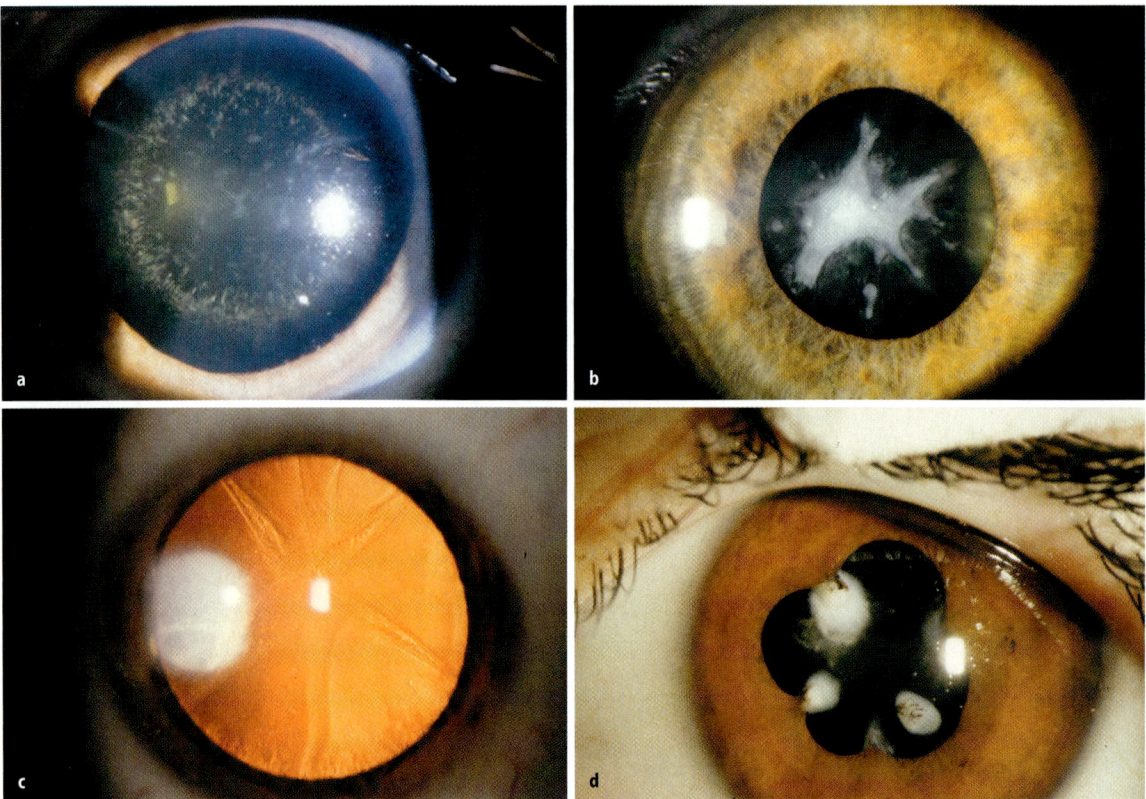

Fig. 5.5.20. Cataracts associated with systemic disorders. **a** Cataracta diabetica. **b** Cataracta syndermatotica. **c** Cataracta myotonica. **d** Cataract with juvenile rheumatoid arthritis: focal posterior synechiae with plaque of anterior subcapsular pseudometaplasia of the lens epithelium

Lenses from individuals with *Alzheimer's disease* disclose beta-amyloid deposits in the cytoplasm of supranuclear/deep cortical lens fibers. These deposits may be related to the equatorial supranuclear cataracts typically observed in Alzheimer patients (Goldstein et al. 2003). Because cerebral beta-amyloid plaques represent a hallmark of Alzheimer's disease, detection of these specific deposits in the lens might be a means for early diagnosis of Alzheimer's disease.

5.5.5.3.1
Basic Mechanisms of Cataract Formation

Transparency of the lens results from a close, regular packing of anucleate fiber cells and a highly ordered, evenly distributed, spatial arrangement of lens crystallins, causing minimal light scatter. Opacification results from zones of increased light scattering, which may be caused by a breakdown of fiber regularity, by intra- and extracellular fluid accumulations, by products of membrane degradation, by crystalline precipitates, or by

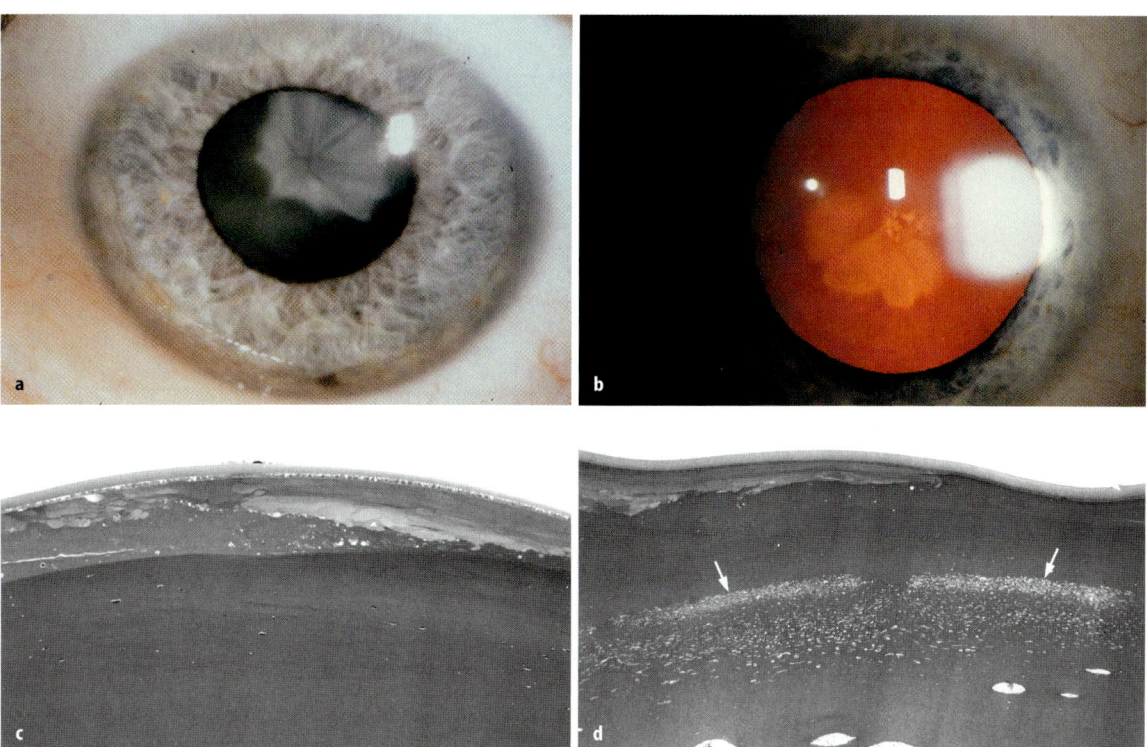

Fig. 5.5.21. Contusion cataract. **a, b** Contusion rosette. **c** Vacuolization of the anterior lens epithelium and swelling of subcapsular lens fibers 4 months after trauma. **d** Lamellar zone of opacification (*arrows*) in the deep anterior cortex 13 years after trauma

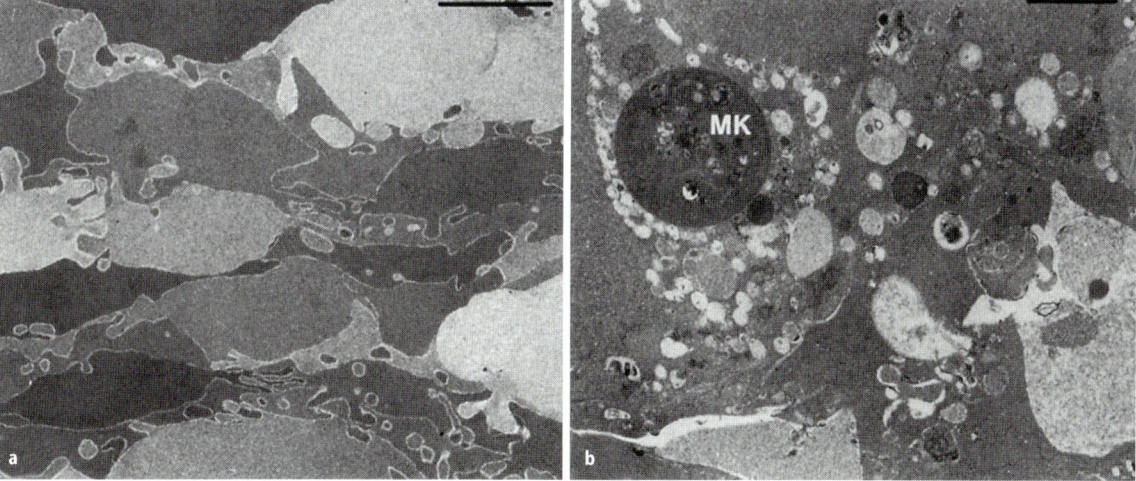

Fig. 5.5.22. Degenerative alterations of cortical lens fibers by transmission electron microscopy. **a** Swelling of lens fibers leading to varying cytoplasmic densities (*scale bar* 5 µm). **b** Globular degeneration of lens fibers into morgagnian droplets (*MK*) (*scale bar* 2 µm). (**c, d** *see p. 238*)

macromolecular protein aggregates within the fiber cells (Figs. 5.5.22, 5.5.23). However, cataracts should be distinguished from physiological aging changes including various degrees of nuclear sclerosis.

Numerous individual causes of cataracts exist, and often multiple factors act together. An association with cataractogenesis has been established for UV-A irradiation, smoking, alcohol consumption, and systemic diseases such as diabetes mellitus, PEX syndrome or myotonic dystrophy. Certain intraocular diseases (uveitis, retinal dystrophies) are associated with "complicated cataracts." Among the most important factors contributing to cataract formation are oxidative and osmotic stress, caused by ultraviolet light and a disturbance in the osmotic balance between the aqueous and the lens substance. In senile cataracts, increased ab-

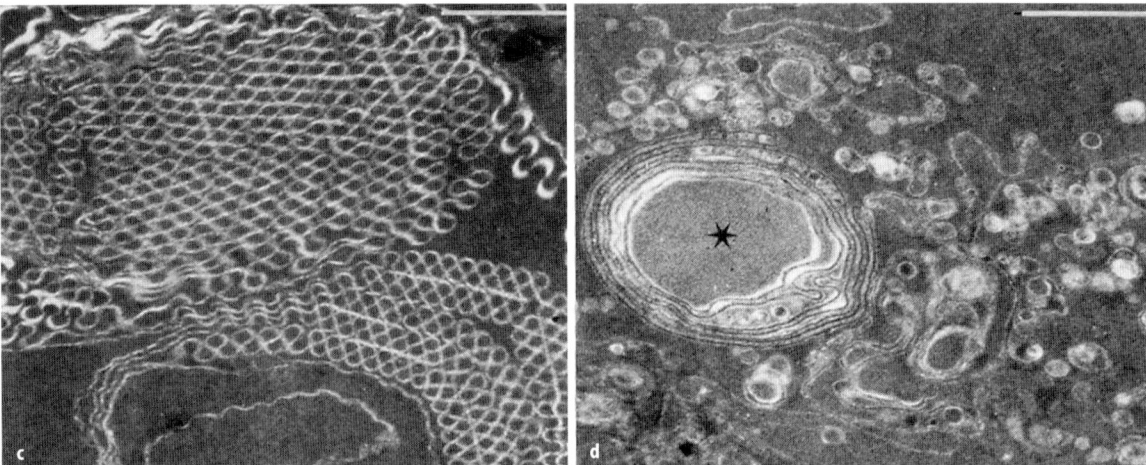

Fig. 5.5.22. c Remnants of fiber membranes forming "figure-of-eight" structures (*scale bar* 1 μm). **d** Remnants of fiber membranes forming multilamellar bodies (*) (*scale bar* 1 μm)

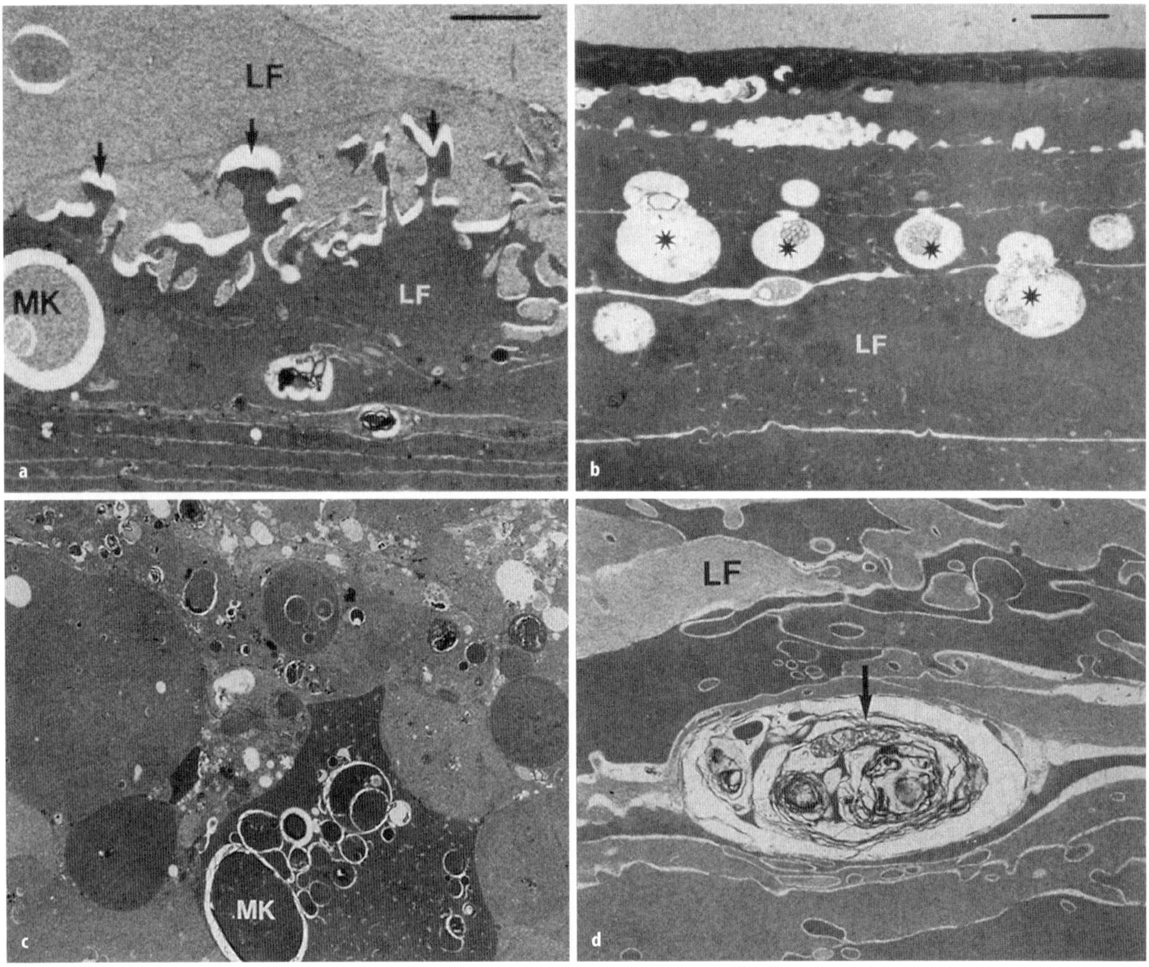

Fig. 5.5.23. Degenerative alterations of cortical lens fibers by transmission electron microscopy. **a** Swelling of lens fibers, enlargement of intercellular spaces by fluid accumulation, and dissociation into morgagnian globules (*MK*) (*scale bar* 3 μm). **b** Increased intercellular spaces and vacuolization (*) by fluid accumulation between lens fibers (*LF*) (*scale bar* 3 μm). **c** Globular degeneration of lens fibers into morgagnian droplets (*MK*) (*scale bar* 5 μm). **d** Remnants of fiber membranes forming multilamellar bodies (*arrow*) between swollen lens fibers (*LF*) (*scale bar* 2 μm)

sorption of light occurs through the formation of nuclear yellow-brown pigments (brunescence). Due to a concomitant decrease in antioxidant activity, lens fibers are more susceptible to oxidative damage and lipid peroxidation of cell membranes and lens proteins. Oxidative damage to cell membranes causes alterations in membrane permeability, leading to osmotic stress. Osmotic stress is believed to apply particularly in diabetic cataract and galactosemic cataract, in which sugars are converted to their respective sugar alcohol by the enzyme aldose reductase in the so-called sorbitol pathway. These sugar alcohols (sorbitol, galactitol) cannot pass through plasma membranes causing water entry and hence swelling of lens epithelial and fiber cells.

The basic tissue alterations occurring in most forms of cataract involve relatively few patterns of histopathologic changes of the lens epithelium, the lens fibers, and the capsule. Finally the development of cataracts may also be induced or accelerated as a side effect of ocular or systemic therapy. As examples we mention other intraocular surgery (e.g. vitrectomy, trabeculectomy, phakic lens implantation) and local or systemic treatment with corticosteroids.

Lens Epithelium

The density of the lens epithelium is significantly *decreased* in age-related cataracts: it is highest in nuclear cataracts, decreases with cortical involvement, and is lowest in hypermature cataracts (Karim et al. 1987; Konofsky et al. 1987; Tseng et al. 1994). This decrease is accompanied by *degenerative* changes, e.g., formation of intracellular vacuoles, particularly in subcapsular and cortical cataracts. Pronounced degenerative or necrotic alterations of the lens epithelium may occur in advanced age-related cataracts, iritis, or after mechanical or chemical injury. Focal areas of epithelial necrosis are frequent complications of acute pupillary block angle closure glaucomas ("*Glaukomflecken*").

However, the epithelium is also susceptible to *active proliferation*. Various insults (e.g., inflammation, trauma, irradiation, systemic diseases) can stimulate the anterior lens epithelium to undergo an increased mitotic and proliferative activity with subsequent formation of atypical lens cells (Fig. 5.5.24). Central epithelial cells may be transformed into spindle-shaped, fibrocyte-like cells producing considerable amounts of extracellular matrix including basement membrane and collagen fibers (Font and Brownstein 1974; Pau and Novotny 1985). This *fibrous pseudo-metaplasia* creates an *anterior subcapsular cataract*, i.e., a connective tissue plaque between the anterior capsule and the epithelium, which commonly develops following eye injury (Fig. 5.5.25). The metaplastic cells express alpha-smooth muscle actin and contain myofilaments typical of myofibroblasts. Contraction of

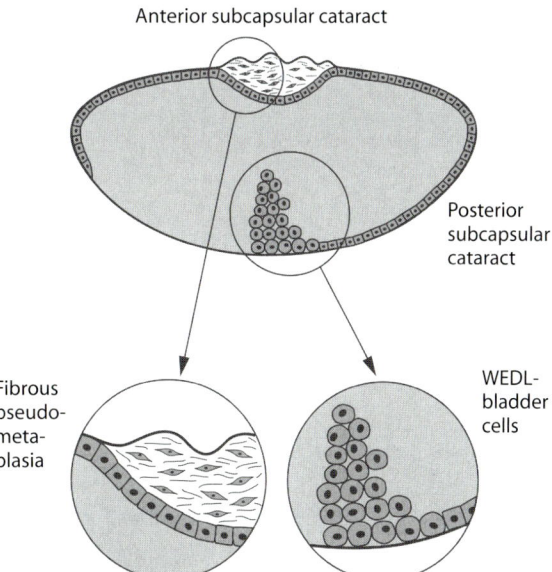

Fig. 5.5.24. Schematic representation of abnormal proliferation of the lens epithelium leading to anterior subcapsular cataract caused by fibrous metaplasia of the anterior epithelium and to the formation of a posterior subcapsular cataract caused by posterior migration of the equatorial epithelium and bladder cell formation

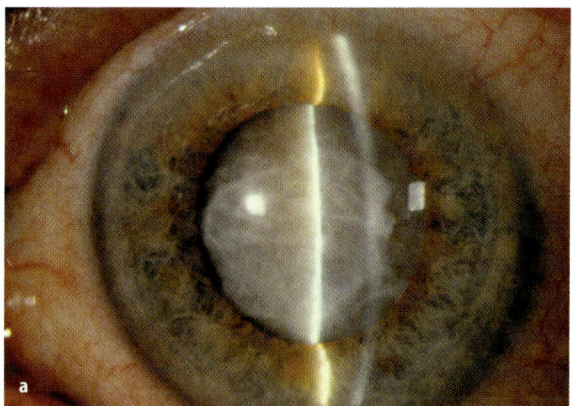

Fig. 5.5.25a–e. Anterior subcapsular cataract. **a** Clinical appearance

these myofibroblasts results in a wrinkling of the anterior capsule.

Another common pathologic response of the germinative lens epithelium is the *proliferation* and *migration* beyond the lens equator toward the posterior pole with bladder cell formation (Fig. 5.5.24). The abnormally differentiating epithelial cells are disorganized and imperfectly rotated and their dysplastic differentiation products migrate posteriorly. These cells often become swollen, measuring up to 120 μm in diameter, and transform into *bladder cells of Wedl*, each representing an abortive fiber cell (Eshagian 1982). These bladder cells move into the posterior cortex and finally may degenerate producing posterior subcapsular cataracts (Fig. 5.5.26).

Fig. 5.5.25. b, c Multilayered connective tissue plaque formed by pseudometaplastic epithelial cells beneath the wrinkled lens capsule (**c**) (* precapsular contracting occlusion membrane). **d, e** Proliferating pseudometaplastic epithelial cells surrounded by basement membranes and embedded in a dense collagenous matrix (**c** lens capsule) (PAS, MASSON)

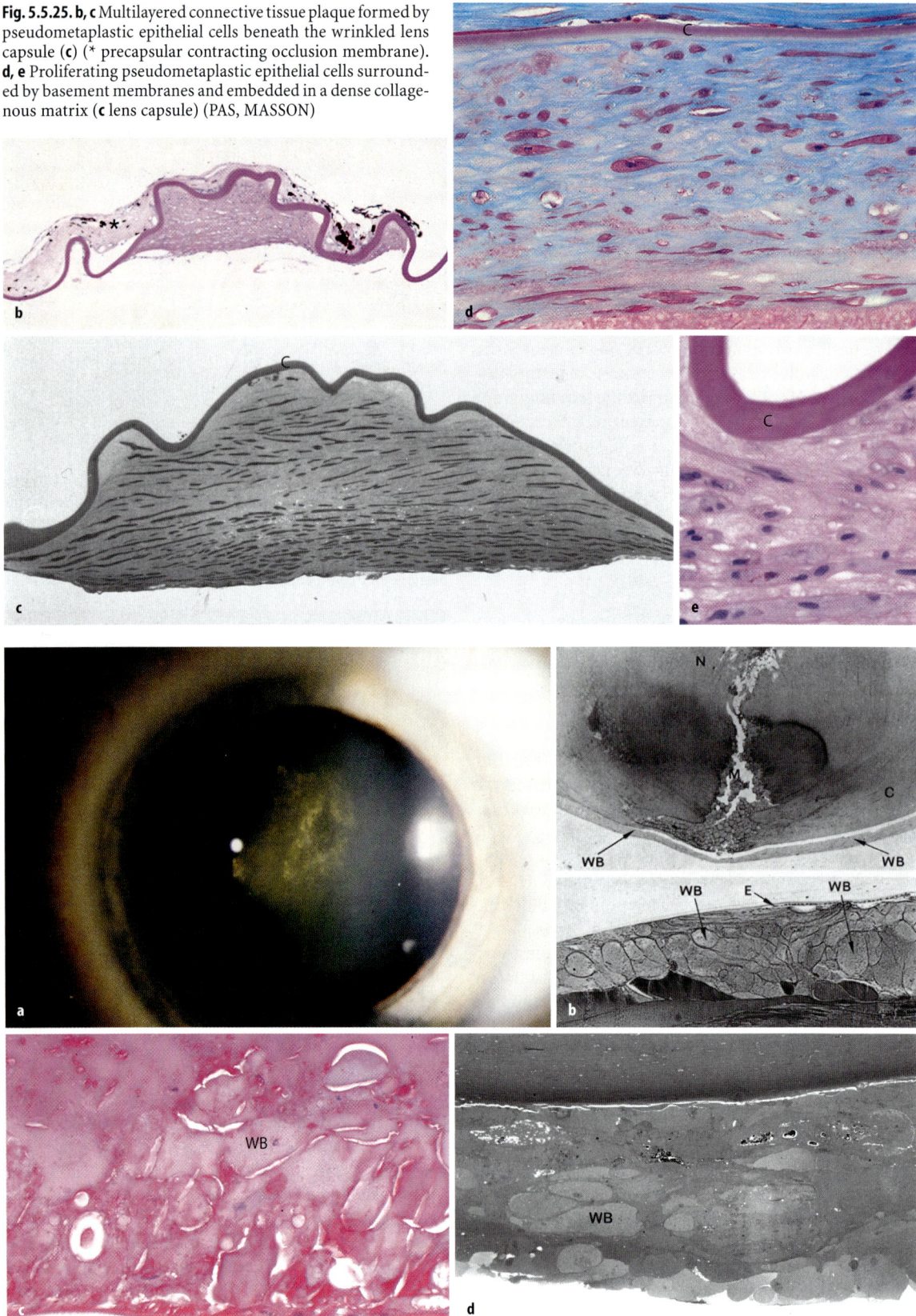

Fig. 5.5.26 (*Legend see p. 241*)

Lens Fibers

Age-related cataracts occur as cortical, nuclear, and subcapsular opacities, with cortical cataract being the most frequent. Cortical and subcapsular cataracts are caused by striking degenerative alterations of lens fibers, whereas nuclear cataracts are characterized by subtle biochemical alterations of lens fiber proteins (Fig. 5.5.27).

Cortical opacifications mostly result from a breakdown of fiber regularity and degenerative liquefaction of lens fiber substance. Disturbances of ion and water regulation lead to swelling, vacuole formation, and vacuolar degeneration of superficial lens fibers (Fig. 5.5.28). Extracellular fluid accumulation manifests as vacuoles and radial water clefts between the fibers. Degradation products of fiber membranes may form complex membrane configurations, such as multilamellar bodies and "figure-of-eight" structures, producing punctate opacifications (Fig. 5.5.22). Liquefaction of lens proteins and fiber breakdown results in the formation of globular bodies termed morgagnian droplets containing degenerated lens substance. After complete liquefaction of the cortex (cataracta matura), the sclerotic lens nucleus may sink inferiorly by gravitation (morgagnian cataract) within the liquefied cortex (Fig. 5.5.29). In long-standing cases, the degenerative lens substance may become calcified (cataracta calcarea). In hypermature cataracts, loss of fluid leads to shrinkage of the lens and wrinkling of the lens capsule (Fig. 5.5.29).

A lamellar cataract forms if the fibers within a particular growth shell are affected. Similarly, if a group of fibers are affected, the appearance is that of a spoke. If the tips of the fibers are affected, the opacity appears in a branching pattern of the suture (e.g., traumatic cataract) (Fig. 5.5.21).

In contrast, by light microscopy no major histological change appears to occur in nuclear cataracts, which can be hardly differentiated from physiological sclerosis of the lens nucleus. Nuclear opacification mostly results from the formation of light-scattering foci in the nuclear fiber cytoplasm by accumulation of large high-molecular-weight protein aggregates. A special feature of nuclear cataracts are *spheroliths*, which represent roundish bodies (80–500 µm in diameter) consisting of calcium oxalate, calcium phosphate, or calcium carbonate crystals. The latter light up under the polarizing microscope (Fig. 5.5.30).

◁
Fig. 5.5.26. Posterior subcapsular cataract. **a** Clinical appearance. **b** Complicated cataract with bladder cell formation (*WB*), central liquefaction of lens fibers and formation of morgagnian droplets (*M*) at the posterior pole (*C* lens cortex, *E* epithelial cells, *N* lens nucleus). **c, d** Formation of bladder cells (*WB*) at the posterior pole of the lens

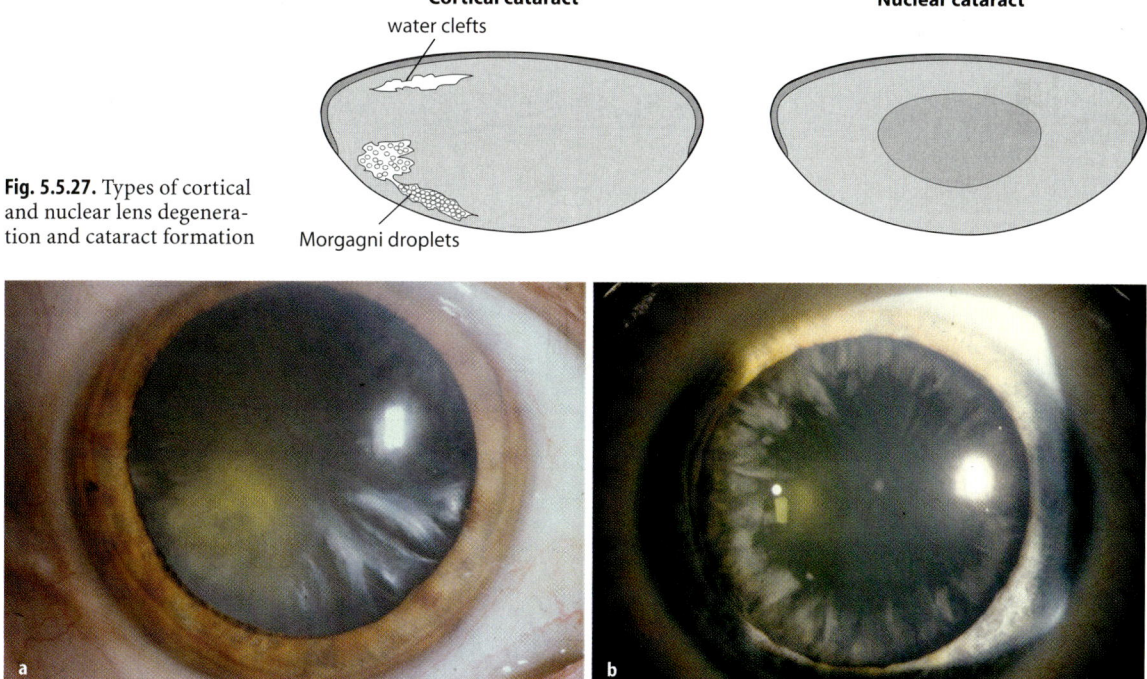

Fig. 5.5.27. Types of cortical and nuclear lens degeneration and cataract formation

Fig. 5.5.28a–e. Age-related cortical cataract. **a, b** Clinical appearance of water clefts and spokes in the equatorial region of the lens cortex

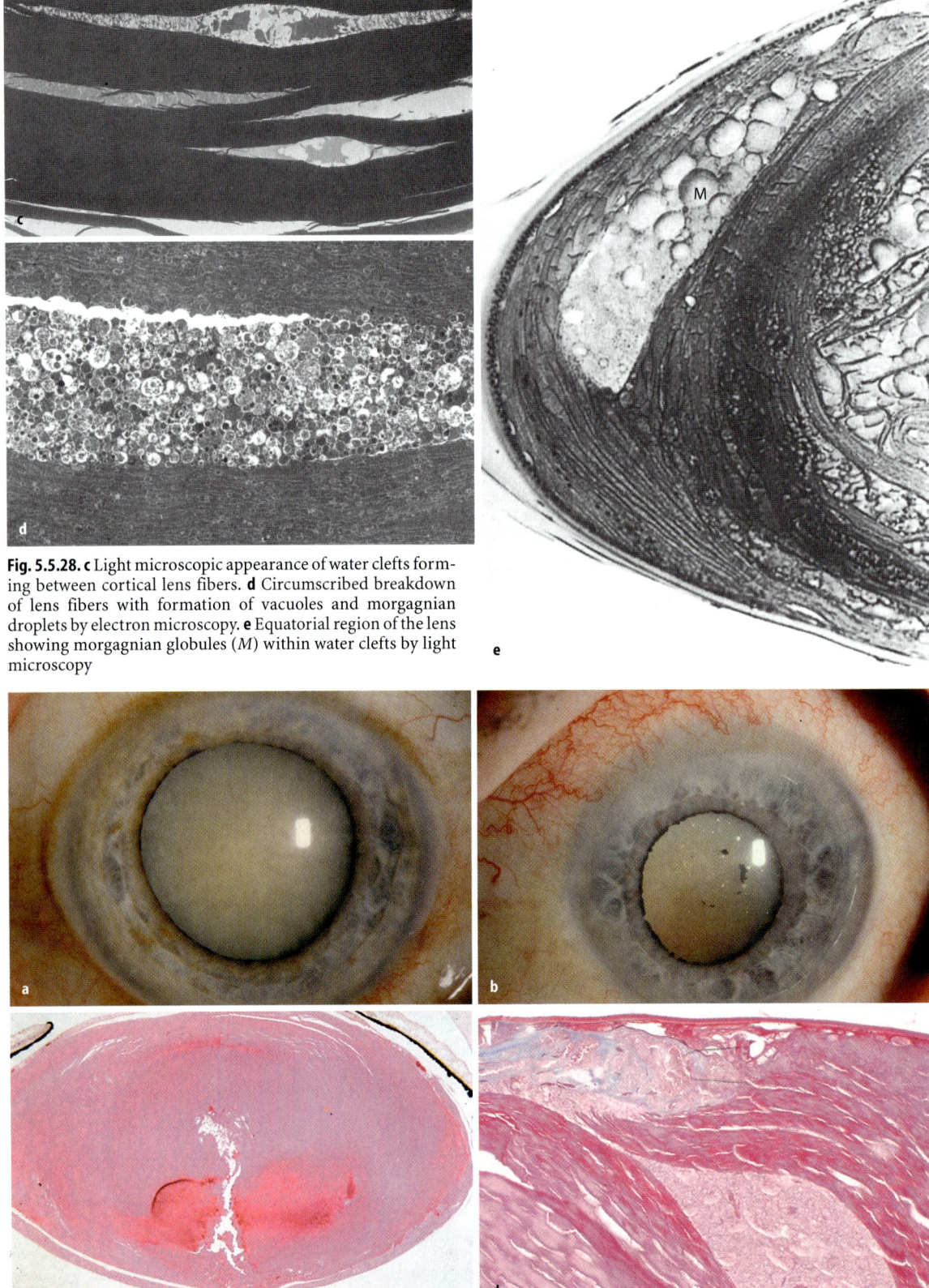

Fig. 5.5.28. c Light microscopic appearance of water clefts forming between cortical lens fibers. **d** Circumscribed breakdown of lens fibers with formation of vacuoles and morgagnian droplets by electron microscopy. **e** Equatorial region of the lens showing morgagnian globules (*M*) within water clefts by light microscopy

Fig. 5.5.29. Cataracta matura, cataracta hypermatura (Morgagni). **a** Cataracta matura. **b** Morgagnian cataract showing a sunken lens nucleus. **c–e** Cataracta intumescens with thickened lens showing water clefts (**c**), swelling of lens fibers (**d**), ...

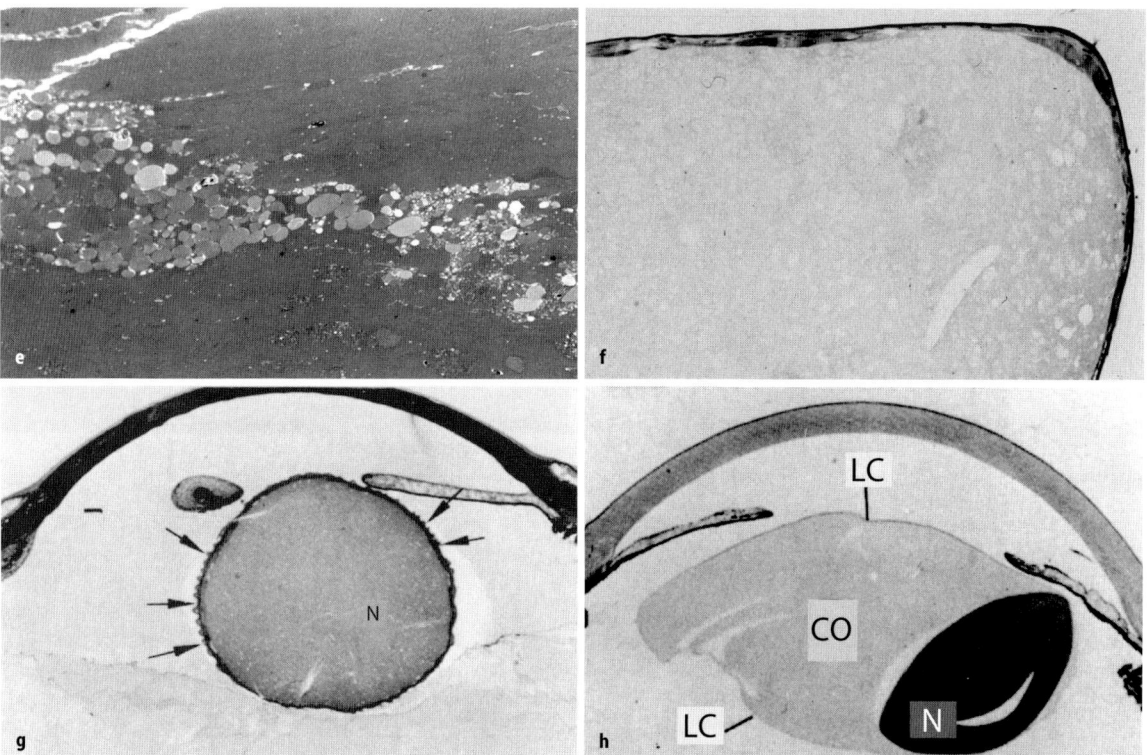

Fig. 5.5.29. (*Cont.*) ... and fiber breakdown in morgagnian droplets (**e**). **f, g** Cataracta hypermatura with complete liquefaction of the lens cortex (**f**), shrinkage of the lens and wrinkling of the lens capsule (*arrows*) (*N* nucleus) (**g**). **h** Morgagnian cataract with a sunken nucleus (*N*) within the liquefied cortex (*CO*) surrounded by an intact lens capsule (*LC*)

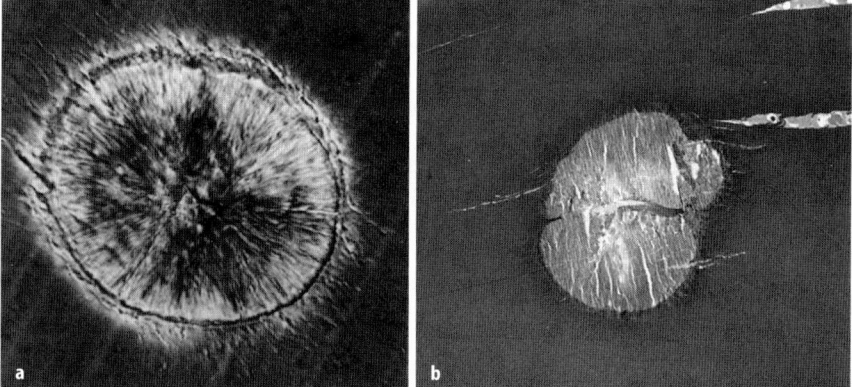

Fig. 5.5.30. Spheroliths. **a** Calcium oxalate crystal within a nuclear cataract as viewed with polarized light. **b** Spherolith in the lens nucleus by normal light microscopy

Lens Capsule

Although the capsule may be ruptured after perforating injuries, it is in general extremely resistant to pathologic insults including intraocular inflammations. However, in hypermature cataracts, the lens capsule can form minute perforations and crystallin fragments may leak into the anterior chamber inducing macrophage activity and secondary *phacolytic open-angle glaucoma*.

In *true exfoliation* of the lens capsule, today a rare disease related to excessive exposure to infrared light (glassblower's cataract), lamellar splitting and peeling of the superficial capsular layers occurs (Karp et al. 1999) (Fig. 5.5.31a, b). Such a true exfoliation of the capsule has also been described to occur idiopathically in elderly individuals (Cashwell et al. 1989). In lenticonus anterior and posterior, the lens capsule is markedly thinned (Khalil and Saheb 1984). In contrast, the very common systemic disorder of *PEX syndrome* is not associated with a true exfoliation of capsular layers, but rather with *depositions* of an abnormally produced extracellular material on the surface of the anterior lens capsule and other structures of the anterior segment (see Chapter 6.3) (Fig. 5.5.31c, d).

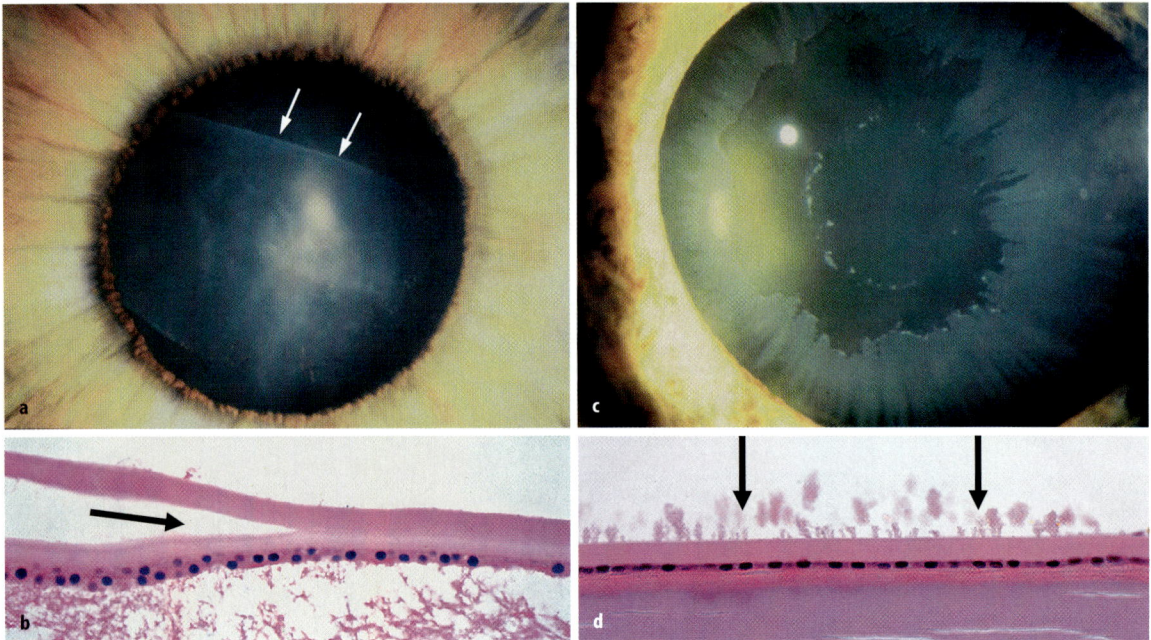

Fig. 5.5.31. True exfoliation and pseudoexfoliation of the lens capsule. **a, b** True exfoliation of the lens capsule (glassblower's cataract) with partial lamellar splitting of the central anterior lens capsule (*arrows*) (courtesy M. Küchle). **c, d** Pseudoexfoliation syndrome with deposition of an abnormal extracellular material (*arrows*) on the intact anterior lens capsule

By-products of abnormal metabolism or intraocular foreign bodies may accumulate in the lens capsule, e.g., silver inclusions in exogenous or endogenous siderosis lentis, gold particles in ocular argyrosis, or copper inclusions in morbus Wilson. Drugs and their metabolites may also accumulate as fine granules, usually anteriorly in the capsule or in the superficial cortex.

5.5.6
Basic Aspects of Cataract Surgery

5.5.6.1
Preoperative Examinations

The diagnosis of cataract can easily be made with the slit lamp in advanced cases or with torchlight. Further diagnostic procedures are indicated if the lens is decentered or dislocated or to rule out additional pathology in the vicinity of the lens such as intraocular tumors [abnormalities of the anterior segment by ultrasound biomicroscopy (UMB) and optical coherence tomography (OCT); damage to the blood-aqueous barrier by laser tyndallometry] and by A- and B-echography to exclude tumor or other pathology of the posterior part of the eye.

Another important factor of preoperative examination is the exact measurement of the refractive status to select the desired power of the IOL implant.

5.5.6.2
Indications for Removal of the Lens and Artificial Lens Implantation

Like in other areas of clinical medicine, the pros and cons of the planned surgical procedure need to be discussed in detail with the patients and/or their relatives (Table 5.5.6). Most of the time the indications for surgery are relative and depend on the individual needs (Jünemann et al. 1998). However, there are absolute indications for lens extraction, e.g., in persisting acute glaucomas caused by fluid lens material of hypermature (*phacolytic glaucoma*) cataracts or by pupillary or ciliary block. In cases of phakogenic uveitis or "*endophthalmitis phacoanaphylactica*", caused by a granulomatous reaction against the lens nucleus after traumatic rupture (Fig. 5.5.32), the lens nucleus must be removed

Table 5.5.6. Indications for cataract extraction

Intra-capsular:	Calcified cataract
	Extensive anterior subcapsular fibrous pseudometaplasia
	Shrunken hypermature cataract, dislocated
Extra-capsular:	Standard situation
	Dis- and subluxated lenses
Lens implantation:	
	All
	Exceptions:
	Acute inflammatory intraocular processes
	Infants in first year

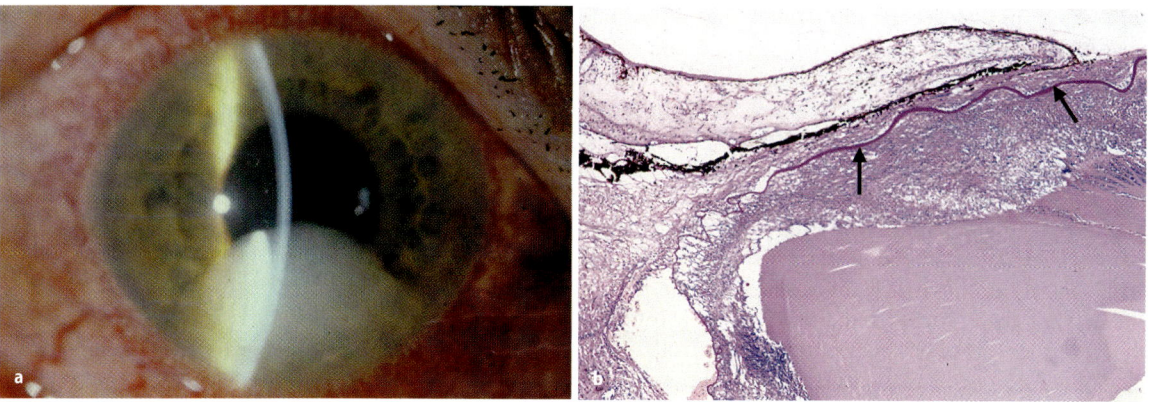

Fig. 5.5.32. a Phacogenic uveitis. **b** Beginning of "endophthalmitis phacoanaphylactica" with foreign body giant cells; the *arrows* mark the lens capsule (PAS)

because the persisting ocular hypotony can be only cured by removal of the lens. The concept of waiting until the intraocular pressure has been raised by medical means is not effective.

Opacities of the lens are the main indication: In the industrialized countries, such lens opacities are partial or are immature; in the developing world, advanced stages of mature or hypermature cataracts are frequent.

Today, removal of the crystalline lens in the sense of a refractive lens exchange in high myopia and/or hyperopia is under debate. There is even discussion about removal of the clear lens to meet presbyopia by implantation of a device achieving pseudo-accommodation.

Congenital hereditary and acquired lens dislocations are relatively rare but are treated by phacoemulsification and anterior vitrectomy. If the dislocated lens contains a very hard nucleus, an intracapsular cataract extraction is indicated.

5.5.6.2.1
Extracapsular Cataract Extraction

The treatment of choice for most variants of cataracts in children and adults is extracapsular cataract extraction with the device for phacoemulsification (Kelman 1974) with consecutive IOL implantation. In the second half of the last century extracapsular cataract extraction replaced the intracapsular cataract extraction and facilitated the fixation of artificial lens implants in the eye behind the pupil, either endocapsular inside the lens capsule or between the lens capsule remnants and the iris root in the sulcus ciliaris (Fig. 5.5.33).

The choice of material of the lens implant depends on the overall situation of the anterior and posterior segment of the eye. In the last 50 years the advance of

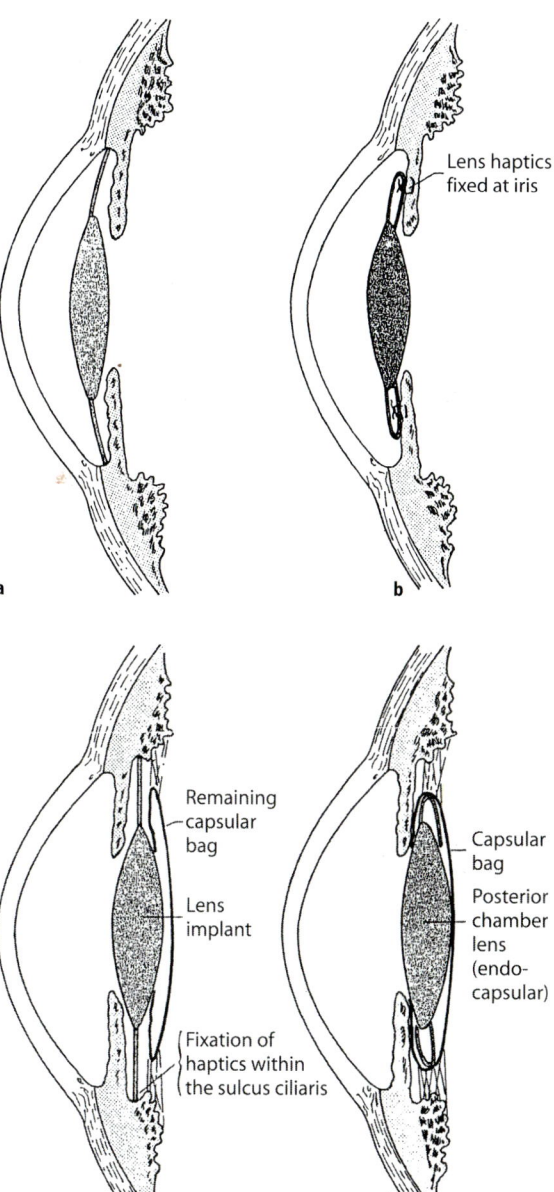

▷

Fig. 5.5.33. Schematic representation of main loci of fixation of artificial lenses: anterior chamber lens (**a**)

techniques and the opportunities for any indication have been spectacular. Today, IOL implantation after extracapsular cataract extraction is indicated and possible in most situations. However, after severe trauma, lens implantation might be postponed as a second procedure after cataract extraction as soon as the anterior segment of the eye is less inflamed.

Moreover, patients suffering from juvenile uveitis as part of a juvenile rheumatoid arthritis may be treated with special caution. Any form of lens implantation in these eyes may be considered only if the basic inflammatory process is under pharmacologic control.

Patients need to be made aware of special risks in diabetes, pseudoexfoliation syndrome and other intraocular pathology.

All variants of cataract extraction require access to the intraocular space by introduction of instruments and implantation of rigid or foldable lens implants and therefore share the risks of all intraocular procedures (see Chapters 2, 4) (Fig. 5.5.33).

5.5.6.2.2
Intracapsular Cataract Extraction

Removal of the intracapsular lens has advantages and disadvantages (Table 5.5.7). When the lens is removed in toto, secondary cataract cannot develop, and ophthalmoscopic examination of the fundus of the eye is not disturbed. The main disadvantage is an increased frequency of retinal detachment and the difficulty of fixing the artificial lens implant. It requires suturing to the iris or transscleral sutures for placing the haptic into the chamber angle. Even if the surgeon is successful in preserving the anterior vitreous face during intracapsular cataract extraction, this structure frequently breaks leading to a prolapse of vitreous into the anterior chamber. As the removal of the lens in one piece requires a larger corneal or corneoscleral wound, loss of corneal endothelial cells is more pronounced than in extracapsular cataract extraction.

5.5.7
Complications After Cataract Surgery and Wound Healing

Cataract surgery is the most commonly performed type of ocular surgery. In the vast majority of cases, the surgery is uncomplicated. However, cataract surgery should never be trivialized. In a *small* percentage of patients, complications can occur (Table 5.5.8).

Table 5.5.8. Cataract surgery: risks and complications

A. Risks
1. Blepharitis
2. Extremely deep anterior chamber in high myopes
3. Relative anterior microphthalmus (RAM) ("crowded" anterior chamber)
4. Zonular weakness (PEX)
5. Poor mydriasis and "intraoperative floppy iris syndrome" (IFIS)
6. Globe perforations by local injection anesthesia
7. Massive "vis a tergo" with nanophthalmus
B. Complications
1. Posterior capsule rupture (1–3%)
2. "Toxic anterior segment syndrome (TASS)" due to irrigation, medication, sterilizing problems
3. Clear cornea incision (CCI) without suture: "silent epidemic" of infectious endophthalmitis
4. Suprachoroidal hemorrhage
5. Lens nucleus descending, more in posterior polar cataract (PPC)
6. Vitreous incarceration in wound: Hruby-Irvine-Gass syndrome
7. Chronic postoperative endophthalmitis (originally confused with "toxic lens syndrome")
8. Cystoid macula edema
9. Age related macular degeneration (threefold increase over 10 years)
10. Retinal detachment (fourfold increase over 20 years)
11. Corneal decompensation ~2‰
12. Late "surgically induced necrotizing scleritis (SINS)"

Table 5.5.7. Advantages and disadvantages of intra- and extracapsular cataract extraction

	Advantages	Disadvantages
Intracapsular CE	*No secondary cataract*	Large incision More corneal endothelial cell loss Loss of iris-lens diaphragm More retinal detachment More cystoid macular edema
Extracapsular CE	Small incision Intact iris-lens diaphragm, less retinal detachment Less corneal endothelial cell loss Mini incisions with minimal blood-aqueous barrier	*Secondary cataract*

5.5.7.1
Complications

5.5.7.1.1
Corneal Endothelial Cell Loss

Cataract surgery has direct traumatic effects on the corneal endothelium leading to a significant loss of endothelial cells varying from 4% to 25%.

No significant differences in overall corneal endothelial cell loss have been reported between extracapsular cataract extraction and phacoemulsification surgery (Bourne et al. 2004) nor between small-incision surgery and standard techniques (Mencucci et al. 2006).

5.5.7.1.2
Iris Damage

Cataract surgery may cause possible direct damage to the iris, e.g., by iris prolapse out of the incision, by phacoemulsification tip suction (Fig. 5.5.37a), by mechanical mydriasis with iris hooks for small pupils, or in intraoperative floppy iris syndrome (IFIS) (see Sect. 5.3). All surgical procedures are invariably followed by a marked disruption of the blood-aqueous barrier (Ferguson and Spalton 1992).

5.5.7.1.3
Retinal Damage

Cataract surgery has been known to cause retinal damage in approximately 1.5% of patients.

Cystoid maculopathy following cataract surgery may be detected by OCT in up to 60%. Older estimates range from 1% to 19% and may be associated with more subtle symptoms of contrast sensitivity, reading speed, or deficits in color perception (Donnenfeld 2007).

Late risks after uneventful extracapsular cataract extraction with lens implants are:

1. The cumulative probability of *retinal detachment at 20 years after uneventful extracapsular cataract extraction and phacoemulsification leading to unremarkable pseudophakia was fourfold higher* than would be expected in patients not undergoing cataract surgery (Erie et al. 2006). However, there was no significant difference in the probability of retinal detachment between extracapsular cataract extraction with nuclear expression and phacoemulsification.
2. Moreover, cataract surgery in older persons may be associated with an increased risk for developing late-stage age-related macular degeneration (AMD), particularly neovascular AMD (Wang et al. 2003). Nonphakic (aphakic or pseudophakic) eyes had a *threefold increased risk of developing late AMD* compared with phakic eyes over 10 years (Cugati et al. 2006), which may be related to the increased exposure of the retina to short-wavelength light. These eyes did not show any signs of macular disease pre- and immediately postoperatively. The rate of these complications with refined current methods of extracapsular cataract extraction is not known.

5.5.7.1.4
Endophthalmitis

Acute postoperative endophthalmitis is a rare but still one of the most serious complications of cataract surgery (Fig. 5.5.37b), occurring at a rate of up to 0.2–0.3% (Taban et al. 2005).

The incidence of postoperative endophthalmitis is reported to have increased over the last decade, which coincides with the development of sutureless clear corneal surgery of 2,8 mm particularly if located temporally (Taban et al. 2005). McDonnel therefore has warned of a *"silent epidemic of postoperative endophthalmitis following cataract extraction."* The rate of endophthalmitis after cataract surgery can be reduced by prophylactic addition of antibiotics to the irrigation fluid. Lundström et al. (2007) consider the low frequency (0,048% of postoperative endophthalmitis in a nationwide prospective study in Sweden as a consequence of the use of prophylactic intracameral cefuroxime. Acute postoperative endophthalmitis requires immediate intervention – often pars plana vitrectomy.

Chronic postoperative endophthalmitis by less aggressive bacteria and fungi initially was confused with the "toxic lens syndrome" caused by sterilizing procedures using toxic substances, e.g., lyes or acids (Naumann et al. 1971; von Below et al. 1991). Removal of the lens implant only rarely can be avoided. The classic toxic lens syndrome may respond to local steroid therapy, while chronic endophthalmitis deteriorates. The toxic anterior segment syndrome (TASS) represents a more severe form of the toxic lens syndrome (see Chapter 4).

"Surgically induced necrotizing scleritis" (SINS) develops after an unremarkable interval of several months causing loss of corneal and scleral tissue in the limbus region leading to a furrow. General collagen diseases must be ruled out (Fig. 4.18).

5.5.7.2
Secondary Cataract After Extracapsular Cataract Surgery

Secondary cataract, predominantly posterior capsule opacification (PCO), is a significant late complication of extracapsular cataract extraction. It does occur in *all* eyes after extracapsular cataract surgery, but may be invisible with the slit lamp because it is hidden behind the peripheral iris originating from the equatorial lens capsule. PCO in the visual axis develops in up to 50% of patients between 2 months and 5 years after the initial surgery. The frequency of PCO is age related. Almost all children develop PCO after cataract extraction, but in adults the incidence is much lower. This is thought to be because of the higher proliferative capacity of lens epithelial cells in the young compared with the old. PEX syndrome is associated with a higher frequency of PCO, whereas lenses from patients with diabetes mellitus are less frequently affected (Küchle et al. 1997).

After cataract extraction, residual epithelial cells that were not removed at the time of surgery still possess the capacity to proliferate, differentiate, and undergo fibrous metaplasia (Frezzotti et al. 1990). Migration of these cells toward the center of the previously acellular posterior capsule together with the synthesis of matrix components results in light scatter, and the associated opacification in the visual axis reduces visual acuity. The cells move posteriorly along the intact capsule and form bladder cells and fibrous plaques. The two morphological distinct types of PCO are *fibrosis* and Elschnig's *pearls*, which occur independently or in combination. In addition, cataract extraction procedures may result in the formation of an equatorial Soemmerring's ring.

5.5.7.2.1
Fibrosis-Type PCO

Residual lens epithelial cells that are still attached to the anterior capsule after cataract extraction are thought to be the predominant cells involved in the formation of fibrous membranes. Remnant epithelial cells on the anterior capsule differentiate under the influence of growth factors in the aqueous and vitreous into *spindle-shaped, fibroblast-like cells* (myofibroblasts), which express alpha-smooth muscle actin and become contractile. These fibroblastic cells proliferate and migrate onto the posterior capsule to form a multilayered cellular layer that secretes extracellular matrix components and basal lamina-like material. Cellular contraction results in the formation of numerous folds and wrinkles in the posterior capsule. No significant visual loss occurs until the cells migrate into the visual axis (Fig. 5.5.34).

Transdifferentiation of lens epithelial cells into fibroblast-like cells also can cause opacification of the anterior capsule (anterior capsule fibrosis). In some cases of anterior capsule fibrosis, the anterior capsule contracts centrifugally, which enlarges the capsular opening. Contraction of the anterior capsule, however,

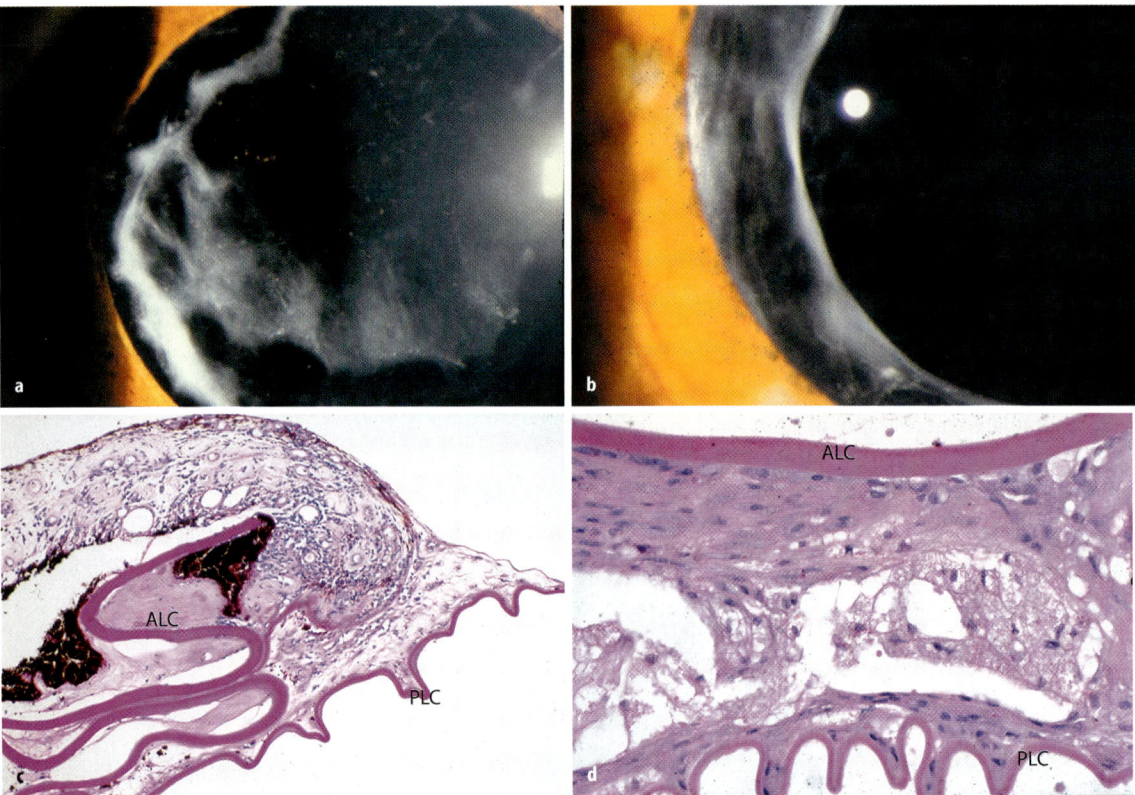

Fig. 5.5.34. Fibrosis of the posterior and anterior capsule following extracapsular cataract surgery. **a** Fibrous-type posterior capsule opacification. **b** Anterior capsule fibrosis. **c, d** Fibrous metaplasia of the equatorial lens epithelium with formation of collagenous connective tissue between anterior and posterior lens capsule with posterior synechiae (*ALC* anterior lens capsule, *PLC* posterior lens capsule) (PAS) (see also Fig. 5.5.5)

normally is centripetal, which shrinks the anterior capsular opening (capsule contraction syndrome). Vision is reduced only if the anterior capsular flap obscures the visual axis, but this can be corrected by making small radial incisions in the anterior capsule. Opening of these fibrotic plaques with the Nd:YAG laser requires higher energy because of their firm consistency.

5.5.7.2.2
Pearl-Type PCO

The pearls formed in this type of PCO are identical in appearance to Wedl bladder cells involved in the formation of posterior subcapsular cataracts. It is believed that residual lens epithelial cells in the equatorial region of the capsule are the predominant cells involved in the formation of pearls. Clinically, cases of pearl formation occur somewhat *later* (up to 5 years postoperatively) than those of fibrosis (2–6 months postoperatively). Pearls were first observed by Elschnig in 1911 and are referred to as *Elschnig's pearls*. Newly formed lens fibers form a mass of large, globular nucleated cells, loosely connected and piled on top of each other. The diameters of these cells are in the range of 5–120 μm. Each pearl represents the aberrant attempt of one epithelial cell to differentiate into a new lens fiber. Visual acuity is affected only if the pearls protrude into the center of the posterior capsule (Fig. 5.5.35).

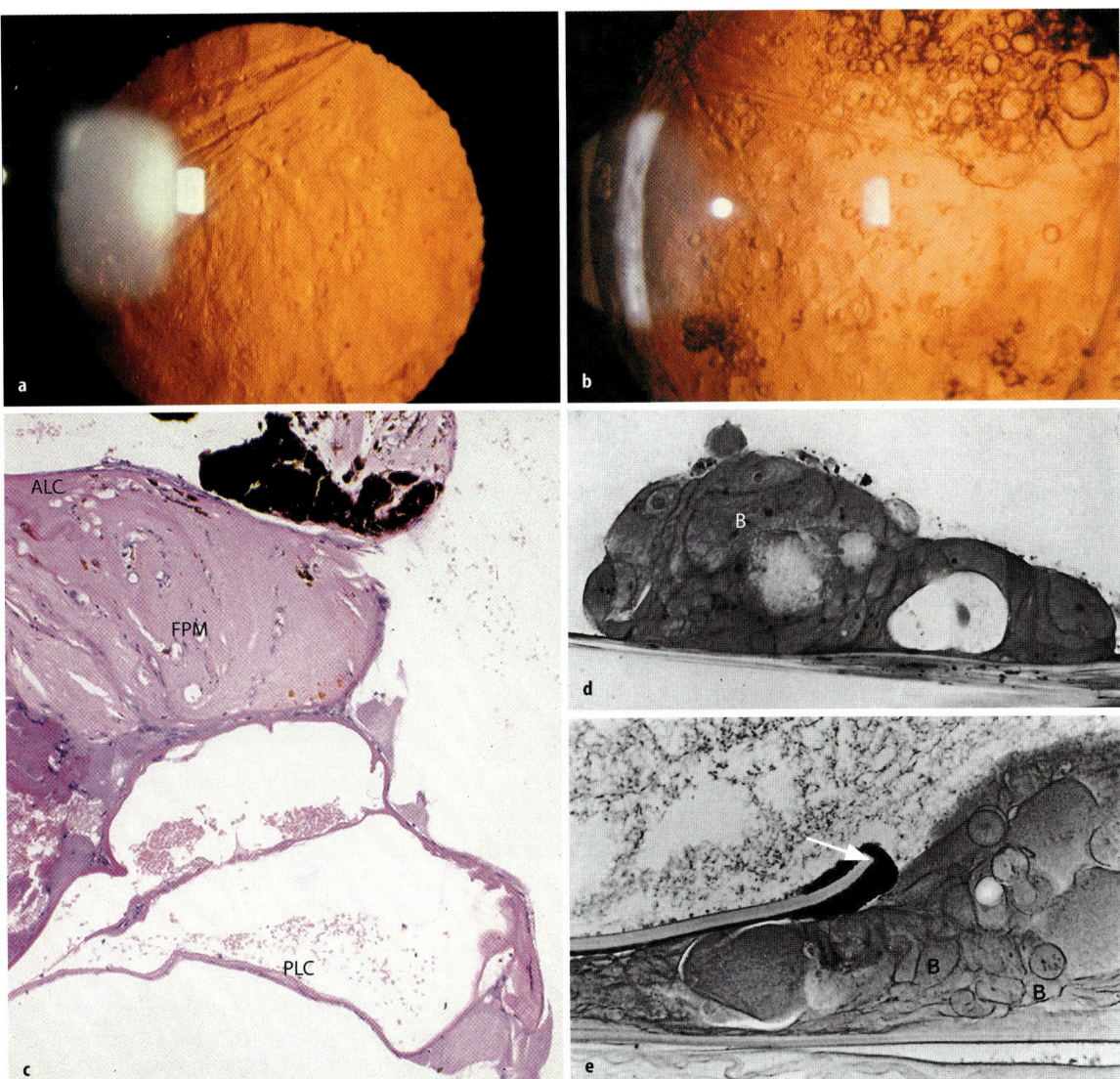

Fig. 5.5.35. Pearl-type posterior capsule opacification. **a, b** Elschnig's pearls on the posterior capsule. **c** Secondary cataract showing a mixture of bladder cells and fibrosis between anterior (*ALC*) and posterior (*PLC*) lens capsule. **d, e** Accumulation of proliferating lens epithelial cells and bladder cells (*B*) on the posterior lens capsule; iris pigment epithelium has entered the lens through the opening of the anterior lens capsule (*arrow*). Fibrous pseudometaplasia (*FPM*)

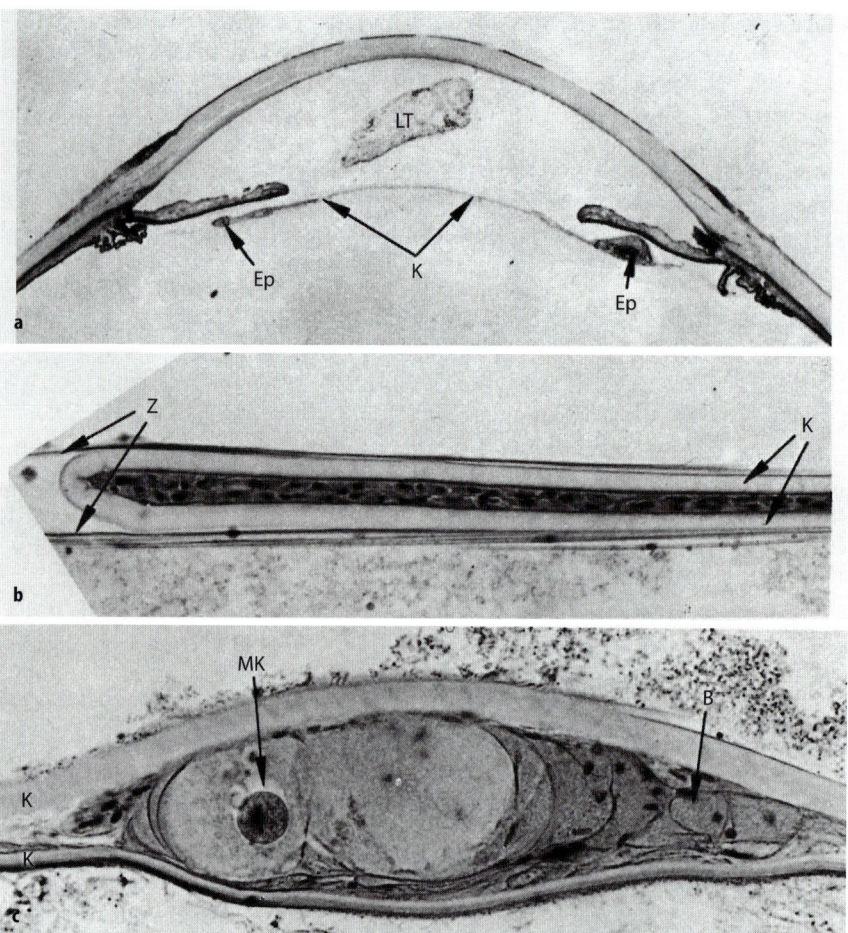

Fig. 5.5.36. Soemmerring's ring cataract. **a** Advanced proliferation of the lens epithelium (*Ep*) in the equatorial region and bare lens capsule (*K*) crossing the pupillary aperture; lens tissue in anterior chamber (*LT*). **b** Double layer of lens epithelium between the anterior and posterior lens capsule (*K*) in the equatorial region (*Z* zonular fibers). **c** Bladder cells (*B*) and morgagnian droplets (*MK*) between the anterior and posterior lens capsule (*K*) in the equatorial region

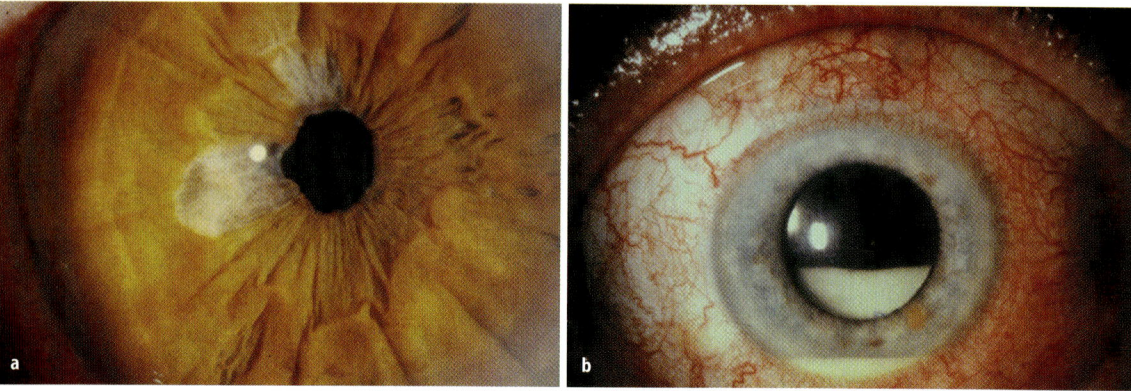

Fig. 5.5.37. Potential complications of cataract surgery. **a** Damage to the iris stroma by phacoemulsification tip suction. **b** Postoperative chronic endophthalmitis with hypopyon in anterior chamber and between pseudophakos and posterior lens capsule (courtesy: H. Wenkel)

5.5.7.2.3
Soemmerring's Ring

Soemmerring first noticed PCO in humans in 1828. After cataract extraction, the cut edge of the remaining anterior capsular flap may attach itself to the posterior capsule within approximately 4 weeks postoperatively, through the production of fibrous tissue. Any residual cortical fibers and epithelial cells, therefore, are trapped within this sealed structure. The equatorial cells retain the capacity to proliferate and differentiate into lens fibers and to produce matrix components filling the space between the anterior and the posterior capsule. This results in the formation of a ring. Because the ring forms at the periphery of the lens, vision is not affected. The true seal needed for the formation of Soemmerring's ring occurs only if the cut edge of the anterior capsule comes into contact with the posterior capsule, because either the IOL optic is smaller than the opening or the capsule has retracted beyond the edge of the optic (Fig. 5.5.36).

The ring has two important functions. First, the haptics of an implanted IOL, which extend to the equator of the capsular bag, are held in place, which prevents decentration. Second, the early fibrosis which is known to seal the capsular surfaces may help to contain the Elschnig's pearls by enhancing the seal between these two surfaces. Some surgeons, therefore, believe that to keep the cut edge of the anterior capsular flap in *front of the optic* will ensure that the residual cells are kept further away from the center of the posterior capsule and thus reduce the incidence of PCO.

5.5.7.2.4
Other Causes of PCO

Cell types other than lens epithelial cells may be involved in PCO formation. Cataract surgery is associated with a breakdown of the blood-aqueous barrier, allowing inflammatory cells, erythrocytes, and many other components to be released from the blood into the aqueous humor. This elicits an inflammatory response of variable severity, which may be increased by the implantation of an IOL. This foreign body reaction elicits an immune response that involves many different cell types including polymorphonuclear leukocytes, giant cells, and fibroblasts. As a result, collagen is deposited onto the IOL and the capsule, which causes opacities, and fine wrinkles may form in the posterior capsule. In most cases, however, this inflammatory response is clinically insignificant.

5.5.7.2.5
Prevention and Treatment of PCO

As yet there is *no reliable treatment* to prevent PCO. Experimental approaches being assessed include refinement of surgical technique, changes to the IOL design, modifications of the IOL surface, and the development of pharmacological strategies either to kill all residual epithelial cells or to prevent their proliferation and migration. Ideally, the best way to prevent PCO would be to remove all the lens epithelial cells and the cortical remnants at the time of surgery. Many different approaches have been used with variable success. Infusion of sterile saline or water under the capsule ruptures many, if not all, of residual epithelial cells (Maloof et al. 2005). Anterior capsule cleaning with an ultrasonographic irrigating scratcher removes all fibers and reduces the number of residual epithelial cells. Pharmacologic agents, antimetabolites, and other agents have been used to try to reduce the proliferative capacity of lens epithelial cells and hence PCO.

An anterior capsulectomy can be considered an *epithelial wound* creating a stimulus to close the defect by lens epithelial proliferation, migration and pseudometaplasia. Originally the consensus was, that to remove more of the anterior capsule would remove more lens epithelial cells and therefore reduce the risk of PCO. It is now thought that the wider the opening, the greater the number of epithelial cells released from contact inhibition, and therefore the greater the number of cells capable of proliferation and migration onto the posterior capsule. Cases of PCO are less prevalent in patients who undergo a circular capsulorrhexis, because this technique enhances the efficiency of hydrodissection, subsequent cortical clean-up and shortens the lens of the "capsule wound." The implantation of a posterior chamber IOL into the capsular bag after cataract extraction is known to reduce the likelihood that a patient will develop PCO, because the IOL acts as a mechanical barrier and may delay the migration of cells around and into the center of the posterior capsule.

Patients who develop PCO with significantly impaired vision need a posterior capsulotomy achieved by Nd:YAG laser. Complications of this procedure include transient and long-term IOP rise, dislocation of the lens implant, rupture of the anterior vitreous face and anterior displacement of the vitreous, retinal detachment, and cystoid macular edema. The incidence of retinal detachment after Nd:YAG laser capsulotomy is approximately 1%.

5.5.7.3
Pseudophakia and Complications

Correction of aphakia after cataract extraction has long been a dream of mankind which was only recently fulfilled after a long period of trial and error between the secular breakthrough of implantation of the first artificial lens (by Ridley in 1949) and today's standardized extracapsular cataract extraction usually with phakoemulsification avoiding a large corneoscleral wound or after nuclear expression with IOL implantation.

Aside from multiple steps in technical details regarding lens design, medications, instrumentation, microscopes, temperature of the infusion fluid (Machemer, see chapter 4), *two pioneering breakthroughs* enabled the current state of the art:

Kelman (1967) modified the aspiration/irrigation system of the Fuchs' syringe by developing the technique of *phacoemulsification* in the 1960s. Fankhauser et al. (1981) pioneered the use of the *YAG laser* for clearing the opacities created by axial secondary cataract without opening the eye.

In the first 20 years after Ridley, the problem of fixation of the IOL implant had to be explored: Mobile lens implants caused secondary glaucomas with open and closed angle, corneal endothelial decompensation and retinal complications. During the same time methods to sterilize the IOL implant were developed. Initially, sterilization was achieved by acid, lye and other toxic substances. Remnants of this toxic material caused severe inflammation inside the eye, a so-called *toxic lens syndrome*. This can be avoided by using radiation for sterilization of the lens implant. However, the "toxic anterior segment syndrome (TASS)" still may represent a problem today.

Later on we learned that infectious agents may cause a syndrome that resembles "toxic lens syndrome" but originates from *infection with slow growing bacteria and fungi and in fact is a "subacute or chronic postoperative endophthalmitis"* that becomes worse after treatment with corticosteroids and nonsteroidal inflammatory agents.

Today, fixation of the IOL implant inside the lens capsule is standard; sterilization is achieved by radiation and the transparency of the IOL implants intraocularly appears to be stable even after decades. New materials always have the risk of creating new surprises and require careful preclinical and clinical studies before their general introduction into clinical practice.

Current clinical research is focusing on methods to reduce the occurrence of secondary cataract and to achieve the dream of true pseudophakic accommodation by multifocal or refractive IOL implants in order to address the problems of presbyopia. However, the progressive age-related fibrosis of the ciliary muscle – as the engine of accommodation – implies a certain skepticism as to whether this can be achieved (Weale 2005). On the other hand the potential of new nanotechnology to develop miniature accommodative devices to be placed intraocularly may be promising in the future.

5.5.7.3.1
True Pseudophakic Accommodation and Pseudoaccommodation

These two entities need to be distinguished: *Pseudoaccommodation* may be achieved by a very narrow pupil, or myopic astigmatism and can occur in aphakic, phakic and pseudophakic eyes. *True pseudophakic accommodation* would depend on the residual action of the ciliary muscle (Fig. 5.4.3) on the pseudophakos to contribute to an alteration of the optical surfaces of the pseudophakos and/or an "axial shift." The former so far has not been proven objectively.

In the future extreme miniaturization of optical devices within the pseudophakos potentially might allow new approaches to compensate for the loss of accommodation after cataract surgery in ways that we cannot imagine today.

5.5.7.4
Complications After Intracapsular Cataract Extraction

The only advantage of intracapsular cataract surgery is the absence of secondary cataract. All other risks – loss of corneal endothelial cells, rate of retinal detachment or wound rupture, cystoid maculopathy, secondary glaucomas, are worse. In addition fixation of the pseudophakos cannot be anchored to the lens capsule and visual rehabilitation is slower.

References (see also page 379)

Apple DJ. Über angeborene Kolobome. Klin Mbl Augenheilk 1979; 174:649–651
Asano N, Schlötzer-Schrehardt U, Dörfler S, Naumann GOH. Ultrastructure of contusion cataract. Arch Ophthalmol 1995; 113:210–215
Assia EI, Apple DJ, Morgan RC, Legler UF, Brown SJ. The relationship between the stretching capability of the anterior capsule and zonules. Invest Ophthalmol Vis Sci 1991; 32: 2835–2839
Assia EI, Apple DJ. Side-view analysis of the lens. I. The crystalline lens and the evacuated bag. Arch Ophthalmol 1992a; 110: 89–93
Assia EI, Apple DJ. Side-view analysis of the lens. II. Positioning of intraocular lenses. Arch Ophthalmol 1992b; 110: 94–97
Barraquer J. Enzymatic zonulolysis in lens extraction. Arch Ophthalmol 1961; 66: 6–11
Barraquer RI, Michael R, Abreu R, Lamarca J, Tressera F. Human lens capsule thickness as a function of age and location along the sagittal lens perimeter. Invest Ophthalmol Vis Sci 2006; 47: 2053–2060
Bartholomew RS. Lens displacement associated with pseudocapsular exfoliation. A report on 19 cases in the southern Bantu. Br J Ophthalmol 1970; 54:744–750
Benedek GB. Why is the lens transparent? Nature 1983; 302:383–384
Berman ER. Biochemistry of cataracts. In: Garner A, Klintworth GK, Eds. Pathobiology of Ocular Disease. A Dynamic Approach. New York: Marcel Dekker Inc, 1994
Bourne RR, Minassian DC, Dart JK, Rosen P, Kaushal S, Wingate N. Effect of cataract surgery on the corneal endothelium: modern phacoemulsification compared with extracapsular cataract surgery. Ophthalmology 2004; 111: 679–685
Bron AJ, Vrensen GFJM, Koretz J, Maraini G, Harding JJ. The ageing lens. Ophthalmologica 2000; 214: 86–104
Burian HM, von Noorden GK, Ponseti IV. Chamber angle anomalies in systemic connective tissue disorders. Arch Ophthalmol 1960; 64: 671–680
Cashwell LF Jr, Holleman IL, Weaver RG, van Rens GH. Idiopathic true exfoliation of the lens capsule. Ophthalmology 1989; 96: 348–351
Cross HE, Jensen AD. Ocular manifestations in the Marfan syndrome and homocystinuria. Am J Ophthalmol 1973; 75:405–420
Cruysberg JR, Pinckers A. Ectopia lentis et pupillae in three generations. Br J Ophthalmol 1995; 79: 135–138
Cugati S, Mitchell P, Rochtchina E, Tan AG, Smith W, Wang JJ. Cataract surgery and the 10-year incidence of age-related maculopathy: the Blue Mountains Eye Study. Ophthalmology 2006; 113: 2020–2025

Dawczynski J, Strobel J. "The aging lens" – neue Konzepte zum Alterungsprozess der Linse. Ophthalmologe 2006; 103: 759–764

Donnenfeld ED. Eyenet (Feb) 2007, 29–30

Erie JC, Raecker MA, Baratz KH, Schleck CD, Burke JP, Robertson DM. Risk of retinal detachment after cataract extraction, 1980–2004: a population-based study. Ophthalmology 2006; 113: 2026–2032

Eshagian J. Human posterior subcapsular cataracts. Trans Ophthalmol Soc UK 1982; 102:364–368

Fankhauser F, Roussel P, Steffen J, van der Zypen E, Chrenkova A. Clinical studies on the efficiency of high power laser radiation upon some structures of the anterior segment of the eye. First experiences of the treatment of some pathological conditions of the anterior segment of the human eye by means of a Q-switched laser system. Int Ophthalmol 1981; 3: 129–139

Farnsworth PN, Shyne SE. Anterior zonular shifts with age. Exp Eye Res 1979; 28: 291–297

Ferguson VM, Spalton DJ. Continued breakdown of the blood aqueous barrier following cataract surgery. Br J Ophthalmol 1992; 76: 453–456

Fisher RF, Pettet BE. The postnatal growth of the capsule of the human crystalline lens. J Anat 1972; 112: 207–214

Font RL, Brownstein S. A light and electron microscopic study of anterior subcapsular cataracts. Am J Ophthalmol 1974; 78:972–984

Freissler K, Küchle M, Naumann GOH. Spontaneous dislocation of the lens in pseudoexfoliation syndrome. Arch Ophthalmol 1995; 113: 1095–1096

Frezzotti R, Caporossi A, Mastrangelo D, Hadjistilianou T, Tosi P, Cintorino M, Minacci C. Pathogenesis of posterior capsular opacification. Part II: Histopathological and in vitro culture findings. J Cataract Refract Surg 1990; 16: 353–360

Gibbs ML, Jacobs M, Wilkie AOM, Taylor D. Posterior lenticonus: clinical patterns and genetics. J Pediatr Ophthalmol Strabismus 1993; 30:171–175

Goldberg MF. Persistent fetal vasculature (PFV): an integrated interpretation of signs and symptoms associated with persistent hyperplastic primary vitreous (PHPV). LIV Edward Jackson Memorial Lecture. Am J Ophthalmol. 1997 Nov; 124(5):587–626

Goldstein LE, Muffat JA, Cherny RA, Moir RD, Ericsson MH, Huang X, Mavros C, Coccia JA, Faget KY, Fitch KA, Masters CL, Tanzi RE, Chylack LT, Bush AI. Cytosolic beta-amyloid deposition and supranuclear cataracts in lenses from people with Alzheimer's disease. Lancet 2003; 361(9365): 1258–1265

Guggenmoos-Holzmann I, Engel B, Henke V, Naumann GOH. Cell density of human lens epithelium in women higher than in men. Invest Ophthalmol Vis Sci 1989; 30:330–332

Guzek JP, Holm M, Cotter JB, Cameron JA, Rademaker WJ, Wissinger DH, Tonjum AM, Sleeper LA. Risk factors for intraoperative complications in 1000 extracapsular cataract cases. Ophthalmology 1987; 94: 461–466

Hagee MJ. Homocystinuria and ectopia lentis. J Am Optom Assoc 1984; 55: 269–276

Halbert SP, Manski W. Biological aspects of autoimmune reactions in the lens. Invest Ophthalmol 1965; 4:516–530

Hayashi H, Hayashi K, Nakao F, Hayashi F. Anterior capsule contraction and intraocular lens dislocation in eyes with pseudoexfoliation syndrome. Br J Ophthalmol 1998; 82: 1429–1432

Hockwin O. Scheimpflug photography of the lens. Fortschr Ophthalmol 1989; 84: 304–311

Hockwin O. Biochemistry of the lens. Retrospect of thematic and methodologic developments, prospects for future research. Klin Monatsbl Augenheilkd 1993; 202: 544–551

Hyams M, Mathalone N, Herskovitz M, Hod Y, Israeli D, Geyer O. Intraoperative complications of phacoemulsification in eyes with and without pseudoexfoliation. J Cataract Refract Surg 2005; 31: 1002–1005

Jehan FS, Mamalis N, Crandall AS. Spontaneous late dislocation of intraocular lens within the capsular bag in pseudoexfoliation patients. Ophthalmology 2001; 108: 1727–1731

Jensen AD, Cross HE, Paton D. Ocular complications in the Weill-Marchesani syndrome. Am J Ophthalmol 1974; 77: 261–269

Jünemann A, Küchle M, Händel A, Naumann GOH. Kataraktchirurgie bei Nanophthalmus mit einer Bulbuslänge unter 20,5 mm. Klin Monatsbl Augenheilkd 1998; 212: 13–22

Kainulainen K, Karttunen L, Puhakka L, Sakai L, Peltonen L. Mutations in the fibrillin gene responsible for dominant ectopia lentis and neonatal Marfan syndrome. Nat Genet 1994; 6: 64–69

Karim AKA, Jacob TJC, Thompson GM. The human anterior lens capsule: cell density, morphology, and mitotic index in normal and cataractous lenses. Exp Eye Res 1987; 45:865–874

Karp CL, Fazio JR, Culbertson WW, Green WR. True exfoliation of the lens capsule. Arch Ophthalmol 1999; 117: 1078–1080

Kelman CD. Phaco-emulsification and aspiration. A new technique of cataract removal. A preliminary report. Am J Ophthalmol 1967; 64: 23–35

Kelman CD. Symposium: Phacoemulsification. History of emulsification and aspiration of senile cataracts. Trans Am Acad Ophthalmol Otolaryngol 1974; 78: OP5–13

Khalil M, Saheb N. Posterior lenticonus. Ophthalmology 1984; 91: 1429–1430

Konofsky K, Naumann GOH, Guggenmoos-Holzmann I. Cell density and sex chromatin in lens epithelium of human cataracts. Quantitative studies in flat preparation. Ophthalmology 1987; 94:875–880

Krag S, Olsen T, Andreassen TT. Biomechanical characteristics of the human anterior lens capsule in relation to age. Invest Ophthalmol Vis Sci 1997; 38: 357–363

Krag S, Andreassen TT. Mechanical properties of the human posterior lens capsule. Invest Ophthalmol Vis Sci 2003; 44: 691–696

Küchle M, Amberg A, Martus P, Nguyen NX, Naumann GOH. Pseudoexfoliation syndrome and secondary cataract. Br J Ophthalmol 1997; 81: 862–866

Kuszak JR, Ennesser CA, Umlas J et al. The ultrastructure of fiber cells in primate lenses: A model for studying membrane senescence. J Ultrastruct Mol Struct Res 1988; 100:60–74

Kuwabara T. The maturation of the lens cell: a morphologic study. Exp Eye Res 1975; 20:427–443

Lang GK, Naumann GOH. Zur Klinik und Differentialdiagnose des Lentiglobus posterior (Bericht über vier Kinder). Klin Monatsbl Augenheilkd 1983; 183: 489–492

Lee B, Godfrey M, Vitale E et al. Linkage of Marfan syndrome and a phenotypically related disorder to two different fibrillin genes. Nature 1991; 352:330–334

Lundström M, Wejde G, Steveni U et al. Endophthalmitis after Cataract Surgery: A Nation-wide study. Ophthalmology 2007; 114:866–870

Malbran ES, Croxatto JO, D'Alessandro C, Charles DE. Genetic spontaneous late subluxation of the lens. A study of two families. Ophthalmology 1989; 96: 223–229

Maloof AJ, Pandey SK, Neilson G, Milverton EJ. Selective death of lens epithelial cells using demineralized water and Triton X-100 with PerfectCapsule sealed capsule irrigation: a histological study in rabbit eyes. Arch Ophthalmol 2005; 123: 1378–1384

Marak GE Jr. Phacoanaphylactic endophthalmitis. Surv Ophthalmol 1992; 36:325–3

Marshall J, Beaconsfield M, Rothery S. The anatomy and development of the human lens and zonules. Trans Ophthalmol Soc UK 1982; 102 Pt 3: 423–440

Maumenee IH. The eye in the Marfan syndrome. Trans Am Ophthalmol Soc 1981; 79:684

Mencucci R, Ponchietti C, Virgili G, Giansanti F, Menchini U. Corneal endothelial damage after cataract surgery: Microincision versus standard technique. J Cataract Refract Surg 2006; 32: 1351–1354

Mohan PS, Spiro RG. Macromolecular organization of basement membranes. Characterization and comparison of glomerular basement membrane and lens capsule components by immunochemical and lectin affinity procedures. J Biol Chem 1986; 261:4328–4336

Moroi SE, Lark KK, Sieving PA, Nouri-Mahdavi K, Schlötzer-Schrehardt U, Katz GJ, Ritch R. Long anterior zonules and pigment dispersion. Am J Ophthalmol 2003;136:1176–1178

Mudd SH, Finkelstein JD, Irreverre F et al. Homocystinuria: an enzymatic defect. Science 1964; 143:1443–1445

Naumann GOH, Ortbauer R, Witzenhausen R. Candida albicans-endophthalmitis nach Kataraktextraktion. Ophthalmologica 1971; 162: 160–166

Naumann GOH, Küchle M, Schönherr U. Pseudoexfoliation syndrome as a risk factor for vitreous loss in extracapsular cataract extraction. Fortschr Ophthalmol 1989; 86: 543–545

Nelson LB, Maumenee IH. Ectopia lentis. Surv Ophthalmol 1982; 27: 143–160

Nemet AY, Assia EI, Apple DJ, Barequet IS. Current concepts of ocular manifestations in Marfan syndrome. Surv Ophthalmol 2006; 51: 561–575

Ohrloff C, Hockwin O. Lens metabolism and aging: enzyme activities and enzyme alterations in lenses of different species during the process of aging. J Gerontol 1983; 38: 271–277

Pau H, Novotny GEK. Ultrastructural investigations on anterior capsular cataract. Cellular elements and their relationship to basement membrane and collagen synthesis. Graefes Arch Clin Exp Ophthalmol 1985; 223:41–46

Raviola G. The fine structure of the ciliary zonule and ciliary epithelium. With special regard to the organization and insertion of the zonular fibers. Invest Ophthalmol 1971; 10: 851–869

Resnikoff S, Pascolini D, Etya'ale D, Kocur I, Pararajasegaram R, Pokharel GP, Mariotti SP. Global data on visual impairment in the year 2002. Bull World Health Organ 2004; 82: 844–851

Rohen JW. Scanning electron microscopic studies of the zonular apparatus in human and monkey eyes. Invest Ophthalmol Vis Sci 1979; 18:133–144

Saber HR, Butler TJ, Cottrell DG. Resistance of the human posterior lens capsule and zonules to disruption. J Cataract Refract Surg 1998; 24: 536–542

Sakabe I, Oshika T, Lim SJ, Apple DJ. Anterior shift of zonular insertion onto the anterior surface of human crystalline lens with age. Ophthalmology 1998; 105: 295–299

Schlötzer-Schrehardt U, Naumann GOH. A histopathologic study of zonular instability in pseudoexfoliation syndrome. Am J Ophthalmol 1994; 118:730–743

Schneider H, Guthoff R. Evidenzbasierte Beobachtungen zu akkommodativen Kunstlinsen. Klin Monatsbl Augenheilkd 2005: 222: 357–360

Seland JH. The lens capsule and zonulae. Acta Ophthalmol Suppl. 1992; 205: 7–12

Skuta GL, Parrish RK 2nd, Hodapp E, Forster RK, Rockwood EJ. Zonular dialysis during extracapsular cataract extraction in pseudoexfoliation syndrome. Arch Ophthalmol 1987; 105: 632–634

Sommer A. Cataracts as an epidemiologic problem. Am J Ophthalmol 1977; 83:334–339

Stark WJ, Streeten BW. The anterior capsulotomy of extracapsular cataract extraction. Ophthalmic Surg 1984; 15: 911–917

Stirling RJ, Griffiths PG. Scanning EM studies of normal human lens fibres and fibres from nuclear cataracts. Eye 1991; 5:86–9

Streeten BW, Robinson MR, Wallace R, Jones DB. Lens capsule abnormalities in Alport's syndrome. Arch Ophthalmol 1987;105:1693–1697

Taban M, Behrens A, Newcomb RL, Nobe MY, Saedi G, Sweet PM, McDonnell PJ. Acute endophthalmitis following cataract surgery. Arch Ophthalmol 2005; 123: 613–620

Thylefors B. Avoidable blindness. Bull World Health Organ 1999; 77: 453

Tripathi RC, Tripathi BJ. Lens morphology, aging, and cataract. J Gerontol 1983; 38:258–270

Tseng SH, Yen JS, Chien HL. Lens epithelium in senile cataract. J Formos Med Assoc 1994; 93:93–98

Völcker HE. Kontusionskatarakt und Linsenluxation. Fortschr Ophthalmol 1984; 81:308–311

von Below H, Wilk CM, Schaal KP, Naumann GOH. Rhodococcus luteus and Rhodococcus erythropolis chronic endophthalmitis after lens implantation. Am J Ophthalmol 1991; 112: 596–597

von Sallmann L, Grimes P, McElvain N. Aspects of mitotic activity in relation to cell proliferation in the lens epithelium. Exp Eye Res 1962; 1:449–456

Vrensen GF. Aging of the human eye lens – a morphological point of view. Comp Biochem Physiol A Physiol 1995; 111: 519–532

Vrensen GF, Kappelhof J, Willekens B. Morphology of the aging human lens. Lens Eye Tox Res 1990; 7: 1–30

Wallace RN, Streeten BW, Hanna RB. Rotary shadowing of elastic system microfibrils in the ocular zonule, vitreous, and ligamentum nuchae. Curr Eye Res 1991; 10: 99–109

Wang JJ, Klein R, Smith W, Klein BE, Tomany S, Mitchell P. Cataract surgery and the 5-year incidence of late-stage age-related maculopathy: pooled findings from the Beaver Dam and Blue Mountains eye studies. Ophthalmology 2003; 110: 1960–1967

Weale RA. The accommodation of lens implants. Ophthalmic Res 2005; 37: 156–158

Retina and Vitreous

A.M. Joussen and G.O.H. Naumann
with Contributions by S.E. Coupland, E.R. Tamm, B. Kirchhof, N. Bornfeld

5.6.1
Surgical Anatomy

5.6.1.1
Vitreous Attachments at the Base of the Ora Serrata and Martegiani's Ring

The vitreous body is the largest structure in the eye and comprises about 80% of its volume (Hogan 1971). The fully developed human vitreous consists of a "solid" cortex and a more "fluid" central part. Solid septa extend from the cortex into the vitreous center (Fig. 5.6.1).

During embryonic development the primary vitreous is vascularized and is formed by the ectodermal components derived from the lens epithelial cells, neuroectodermal tissue from the eyecup and mesodermal tissue derived from the hyaloid vasculature.

The primary vitreous is substituted by the secondary vitreous during the early embryogenic phase. A tight contact persists between the vitreous, the posterior lens capsule and the macular area, and to a lesser degree with the major retinal vessels.

In the anterior-posterior direction the vitreous is demarcated by the bursa retrolentalis (room of Berger) between the posterior lens capsule and the anterior vitreous lamina. It is a previtreal and not an intravitreal structure. In the young eye, Berger's space is a potential space since the surfaces of the anterior vitreous lamina and posterior lens capsule are intimately connected. Aging changes cause a gradual separation of the two.

Berger's space is separated from Petit's canal by a circular adhesion band between the anterior vitreous lamina, the posterior lens capsule, and the hyaloideocapsular ligament (ligamentum hyaloideocapsulare) (Wieger 1883).

The hyaloid vessels begin to atrophy at an embryonic length of 40 mm. The only remnant of the primary vitreous is Cloquet's canal, which in the fetal eye accommodates the hyaloid artery. Cloquet's canal was first described in 1818 (Duke Elder 1968), and runs through the central vitreous, originating retrolentally, continuing in an S-shaped, slightly spiralling course through the vitreous and being inserted around the optic nerve head at "Martegiani's ring." Martegiani (1814) noted the absence of vitreous substance at the posterior

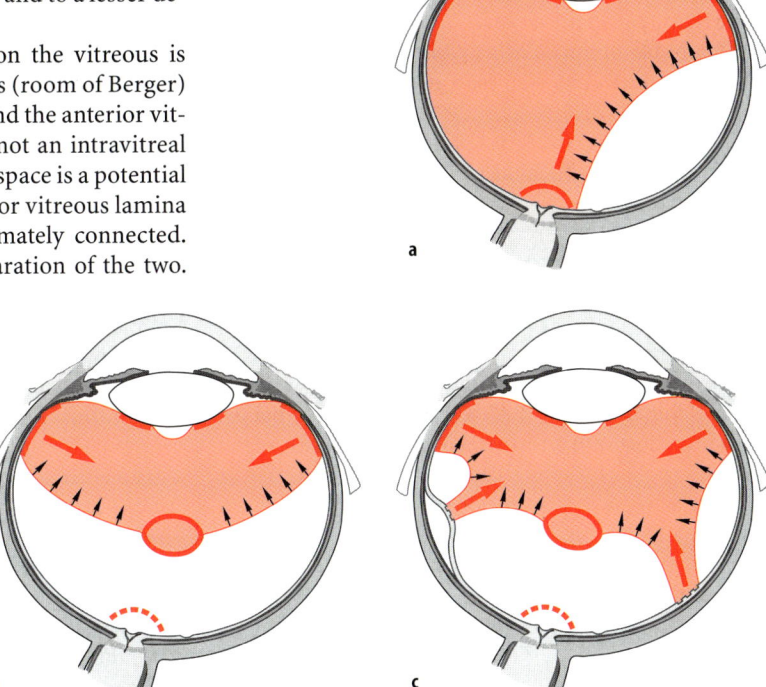

Fig. 5.6.1. Variants of posterior vitreous detachment: **a** Incomplete. **b** Complete with detachment of the Martegiani ring. **c** Incomplete with vitreomacular traction

part of the hyaloid canal. This corresponds with the absence of vitreous cortex at the optic nerve head (Worst 1975).

The tertiary vitreous results from further differentiation. The expansion of the vitreous and the resulting tractional forces are a prerequisite for the development of the retinal pigment epithelium (RPE).

With ageing (particularly in myopic eyes), the vitreous rarely persists as a transparent sphere and there is often a separation from the inner retinal surface, i.e., "detachment of the posterior vitreous face" with "fluid in the subhyaloidal space." After retinal detachment, the vitreous may remain attached to the disc, but if this tears, the vitreous separates and collapses to form a condensed mass which exerts traction on the equatorial retina. Traction may also separate the non-pigmented layer of the ciliary epithelium from the pigmented epithelial layer.

5.6.1.2
Bursa Macularis

Various observations indicate the presence of an area in front of the macula, which has few tissue elements. The extreme fragility of the prefoveal area is apparent from the frequency with which a premacular hole is formed during isolation of the vitreous-lens specimen (Eisner 1971; Sebag 1985; Worst 1975). Sebag and Balazs (Sebag et al. 1985, 1989) found a circular premacular hole in isolated vitreous specimens. Similarly, Kishi and Shimizu (Kishi 1990; Worst 1991) described a pocket in front of the macula. They found a precortical vitreous lacuna in all eyes in which the vitreoretinal attachment was at least partly preserved.

This bursa premacularis (Worst 1975) resembles a vitreoschisis and can suggest a posterior vitreous detachment.

The relevance of the bursa premacularis for macular hole formation has been the subject of controversy (see Sect. 5.6.2.5).

5.6.1.3
Bergmeister Disc

The primary vitreous forms the hyaloid vessels that extend from the optic disc to form the tunica vasculosa lentis. Remnants of the hyaloid vasculature can persist as a Mittendorf spot, mostly seen at the nasal side of the posterior pole of the lens capsule (anterior persistent primary vitreous). A posterior persistent primary vitreous is a cluster of ectodermal glia cells, which normally form the primitive epithelial papillae and enclose the hyaloid artery, covering the surface of the optic disc as a veil of juxtapapillary retinal folds may develop.

5.6.1.4
Potential Subretinal Spaces: Foveolar and Ora Clefts

The retinal photoreceptors and the RPE are bound by acid mucopolysaccharides (which are resistant to hyaluronidase) and the "mechanical" interdigitation like two combs clinging together. These connections are weakened in two areas.

Both predispose to separation of neuroretina and RPE leading to disciform detachments of the macula or rhegmatogenous or exudative detachments.

5.6.1.4.1
Potential "Ora Cleft"

In the retro-ora serrata region rudimentary rods do not strengthen the contact between sensory retina and RPE. This facilitates accumulation of subretinal fluid peripherally, although this does not usually limit visual function. Nevertheless, normal variations, including meridional folds and complexes, enclosed ora bays, or developmental abnormalities such as zonular traction tufts, and other peripheral degenerations (e.g., peripheral cystoid degeneration, paving stone degeneration, pearls of the ora serrata, and pars plana cysts), should be distinguished from lesions prone to rhegmatogenous detachment (see Sect. 5.6.2.1). The above-described normal variations and developmental abnormalities are not of clinical significance.

5.6.1.4.2
Potential "Foveola Cleft"

By a different mechanism in the area of the potential foveola cleft, cones are predominant and these are less intertwined with the RPE than rods.

In contrast to peripheral processes, opened subretinal spaces may be relevant to visual function if they are located in the foveal area. In central serous retinopathy involving the center of the fovea, there is an early decrease in visual acuity (see Sect. 5.6.2.3). In eyes with macula-off retinal detachments, a complete foveal reattachment subsequently occurs without delay following vitrectomy. In contrast, subfoveal fluid may persist subclinically for several months in patients with an encircling buckle who have been operated on (Wolfensberger et al. 2004).

Subretinal fluid in a preoperatively uninvolved macula can be found after successful treatment of rhegmatogenous retinal detachment in eyes in which the fovea initially appeared to be attached on fundoscopy. Foveal detachments postoperatively associated with reduced visual acuity may develop after successful retinal reattachment surgery in eyes with previously attached macula (Gibran et al. 2005). The visual acuity does not reach the preoperative levels and may explain, in part, the delayed improvement in visual acuity after successful scleral buckling (Hagimura et al. 2002; Theodossiadis et al. 2003).

5.6.1.5
Horizontal Barriers ("*Leitstrukturen*")

The retina consists of a complex structure of neuronal and vascular cells separated and organized by different barriers (Fig. 5.6.2). Pathological processes usually extend along the planes of anatomical barriers. The retina is separated by different "horizontal" and vertical structures that explain the extent and shape of exudate hemorrhages or infarcts that we can analyze with the ophthalmoscope (Fig. 5.6.3).

The *inner limiting membrane* (ILM) separates the vitreous cavity from the retinal layers. Essentially it represents the basement membrane of the Müller cells.

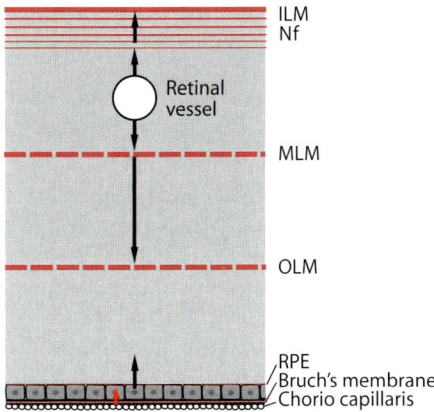

Fig. 5.6.3. Horizontal barriers (*Leitstrukturen*) and the preformed spaces

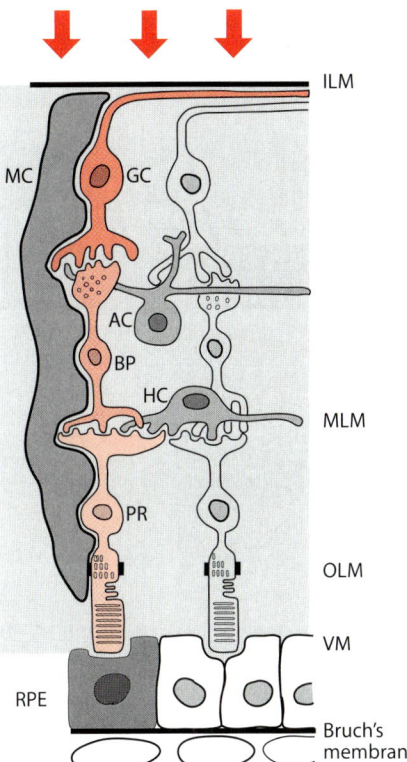

Fig. 5.6.2. Extremely simplified structural elements of the extraordinarily complex retina: photoreceptors (*PR*), bipolar cells (*BC*), ganglion cells (*GC*) with axons to optic nerve (*thin arrow*), Müller cells (*MC*), retinal pigment epithelium (*RPE*). True basement membranes: internal limiting membrane (*ILM*) of MC, Bruch's membrane of RPE. So-called membranes formed by intercellular connections: "Verhoeff membrane" (*VM*) consisting of zonular occludentes of apical region of RPE, outer limiting membrane (*OLM*) by outer segments of PR and Müller cells, middle limiting membrane (*MLM*), amacrine cells (*AM*), horizontal cells (*HC*). *Neuronal convergence* from 100 million photoreceptors to 1 million GC. *Double vascular supply* of retina from choroid (100 times higher) and retinal vessels nourishing only inner retinal layers

The structure and development of the ILM are discussed in Sect. 5.6.3.3.

Histologically, both the *intermediate (middle) limiting membrane* (MLM) and the *outer limiting membrane* (OLM) of the retina can be recognized. However, these are not true membranes in the strict sense, but intercellular connections: The so-called MLM results from the synaptic connection from photoreceptors to the bipolar layer, and the OLM from the zonulae occludentes binding the inner segments of photoreceptors and Müller cells. By virtue of their structural organization, they act as barriers against the spread of pathological processes throughout the retina (e.g., hemorrhage, exudates).

A horizontal barrier is also formed by the embryonic optic ventricle between the RPE and photoreceptors. This potential space reopens in retinal detachment (see Sect. 5.6.2.3).

The retina is separated from the choroid by the retinal pigment epithelial cells (RPE cells), which form a monolayer linked by the formation of tight junction molecules resembling the outer blood-retinal barrier (Verhoeff membrane; see Sects. 5.6.3.6, 5.6.4.1). They are separated from the choroid by the multilayered Bruch's membrane.

Clinically, horizontal barriers are relevant in interpreting the phenotype in disciform processes, e.g., in RPE detachments as seen in age-related macular degeneration; intraretinal hemorrhages and/or exudates along the axonal structures as seen in central retinal vein occlusion; and circinate lipid assembly along the Henle fibers. In X-linked retinoschisis, a star like cleft forms between the radial Henle fibers (see Chapter 12 of Naumann et al. 1980).

5.6.1.6
Vertical Barriers ("*Leitstrukturen*") (Fig. 5.6.4)

Vertically, the retina is separated by the neuronal chain consisting of photoreceptor neuronal cells of the bipolar layer and finally ganglion cells. The Müller cells extending between the ILM and OLM further contribute to a vertical orientation.

Due to lack of a large intercellular space, the vertical "barriers" limit expansion of pathological processes such as hemorrhages or cystic degeneration. They appear as round cavities and holes.

In the fovea, bipolar and ganglion cells are pulled to the side and the vertical barriers in the perifovea are narrowed, building the radial Henle's layer. Henle's layer leads to the characteristic star-like appearance of degenerative processes of the macula and also to dystrophic entities such as juvenile retinoschisis.

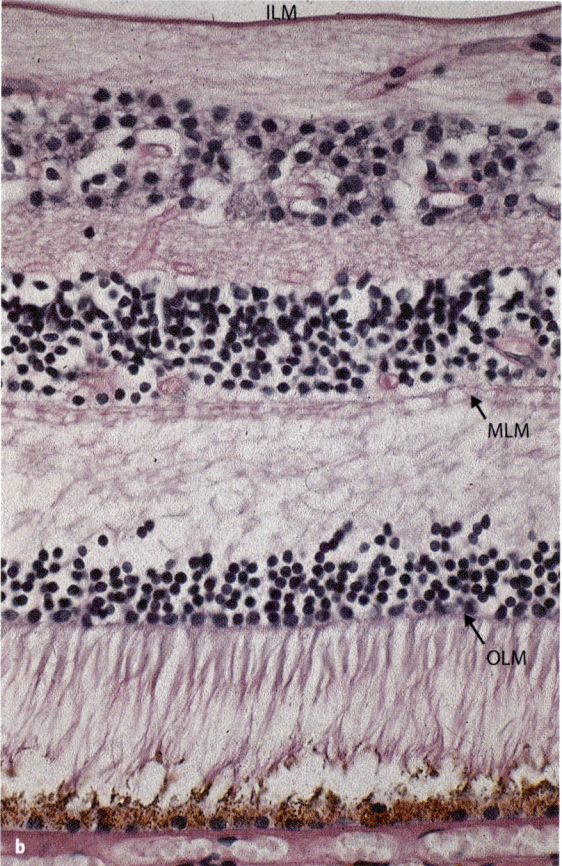

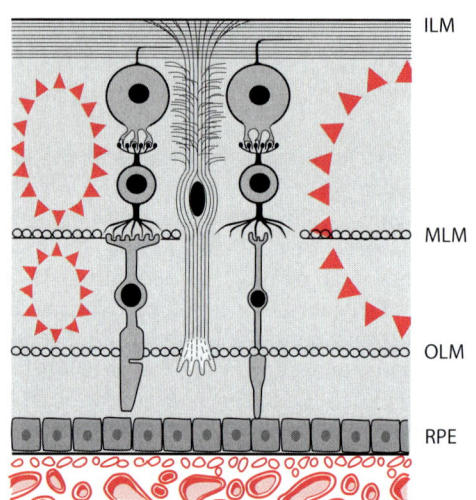

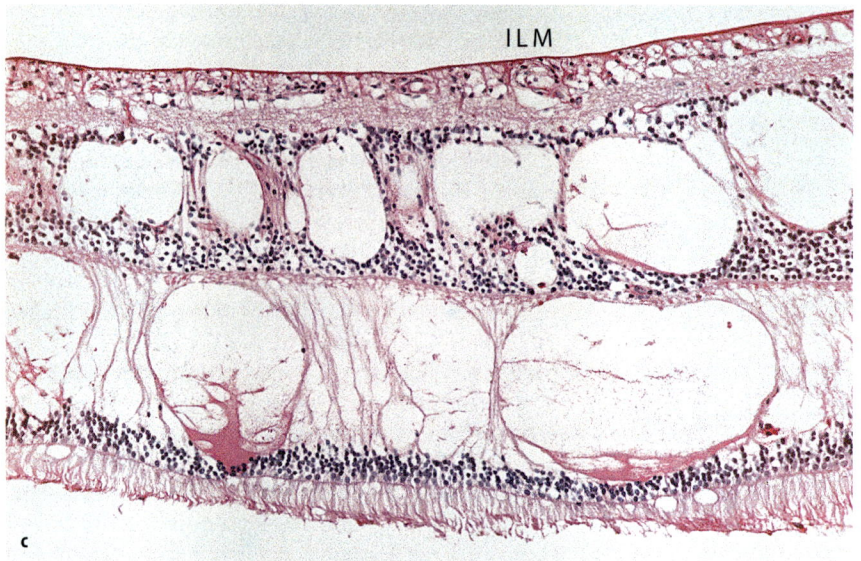

Fig. 5.6.4. a Vertical barriers (*Leitstrukturen*). Red *arrows* indicate in which preformed spaces processes can expand. **b** Horizontal *Leitstrukturen*: internal limiting membrane (*ILM*), so-called middle limiting membrane (*MLM*) and outer limiting membrane (*OLM*). **c** Cystoid degeneration limited by middle limiting membrane and outer limiting membrane and Müller cells

5.6.1.7
Subretinal Immune Privilege

The subretinal space, better termed the "photoreceptor-pigment epithelial interface," has gained great importance with the expanding field of RPE cell transplantation. Despite the existence of ocular immune privilege, immune rejection may be a barrier to successful retinal transplantation.

Interestingly, the immune privilege of the subretinal space is closely correlated to the immune privilege at other ocular sites. Various parameters of immune privilege, originally described for the anterior chamber, are characteristic of immune privilege within the subreti-

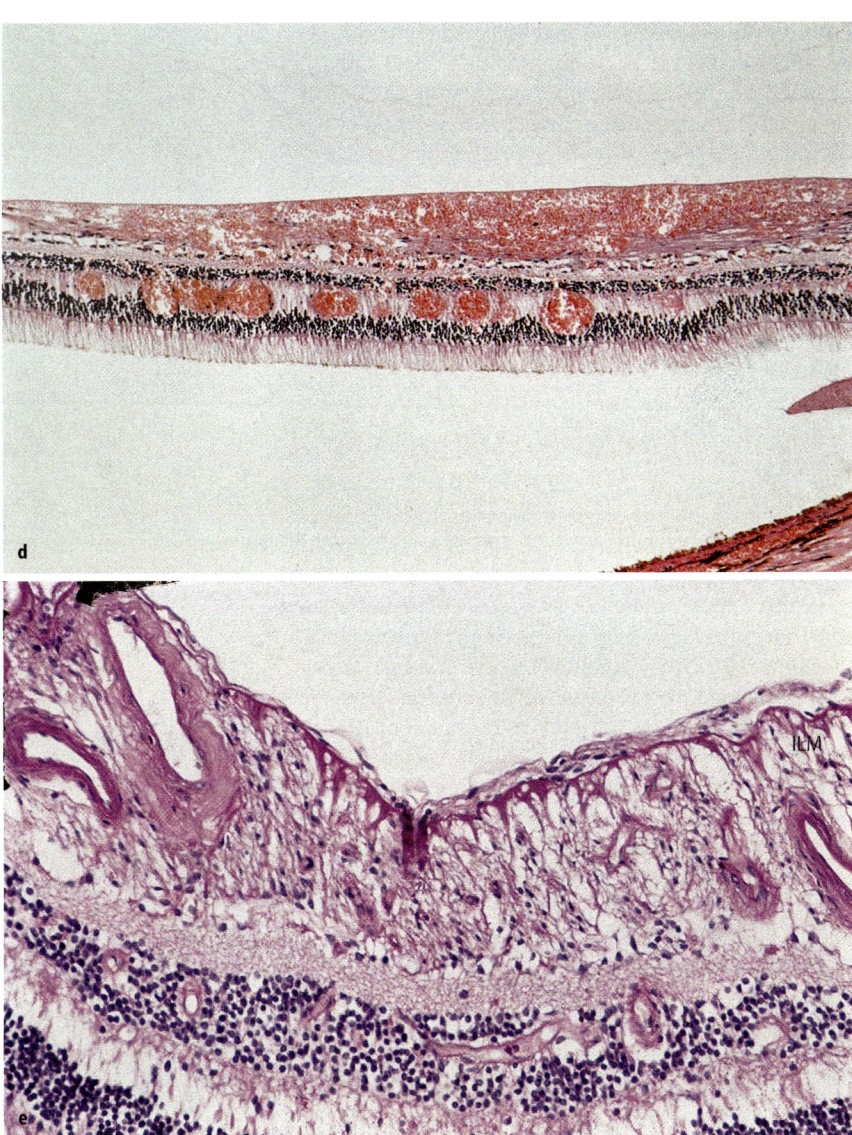

Fig. 5.6.4. d Hemorrhage in the inner and outer retinal layers beyond middle limiting membrane. Beginning of preretinal vascular layer formation. **e** Shrinking preretinal membrane leads to foldings of the internal limiting membrane (*arrows*) (PAS)

nal space. The subretinal space can extend immune privilege to allogeneic tumor cell grafts that do not possess their own inherent immune privilege, and thus immune privilege in the subretinal space can be distinguished from immune privilege in the anterior chamber (Wenkel et al. 1999). Experimentally the subretinal space supports immune deviation for histoincompatible tumor cells and soluble protein antigens by actively suppressing antigen-specific delayed-type hypersensitivity. Acute loss of immune privilege in the subretinal space and the vitreous cavity does not cause loss of privilege in the anterior chamber. However, abolition of immune privilege in the anterior chamber eliminates the capacity of the subretinal space and the vitreous cavity to support immune deviation to antigens injected locally (Wenkel et al. 1998).

Similarly, the immune privilege of the eye is different from brain-associated immune deviation. For brain-associated immune deviation, in contrast to immune deviation elicited via the eye, an intact spleen is not required. This indicates that immune privilege in the brain is actively maintained and is mediated by an immune deviation mechanism that differs from the eye-derived immune deviation (Wenkel et al. 2000a).

Through constitutive expression of CD95 ligand (FasL), allogeneic neonatal RPE grafts promote their own survival at heterotopic sites. Paradoxically, these grafts also display immunogenicity. Thus, neonatal RPE tissue owes its immune privilege to the capacity to prevent immune rejection rather than to inhibit sensitization (Wenkel 2000b). This is in agreement with the hypothesis that tissues derived from immune-privileged sites sometimes possess special characteristics that promote their own survival when transplanted to a non-privileged site.

From the data available, it can be concluded that: (1) the subretinal space is an immune privileged site; (2) neonatal RPE is an immune privileged tissue; (3) neuronal retina is a partially immune privileged tissue; and (4) microglia within neonatal neural retina grafts promote photoreceptor differentiation, become activated, and induce sensitization of the recipient and serve as targets of immune rejection (Streilein 2000).

5.6.2
Surgical Pathology

5.6.2.1
Peripheral Retinal Degenerations and Vitreous Traction (Fig. 5.6.5)

Idiopathic retinal detachment has an incidence of 1:10,000 per year (Heimann et al. 1982; Meyer-Schwikkerath et al. 1975; Wilkes et al. 1982). In pseudophakic eyes, this number increases to 1–3% (Heimann et al. 1982; Tielsch 1996). Patients suffering from a rhegmatogenous retinal detachment in one eye and a predisposing peripheral degeneration in the contralateral eye have an increased risk of retinal detachment of 10% in this eye (Beyer 1979; Hovlang 1978; Rosengren 1976).

The pathogenesis of a rhegmatogenous retinal detachment includes vitreous syneresis followed by posterior vitreous detachment resulting in vitreoretinal traction with formation of retinal defect break(s). Intraocular fluid currents separate the neurosensory retina from the RPE resulting in a retinal detachment.

Degenerative conditions of the peripheral retina can lead to the formation of atrophic retinal holes or tractional retinal tears, and thus predispose to the development of a rhegmatogenous retinal detachment. Atrophic retinal *holes* within areas of peripheral retinal degenerations rarely cause a retinal detachment when the liquid vitreous passes through the atrophic hole and separates the neurosensory retina from the RPE. This process can occur even in the absence of a posterior vitreous detachment. Tractional retinal *tears* are more likely to occur in areas of abnormal vitreoretinal adhesions within peripheral retinal degenerations. As the posterior vitreous detaches from the retina, the vitreous exerts traction on the abnormal vitreoretinal attachment, which can lead to a retinal tear and subsequent retinal detachment. Most of the peripheral retinal degenerations may not require treatment except in rare, high-risk situations. According to current knowledge, there is no increased risk of a secondary pucker or other side effects after laser coagulation. Therefore, generous laser treatment is recommended if risk factors apply.

Degenerative changes of the peripheral retina can be divided into degenerations more prone to rhegmatogenous detachment and others that usually remain clinically insignificant (Table 5.6.1; Beyer 1999). We concentrate on degenerations potentially requiring treatment and disregard the clinically insignificant ones.

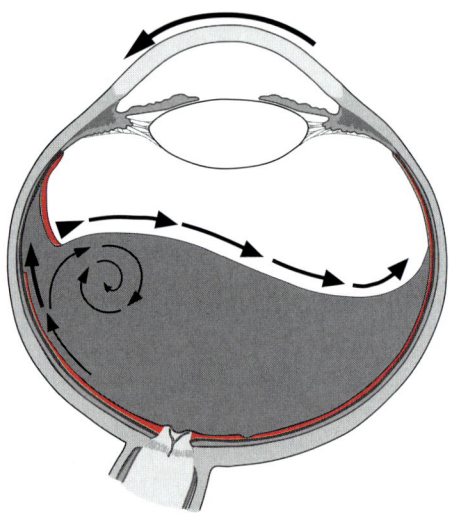

Fig. 5.6.5. Vitreous detachment. Eye movements toward the left-hand side result in a spin of the vitreous toward the right and may result in tearing of the retina at the sides of the vitreoretinal adhesion

Table 5.6.1. Common findings in the retinal periphery

Clinically insignificant findings	Clinically significant rhegmatogenous lesions

A. Normal variations
  1. Meridional folds and complexes
  2. Enclosed ora bays
B. Developmental abnormalities
  1. Non-cystic retinal tufts
  2. Zonular traction tufts
C. Various peripheral degenerations and other findings
  1. Peripheral cystoid degeneration
  2. Paving stone degeneration
  3. Pearl of the ora serrata
  4. Pars plana cyst
  5. White-with-pressure sign
	A. Lattice degeneration
	B. Cystic retinal tufts
	C. Degenerative (senile) retinoschisis
	D. Asymptomatic retinal breaks[a]
	E. Multiple risk factors for retinal detachment

[a] Distinction hole – horseshoe tear is clinically important: a round hole does not suffer from vitreous traction. In tears the tongue is still threatened by vitreous pull at the edges

5.6.2.1.1
Lattice Degeneration

Clinical and pathological observations on this bilateral disease have stressed its importance as a predisposing factor in rhegmatogenous detachment (Gonin 1920; Straatsma et al. 1974). Lattice degeneration can occur early in life and peaks in the 2nd decade of life. In high myopes the incidence of lattice degeneration is said to be high (10%) after the 5th decade. The lesions are usually located slightly anterior to the equator, but they can be present posterior to the equator where they are frequently more radially oriented (Beyer 1979). These may also be present at a similar frequency in pilots with full visual acuity (Lang GK: KMA 1980; Chaps. 11/12).

Lattice degeneration is typically characterized by sharply demarcated, circumferentially oriented, oval or round areas of retinal thinning (1–3 mm diameter) with overlying vitreous liquefaction and exaggerated vitreoretinal attachments along its edges. Other features that can be but are not always present include fine white lines (lattice-like) in the crossing of white hyalinized retinal vessels, speckled foci of proliferating retinal pigment epithelial cells, small white-yellow particles at the margin of the surface of the lesion, punched out areas of extreme retinal thinning or excavations and atrophic retinal holes. Retinal tears can occur at the posterior or lateral margin of the lesion from vitreous traction following posterior vitreous detachment.

The pathogenesis of hole formation as a consequence of lattice degeneration leading to a tear at the junction between the anterior part of the atrophic strip and the adjacent normal retina is a consequence of simple mechanical forces exerted from the vitreous base by ocular movements. Careful study of the disease does not always reinforce the accepted dogma.

The etiology of lattice degeneration is uncertain. Several theories have been proposed including developmental anomalies of the internal limiting membrane, vitreous traction, embryologic vascular anastomosis and choroidal abnormalities (Beyer 1979; Tolentino 1976; Ricci 1969), as well as ischemic atrophy in the retina due to hyalinization in the peripheral vascular arcades (Straatsma et al. 1974).

The most interesting histological feature, which is best demonstrated with Alcian blue or colloidal iron, is an overlying zone in the vitreous with condensations and liquefactions. Sometimes, an obvious hole will be identified or microcystic nodules may appear.

Lattice degeneration is the most important peripheral retinal degeneration that predisposes to a rhegmatogenous retinal detachment. Most rhegmatogenous retinal detachments with lattice degeneration are due to tractional retinal *tears* following posterior vitreous detachment. However, atrophic retinal *holes* within lattice lesions can cause a localized retinal detachment and only rarely a progressive retinal detachment. Retinal tears, due to vitreous traction to the strongly adherent posterior and lateral vitreoretinal margins of lattice lesions, follow a posterior vitreous detachment. The prevalence of posterior vitreous detachment and retinal tears is higher in eyes with lattice degeneration. In a large clinical series, 30% of eyes with acute retinal detachment and retinal breaks had lattice degeneration (Dumas et al. 1966). In 83% of these cases, the retinal tear was associated with a lattice lesion.

The 3- to 10-year incidences of retinal detachment in phakic eyes with lattice degeneration and a history of retinal detachment in the fellow eye are 6–15% (Schepens 1952). The prevalence of lattice degeneration of the retina in the fellow eye of patients with rhegmatogenous retinal detachment ranges from 9.2% to 35% (Tillery et al. 1976; Davis et al. 1974).

Although lattice degeneration is a risk factor for development of a rhegmatogenous retinal detachment, the great majority of patients with lattice degeneration do not develop a retinal detachment, and up to 80% of rhegmatogenous retinal detachments are not associated with lattice degeneration of the retina (Beyer 1979). Only approximately 2.8% of rhegmatogenous retinal detachments are due to retinal holes within lattice degeneration (Dumas et al. 1966; Schepens 1952; McPerson et al. 1981). Because lattice degeneration is present in 30% of phakic rhegmatogenous retinal detachments, these lesions have been frequently considered for prophylactic therapy.

In order to determine if prophylactic treatment of eyes with lattice degeneration with or without retinal holes is beneficial, it is necessary to design a study with appropriate statistical methods and power to produce either statistical significant results or to show no difference. Currently, there is no scientific evidence to suggest that prophylactic treatment of lattice degeneration with or without retinal holes in phakic, non-fellow eyes is beneficial.

In a retrospective study, Folk and colleagues (1989) studied 388 consecutive patients with lattice degeneration in one eye and a history of rhegmatogenous retinal detachment associated with lattice degeneration in the fellow eye. Based on this study, retinal detachments were prevented in only 3% of the eyes with lattice degeneration that were treated in a phakic fellow eye and a history of retinal detachment in the other eye.

Prophylactic treatment might be considered in patients with lattice degeneration in the fellow eye of a patient with a history of rhegmatogenous retinal detachment in the first eye. This would particularly be the case if the visual function is poor in this eye, if the patient does not have or has minimal access to ophthalmic care, or if they are mentally retarded and might not recognize the symptoms of a posterior vitreous separation. Prophylactic cryotherapy or photocoagulation is further recommended when lattice degeneration is associated with myopia, if the patient has symptoms or abnormalities are identified in the peripheral retina (see Table 5.6.2).

5.6.2.1.2
Cystic Retinal Tuft

The retinal lesion that Foos and Allen named *cystic retinal tuft* in 1967 was first illustrated in 1936 by Vogt (Foos 1967; Vogt 1936). Cystic retinal tuft is a congeni-

Table 5.6.2. Recommendations for prophylactic laser coagulation in patients with lattice degeneration with and without retinal holes

	Emmetropic	Myopic >4 dpt	Aphakic	Fellow eye with detachment	Old horseshoe tear	Vitreoretinal dystrophy (e.g., m. Wagner)
With symptoms						
Phosphenes	Photocoagulation	Photocoagulation	Photocoagulation	Photocoagulation	Photocoagulation	Photocoagulation
Phosphenes, fresh posterior vitreous detachment	Photocoagulation	Photocoagulation	Photocoagulation	Photocoagulation	Photocoagulation	Photocoagulation
Without symptoms						
Patient against treatment	Wait and watch	Wait and watch	Wait and watch	Photocoagulation	Wait and watch	Wait and watch
Patient neutral	Wait and watch	Photocoagulation	Photocoagulation	Photocoagulation	Photocoagulation	Photocoagulation
Patient wants safety	Photocoagulation	Photocoagulation	Photocoagulation	Photocoagulation	Photocoagulation	Photocoagulation
Reduced compliance	Photocoagulation	Photocoagulation	Photocoagulation	Photocoagulation	Photocoagulation	Photocoagulation

tal vitreoretinal abnormality in the development of the peripheral retina associated with firm vitreoretinal adhesions. Cystic retinal tufts are present at birth, and affect approximately 5% of the population (Straatsma et al. 1986). This is in accordance with the finding that cystic retinal tufts are present in 5% of autopsy cases (Beyer 1981).

The cystic retinal tuft is a round or oval, elevated vitreoretinal lesion which is small, discreet, sharply circumscribed, and has a chalky-white color. Vitreous condensations are attached to its surface and its base may have pigmentary changes. The dense vitreoretinal adherence present in cystic retinal tufts explains why they are commonly associated with retinal tears which can have either a flap or an operculum and can occur with or without a posterior vitreous detachment (Foos 1974a, b; Byer 1981). The lesion occurs most frequently (78%) in the extrabasal or equatorial zone of the eye, is single in most cases, and unilateral in 80% of the patients (Straatsma et al. 1986).

Histologically, accumulations of glial tissue form in nodules on the retinal surface, which enclose crypts of formed vitreous within the lesion. Large tufts demonstrate an absence of photoreceptors (Foos et al. 1974a, b).

In association with cystic retinal tufts, two types of retinal breaks have been found, i.e., horseshoe- or crescent-shaped flap tears and round opercular tears. Flap tears were found more frequently, which were located at the juxtabasal zone of the equator and induced acute, highly elevated detachments. Opercular tears were located at the extrabasal zone of the equator and caused relatively slowly developing, shallow detachments. It was concluded that the cystic retinal tuft is an important vitreoretinal abnormality predisposing to rhegmatogenous retinal detachment (Murakami-Nagasako et al. 1982; Byer et al. 1981).

Of 200 consecutive cases with phakic non-traumatic rhegmatogenous retinal detachment, 15 (7.5%) were causally related to retinal tears in areas of cystic retinal tufts. The risk of a cystic retinal tuft leading to retinal detachment was computed to be less than 1% (range 0.18–0.28%). Rarely, atrophic retinal holes in an area of chronic vitreoretinal traction can be the cause of rhegmatogenous retinal detachment.

Since the natural history and the results of treatment of cystic retinal tufts have not been studied, and knowing that the risk of developing a rhegmatogenous retinal detachment from a cystic retinal tuft is 0.28%, prophylactic treatment is not usually indicated (Foos 1967; Wilkinson 2000).

5.6.2.1.3
Peripheral Microcystoid Degeneration

This abnormality is commonly seen macroscopically as a "honeycomb"-like band at the retinal periphery (O'Malley and Allen 1967). Histologically, the disorder takes the form of cystic degeneration in the outer plexiform layer with compression of the bipolar and photo-

Table 5.6.3. Peripheral microcystoid degeneration in degenerative retinoschisis

Microcystoid degeneration	Retinoschisis
Typical (Blessing-Iwanoff type)	Degenerative • Typical • Reticular
Reticular	Juvenile (X-chromosome) Tractive • Vasoproliferative • Trauma • Uveitis

receptor nuclei and some sparing of Müller cells, which later are the only cells to surround the cystic spaces (Blessig-Ivanoff cysts). Microcystoid degeneration rarely has serious consequences, but sometimes the pillars of Müller cells break down and a split extends posteriorly to separate the two layers to form a retinoschisis. It is not uncommon for tears to occur in either the inner or the outer layers, or both, and this can lead to retinal detachment (see Sect. 5.6.2.4).

Degenerative senile retinoschisis is listed under Sect. 5.6.2.4.

5.6.2.2
Peripheral Retinal Holes and Tears (Fig. 5.6.6)

Simple innocuous holes in the retina are sometimes based on lattice degeneration, but they often occur for no obvious reason. The fact that holes can be present within an attached retina indicates the belief that vitreous liquefaction with condensation and traction is involved in the accumulation of fluid into the subretinal space. Clinically, the dilemma is whether or not to treat a simple hole with cryotherapy or laser.

Cases 1–7 (Fig. 5.6.7) are shown to help decision-making in typical constellations.

The authors believe that retinal *tears* should be generally treated by a double row of argon laser coagulation spots. If the periphery cannot be successfully coagulated, the hole should be demarcated up to the ora serrata (Case 3), or the edges sealed by cryotherapy. In general, fresh horseshoe tears should be without exception treated by laser photocoagulation (Table 5.6.4).

Although there are concerns discussing the increased risk of pucker formation after laser photocoagulation, it is in fact the retinal hole which is associated with pucker formation not the treatment thereof. Patients following panretinal photocoagulation for proliferative diabetic retinopathy do not usually demonstrate pucker formation. Thus, the indication for laser photocoagulation should be made rather generously as there is no increased proven risk for pucker formation.

Folk and coworkers investigated 388 patients with lattice degeneration in one eye and a history of rhegmatogenous detachment in the contralateral eye (Folk et al. 1989). During a follow-up of 7 years, new holes without detachment were detected in 6.6% of the eyes, in 9.6% of partially prophylactically treated eyes, and in 3% of the completely treated eyes. The prevalence was 5.9% in untreated eyes, and 6.8% and 1.8% of prophylactically treated eyes. As indicated above, this results

Table 5.6.4. Recommendations for a prophylactic laser photocoagulation in patients with fresh horseshoe tears

Clinical situation	Treatment
Patient against treatment	Laser photocoagulation
Patient neutral	Laser photocoagulation
Patient wants safety	Laser photocoagulation
Reduced compliance	Laser photocoagulation

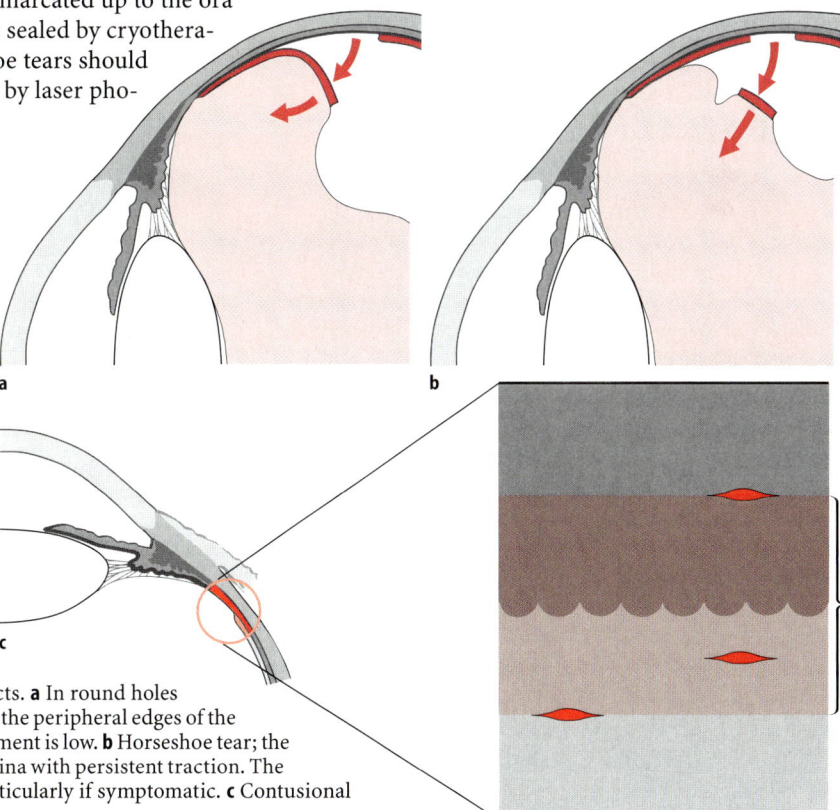

Fig. 5.6.6. Peripheral retinal defects. **a** In round holes (foramen) there is no traction on the peripheral edges of the hole and thus the risk of a detachment is low. **b** Horseshoe tear; the vitreous is still attached to the retina with persistent traction. The risk of a detachment is high, particularly if symptomatic. **c** Contusional pre-, intra- and retrobasal tears

Fig. 5.6.7. Seven types of retinal process with treatment recommendation

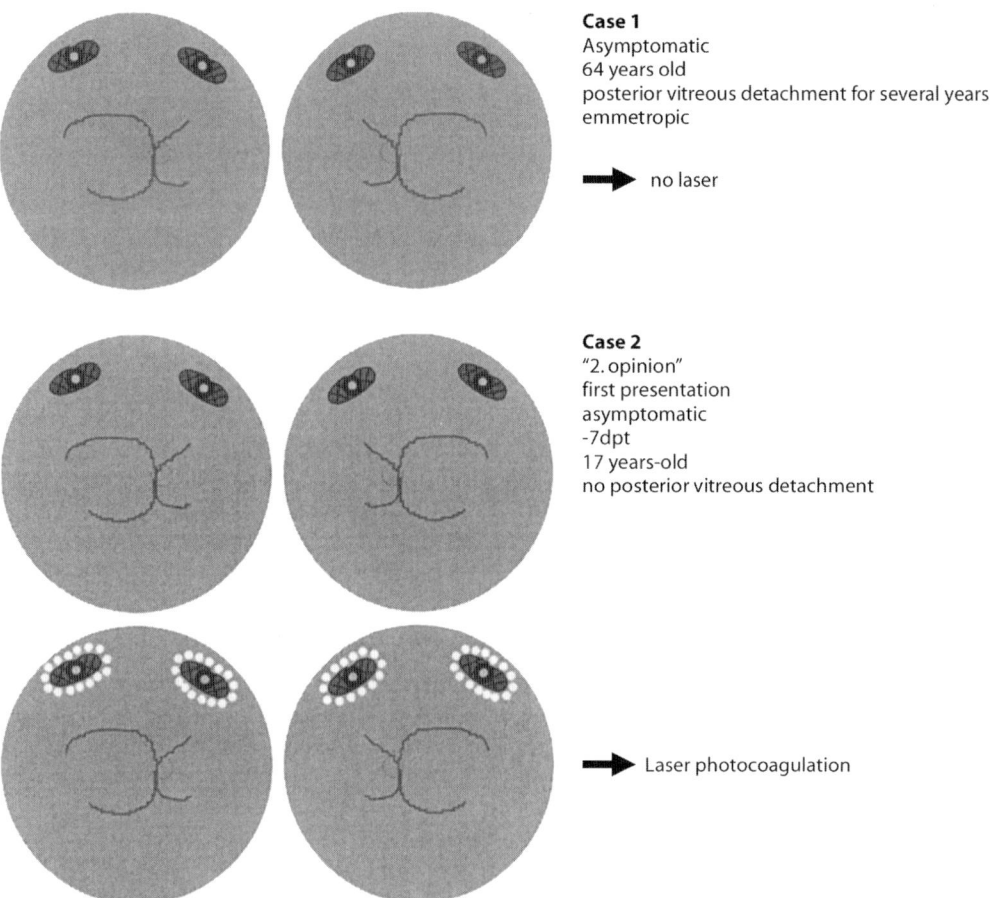

Case 1
Asymptomatic
64 years old
posterior vitreous detachment for several years
emmetropic

➡ no laser

Case 2
"2. opinion"
first presentation
asymptomatic
-7 dpt
17 years-old
no posterior vitreous detachment

➡ Laser photocoagulation

Case 3: more "floaters", 64 years-old, posterior vitreous detachment several weeks ago, emmetropic

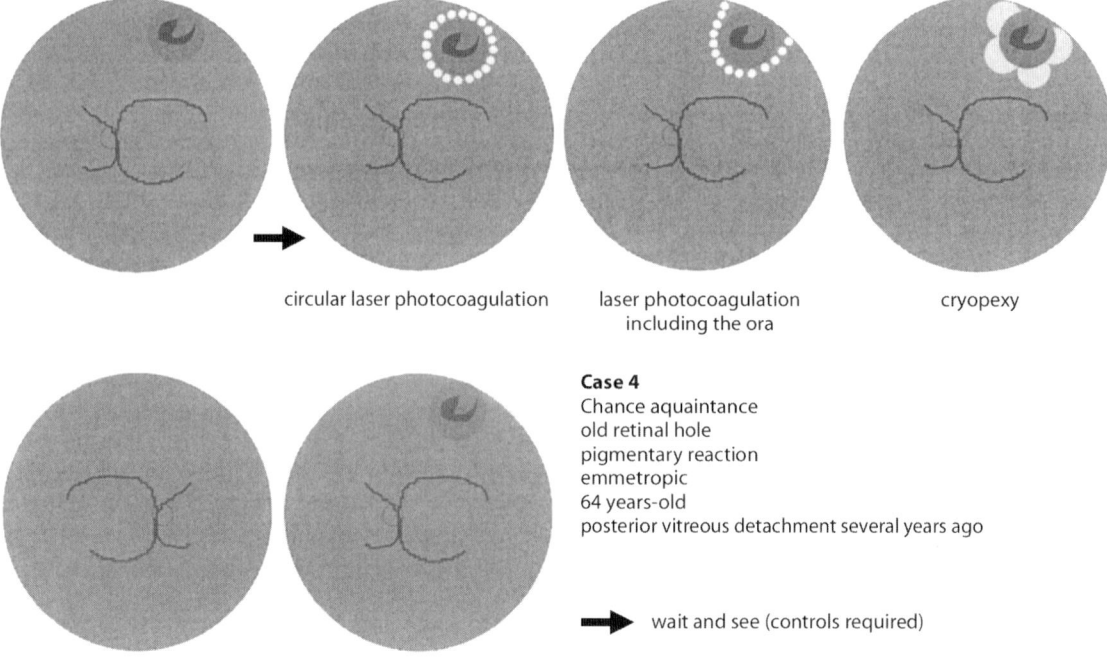

circular laser photocoagulation   laser photocoagulation including the ora   cryopexy

Case 4
Chance aquaintance
old retinal hole
pigmentary reaction
emmetropic
64 years-old
posterior vitreous detachment several years ago

➡ wait and see (controls required)

Fig. 5.6.7. (*Cont.*)

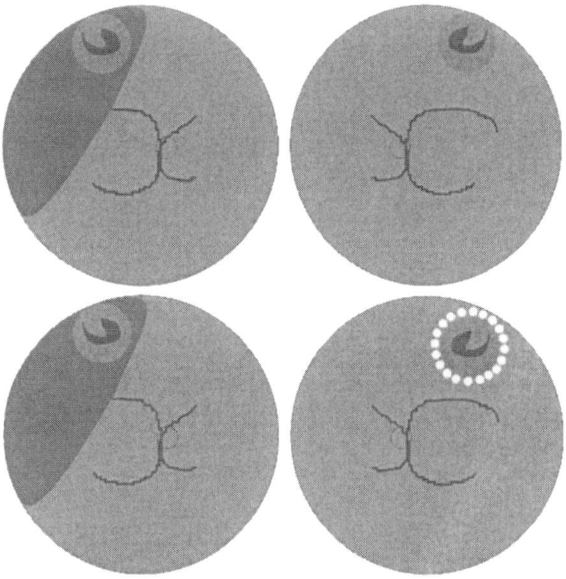

Case 5
OD fresh detachment
OS old retinal hole with pigmentary reaction
emmetropic
64 years-old
posterior vitreous detachment several years ago

→ OD buckling procedure
OS laser-photocoagulation

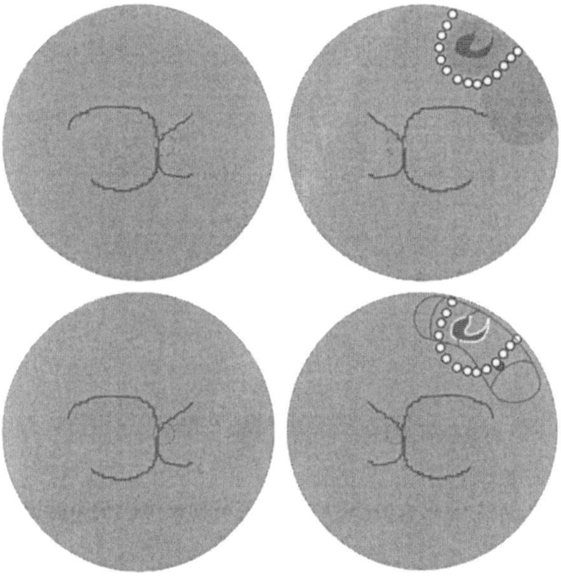

Case 6
OS detachment
7 months after photocoagulation
emmetropic
64 years-old
posterior vitreous detachment several years ago

→ buckling procedure

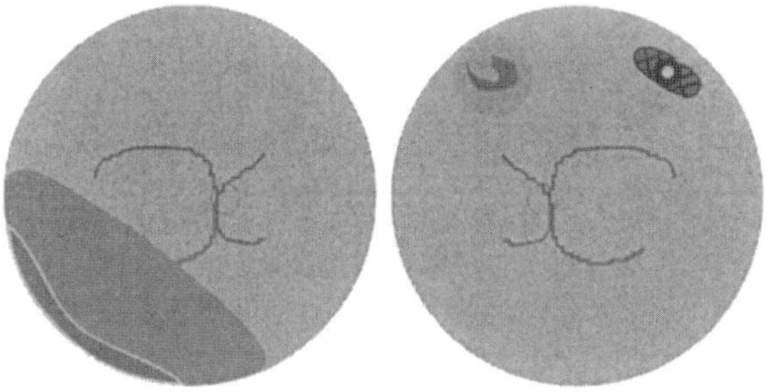

Case 7
OD: traumatic dialysis at the ora
OS: old retinal tear and degeneration

→ OD observation
OS no treatment

Table 5.6.5. Differential diagnosis of peripheral retinal defects

Atrophic holes
Tractional tears
• Round tears with lid
• Horseshoe tear
• Giant tears
Oral dialysis
Defects in the outer layer of retinoschisis

in a positive prophylactic effect of the laser treatment in 3 of 100 eyes with lattice degeneration. Thus, we believe that prophylactic photocoagulation is important in eyes with a high risk for detachment. However, detachment will occur in previously unaffected areas in 5% of the patients (Smiddy 1991).

It is unlikely that the currently available retrospective studies on peripheral degenerations by Straatsma, Byer and others (Straatsma 1986; Byer 1989) will be supplemented by evidence-based data in the future. A reason is the high cost of those trials compared to the small effects of prophylactic retinopexy.

What has been established on clinical and experimental grounds is that any retinal defect (e.g., a tear or hole) that allows fluid movement from the vitreous into the photoreceptor-pigment epithelial interface can progressively separate the layers (so called rhegmatogenous detachment). It is equally possible that a retina can reattach spontaneously, when the fluid is reabsorbed, but frequently the loss of the normal relationship between photoreceptors and the RPE results in photoreceptor atrophy and misalignment and reactive proliferation in the RPE.

Conversely, it is now accepted that flat holes can occur at the macula and at the periphery, and that their presence may not lead to separation. It seems likely that some form of traction by condensed vitreous is essential for maintaining an eversion of the lip of the hole to promote fluid movement from the vitreous (Foos and Allen 1967).

Prevention of detachment is the major aim as the functional result frequently remains poor despite good anatomical attachment rates. Patients with peripheral retinal degenerations associated with a higher risk of retinal detachment should be aware of possible symptoms, such as phosphenes and the increase of "*mouches volantes*." If these symptoms occur, photocoagulation should be considered. Patients with detachments in the first eye usually have a good functional result in the contralateral eye as symptoms are noticed early in the course of time.

5.6.2.3
Retinal Detachment

Retinal detachment is a separation between the neural retina and the RPE; thus it is a reopening of the embryonic optic ventricle between the inner and outer layers of the optic cup. Therefore, "retinal detachment" is a misnomer because it implies a separation of the retina from the choroid (Lee 2002).

The subretinal space (better termed "photoreceptor-pigment epithelial interface") between the photoreceptors and the RPE is the remnant of the embryonic optic vesicle. Before considering the etiology and pathogenesis of separation of the two embryonic layers – which are in contact only where the outer segments of the photoreceptors are surrounded by processes from the pigment epithelium – it is relevant to consider the mechanisms which maintain their apposition. In the developed eye, the subretinal space is of minimal size. One might assume that the processes of the RPE cells would connect with the photoreceptors, but no tissue junctions exist and the subretinal space can reopen under pathological conditions of retinal detachment.* Ocular pump mechanisms are necessary to prevent an accumulation of fluid, and to remove it under conditions of stress or disease (Marmor 1990).

"*Rhegmatogenous*" detachment occurs when fluid passes from the vitreous cavity through a retinal defect into the "subretinal space." The "hole" or "tear" is most commonly secondary to degenerative disease in the retina and vitreous (e.g., lattice degeneration), and is probably precipitated by minor trauma. The vitreous is attached at the base to the pars plana and at the inner surface of the peripheral retina so that a vitrectomy is an integral part of the surgical attempt to abolish vitreous traction and to reattach the retina. Vitrectomy is not always required and successful reattachment may also be achieved by a simple scleral buckle (see Sect. 5.6.3.1).

"*Exudative*" detachment, in contrast, refers to accumulation of fluid under the neural retina in situations in which there is abnormally excessive permeability of the blood-retinal barrier in the retinal and in the choroidal vessels and Verhoeff's membrane of the RPE. This process is encountered in inflammation or neoplasia and in retinal or choroidal vasculopathy with loss of endothelial cell integrity, and in this event the subretinal space is filled with more viscous proteinaceous exudates.

"*Traction*" detachment occurs when there is condensation or disorganization of the vitreous, e.g., by trauma or neovascularization. In severe trauma, the vitreous gel may be invaded by contractile cells (fibroblasts from the scleral coat), which form traction bands and pull the retina internally. In all types of proliferative vitreoretinopathy (trauma, both surgical and non-

---

* Please note that the connection between sensory retina and RPE is so loose that in histologic sections of whole eyes the artificial separation of the two layers often cannot be avoided. Melanin granula of the RPE are torn to the photoreceptor. The detachments show subretinal exudate and atrophy of the outer segment.

surgical as well as idiopathic cases), the retina is lined by cells derived from retinal glial cells (see Sects. 5.6.4.2, 5.6.4.3). In vasoproliferative retinopathy, the membranes contain glial cells, fibroblasts and macrophages, in addition to vessels possessing endothelial cells and pericytes.

5.6.2.3.1
Effects of Detachment of the Ocular Tissues

Retinal detachment as seen in the laboratory can vary from a funnel shape to such an extreme form that the retina is totally engulfed by a vitreoproliferative mass and the normal anatomy is disturbed. The structure of sensory retina and optic disc is often surprisingly well preserved (Cursiefen et al. 2001). It is of note that during preparation of the tissue for histopathology *artificial retinal detachment* often occurs, particularly if the globe is fixed in formalin. This is easily recognizable on light microscopy as the photoreceptors maintain their normal structure and are not atrophic and show melanin granules of RPE. In contrast, in long-lasting preexisting retinal detachments, the photoreceptor processes are shortened and rounded with more degenerative changes in the adjacent photoreceptor layer outer segment, later in the inner segment, then loss of nuclei in the outer nuclear layer (see Machemer 1968).

The early effects of separation of the outer part of the neural retina from the RPE are best studied in collateral exudative detachments secondary to choroidal melanomas in routine specimens. The photoreceptor atrophy commences with swelling of the outer segment, followed by degeneration in the inner segment and the outer nuclear layer. Müller cells proliferate in the outer retina and form membranes on the outer surface. This is one factor in the failure of photoreceptors to regenerate (Lewis and Fischer 2000). Irreparable damage is said not to occur until about 6 weeks. The outer nuclear layer may remain well preserved up to 3–4 months, but after this time period atrophy and gliosis occur progressing on to cyst formation. Ultimately, large cysts are formed on the outer surface of the funnel-shaped detached retina.

The cells in the inner two-thirds of the retina have a preserved blood supply and are able to survive and there are usually plentiful axons in the stalk of the funnel and in the disc and optic nerve – as long as there is no secondary or primary glaucoma. Nevertheless, preretinal membrane formation will be a prominent feature due to the associated primary or secondary degenerative disease in the retinal vessels. Glial cells or fibrovascular membranes cause marked wrinkling of the inner retina as do cells of RPE origin when a hole in the retina provides access. Gliosis may predominate at the end stage and "pseudogliomas" are formed by proliferating glial cells within a totally disorganized and barely recognizable retinal tissue.

Interestingly, apart from alterations in the detached retina, glial cell changes occur even in parts of the retina which are still attached. In addition to the well-known degeneration of photoreceptor cells in the detached retina, there is considerable ganglion cell death, particularly in the detached area. Small adherent groups of photoreceptor cells in the attached retina *distant* from the detachment degenerate in an atypical sequence, with severe destruction of somata and inner segments but well-maintained outer segments (Faude et al. 2001; Lewis et al. 1995, 2000).

Whether or not Müller cells are involved in the process of retinal degeneration is a matter of controversy. Faude and Lewis did not find retinal degeneration to be accompanied by any significant loss of Müller (glial) cells. In contrast, Franke and coworkers suggested that the inverse mode of photoreceptor cell degeneration in the attached tissue suggests a disturbed support of the photoreceptor cells by Müller cells which show various indications of gliosis (increased expression of intermediate filaments, cell hypertrophy, decreased plasma membrane K^+ conductance, increased Ca^{2+} responsiveness to purinergic stimulation) in both detached and attached tissues. The downregulation of the K^+ conductance of Müller cells may prevent effective retinal K^+ and water clearance, and may favor photoreceptor cell degeneration and edema development (Francke et al. 2005).

5.6.2.3.2
Histopathology of Rhegmatogenous Detachment

Untreated or uncomplicated primary rhegmatogenous detachment due to a hole or tear is rarely encountered in the ophthalmic pathology laboratory today.

In rhegmatogenous detachment, a history of severe trauma is unusual and the clinical symptoms take the form of premonitory flashes and light (photopsia) before the visual field is progressively reduced by an opaque descending veil or curtain, as subretinal fluid separates the inferior neural retinal pigment epithelium from the RPE.

Should a retinal hole be detected on macroscopic and microscopic examination, it may appear to have a lid (operculum) with an anterior traction or it may be flat.

Serial sections will show that the edges of the hole are rounded and that there is glial cell replacement of the inner retinal neurons with an accompanying microcystic degeneration (Lee 2002). An intriguing feature is the presence of vitreous condensation with an apparent anterior traction on the "lid" formed by the horseshoe-shaped tear (see Sect. 5.6.2.2).

The enucleated eye should be subject to a careful search for the primary hole or tear after a rhegmatogenous retinal detachment. Sometimes the presence of retinal pigment epithelial cells on the inner surface of the retina ("tobacco dust"), or in the vitreous, may be the only indication of a preexisting retinal hole. In the later and complicated stages, identification of the hole or defect may be impossible because the opaque peripheral vitreous becomes condensed and may obscure the inner surface of the retina. Secondary pre-retinal membranes distort the funnel-shaped detachment and may overlie the preexisting hole. On the other hand, a hole may enlarge as a detachment progresses.

Post-traumatic tears – mostly after severe contusion – in an otherwise normal retina are more likely to be found in histopathological specimens. These can occur at any anatomical location in the tissue and may complicate penetrating wounds or follow concussion or compression injury. Large peripheral defects, expanding for more than 3 clock-hours, should be referred to as "*giant retinal tears*." Prior to the pars plana vitrectomy era, giant retinal tears have been associated with a high risk of proliferative vitreoretinopathy (PVR) and a poor prognosis. In this event, vitreous may remain attached to the retina behind the tear, which interferes with surgical attempts to reattach the retina. In contrast, the term "retinal dialysis" is used for separation of the retina from the RPE at the ora, which may occur spontaneously or bilateral in the inferior temporal quadrant and has a better prognosis.

Table 5.6.6. Causes of exudative retinal detachments

General diseases
Malignant arterial hypertension
Renal insufficiency
Eclampsia
Collagen disease
Rare hematologic disease
Uveitis
Vogt-Koyanagi-Harada
Scleritis
Other severe infectious and other uveitis
Neoplastic disease
Malignant melanoma of choroid
Metastasis
Retinoblastoma
Lymphoma
Retinal vascular disease
Coats'
Angiomatosis retinae
Retinopathy of prematurity
Familial exsudative vitreoretinopathy (FEVR)
Idiopathic or with congenital anomalies
Uveal effusion
Pit of the optic disc
Colobomatous detachment (morning glory)
Others
Subretinal neovascularization
Excessive laser or cryocoagulation
Ocular hypotony

5.6.2.3.3
Exudative Detachment

The delicate balance of fluid movement within the globe is easily disturbed and the mechanisms involved in metabolic control of water and solute transfer are sensitive to inflammatory mediators. Exudative detachments are most often seen in collateral to malignant melanoma of choroid. The choroid contains a permeable vasculature and the choroidal stroma exerts osmotic pressure on the water which passes through the retina and through the photoreceptor retinal pigment epithelial interface. Fluid movement is probably impeded or modulated by the retinal pigment epithelial monolayer, which consists of hexagonal cells attached by zonulae occludentes. The architecture of the RPE cell, with its apical processes and basal infoldings, suggests a capacity for "ion" transport (see Sect. 5.6.2.3.1).

A convincing explanation for the pathogenesis of exudative retinal degeneration could be leakage of protein-rich fluid from a diseased retinal circulation as seen in congenital vascular malformations, e.g., retinal *angiomas* or in exudative retinal *vasculopathy* [Coats' disease, familial exsudative vitreoretinopathy (FEVR)]. Furthermore, granulomatous and non-granulomatous *inflammatory* disease cause exudative detachment. Similarly, exudation through the walls of choroidal vessels occurs in persisting *ocular hypotony*.

A primary or secondary neoplasm in the choroid can disturb the function of the choriocapillaris and lead to plasma leakage. Neovascularization in age-related macular degeneration will inevitably lead to subretinal exudation.

The *uveal effusion syndrome* is a rare entity and results in a ring-like detachment of anterior choroid and retina, simulating a malignant melanoma. Uveal effusion syndrome can be idiopathic or associated with rheumatoid scleritis (>50% of cases).

The histological features of exudative retinal detachment are usually investigated in choroidal tumors with associated detachment. The retinal structure remains intact better in the region with the smallest distance to the choriocapillaris.

5.6.2.3.4
Central Serous Retinopathy

Central serous retinopathy is a form of exudative detachment of the macula, which is usually self healing, and which occurs in the macular region in young adults and may be recurrent. There is fluid accumulation both in the subretinal space and/or in the sub-RPE space.

The etiology of central serous retinopathy is poorly understood and pathological material is sparse (Mazzuca and Benson 1986; Smiddy et al. 1990). The four published descriptions show a simple accumulation of fluid between the photoreceptors and the pigment epithelium (Gass et al. 1973) and an inconspicuous choroidal disturbance in RPE fluid transport mechanisms.

It is noteworthy that a similar effusion is observed in aphakia or as an agonal event in eyes removed at autopsy (Lee 2002).

Optical coherence tomography (OCT) may provide additional information (Montero et al. 2005) (Fig. 5.6.16). These authors describe the characteristic features observed in patients with a clinical diagnosis of central serous retinopathy using the OCT ophthalmoscope. In a study by van Velthofen, the characteristics of active CSR ($n=29$) included large neurosensory detachment (23/29), subretinal hyperreflective deposits (20/29), and pigment epithelial detachment (15/29) (van Velthofen 2005).

Interestingly, high-resolution OCT demonstrates changes in the foveal photoreceptor layer in CSR that are highly correlated with visual acuity loss and may predict visual recovery after macular reattachment (Piccolino et al. 2005).

5.6.2.3.5
Traction Detachment

Today, traction detachment is rarely seen in the ophthalmo-pathological laboratory, although many experimental studies are available (Hui et al. 1988). Nevertheless, surgically excised membranes are obtained from surgical specimens, e.g., in proliferative diseases or PVR (detailed in Sect. 5.6.4.2).

A severe form of PVR with traction detachment occurs frequently following trauma. Fibrous ingrowth from any form of scleral and uveal perforation incorporates spindle cells which originate from scleral or choroidal fibroblasts. Traction exerted in this manner can displace the retina across the pars plana. In rare cases, the posterior retina remains attached. Traction detachment may also occur in pseudophakic or aphakic patients, when the vitreous prolapses and there is kinking and distortion of the retinal periphery behind the vitreous base. This sometimes gives the impression that there is sufficient strength in the condensed vitreous to exert traction (Lee 2002).

Furthermore, traction is a dominant feature of preretinal neovascularization in ischemic disease of the retina (particularly diabetic vasoproliferative retinopathy) (see Sect. 5.6.2.7). Hemorrhage, due to any cause, stimulates macrophagic infiltration and fibrovascular ingrowth.

5.6.2.3.6
Special Forms of Retinal Detachment

The pathology of *inherited vitreoretinopathy* resembles peripheral reticular degeneration. It takes the form of atrophy and schisis in the inner retina, which is associated with vitreous condensation and traction on the retina and disc (see Lang 1990).

For differentiation of inherited disorders both clinical examination and linkage analysis of markers flanking the *COL2A1* gene associated with Stickler syndrome type 1, the loci for Wagner disease/erosive vitreoretinopathy (5q14.3), high myopia (18p11.31 and 12q21-q23), and non-syndromic congenital retinal non-attachment (10q21) can be used (van Velthofen 2005).

Hereditary X-linked retinoschisis may also be due to abnormalities in the vitreous, but the current hypothesis favors an abnormality in the Müller cells in the inner part of the retina (Condon et al. 1986; George et al. 1996). There is severe visual loss in males at an early age, and this is due to splitting in the nerve fiber layer which progresses to cyst formation. The abnormal gene (*XRLS1*) in this condition is coated on chromosome 22 at the Xp22.2 locus (see Sect. 5.6.2.4).

Hereditary progressive arthro-ophthalmopathy (Stickler syndrome) is an autosomal dominant condition due to a point mutation at the gene locus (*COL2A1*) on chromosome 12, where the control of the normal synthesis of type II collagen occurs. Since this collagen type is found in cartilage, abnormalities are found in the cartilage of joints and the ossicles in the middle ear. Myopia and paravascular lattice degeneration feature in the ocular manifestations, but the salient feature is the presence of condensed vitreous strands at the periphery with optically empty spaces in the central vitreous.

Familial exudative vitreoretinopathy is an inherited, bilateral peripheral vascular disease in children, with no association with prematurity (see Sect. 5.6.2.6). The pattern of inheritance is autosomal dominant. Unlike other inherited diseases, expression of FEVR may be asymmetrical between the two eyes. The clinical course is slowly progressive and rarely stable. Its presentation may be confined to a peripheral avascular zone and a reduced angle kappa or it may lead to a falciform or a rhegmatogenous retinal detachment. The presence of hyalinized preretinal membranes and hyalinized blood vessels surrounded by astrocytes may be an important diagnostic histological feature (Boldreay et al. 1985; Glazer et al. 1995). Retinal exudates and a peripheral fibrovascular mass result from the leakage of peripheral vessels, forming aneurysms, tubular dilatation, and neovascularization, indicating a progressive disease. Such abnormalities must be treated by laser or cryotherapy to stop exudation. Usually, repetitive applications of retinopexy are necessary. The main goal of treatment is the occlusion of abnormal retinal vessels to avoid complications such as tractional retinal detachment and the re-growth of vitreous membranes. The involvement of Wnt signaling in the pathogenesis of FEVR is currently the subject of discussion. Frizzled-

4 (Fz4), a presumptive Wnt receptor, and Norrin, the protein product of the Norrie's disease gene, function as a ligand-receptor pair.

5.6.2.4
Retinoschisis (Fig. 5.6.8)

A schisis of the retina is found in two distinct entities: frequently as a degenerative change, a consequence of traction from neovascular disease, and as a consequence of trauma or uveitis (Zimmerman and Naumann 1968) and rarely in X-linked juvenile retinoschisis.

Degenerative retinoschisis was first described by Bartels (1933). Straatsma and Foos described two forms based on histopathology, *typical* or flat retinoschisis and *reticular or bullous retinoschisis* (Straatsma et al. 1973). A *schisis detachment* follows the clinically more severe reticular form (Byer 1986).

In degenerative retinoschisis, there is a coalescence of microcystoid intraretinal lesions as a result of degen-

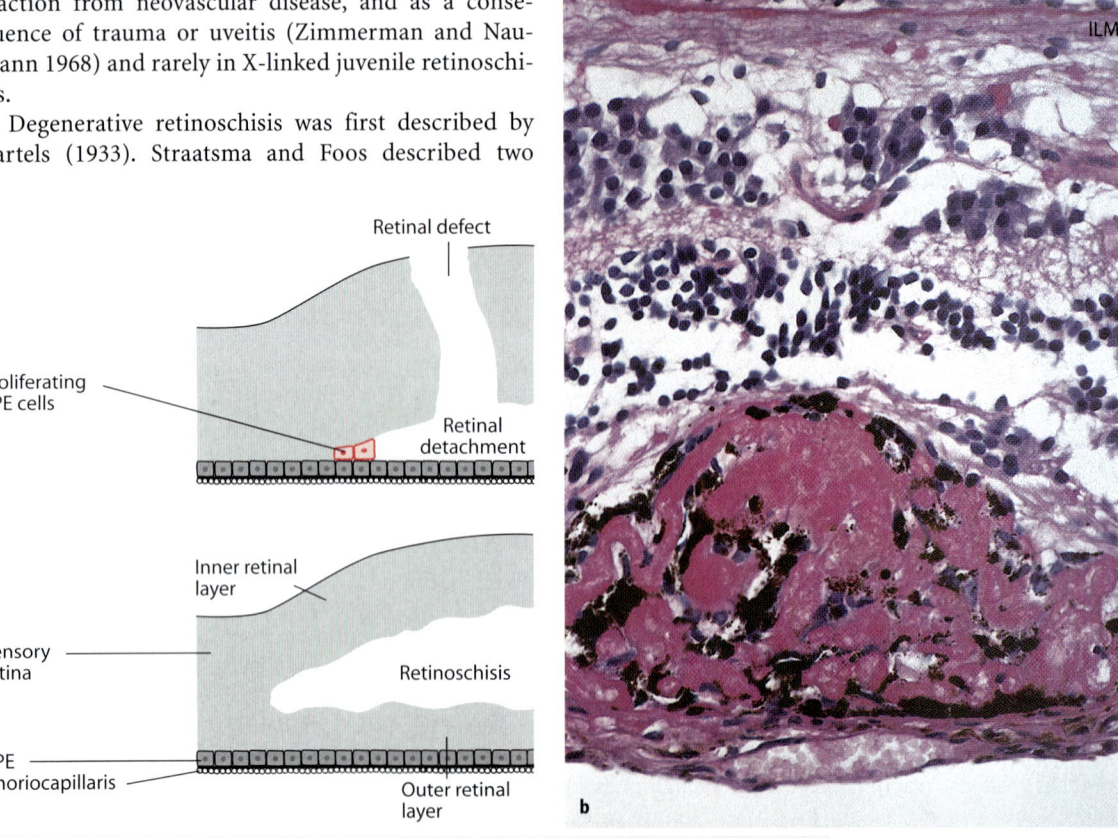

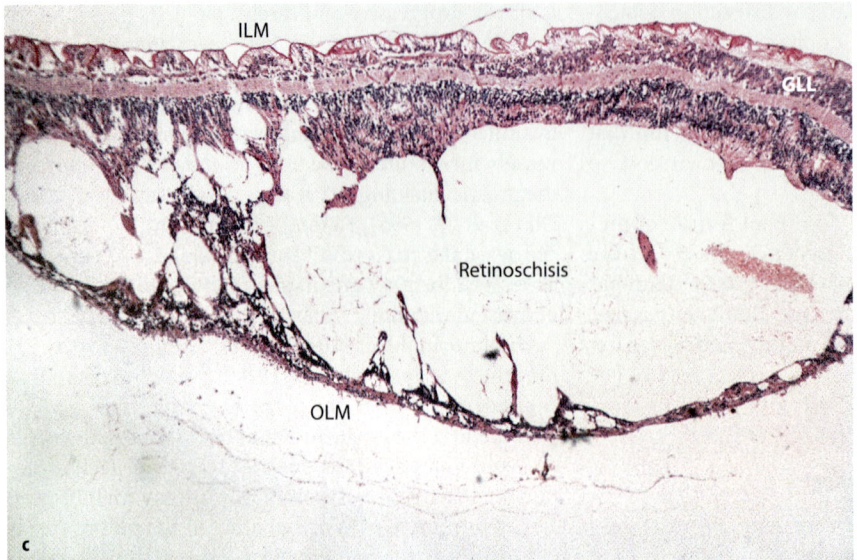

Fig. 5.6.8. a Retinal detachment and retinoschisis. Together with an old detachment additional schisis may develop. Much more rarely a detachment develops from a schisis with holes in the inner and outer layer. **b** RPE proliferation clump behind detached retina. **c** Retinoschisis in old detachment

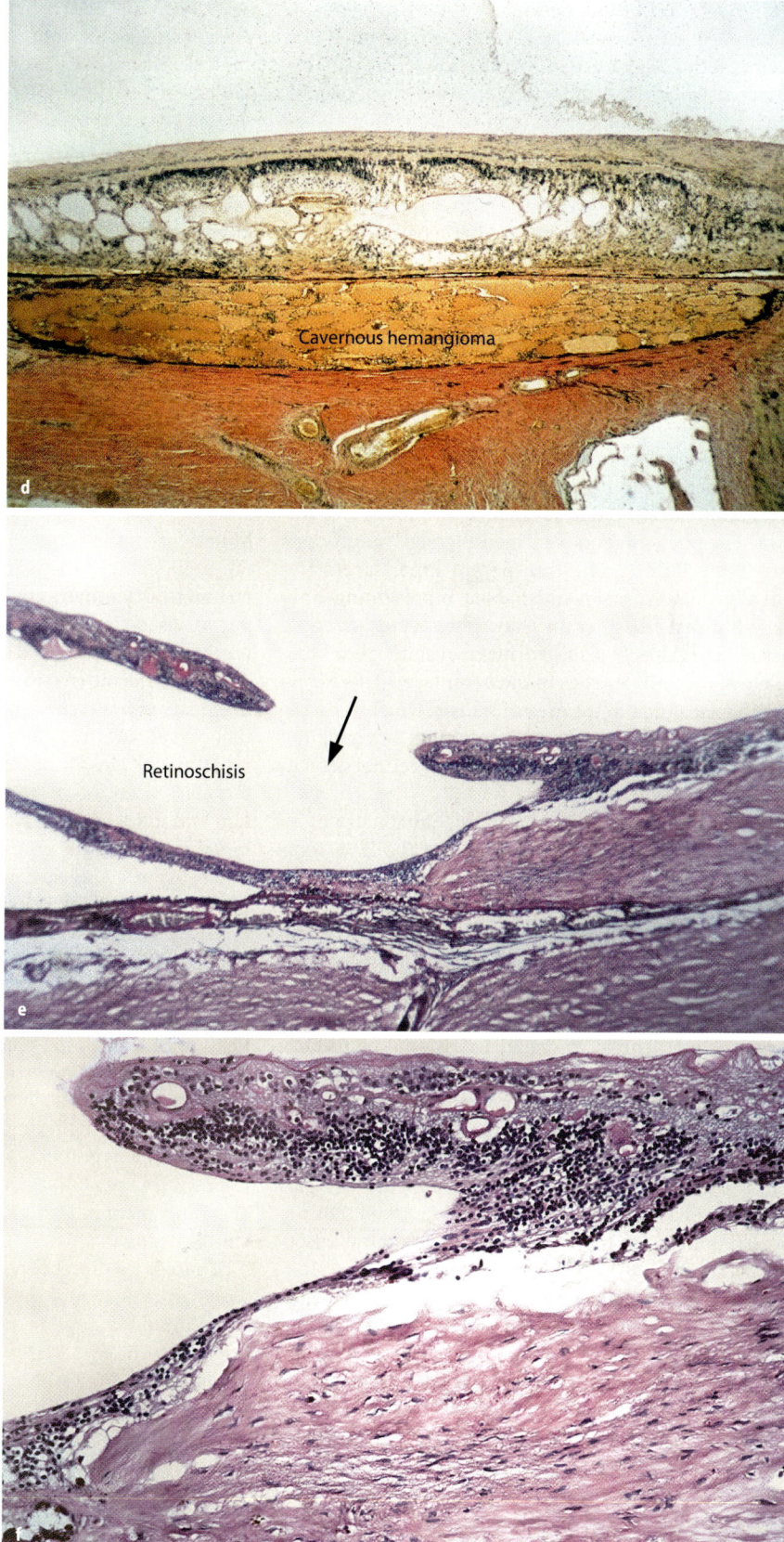

Fig. 5.6.8. d Secondary retinoschisis overlying cavernous hemangioma of the choroid. **e, f** Long-standing retinal detachment. Disciform fibrous macular degeneration with inner hole of the retinoschisis (*arrow*)

eration of neuroretinal and glial supporting elements in the periphery (Lewis 2003). This area enlarges slowly accumulating acid mucopolysaccharide sensitive to hyaluronidase (Zimmermann 1960). As a consequence, separation or splitting of the retina into an inner and an outer layer occurs with severing of neurons and ruptures of Müller cells leading to irreversible loss of visual function – relevant if it extends more centrally.

In *typical* retinoschisis, the retinal separation occurs deeper in the retina (at the level of the outer plexiform layer) as compared to *reticular* retinoschisis (inner plexiform layer). Thus, histopathology of typical retinoschisis shows that the inner layer contains the ILM, retinal vessels, and inner plexiform layer, while the outer layer has portions of the outer plexiform, outer nuclear, and photoreceptor layers.

Cyst formation in typical retinoschisis (or typical cystoid degeneration) begins in the outer plexiform layer and was referred to as "edema" by Blessig and Ivanoff. The phenomenon is termed Blessig-Ivanoff cysts (see Sect. 5.6.2.1). The transparent inner layers frequently demonstrate whitish dots representing lipid carrying glial cells after they have phagocytosed retinal tissue. The aspect of forged metal results from remnants of torn Müller cells in the outer layer. There is an absolute scotoma in the area of schisis, which is due to the interruption between photoreceptors and ganglion cells (while a relative scotoma occurs in retinal detachment).

In contrast, *reticular* retinoschisis demonstrates an extremely thin inner wall consisting of the ILM, remnants of the nerve fiber layer, attenuated blood vessels, and a complete loss of the supporting radial pillars. Of note, the schisis is mainly located vitreal to the neuronal layer. Holes in the outer layer can progress to schisis detachment.

Degenerative retinoschisis is "idiopathic" with no relation to a genetic, vascular, nutritional or tractive etiology. Typical retinoschisis occurs in 1% of patients, and reticular retinoschisis in 1.6% of the analyzed autopsy eyes (Straatsma 1973, 1986). There is an increasing incidence of 3.7% in patients older than 10 years, but 7% in patients above age 40 years. Eighty-two percent of the cases are bilateral (Straatsma 1968). Retinoschisis is most commonly found in the temporal-inferior quadrant.

A rhegmatogenous retinal detachment rarely occurs in eyes with retinoschisis and retinal breaks. Retinoschisis without retinal breaks in either layer does not cause retinal detachment. In retinoschisis, inner retinal holes are rare and probably occur in less than 4% of cases (Byer 1968, 1986). The incidence of tractional retinal tears in retinoschisis is extremely low. However, retinal tears, secondary to posterior vitreous detachment, may be important in causing progressive rhegmatogenous retinal detachment. Outer retinal holes are more common than inner retinal breaks, and they are present in 23% of autopsy cases and in up to 17% of clinical series (Byer 1986; Zimmermann 1960). They can be single or multiple, can be very large in size, and show a prominent rolled posterior border.

There are two types of retinal detachment associated with retinoschisis: a localized and relatively stable form with outer retinal holes only, and a symptomatic, rapidly progressive detachment with retinal breaks in *both* layers.

In advanced cases, occlusive vascular changes over areas of acquired retinoschisis were observed. There was intraretinal leakage of the dye from deep capillaries and pooling of the dye in cystic cavities near the margin of the retinoschisis (Tolentino et al. 1976).

5.6.2.4.1
X-Linked Retinoschisis

Mutations in the retinoschisin gene, *RS-1*, cause juvenile X-linked retinoschisis (XLRS), a dystrophy characterized by delamination of the inner retinal layers, leading to visual impairment. Although the *retinoschisin protein* (RS) is expressed most abundantly in photoreceptors in the outer retina, XLRS disease affects the innermost retinal layers, including the nerve fiber layer that contains retinal ganglion cells (RGCs).

All major classes of adult retinal neurons, with the possible exception of horizontal cells, express RS protein and mRNA, strongly suggesting that retinoschisin in the inner retina is synthesized locally rather than being transported, as earlier proposed, from distal retinal photoreceptors (Takada et al. 2004).

Foveal lesions vary from predominantly radial striations, microcystoid lesions, honeycomb-like cysts, or their combinations to non-cystic-appearing foveal changes, such as pigment mottling, loss of the foveal reflex, or an atrophic-appearing lesion. Evidence of smaller perifoveal cysts on OCT imaging suggests their location being primarily within the inner nuclear layer of the retina. The findings on OCT images are consistent with the hypothesis of a primary Müller cell defect (Apushinkin et al. 2005a, b). In view of their more radial arrangement in Henle's layer, this fits with perifoveal slitlike changes.

There is no direct correlation between visual acuity, foveal thickness, and the cystic area.

A limited change in visual acuity was observed in our cohort of 38 patients with XLRS even over an extended period. However, patients with pigment mottling or an atrophic-appearing lesion have a more visual impairment compared to those with a cystic-appearing foveal change (Apushinkin et al. 2005a, b).

Surgical or medical treatment for X-linked retinoschisis is not available.

Table 5.6.7. Differential diagnosis of macula hole and its early stages

Preretinal:	Macular pucker with pseudoforamen
Intraretinal:	Cystoid maculopathy
Subretinal:	Central serous macular detachment
	Solar retinopathy
	Central drusen

5.6.2.5 Macular Hole

A macular hole seriously affects visual acuity. Until recently a satisfactory form of treatment was not available. This topic requires detailed discussion. While only 5–15% of the macular holes are a result of blunt trauma or a consequence of high myopia (Reese et al. 1967; McDonnell et al. 1982), 83% of the macular holes in clinical practice are "idiopathic" (Freemann 1993). Ten percent of the macular holes are bilateral (Aaberg 1970). Several hypotheses for the pathogenesis of full thickness macular holes have been suggested including cystoid foveal degeneration and systemic vascular disease. From early investigations of the fine structure of the vitreous (Sect. 5.6.1.2), it was suggested that a premacular bursa in the vitreous leads to the formation of a hole by mechanical forces due to fluid motion and countercurrents in the premacular bursa during ocular movements (McDonnel 1982; James 1980; Aaberg 1970; Yaoeda 1967; Noyes 1971; Collins 1900). In some cases, an apparent operculum containing fibrous astrocytes and Müller cells over the macular hole was confirmed (Ho et al. 1998) and removal of this membrane led to a marked visual improvement.

The frequent association between cellophane membranes and macular holes indicates a possible common pathogenic pathway. Macular hole without evidence of an epiretinal membrane and macular pucker possibly represent two aspects of the same disease, which can be termed traction maculopathy or "*vitreomacular traction syndrome.*" (Fig. 5.6.9). Various intermediate stages between macular hole and macular pucker are in favor of the hypothesis that the condition of the vitreous and the activity of cellular proliferation modulate the disease (see Sect. 5.6.2.6) (Fig. 5.6.10). It is important to distinguish idiopathic macular holes and their initial stages from other diseases such as central serous retinopathy, solar retinopathy, cystoid macular edema, central drusen and macular pucker with pseudo-holes (Fig. 5.6.11–5.6.17).

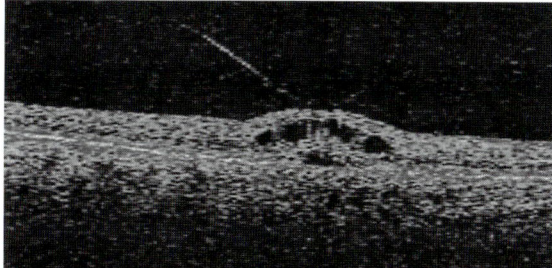
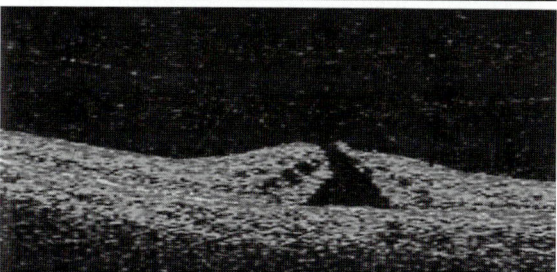
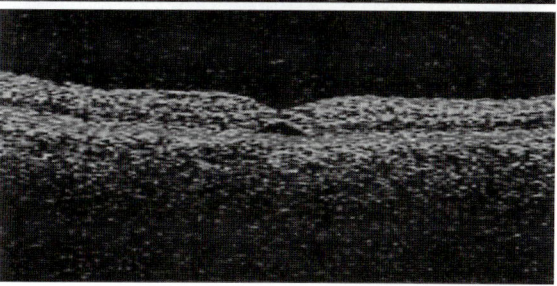

Fig. 5.6.10. Optical coherence tomography (OCT) demonstrating *vitreomacular traction* (*upper*) leading to an impending hole characterized by foveal cyst formation, with the presence of a cystic cavity beneath the elevated retina, *a stage 2 macular hole* (*middle*), and spontaneous closure of the hole after vitreous detachment; a small cystic cavity beneath the elevated retina is still present

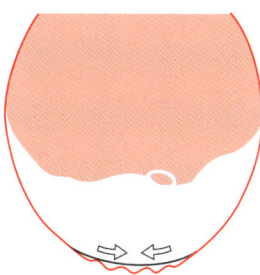
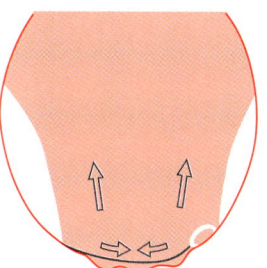
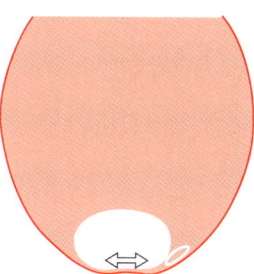

Fig. 5.6.9. Manifestations of vitreomacular traction. "Pucker" (*left*): tangential macular traction with epiretinal contractile membranes with detached vitreous. "Vitreomacular traction syndrome" (*middle*): anterior macular traction with partially detached, but posteriorly attached vitreous (with and without contractile epiretinal membranes). "Impending hole" (*right*): tangential and radial macular traction, e.g., via movements of the bursa macularis with attached posterior vitreous and/or discrete contractile membranes

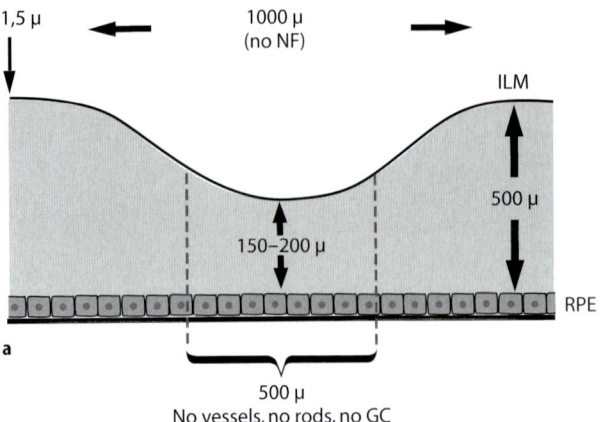

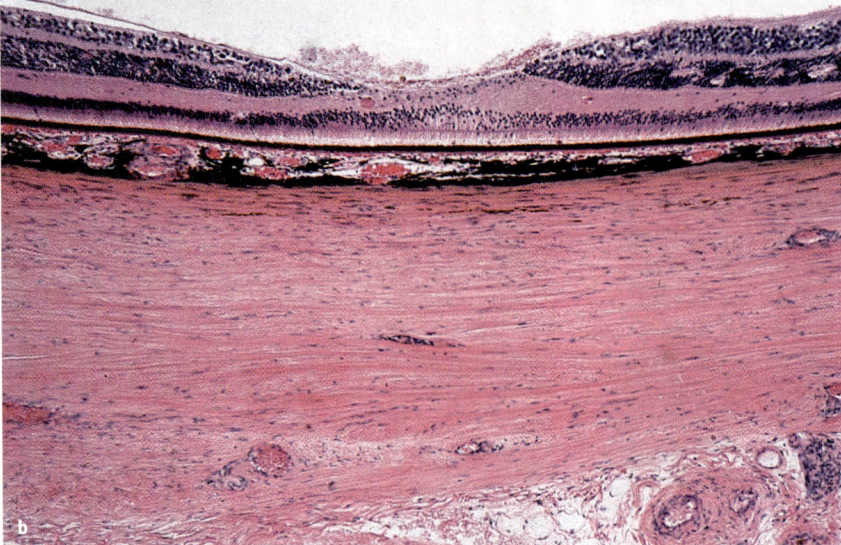

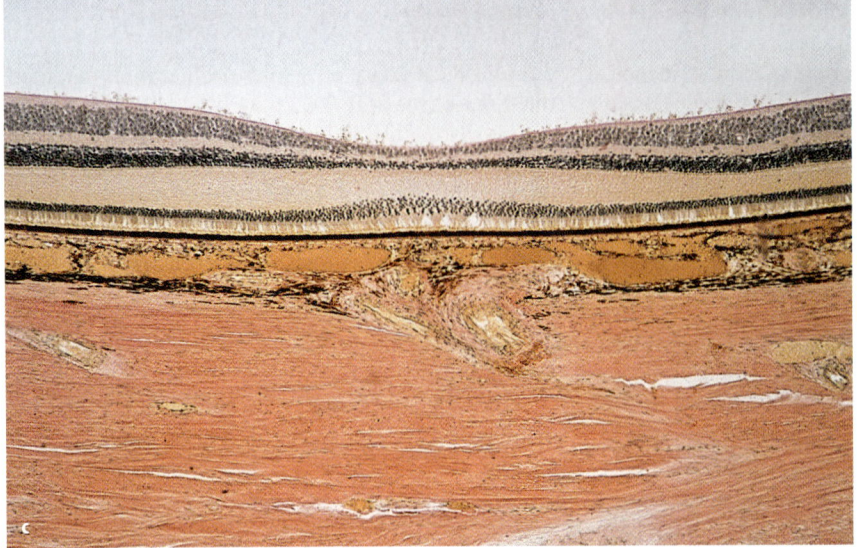

Fig. 5.6.11a–d. Cross sections through macular regions close to the foveola. **a** Scheme with dimensions: Ganglion cells (*GC*), Nerve-fiber-layer (*NF*), retinal pigmentepithelium (*RPE*) **b** Retinal ganglion cells bare the foveola region. **b–d** From different eyes

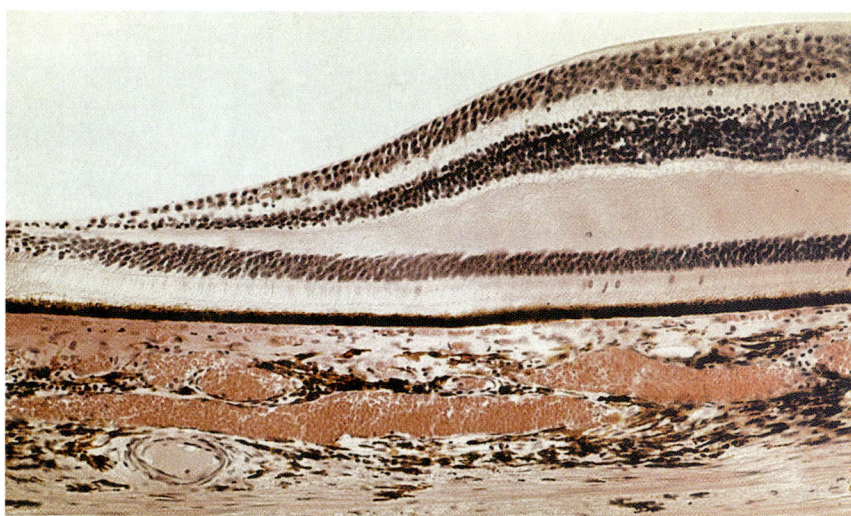

Fig. 5.6.11d

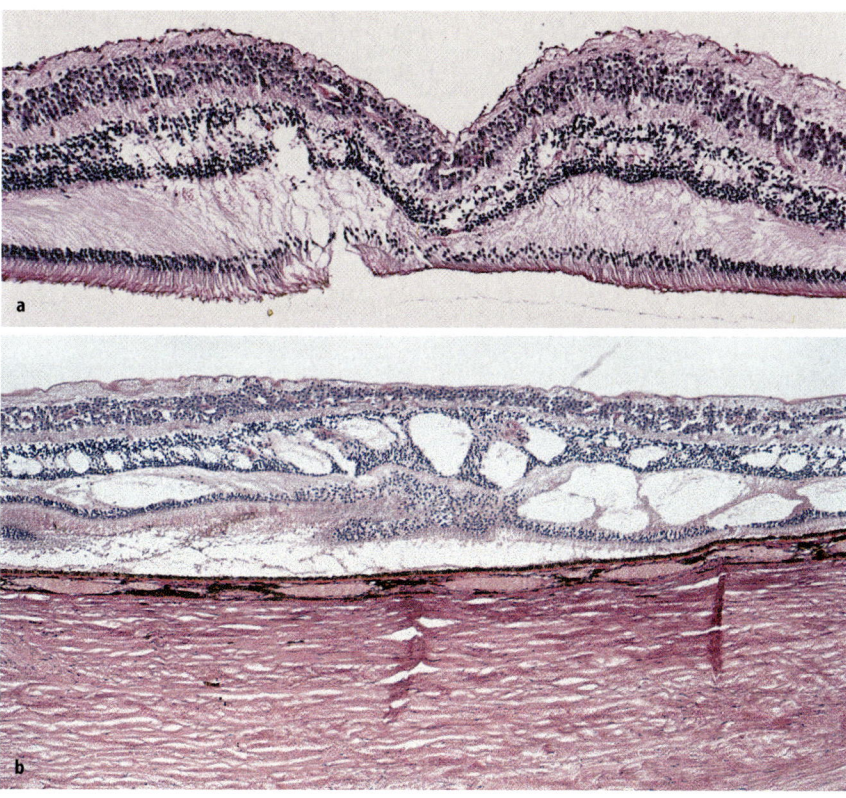

Fig. 5.6.12a, b. Cystoid macular edema. Confluent cystoid spaces. Note the preserved layer of photoreceptors (PAS)

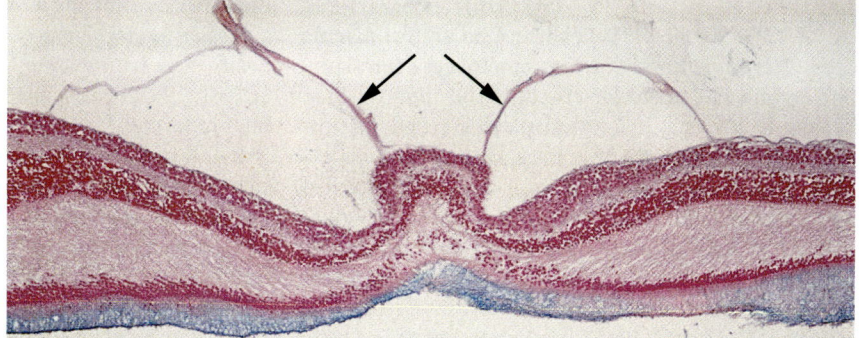

Fig. 5.6.13. Cystoid maculopathy with macular folds. Detachment of the internal limiting membrane (*arrows*), Alcian blue

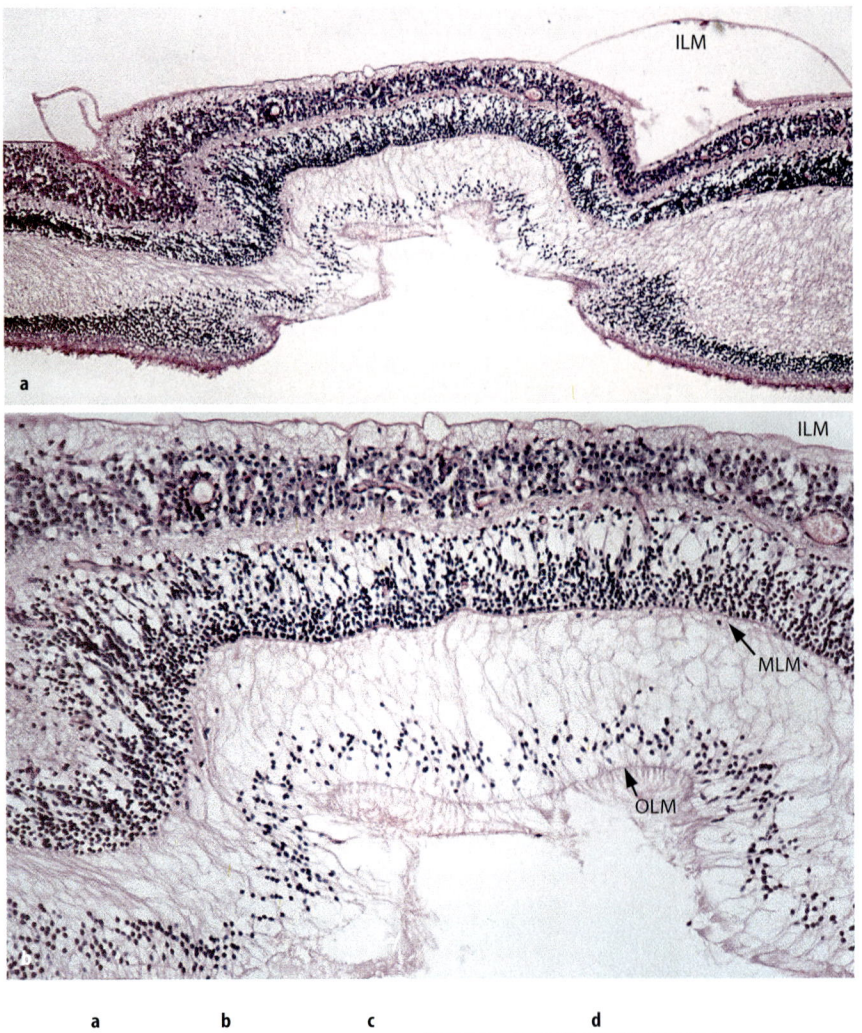

Fig. 5.6.14. Cystoid maculopathy. **a** Cross sections close to foveola. **b** Cystoid spaces in the inner and outer plexiform layer. Inner limiting membrane (*ILM*), outer limiting membrane (*OLM*), middle limiting membrane (*MLM*) (PAS)

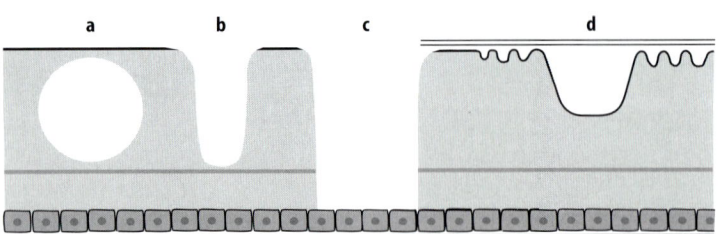

Fig. 5.6.15. Schematic drawing hole and pseudohole: **a** Cystoid space. **b** Incomplete hole. **c** Full thickness hole. **d** Pseudohole

According to Gass, four stages of macular hole are distinguished (Gass 1988, 1995) (Fig. 5.6.18). Characteristic of stage 1a are a yellowish spot at the macula (100–200 µm diameter), a lack of a foveal depression, and an attached posterior vitreous. The spot can then expand to 200–300 µm, forming a ring visible on funduscopy (stage 1b). While in the early stages of macula hole no histology is available, OCT has contributed to a better understanding of the delicate structural changes in macular hole formation. According to Gass, the yellowish spot may be due to the xanthophyll enrichment in *photoreceptors* and is more visible after a foveal detachment (Gass et al. 1995). It is a matter of debate as to whether it is located in the inner or outer retinal layers (Tso 1980). Following a retinal dehiscence at the umbo, a passive enlargement of the "occult" hole occurs beneath the semiopaque, contracted vitreous cortex bridging the edges of the hole. The radial retraction of the photoreceptors results in the ring phenomenon. It is well recognized that 30–50% of stage 1a and 1b lesions will arrest or resolve spontaneously often with resolution symptoms in some eyes (Gass 1988; Johnson 1988; Kokame et al. 1995). In such cases, arrest usually occurs following vitreofoveal separation (Kokame et al. 1995), although some authors have suggested that anterior vitreofoveal traction occurs as a result of shrinkage

5.6.2 Surgical Pathology

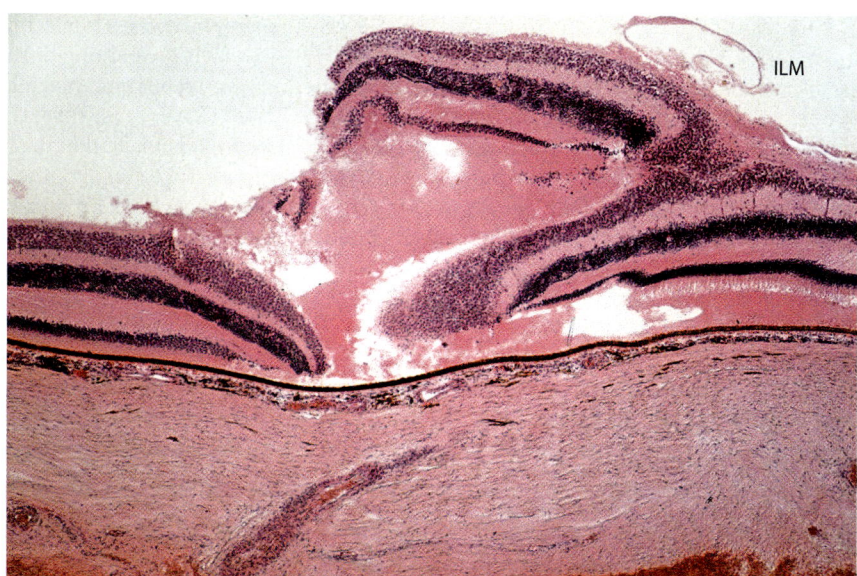

Fig. 5.6.16. Macular hole after severe contusion

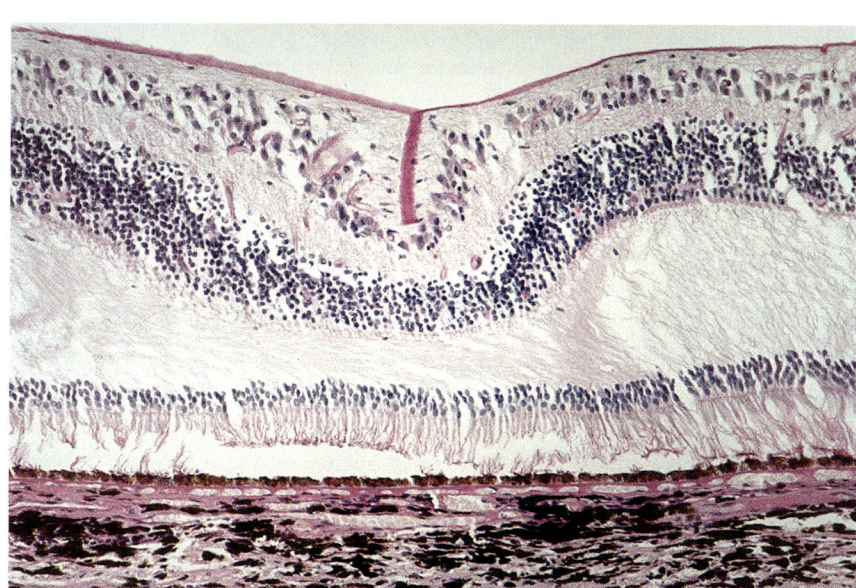

Fig. 5.6.17. Fixed macular folds after reversible ocular hypotony syndrome (PAS stain)

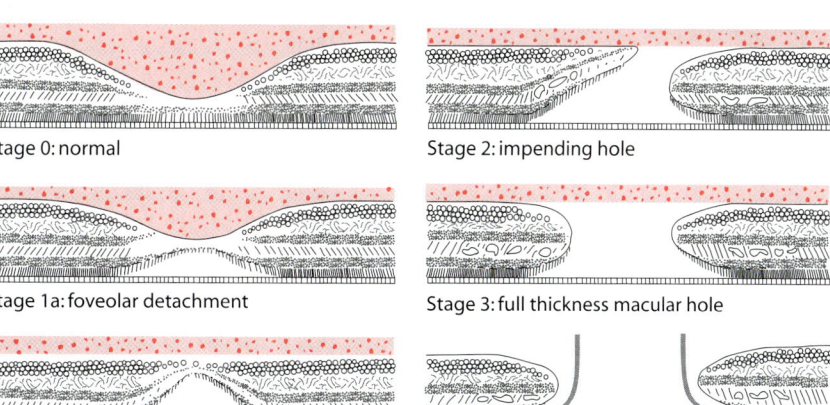

Fig. 5.6.18. Stages of macular holes (modified after Gass)

Stage 0: normal

Stage 1a: foveolar detachment

Stage 1b: foveolar detachment

Stage 2: impending hole

Stage 3: full thickness macular hole

Stage 4: full thickness macular hole with posterior vitreous detachment and elevated edges of vitreous collagen fibers extending from the fovea to the anterior vitreous (Matsomura 2005). However, it seems unlikely that this mechanism accounts for the majority of cases as anterior displacement of the foveal rim forward of the retinal surface is rarely seen: If it does occur, it is associated with an incomplete posterior vitreous detachment at the macula and is termed "vitreomacular traction syndrome" (Matusomura 2005). However, it is now generally accepted that idiopathic full thickness macular holes are caused by vitreofoveal traction.

Recent studies of the early stages of macular holes using OCT have shown that vitreomacular separation may actually occur around the posterior pole *before* hole formation rather than *after* hole formation as proposed by Gass (Fig. 5.6.10). These observations have suggested that an incomplete posterior pole vitreous cortical separation occurs with residual tethering at the fovea and optic disc, and assumes a "trampoline" configuration. Mechanical forces, which are transmitted through the vitreous with eye movements and possibly contraction of the vitreous face between the fovea and the disc and between the fovea and the residual peripheral extramacular temporal attachment, would result in an oblique vector force with both anterior and tangential vectoral components, leading to avulsion of foveal tissue and complete posterior pole vitreous separation.

This is consistent with the presence of radial striae in the majority of cases during the early stages, the presence and progression of the yellow spot and ring during *stage 1*, a relatively high incidence of posterior vitreous detachment (PVD) following the development of full thickness macular hole, and the negligible risk of hole formation in eyes with a preexisting PVD (Ezra et al. 2001). Whether or not vitrectomy and a surgically induced PVD improves prognosis in stage 1 macular holes is still controversial (de Bustros et al. 1994).

A *stage 2* macular hole is the early stage of a full-thickness hole. Frequently, the hole is eccentric and smaller than in the following stages (max. 400 µm; Gass et al. 1995). At this stage, vitrectomy does have a beneficial effect (Kim et al. 1996).

Stages 3 and 4 are full-thickness macular holes of approx. 500 µm which are surrounded by a *halo of detached retina*. In some cases, yellowish drusen are found at the level of the RPE and an operculum floating in the posterior vitreous can be seen. While in stage 3 the posterior vitreous is still attached, stage 4 holes present with a detached vitreous (Gass 1988). The detached retina adjacent to the hole has a microcystoid appearance (Guyer and Green 1992, 2005). Folds in the ILM point to tangential traction forces. Similarly, the ILM is surgically easier to remove and the adhesion between ILM and inner retina seems to be loosened. The ILM is covered by a thin layer of cortical hyaloid and in 68% of cases by a glial membrane with few cells. This membrane can be determined by a lack of indocyanine green (ICG) staining during surgery.

As ideopathic macular holes can spontaneously close (Lewis et al. 1986; Guyer et al. 1990; Bidwell et al. 1988), it is likely that macular holes are a consequence of radial *retraction* of the fovea edges without photoreceptor loss rather than a tissue loss. The assumption is that the preretinal cells around the hole hold the defect open. A release of traction would then allow for a spontaneous hole closure. In contrast, others have suggested that repair takes place by Müller cells growing over the hole and filling the defect (Faude et al. 2004).

The impact of a foveal Müller cell "cone," originally described by Yamada (1969) and Hogan et al. (1971) in histological studies demonstrating that the foveola is composed of an inverted cone of Müller glia with a truncated apex up to the external limiting membrane (ELM) (Yamada et al.1969; Hogan et al.1971), has been discussed in the pathogenesis of macular holes (Gass et al. 1999).

Although previous histological data from light and electron microscopic analyses of prefoveal vitreous cortex, removed at the time of surgery for impending holes, have confirmed the presence of glial cells at this early stage of hole development (Campochiaro et al. 1992; Smiddy et al. 1989), it remains unclear whether these glia initiate foveolar traction by cortical vitreous remodeling or whether they represent an attempted healing response to mechanically induced damage at the fovea due to vitreous traction (Madreperla et al. 1995; Eszra et al. 1997).

Histopathological studies on the ultrastructure of stage 3 macular hole opercula have provided further clues to the pathophysiological mechanisms in full thickness macular hole formation. On immunohistochemical analysis, glial fibrillary acidic protein (GFAP), vimentin, and cellular retinaldehyde binding protein-positive glia have been present in the opercula. All opercula (100%) studied to date have been found to contain *Müller cells* and/or *fibrous astrocytes*. Between 61% and 100% have had identifiable ILM fragments and about 40–50% have contained cone photoreceptors ranging from a few scattered cones to those with densely packed cone photoreceptors (Gass et al 1999; Madreperla et al. 1995; Eszra 1997).

It is difficult on histological grounds to determine whether glial cells within an operculum are avulsed epiretinal glia within a membrane (*pseudo-operculum*), avulsed inner retinal glia (*true operculum*), or both. However, the presence of fragments of ILM in some opercula (Madreperla et al. 1995; Eszra 1997) indicates that a significant number of opercula containing only glia also contain avulsed glial tissue from the inner fovea and are thus "true opercula." The lack of identifiable ILM in some opercula may be explained by sampling of non-serial sections or suggests that these may represent avulsed epiretinal glia rather than inner retinal glia. In these cases "in-situ" disruption of the Müller cell cone may indeed be sufficient to cause an umbo dehiscence (Gass et al. 1999). The variation in cone-photoreceptor density in opercula (40–50% contain photoreceptors) probably reflects the amount of foveal tissue avulsed during hole formation. The extent of foveal neuroretinal tissue loss may affect the outcome of surgery (Ezra et al. 2001).

Although a glial cell activation cannot be neglected, according to the accepted concept of macular hole formation, the most important prerequisite is the *attached posterior vitreous* (Smiddy et al. 1990; Gyer and Green 1992) together with a premacular fluid accumulation (bursa premacularis; Worst 1977; see Sect. 5.6.1.2). Eye movements cause fluid movements in the bursa and tangential traction on the posterior vitreous resulting in macular hole formation.

Traumatic macular holes after blunt trauma may have a different pathogenesis and are likely to be due to a tissue defect by apoptosis of retinal neuronal cells and/or photoreceptors (Weinstock 1976). Contusion leads to loss of receptor outer segments (Berlin's edema without cherry-red spot) via *"contre coupe"* in monkey experiments (Smiddy et al.; see Chapter 11).

A report on a spontaneous closure of traumatic macular hole demonstrated on OCT imaging of a band of tissue linking the inferior edge of the hole to the foveal RPE, and the presence of hyperreflective (glial) material at the bottom of the hole (Carpentino et al. 2005).

Recent work has shown that surgical intervention including vitrectomy, cortical vitreous peeling, and gas tamponade is beneficial in the majority of eyes with full-thickness macular holes in promoting anatomical closure and foveal reapposition with subsequent visual improvement (Kelly 1991; Wendel 1993; Glaser 1992; Lansing 1993; Orrellana 1993; Ruby 1994; Wells 1996; Ryan 1994).

As a spontaneous closure of stage 3 and 4 macular holes is unlikely, surgical intervention in these cases has gained early acceptance. Compared with observation alone, a significant benefit due to surgery was found in the rate of hole closure (4% vs 69%, $p < 0.001$). A significant benefit due to surgery was found in visual acuity after adjusting for baseline visual acuity, hole duration, and maximum hole diameter. However, side effects of the vitrectomy, such as increasing nuclear sclerosis after vitrectomy, should be considered (Freeman et al. 1997). Later reports by Ezra et al. demonstrate a closure rate of 86% after vitrectomy alone (Ezra et al. 2004). The primary closure rate was even improved with gas tamponade (Lai et al. 2003; Couvillion et al. 2005).

A randomized prospective trial evaluated the risks and benefits of vitrectomy surgery in eyes with stage 2 macular holes (Kim et al. 1996). Compared with observation alone, surgical intervention in stage 2 macular holes resulted in a significantly lower incidence of hole enlargement and appeared to be associated with better outcome in some measures of visual acuity.

Nevertheless there is controversy about the necessity of long-term vitreous tamponades and the required positioning. Assuming that a continuous tamponade enforces a sufficient glial wound healing, the significantly higher success rate using C_3F_8 tamponade without positioning compared to SF_6 gas tamponade with positioning suggested that the cumulative tamponade duration is a crucial factor in macular hole surgery (Szurman et al. 2000). In contrast, Sato and coworkers reported the OCT-determined progressive changes in a macular hole following vitreous surgery with a gas tamponade. Small macular holes appeared to be closed as early as 3 days after vitrectomy with gas tamponade. This suggests that the duration of maintenance of a prone position can possibly be shortened (Sato et al. 2003).

With improving visualization techniques (Sect. 5.6.2.8), *ICG-assisted retinal ILM peeling* is used during macular hole repair demonstrating an improvement in anatomic and visual results compared to patients without ILM peeling (DaMata 2004). ILM peeling improved the likelihood of successful macular hole closure to >92% (Al-Abdullah 2004). The technique and rationale of ILM peeling is explained elsewhere (Sect. 5.6.3.3). Vitreous surgery with ILM peeling was effective for macular hole associated with PDR, attaining not only macular hole closure but also resolution of persistent diabetic macular edema (Kurihara et al. 2005).

While autologous serum application does not enhance the results of surgery (Ezra et al. 2004), other adjunctive agents such as autologous platelet concentrate were considered to improve significantly the anatomic success rate of surgery for idiopathic macular holes, but did not improve postoperative visual acuity (Paques 1999). The authors recommend the use of autologous platelet concentrated in patients with persistent macular holes and confirmed ILM peeling.

5.6.2.6
Vitreoschisis and Both Macular and Peripheral Pucker (Figs. 5.6.19)

Epiretinal membranes may occur as a primary idiopathic disorder or secondarily after treatment of retinal tears or after surgery for retinal detachment. Similarly they are found in association with numerous other ocular diseases.

In autopsy eyes there is a prevalence of *idiopathic* epiretinal membranes in patients older than 50 years of 2% increasing to up to 20% in patients of 80 years and older (Roth et al. 1973; Pearlstone 1985). Clinical pre-

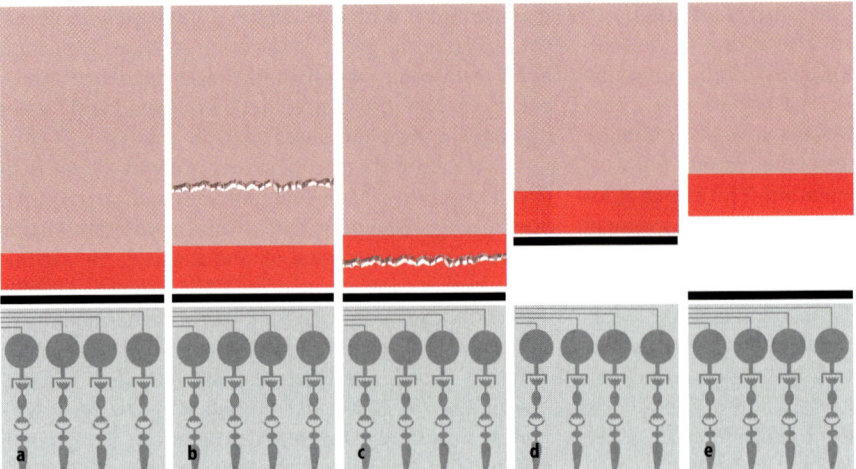

Fig. 5.6.19. Posterior vitreous detachment versus vitreoschisis (from Kirchhof et al. 1986). **a** Attached vitreous. **b** Gap within the vitreous gel. **c** Gap within the posterior vitreous cortex. **d** Complete posterior vitreous detachment including the ILM. **e** Complete posterior vitreous detachment without the ILM

sentation varies from *cellophane-type* to *pucker-type gliosis*. Visual symptoms range from no functional impairment to severe visual deterioration. Idiopathic epiretinal membrane formation usually shows slow progression or may remain stable with minor visual impairment (Fraser-Bell et al. 2003). Epiretinal membranes after surgery for rhegmatogenous detachment are observed in 46–76% of patients (Bonett et al. 1983). In contrast to idiopathic epiretinal membranes, severe *post-detachment pucker* occurs early after surgery and can demonstrate a rapid progression while often being confused with macular edema. Since these conditions can be treated surgically, the pathology and pathogenesis are of particular interest (Smiddy 1990), but the isolated tissue-samples are tiny.

Most histological investigations of epiretinal membrane formation were performed in eyes enucleated for malignancies or autopsy eyes (Bellhorn et al. 1975; Clarkson et al. 1977; Foos et al. 1974; Roth et al. 1971). More recently knowledge has been gained from the examination of surgically excised membranes and their cellular composition (Michels 1982; Smiddy 1990).

In the *adult pucker*, the epiretinal membrane contains *RPE cells* and *collagen* and there is a complete posterior detachment of the vitreous. In children and young adults, the epiretinal membrane contains *myofibroblasts* and *astrocytes* (Smiddy et al. 1992). In the vitreomacular traction syndrome, the vitreous is attached in the macular area and the epiretinal membrane contains *glial cells* and collagen. In *"impending macular hole,"* there is liquefaction of the vitreous anterior to the macula, which is lined on the inner surface by a thin layer of cortical collagen and layers of fibrous astrocytes (Messmer et al. 1998; Ishida et al. 2000). This cellular composition and the vitreoretinal interface with respect to an attached or detached vitreous deserve special attention. With age, the vitreous increasingly liquefies and the adhesion between the vitreous and the ILM loosens, resulting in a PVD. A *complete* PVD results in a clean and smooth retinal surface without vitreous remnants (Foos 1974). If the PVR remains *incomplete*, parts of the vitreous cortex remain on the retinal surface. This happens in cases of vitreous splitting (vitreoschisis), which is common in myopic and diabetic eyes, but can also be seen in emmetropic eyes with idiopathic epiretinal membranes (Sebag 1991, 1997).

The differences in the clinical course of idiopathic and secondary epiretinal membranes are explained by their different morphology. *Idiopathic* epiretinal membranes are mainly composed of glial cell (Müller cells, astrocytes) and newly formed collagen. Surgically ex-

Table 5.6.8. Electron microscopic criteria of periretinal membranes

Cell types	Electron microscopic criteria
1. RPE	Polarized cells with microvilli; junctional complex membranous melanosomes Intracytoplasmatic filaments (diameter 5–7 μm), basal membrane
2. Fibrous astrocytes	Large fusiform cells, intermedia filaments, diameter approx. 10 μm, junctional complex, interdigitating cytoplasmatic processes, basement membrane
3. Fibrocytes	Spindle shaped, no polarity, smooth nuclear contour, rich rough endoplasmatic reticulum, occasional desmosomes
4. Myofibroblasts	Spindle shaped, nuclear infoldings, cytoplasmatic bundles of parallel fibrils resembling small smooth muscle cells Electrodense bodies with attachment sites between the fibrils and the plasma: desmosome maculae adhaerentes
5. Macrophages	Pleomorph cells, no polarity, lobulated nucleus, intracytoplasmatic inclusions, e.g., melanin or hemosiderin in part secondary lysosomes

RPE retinal pigment epithelium

cised membranes demonstrate usually at least parts of ILM together with the epiretinal membrane. None of the histological phenotypes seems to correlate with visual outcome or clinical aspects of the membrane. In contrast, the composition of *secondary* epiretinal membranes, after detachment surgery for example, is more heterogeneous and may contain RPE cells, in addition to the glial cells, macrophages and fibroblasts (Clarkson 1977). These cell types can actively transform, de-differentiate and contract (see Sect. 5.6.4.3). Similarities to PVR may indicate a similar pathogenetic process. Pucker in eyes after coagulation therapy or after retinal detachment surgery is considered as a limited PVR reaction. Macular pucker formation occurs in eyes with retinal defects and subsequent RPE and fibroblast migration into the vitreous. It is not likely to be a result of the photocoagulation or laser treatment alone, as shown by the lack of pucker formation following panretinal laser coagulation (see Sect. 5.6.4.2). These observations are relevant for treatment of epiretinal membranes (see Sect. 5.6.3.3).

5.6.2.7
Retinal Vascular Abnormalities and Neovascularization (Figs. 5.6.20 – 5.6.27)

Retinal neovascularization occurs as a consequence of hypoxia ischemia, inflammation or vascular abnormality. Retinal neovascular disease ultimately leads to secondary glaucoma and is found in eyes which are enucleated to relieve pain in a blind eye (see Sect. 5.2). The primary diagnosis for eyes with these endstages includes central retinal vein occlusion, diabetic retinopathy, long-standing etinal detachment, retinopathy of prematurity and Coats' disease.

Comparing the dual blood supply, the retinal vessels emerging from the central retinal vein and artery seem to be more prone to be involved in vasoproliferative disorders (Fig. 5.6.20). The capillaries connecting arterioles and venules loop down to supply the inner layers of the retina. The outer layers of the retina are maintained via diffusion from the choriocapillaris supplied from the posterior ciliary arteries. Resulting from this dual blood supply, there is a *watershed zone* in the outer plexiform layer and the effects of hypoxic ischemic retinal capillary endothelial damage (blood-retinal barrier breakdown) are seen here as exudates of plasma.

Ischemia can occur in a spectrum ranging from *relative* hypoxia ischemia as seen in diseases presenting with capillary occlusion (diabetic retinopathy, Eales disease, sickle cell disease, central retinal vein occlusion) to a *complete* ischemia as present following occlusion of the central retinal artery.

Relative ischemia is characterized by a progression to neovascular disease with the consequences of blood-retinal barrier breakdown, the development of new capillaries and finally secondary angle closure glaucoma. In contrast, complete retinal ischemia, as seen with central retinal artery occlusion, is less prone to a neovascular response.

Relative ischemia leads to the release of vasoproliferative factors such as vascular endothelial growth factor (VEGF) and basic fibroblast growth factor (bFGF) (Schultz and Grant 1991; Aiello et al. 1995; Poulaki et al. 2003).

Nevertheless, hypoxia via activation of distinct transcription factors may also affect inflammatory processes, which in turn aggravate the inflammatory reaction.

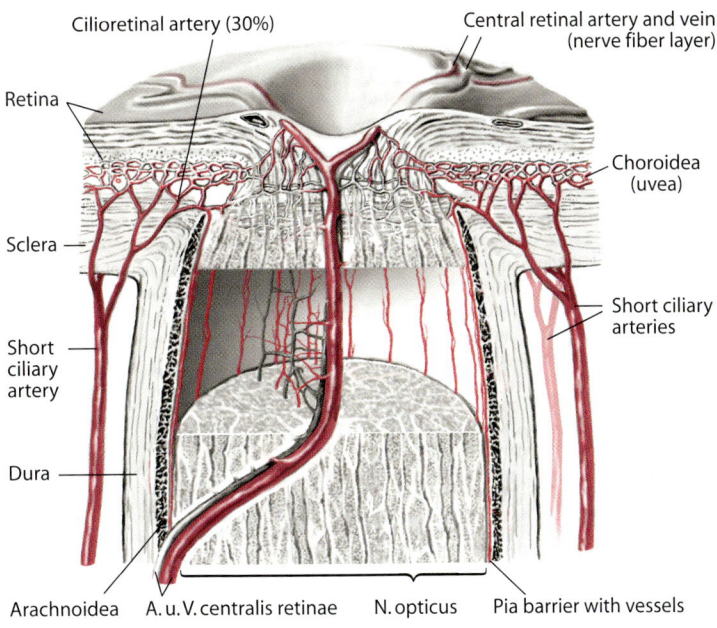

Fig. 5.6.20. Arteria ophthalmica splits into the central retinal artery (retinal circulation) and the short posterior ciliary arteries (choroidal circulation). The central retinal artery enters the eye via the optic nerve about 10 mm behind the globe and spreads on the disc surface in order to supply the quadrants of the peripheral retina. In 30 % of humans, a cilioretinal artery branches off the short posterior ciliary artery and enters the eye beside the optic nerve in order to supply the outer retinal layers, which are seen more often in larger than average disk size

Granulocytes and monocytes/macrophages of the myeloid lineage are the chief cellular agents of innate immunity. Activation of the transcription factor hypoxia-inducible factor (HIF-1alpha) is essential for myeloid cell infiltration and activation in vivo through a mechanism independent of VEGF. When HIF-1alpha is absent, the cellular ATP pool is drastically reduced. The metabolic defect results in profound impairment of myeloid cell aggregation, motility, invasiveness, and bacterial killing. The HIF-1alpha directly regulates the survival and function in the inflammatory microenvironment (Cramer et al. 2003a, b).

Pathological features of focal ischemic retinal disease:

1. Microinfarction ("cotton-wool" spots) (Fig. 5.6.21)
2. Exudation of plasma ("hard exudates") – defect in blood-retinal barrier at level of retinal capillaries (Fig. 5.6.22b)
3. Hemorrhage
4. Microaneurysms
5. Neovascularization (Fig. 5.6.22e)

The earliest response to focal ischemia is microinfarction, fundoscopically visible as "cotton wool" spots. Histologically, the inner retina is thickened by edema and an accumulation of eosinophilic bodies or cytoid bodies, which represent swollen ends of ruptured axons.

Ischemic damage to endothelial cells in the retinal capillaries leads to pooling of plasma in the outer plexiform layer. On macroscopic examination, there is a discrete yellow appearance which histologically stains pink by eosin. On macroscopic examination, there is a discrete yellow appearance which histologically stains the proteinaceous lakes and horizontal and vertical "*Leitstrukturen*" (see above) contained by Müller cells pink by eo-

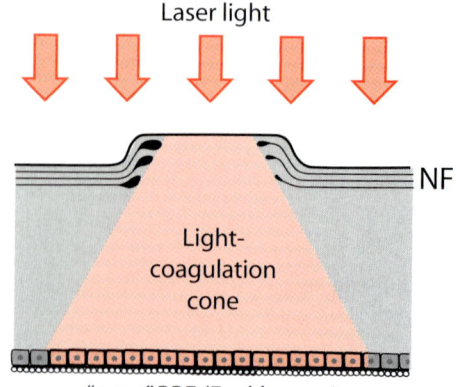

Fig. 5.6.21. Ischemic retinal microinfarct ("cotton-wool spot") following overdose of lasercoagulation: nervefiberlayer (*NF*), retinal pigmentepithelium (*RPE*)

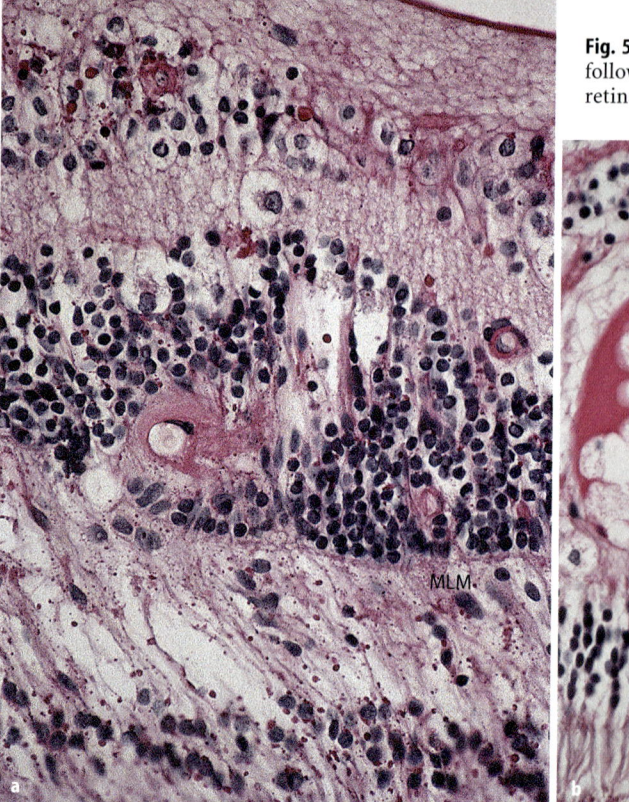

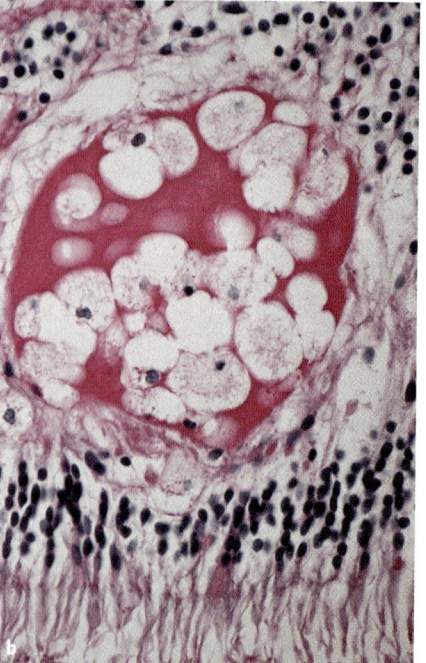

Fig. 5.6.22. Diabetic retinopathy. **a–d** Intraretinal changes: prominent staining of vascular channel wall confined to the tissue behind the internal limiting membrane.

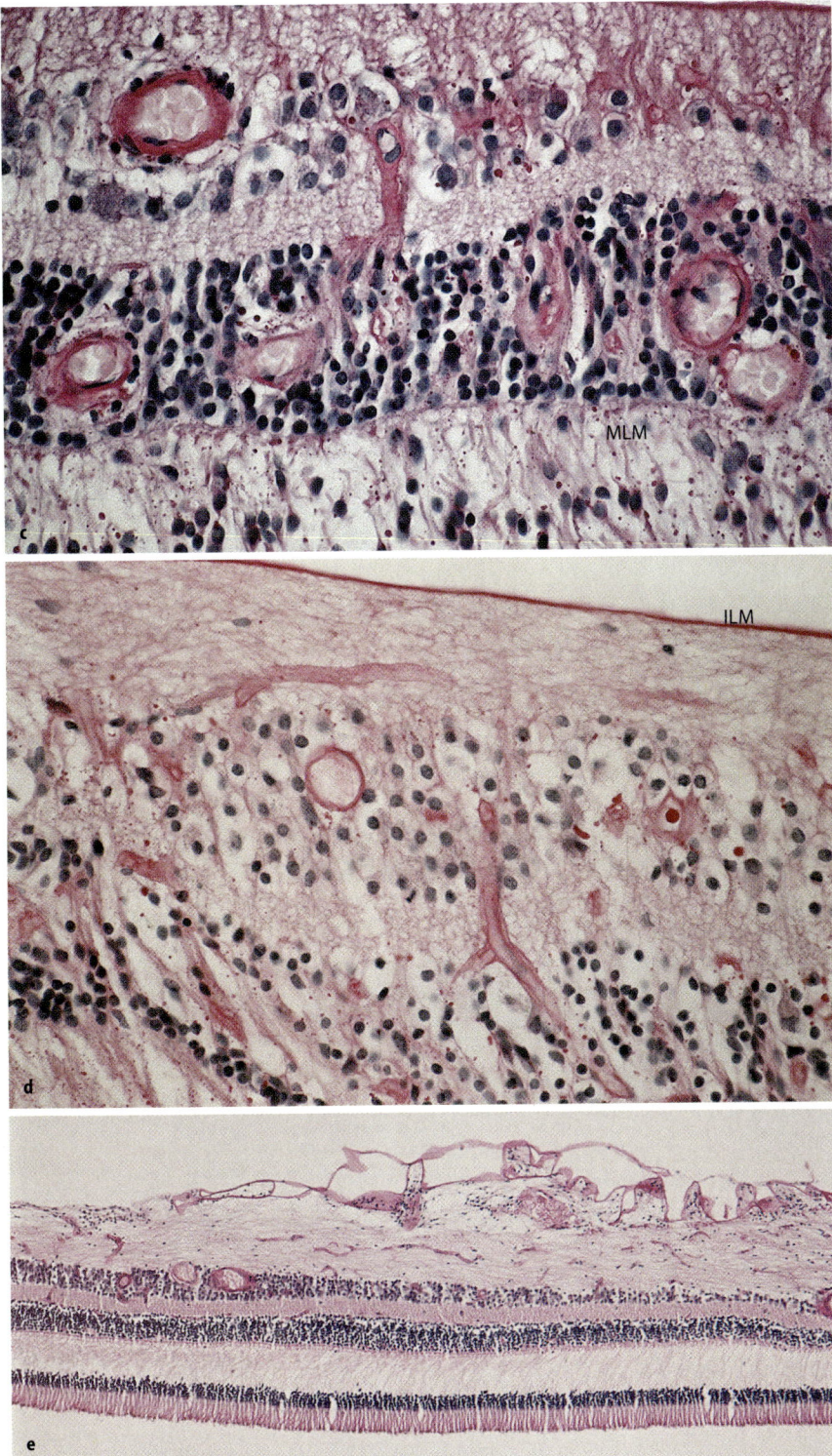

Fig. 5.6.22. (*Cont.*) Hard exudate consisting of lipid laden macrophages and PAS-positive material. **e, f** Capillaries break through internal limiting membrane forming preretinal vascular strands. **g, h** Formation of vascularized collagenous preretinal fibrous tissue (*blue* Masson stain), subretinal exudate (*SRE*) (Abbreviations see Fig. 5.6.4)

sin. Foamy macrophages within the lipoproteinaceous material resemble a self healing reaction (Fig. 5.6.22b).

The shape of *hemorrhages* depends on the source of bleeding and on the site of accumulation (see vertical and horizontal barriers). "Flame hemorrhages" result from bleeding from small arterioles tracking into the nerve fiber layer, while "dot hemorrhages" result from capillary bleedings into the outer plexiform layer. A subhyaloidal hemorrhage develops if the bleeding penetrates the ILM of the retina.

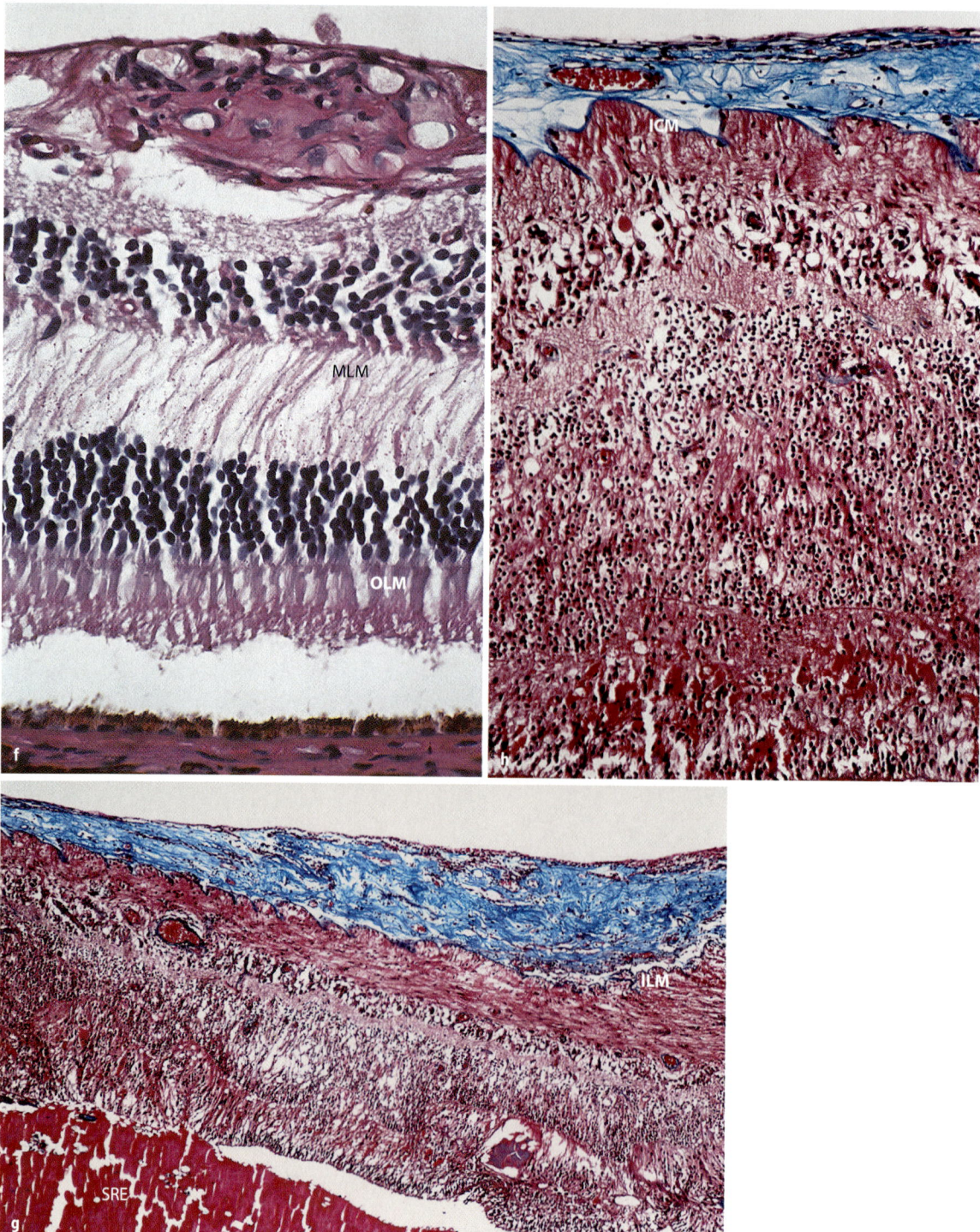

Fig. 5.6.22. (*Cont.*)

Microaneurysms are best evaluated on trypsin digest preparations. Interestingly, in diabetes of humans and experimental animals the most prominent feature of microaneurysms is the *dropout of pericytes* (Fig. 5.6.23), whereas in central retinal vein occlusion (CRVO) and arterial hypertension the number of endothelial cells is reduced (Bek 1998).

Neovascularization most frequently arises at the disc or the capillary bed at the edge of an infarcted area of retina, from the wall of a thickened venule or less

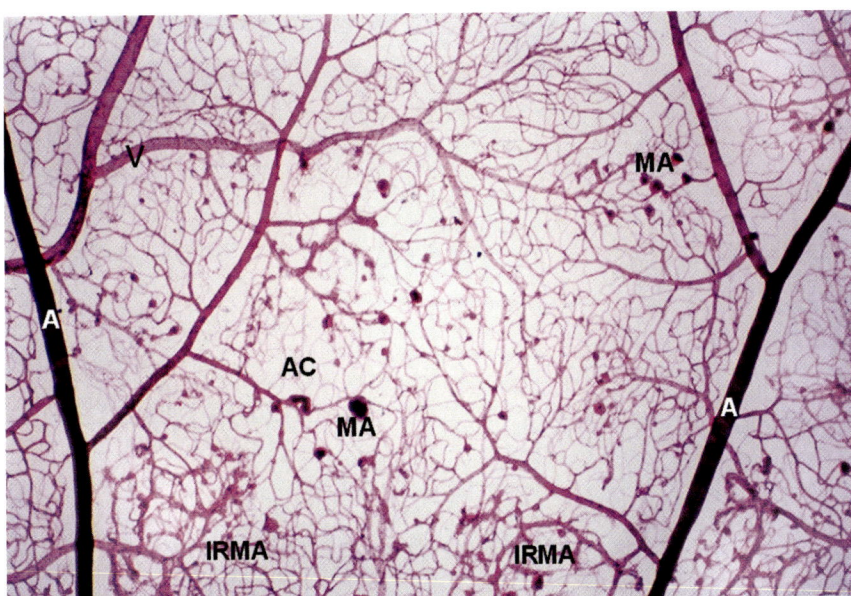

Fig. 5.6.23. Retinal Trypsin digest preparation of a diabetic human (*MA* microneurysms, *AC* acellular capillaries, *IRMA* intraretinal microvascular anomaly). Courtesy of Prof. Desmond B. Archer and Dr. Tom Gardiner, Belfast

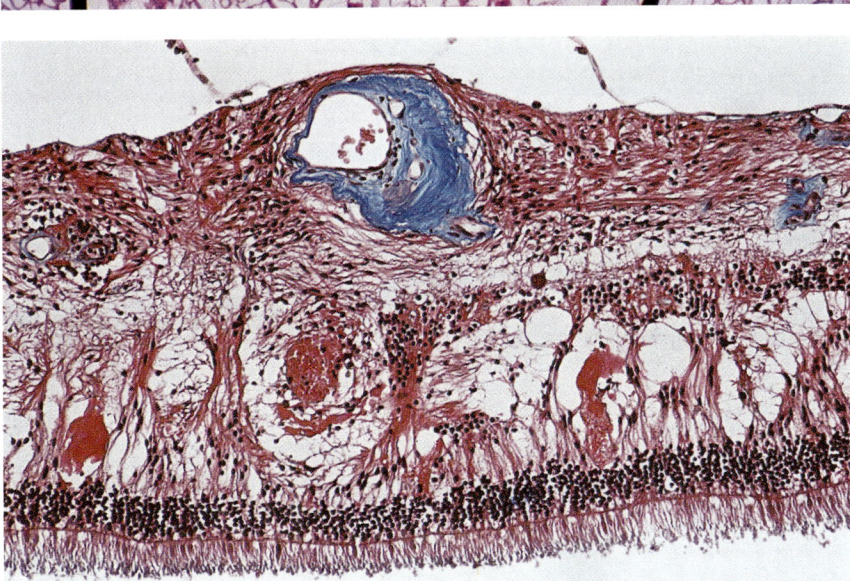

Fig. 5.6.24a, b. Marked thickening of retinal vessel wall by excessive collagen formation. **a** Masson

commonly from the wall of a hyalinized arteriole (Fig. 5.6.24). On histological sections, *endothelial cells stain positive for von Willebrand factor (F:VIII)*, while *glial cells are GFAP (glial fibrillary acidic protein) positive*. Neovascularization growing onto the posterior vitreous surface usually tends to form tight adhesions toward the retina along the vascular arcades developing tree-like proliferation of capillaries and fibroblasts into the vitreous. Rupture of the delicate capillaries releases blood cells which stimulate a macrophagic and fibroblastic reaction to continue the vicious circle. A condensation of sheets of capillaries supported by glial cells and fibroblasts growing on the posterior vitreous surface can cause wrinkling of the ILM and, finally, tractional detachment (Bek 1997a, b; Hofmann 2001) (Fig. 5.6.25).

Neovascularization is a prominent response to relative retinal hypoxia. Not surprisingly therefore the common pattern of retinal neovascularization is similar in different entities. Even though relative hypoxia can be the primary cause of neovascularization such as in CRVO, retinopathy of prematurity (ROP) or hemoglobinopathies, inflammation may play a role in the pathogenesis in diabetic retinopathy or Eales disease, as well as in radiation retinopathy. Vascular abnormalities resulting in relative hypoxia are found in Coats' disease, Norrie's disease, or are causal to FEVR (Table 5.6.9).

Neovascularization originates from the retinal capillaries always toward and beyond the ILM into the vitreous – and not into the outer retinal layer.

Total ischemic infarction of the retina by *central reti-*

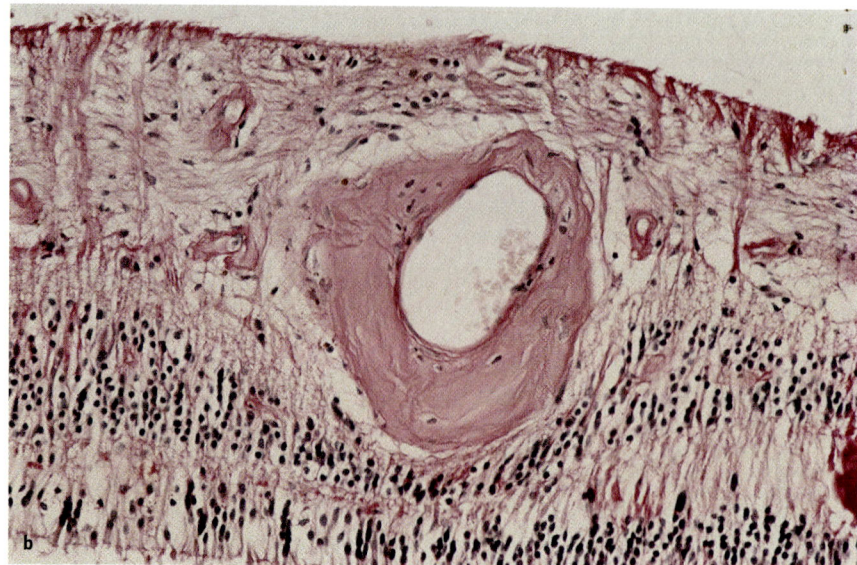

Fig. 5.6.24. b PAS

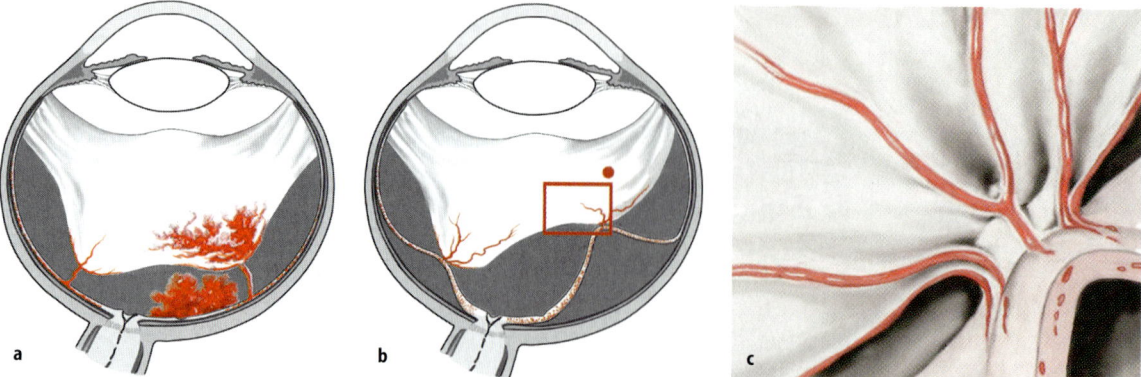

Fig. 5.6.25. Preretinal neovascularization. Schematic drawing of vitreous traction resulting in hemorrhage (**a**) and tractional detachment (**b**). (**c** higher magnification)

No vascularization	Relative hypoxia		Neovascularization
Ischemia (absolute hypoxia)	Relative hypoxia	Inflammation	Vascular abnormalities
Central retinal artery occlusion	Central retinal vein occlusion	Radiation retinopathy	Coats' disease
Posterior ciliary artery occlusion	Retinopathy of prematurity		Norrie's disease
Arterial hypertension	Hemoglobinopathies		Familiar exudative vitreoretinopathy
Disseminated intravascular coagulopathy	Diabetic retinopathy	Diabetic retinopathy	
	Eales disease	Eales' disease	

Table 5.6.9. Neovascularizations originating from relative retinal hypoxia

nal *artery obstruction* does not release vasoproliferative factors. Histologically, the retina consists of the photoreceptors, the outer nuclear layer and a thin layer remnant of cells in the inner nuclear layer at the end stage.

Obstruction of the choroidal blood supply in *posterior ciliary artery occlusion* results in an ischemia of the outer retinal layers which becomes histologically visible as a total loss of the outer nuclear layer. This is evident also in pulseless disease (see Font and Naumann; Founds 1971).

Characteristic features of arterial *hypertension* are described as narrowed vessels, which are occluded by fibrinoid necrosis of the wall with swelling and degeneration of the *endothelium* distal to the occlusion. Choroidal vessels in these patients are often found to be thickened by deposition of PAS-positive material.

5.6.2.7.1
Central Retinal Vein Occlusion

Central retinal vein occlusion is the classic disease leading to relative hypoxia and neovascularization and in the end-stage neovascular glaucoma.

On macroscopic examination the pathologist may see the disease only at the proliferative stage. Hemorrhagic retinopathy is mostly striking early after vein occlusion with blood cell accumulation throughout the retinal layers. Later in the disease the hemorrhagic stage may be more or less resolved. Sections may then demonstrate organized thrombi in the vessels partially undergoing recanalization. A cupped disc may be apparent and an atrophic retina with hyalinized and sclerotic vessels. Histologically preexisting hemorrhage will be identifiable by sectors of gliotic retina which stain positively for iron. Similar changes can be observed in the diseased quadrants after branch vein occlusion.

5.6.2.7.2
Retinopathy of Prematurity (ROP)

In retinopathy of prematurity a relative hypoxia after oxygen treatment in association with a peripheral still avascular retina results in neovascularization (Ben Sira et al. 1986). Today the end stage of the disease with exuberant neovascularization at the periphery with ingrowth into the vitreous and retinal detachment and formation of a white retrolental fibrous membrane (*"retrolental fibroplasia"*) is only rarely seen. Currently it is believed that high tissue oxygen levels in the developing neural retinal suppress the normal process of vascular ingrowth to the periphery. When the external exogenous oxygen supply is terminated, excessive vasoproliferation at the advancing edge of the retinal blood vessels occurs (Ashton 1966). This process is controlled via a VEGF release by astrocytes and ganglion cells and later on by the proliferating endothelial cells themselves (Stone et al. 1996; Gariano et al. 1996a, b). The neovascularization gradually increases from intraretinal arteriovenous shunts to preretinal proliferating endothelial buds to more severe preretinal neovascularization and, finally, tractional detachment.

The International Classification of Retinopathy of Prematurity (ICROP) was published in two parts, the first in 1984 and later an expanded version (An International Classification 1984 and 1987) (Fig. 5.6.26). It emphasizes the location and the extent of the disease in the retina as well as its stages (Fig. 5.6.27). The term "plus" is employed with the stage to denote progressive vascular incompetence. Few modifications were made in 2005 including the introduction of the concept of a more virulent form of retinopathy observed in the tiniest babies (aggressive, posterior ROP), and a description of an intermediate level of plus disease (pre-plus) between normal posterior pole vessels and frank plus disease (An International Classification 2005).

Table 5.6.10. Retinopathy: classification of sickle cell hemoglobinopathy (after Goldberg 1977)

Stage I	Peripheral arterial occlusion
Stage II	Peripheral arteriovenous anastomosis
Stage III	Neovascularization
Stage IV	Vitreous hemorrhage
Stage V	Tractional retinal detachment

5.6.2.7.3
Hemoglobinopathies

Hemoglobinopathies such as sickle cell disease are prone to neovascularization. Heterozygote patients with the genotype HbSC are more prone to neovascularization compared to the homozygote population (HbSS), which present with the more severe general disease (van Meurs 1991, 1992). A possible explanation is an anoxic condition not prone to neovascularization in severe cases of HbSS. In *sickle cell disease*, occlusion of vessels occurs by abnormally rigid red cells combined with blood stasis, hemolysis and subsequent intraretinal and subretinal hemorrhage. Interestingly, extraretinal neovascularization develops in the midperiphery, forming *"sea-fan" like structures* from hyalinized arterioles and venules (McLeod et al. 1997). *"Black sunburst"* lesions are reactive proliferations of RPE cells in response to intraretinal bleeding (Romayananda et al. 1973; Goldberg 1976).

5.6.2.7.4
Diabetic Retinopathy

The end stage is characterized by retinal detachment due to preretinal neovascularization. The clinically most relevant classification for diabetic retinopathy negative treatment is to distinguish between *non-proliferative disease* and the *proliferative forms*.

For histological evaluation of the retinal pathology, trypsin digest flat preparations are a fruitful approach (Cogan and Kuwabara 1984; Archer 1999) (Fig. 5.6.23). For this technique, formalin fixation of the specimen is required. Trypsin digest preparations enable the evaluation of basement membrane thickening, and pericyte and endothelial cell numbers. They show initially a selective loss of pericytes (mural cells) (for table see above). Recently, evidence has emerged that prior to the cellular damage seen on digest preparations *leukocytes with altered adhesion properties* may contribute to endothelial cell damage and capillary occlusion in diabetes (Miyamoto 1999; Joussen 2001, 2003). Thus,

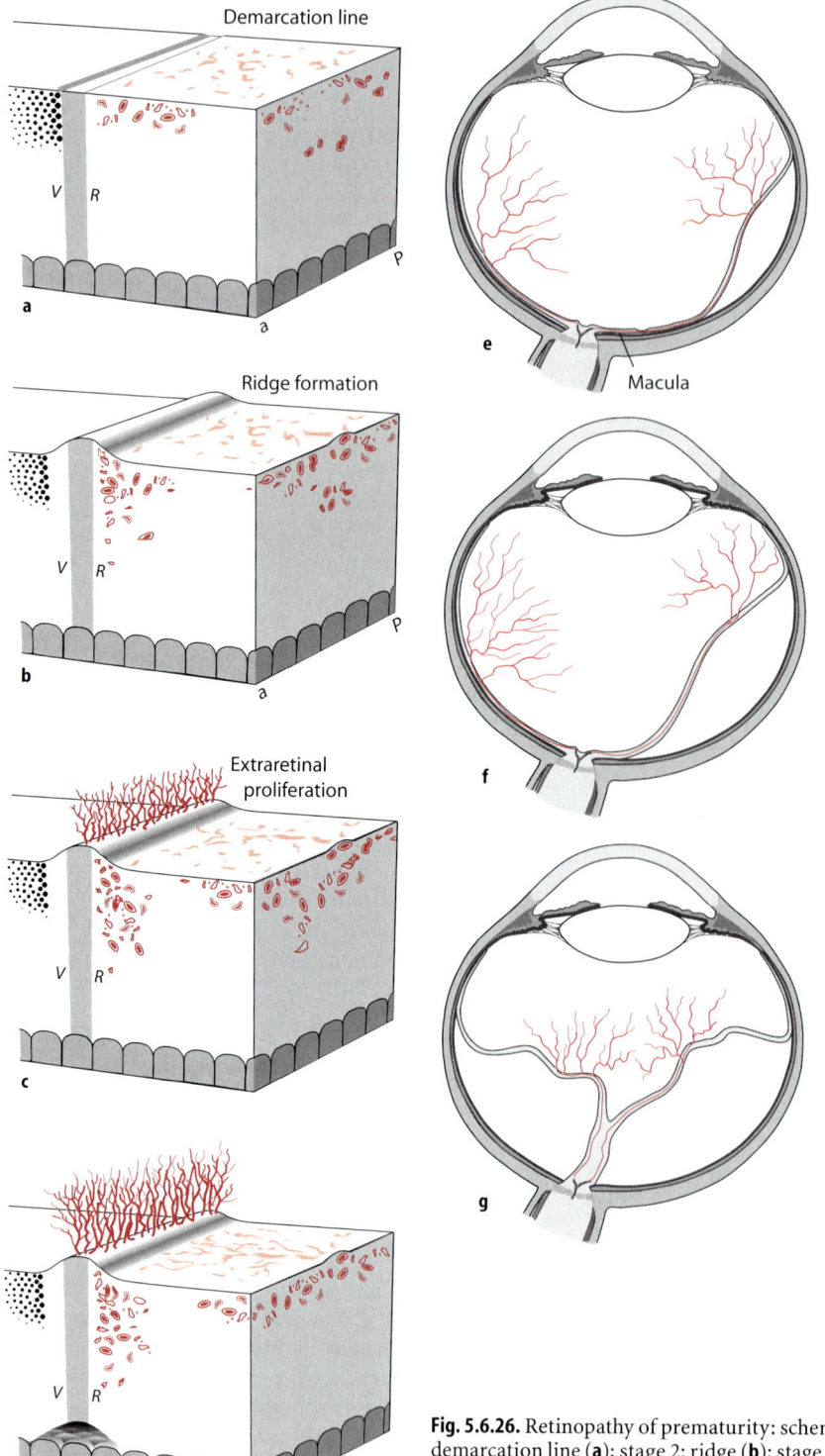

Fig. 5.6.26. Retinopathy of prematurity: schematic drawing of the stages: stage 1: demarcation line (**a**); stage 2: ridge (**b**); stage 3: ridge with preretinal fibrovascular proliferation (**c, d**); stage 4: peripheral tractional detachment with attached fovea (**e**), with foveal detachment (**f**); stage 5: total retinal detachment (**g**)

microvascular ischemia is tightly linked to an inflammatory reaction that precedes histologically and fundoscopically visible damage.

Many of the features of diabetic retinopathy have been described under the general headings of capillary microaneurysms, hemorrhage, exudates, and neovascula-

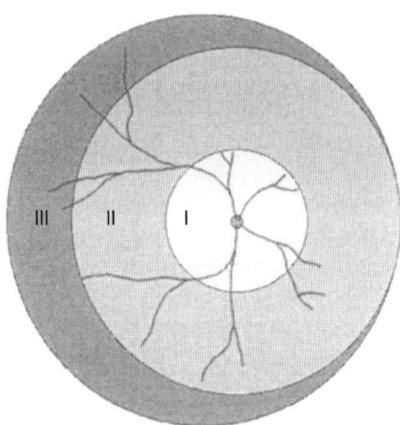

Fig. 5.6.27. International Classification for Retinopathy of prematurity (ICROP) emphasizing location and extent

rization. Traction from epiretinal membranes may lead to secondary retinoschisis (Faulborn et al. 2000). The retinal vessels may be hyalinized later and lipid-laden macrophages may cumulate intravasally. With progressing disease, preretinal neovascularization occurs both at the optic disc and in the midperiphery. When the vitreous detaches, small bridges of neovascularization between the retina and posterior vitreous may tear and cause bleeding either into the vitreous gel or between the vitreous base and the ILM of the retina (subhyaloidal hemorrhage).

5.6.7.2.5
Radiation Retinopathy

Radiation retinopathy appears about 3 years after irradiation, and is basically an ischemic retinopathy in reaction to damage of the endothelium of the retinal arterial bed. Ionizing radiation is used for treatment of choroidal malignant melanomas and orbital and periorbital malignant disease, e.g., in the epipharynx. As the lifespan of capillary endothelial cells in the retina is about 3 years, the *failure of endothelial cells* to replicate after irradiation peaks in cumulative damage in the capillary bed after 3 years. Occasionally capillaries are filled by glial cells (Archer et al. 1993). However, as early as 1 year after irradiation, hemorrhages, microinfarcts and exudates may be present. In response to the focal closure of the capillary bed, there is exudation of lipid-rich plasma into the retina and the subretinal space.

5.6.2.7.6
Eales' Disease

Eales disease is an idiopathic obliterative vasculopathy that usually involves the peripheral retina of young adults. Clinically avascular areas in the retina periphery are seen, followed posteriorly by microaneurysms, dilatation of capillary channels, tortuosity of neighboring vessels, and spontaneous chorioretinal scars. Vascular sheathing with adjacent nerve fiber layer hemorrhages is seen in most patients. The sheathing can manifest as thin white lines, limiting the blood column on both sides of the sheathed vessel to heavy exudative sheathing that can cause vascular occlusion. Although believed to affect primarily the retinal veins, others have reported the same prevalence of both venules and arterioles. Areas of vascular sheathing often leak dye on fluorescein angiography. Neovascularization of *the disc* (NVD) or neovascularization *elsewhere* (NVE) in the retina is observed in up to 80% of patients with Eales disease. The NVE usually is located peripherally, at the junction of the perfused and non-perfused retina. The neovascularization often is the source of vitreous hemorrhage in these eyes, compromising vision. Rubeosis iridis or neovascularization of the iris can develop and may lead to neovascular glaucoma. Fibrovascular proliferation on the surface of the retina may accompany retinal neovascularization. These eyes have associated anteroposterior vitreal traction that could lead to retinal detachment. Cystoid macular edema with significant vision loss can occur in patients with Eales disease due to increased capillary permeability.

The histological appearance of Eales disease is that of an occlusive vasculopathy. Eales disease is believed to be a primary, non-inflammatory disorder of the walls of peripheral retinal vessels, namely the shunt vessels. This often leads to vascular occlusions, peripheral neovascularization, and vitreous hemorrhage. The microvascular abnormalities are seen at the junction of the perfused and non-perfused zones of the retina. Associations with tuberculosis and multiple sclerosis have been suggested, but have not been substantiated in other studies. It is possible that the association of Eales disease with both ocular inflammation and sensitivity to tuberculin protein suggests that this disease may be associated with immunologic phenomena whose mechanisms remain unknown (Gieser 1994; Spitznas 1975). The frequency varies by geography; it is common, e.g., in India (Nagpal 1994). Eales disease is a diagnosis of exclusion, as many other retinal disorders can mimic Eales disease, especially conditions of retinal inflammation or neovascularization.

5.6.2.7.7
Norrie's Disease

Norrie's disease is a rare X-linked inherited disease associated with preretinal neovascularization leading to tractional detachment (Warburg 1965; Anderson 1961). The characteristic feature is *congenital bilateral blindness* with a prominent intraocular mass (pseudoglioma). Noteworthy is a partial avascularity of the retina. The clinical observation that there is a lack of the inner retina and retinal vasculature, which results in retinal hypoxia, led to comparisons with juvenile retinoschisis. However, vice versa, an association between the retinoschisis phenotype and Norrie's disease was not found (Shastry et al. 2000).

In the end stage of the disease, the retina has lost its normal architecture and is severely gliotic with cysts and extensive compact lamellar bone formation (Michaelides 2004). During development there is a delayed maturation of the neuroretina in Norrie's disease. Besides changes of the neuroretina, several mouse models have demonstrated *primary alterations of the retinal vasculature:* Norrie's disease (Ndp(y/–)) mutant mice that are *deficient in norrin* develop blindness, and show a distinct failure of retinal angiogenesis (Richter 1998; Rehm 2002). The retinal vasculature is abnormal by postnatal day 9, with abnormal vessels in the inner retina and few vessels in the outer retina (Richter 1998). However, there are increased numbers of blood vessels in the interface of the ganglion cell layer and the nerve fiber layer and a decrease in the inner and outer plexiform layers in Norrie's disease mice older than 9 days compared with control mice in addition to the previously described alterations of the neuronal retina (Ohlmann 2004, 2005).

Mutations in the Norrie's disease gene (NDP) have been reported in several retinal disorders which are characterized by vascular abnormalities, including Coats' disease, Stage 5 ROP, and X-linked FEVR, suggesting that the protein product of NDP, Norrin, may be involved in normal retinal angiogenesis. The association of ND with peripheral venous insufficiency seen in the family reported here and in a Costa Rican pedigree (Rehm 1997) suggest that Norrin may also play a role in extraocular angiogenesis.

5.6.2.7.8
Coats' Disease

Coats' disease leads to exudative retinal detachment in children, predominantly in boys. The disease is usually unilateral and presents as a sectorial abnormality of the retinal vasculature (Shields et al. 2001). Massive secondary exudation leads to retinal detachment, which in excessive cases may resemble exophytic retinoblastoma. The *sectorial teleangiectasia* of the peripheral vessels is considered to be the basic pathology; secondary changes including the leakage of proteinaceous exudates, fibrin and red cells into the retina result in a destruction of the neuronal components of the retina. Macrophagic infiltration accompanies reactionary gliosis and exudation proceeds to intraretinal cyst formation. The subretinal exudate contains myriads of *cholesterol crystals*, attracting numerous lipid- and melanin-laden macrophages. Pigmented nodules and subretinal strands derived from the RPE may be present.

Histologically, the teleangiectatic vessels appear to be thin-walled and can be found in addition to arterioles and venules showing mural thickening with possible deposition of *PAS-positive material*. The accumulation of fat seen as *cholesterol clefts* and melanin-laden and lipid-laden macrophages in the subretinal space is characteristic of Coats' disease. The neuronal atrophy in the retina is considered to be secondary to ischemia and retinal detachment. Paradoxically, a significant proliferative retinopathy does not occur, even though neovascular glaucoma may be the cause of enucleation.

5.6.2.7.9
Familial Exudative Vitreoretinopathy

Familial exudative vitreoretinopathy (FEVR) is a bilateral disorder of the peripheral retinal vascular development often associated with vitreous traction (Criswick and Schepens 1969; Gow 1971; see Lang and Maumenee). Systemic associations are absent and no association with prematurity is found. Despite earlier theories that emphasized vitreoretinal changes, it is now clear that the fundamental abnormality in FEVR is the *leakiness of the abnormal peripheral retinal vessels* (Canny 1976; Laqua 1980).

Histopathology reveals similarities to other peripheral vasculopathies such as Coats' disease. The vitreous membranes are probably of greatest pathognomic relevance for FEVR. Histopathological characteristics of FEVR include a *thickened retina* containing dilated, teleangiectatic blood vessels. The peripheral vessel walls are thickened and may demonstrate a perivascular infiltrate (Boldrey 1985). Both intraretinal (Boldrey 1985) and subretinal (Nicholson 1984) inflammation may be present. Cellular and acellular vitreous membranes originating from posterior to the ora serrata may attach to the ILM and *throw the retina into folds* (Brockhurst 1981). Nevertheless retinal dysplasia has not been described.

The *failure to vascularize the peripheral retina* is the unifying feature seen in all affected individuals, but, by itself, usually causes no clinical symptoms. The visual problems in FEVR result from secondary complications due to the development of hyperpermeable blood vessels, neovascularization, and vitreoretinal traction. Partial or total retinal detachment occurs in 20% of cases (van Nouhuys 1982, 1989, 1991).

Fibrous proliferation may be the result of chronic peripheral vascular leakage (De Juan 1985). In contrast to this theory, a "regrowth" of onion skin-like vitreous veils can be observed even after full treatment and regression of peripheral neovascularization. Macular traction or retinal detachment occurs with contraction of mesenchymal elements at the avascular border or of the fibrovascular mass that may occur just anterior to it. Mostly traction is located in the temporal periphery, the area with the most apparent ischemia.

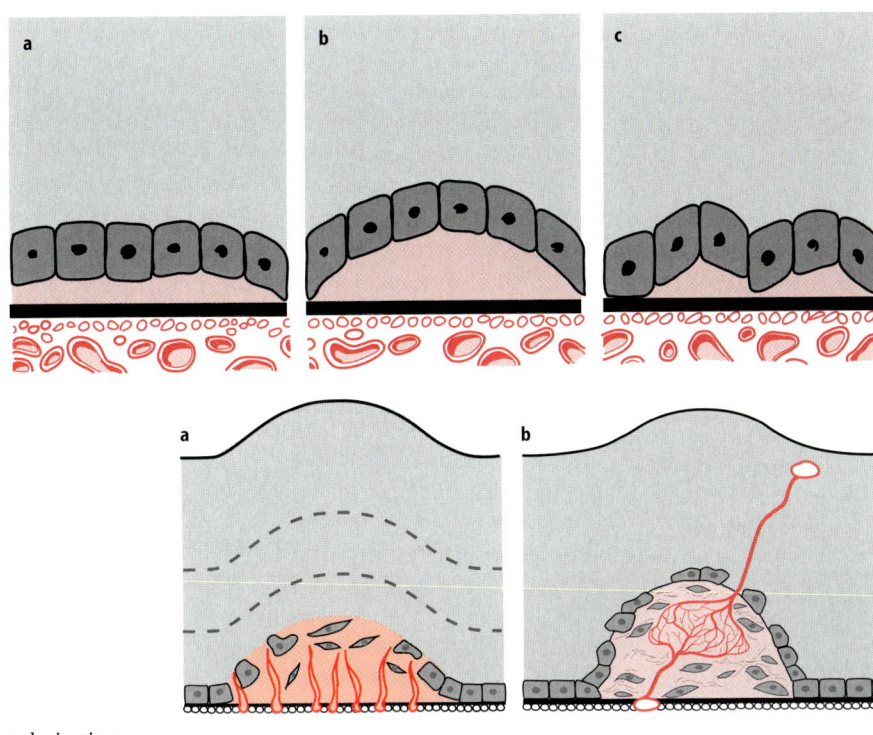

Fig. 5.6.28. Topographic relation of basal laminar deposits (**a**), soft drusen (**b**), and hard drusen (**c**) (from Kirchhof et al.)

Fig. 5.6.29. a Choroidal neovascularization; **b** chorioretinal anastomosis

5.6.2.8
Choroidal Neovascularization (Figs. 5.6.28 – 5.6.32)

Age related macular degeneration (AMD) is clinically seen as an atrophic or exudative process (Sarks et al. 1976; Ryan 1987; Sarks et al. 1988; Schatz et al. 1989; Bressler et al. 1988). Macular pathology evolves fairly symmetrically in both eyes, causing loss of central visual acuity at first in one eye, and soon also in the second eye (Strahlman et al. 1983). The periphery of the retina and the choroid usually remains clinically unaffected; however, peripheral AMD (Delaney et al. 1988) or parapapillary choroidal neovascularization (CNV) is relevant in the differential diagnosis of malignomas.

In "*dry AMD*," the common denominator histologically is atrophy of the inner and outer segment of the photoreceptors and depletion of the outer nuclear layer to a point where this is replacement by glial cells. A variety of changes may be found in the RPE, which may be hypertrophic, hyperplastic, atrophic or completely absent with fusion of the gliotic outer retina with Bruch's membrane (Fig. 5.6.28).

Several types of deposit can be found by light microscopy between the RPE and Bruch's membrane (Abdelsalam et al. 1999; Spraul et al. 1999). "*Hard drusen*" are well circumscribed, in contrast to the granular and vesicular composition with less distinct borders of "*soft drusen*" (Sarks et al. 1994). Soft confluent drusen have been described as "*basal linear deposits*" (Green and Ender 1993). In contrast, the term "*basement membrane deposit*" describes deposits found between the cell membrane and the basement membrane (Loeffler and Lee 1998). Each of the deposits on Bruch's membrane has been the subject of intense speculation in terms of their significance in attracting macrophages, endothelial cells and pericytes, which are the basis of the vasoproliferation in AMD.

According to the current hypothesis, deposits beneath the RPE and in Bruch's membrane stimulate macrophagic migration into the subpigment epithelial space. These cells release VEGF, which induces endothelial cells of the choriocapillaris to penetrate Bruch's membrane. The term *choroidal neovascularization* refers to fibrovascular proliferation, initially between Bruch's membrane and the RPE, and, subsequently, between the RPE and the photoreceptor layer – but never into the choroid itself. Clinically membranes can best be distinguished by fluorescein and ICG angiography. The TAP and VIP studies have identified clear criteria based on fluorescein angiographic features (Barbazetto et al. 2003) (Fig. 5.6.29a, b).

Specimens of surgically excised CNV membranes were available for histopathological confirmation of the clinical grading (Grossniklaus et al. 1998; Lafaut et al. 2000). It is possible to identify fragments of Bruch's membrane, the choriocapillaris or of the deeper choroid in these samples. Depending on the presence and location of photoreceptor outer segments, neovascular

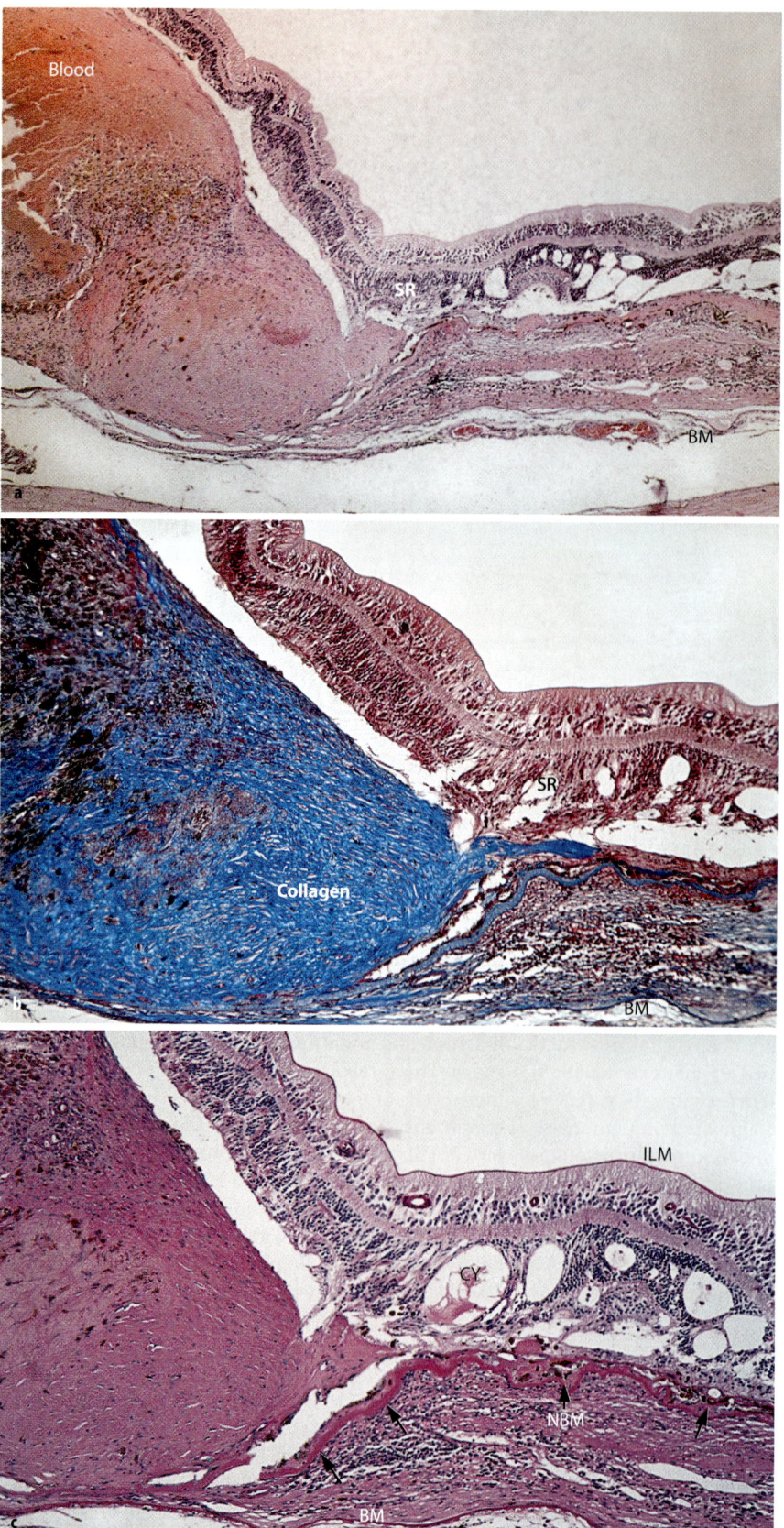

Fig. 5.6.30. Fibrous hemorrhagic disciform macular degeneration: process confined between Bruch's membrane (*BM*) and sensory retina (*SR*). Inner structures of sensory retina recognizable. Outer layers and receptors at the height of the process missing. Cystoid degeneration in outer layers (CY)
a Hematoxylin-eosin stain shows blood and vascularized connective tissue with variable pigmentation.
b Collagen blue (Masson stain). **c** In front of the fibrous plaque a new basement membrane (*NBM*) is formed by proliferating retinal pigment epithelium (*arrows*)

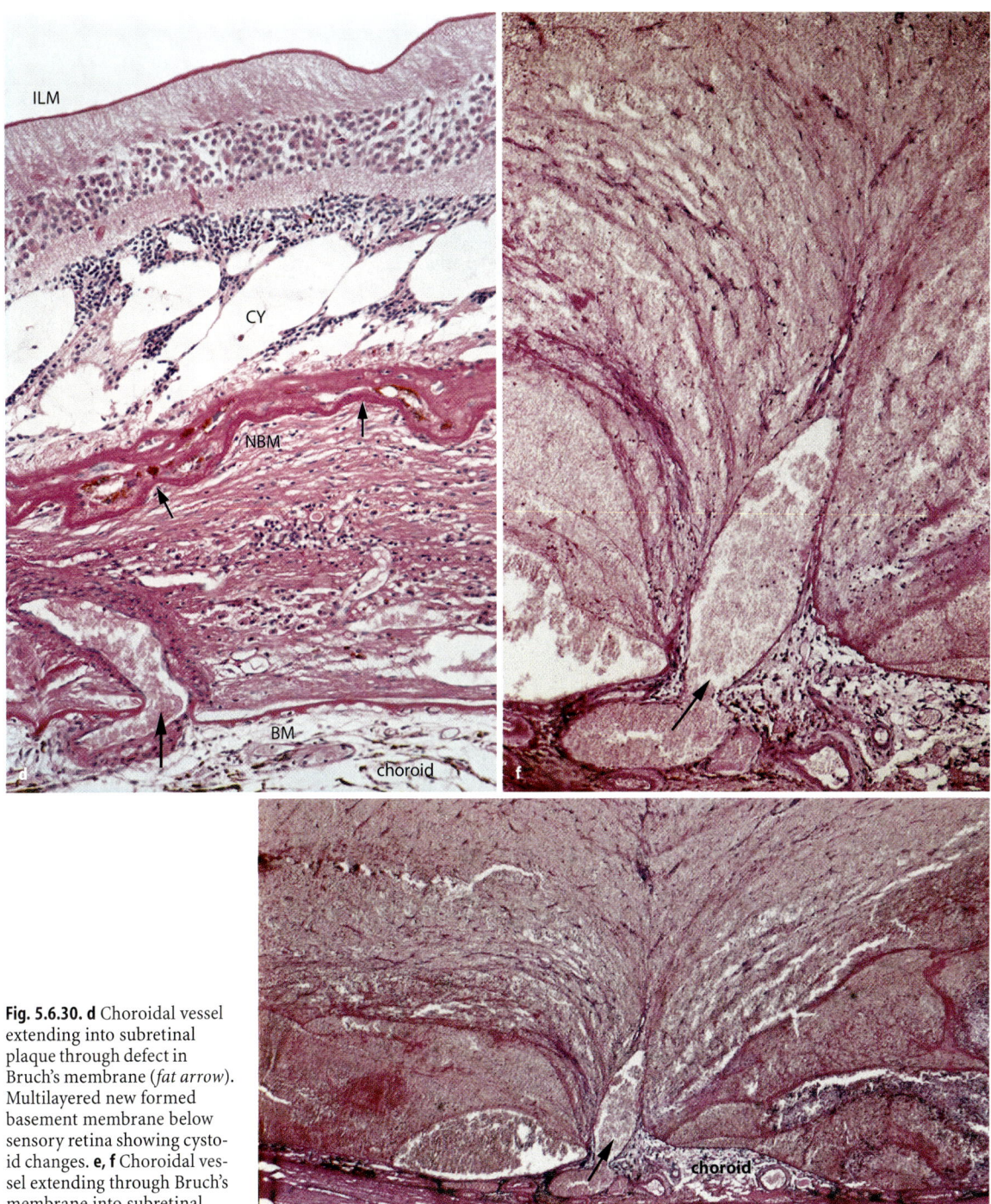

Fig. 5.6.30. d Choroidal vessel extending into subretinal plaque through defect in Bruch's membrane (*fat arrow*). Multilayered new formed basement membrane below sensory retina showing cystoid changes. **e, f** Choroidal vessel extending through Bruch's membrane into subretinal process.

channels and Bruch's membrane, *classic membranes* can be distinguished from *occult membranes*. Specific features to look for within the fibrovascular membranes are lymphocytes, macrophages and fibroblasts derived from metaplastic RPE (Gass 1994; Nasir et al. 1997).

Advanced processes may be dominated by fibrosis. The fibrotic tissue may be pigmented as a consequence of reactive proliferation of RPE cells, lipofuscin and deposition of the breakdown products of blood, free and within macrophages. A close mechanical connection between CNV or fibrosis and the retina can result in inevitable difficulties for surgical approaches when extraction of the membrane becomes traumatic to the overlying retinal tissue (Fig. 5.6.30).

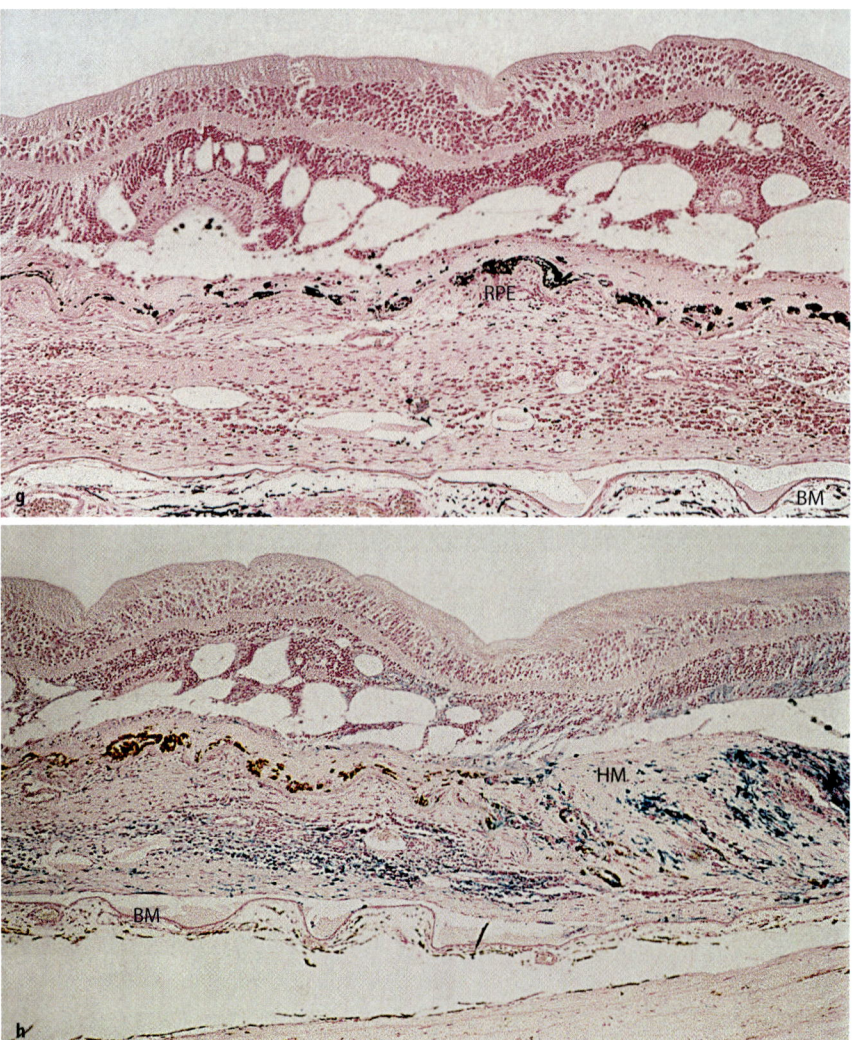

Fig. 5.6.30. g Melanin pigmentation from proliferating pigment epithelium (Fontana stain: black). Pigmentation results from RPE-proliferation and Hemosiderin plus lipofuscin. **h** Hemosiderin laden macrophages (*HM*), Prussian-blue stained

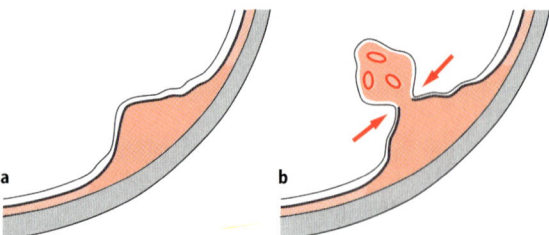

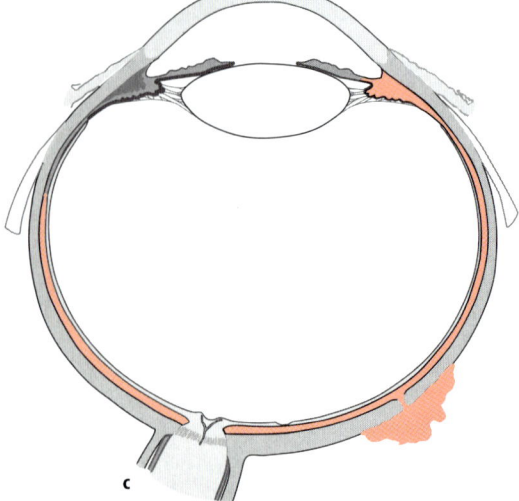

Fig. 5.6.31. Growth pattern of malignant melanoma of the uvea. **a** Choroidal. **b** Choroidal with perforation of Bruch's membrane. **c** Diffuse growth pattern with extrascleral extension, with collateral detachment (see Chapter 4)

5.6.2.9
Tumors of Choroid and Retina

Both benign and malignant uveal tumors arise most commonly from *melanocytes* in the uveal tract. Choroidal malignant melanoma is the most frequently encountered malignant intraocular tumor in the routine laboratory (Fig. 5.6.31). Included in the differential diagnosis are lymphoid and metastatic neoplasms masquarading as a typical uveitis.

Lymphoid neoplasms may occur in both the retina and the uveal tract (Fig. 5.6.32). Those occurring in the retina are very aggressive, may masquerade as a "retinal vasculitis" or as vitritis (Brown et al. 1995), and need to be differentiated from e.g. DD sarcoidosis (Fig. 5.6.33). They are often associated with cerebral manifestation. Those lymphomas of the uvea are considerably rarer.

Vascular tumors of the retina and choroid may be associated with malformation in the central nervous system (von Hippel-Lindau) and skin (Sturge-Weber).

Very rarely seen are tumors of the RPE, or those derived from glial cells (astrocytomas).

Retinoblastoma, a malignant tumor of the retina, is almost exclusively seen in childhood and arises from retinoblasts. Its difficult diagnosis within a group of entities, which can *mimic neoplasms*, emphasizes the importance of this tumor (Fig. 5.6.34).

Below, the histological findings of each of the abovementioned tumors will be briefly discussed.

Choroidal malignant melanoma is associated with leakage of proteinaceous fluid beneath the photoreceptors as they interfere with the function of the choriocapillaris and the fluid pumping capacity of the RPE.

In order to define treatment modalities, it is important to accurately measure the size of the tumor in three dimensions. A mushroom shape of the tumor can occur when the tumor penetrates beyond Bruch's membrane leading to a dilatation of tumor vessels ("turnicat effect"). A pitfall for the surgeon and the radiologist is if the peripheral borders of the tumor are not well defined, and if the tumor infiltrates the adjacent sclera to some degree, which occurs in 90% of serial sections (Donders 1973). Melanoma rarely erodes or penetrates, the retina (Dunn et al. 1988) – with the exception of the Rønne type malignant melanoma free floating tumor cells in the vitreous.

Large tumors can undergo massive spontaneous hemorrhagic necrosis. Widespread endarteritis is the contributory factor for the extensive infarction of all the intraocular tissues.

Similar to transillumination during surgery, a preliminary investigation of the enucleated eye in the

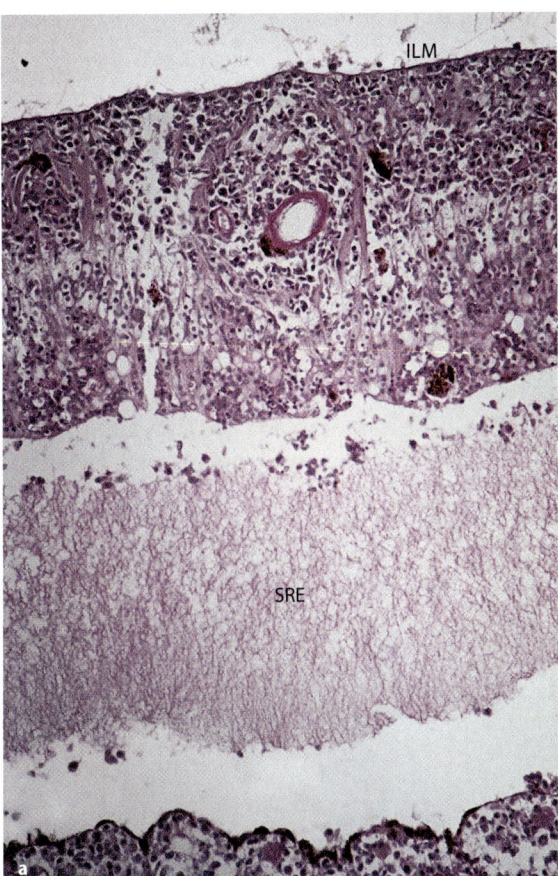

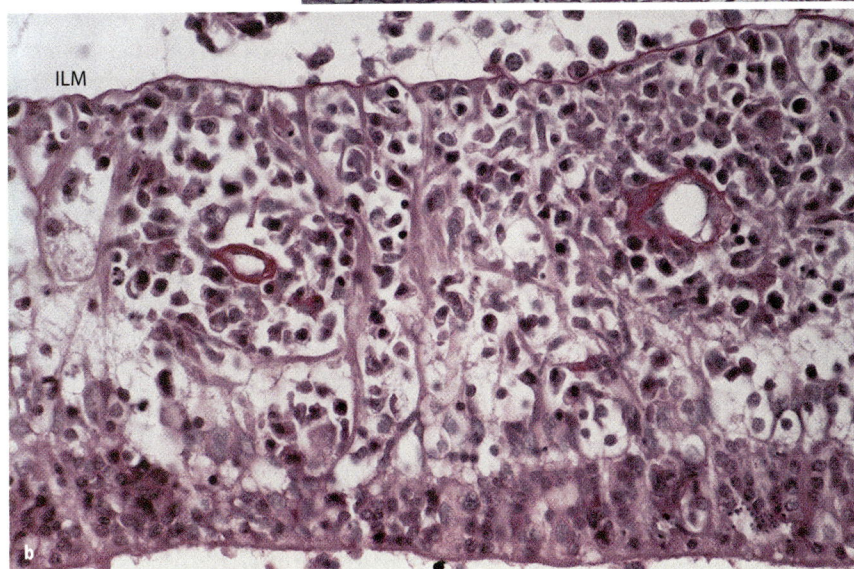

Fig. 5.6.32. Oculocerebral non-Hodgkin lymphoma (NHL). **a** With exudative retinal detachment (*SRE*). **b** Perivascular arrangement of atypical lymphocytes

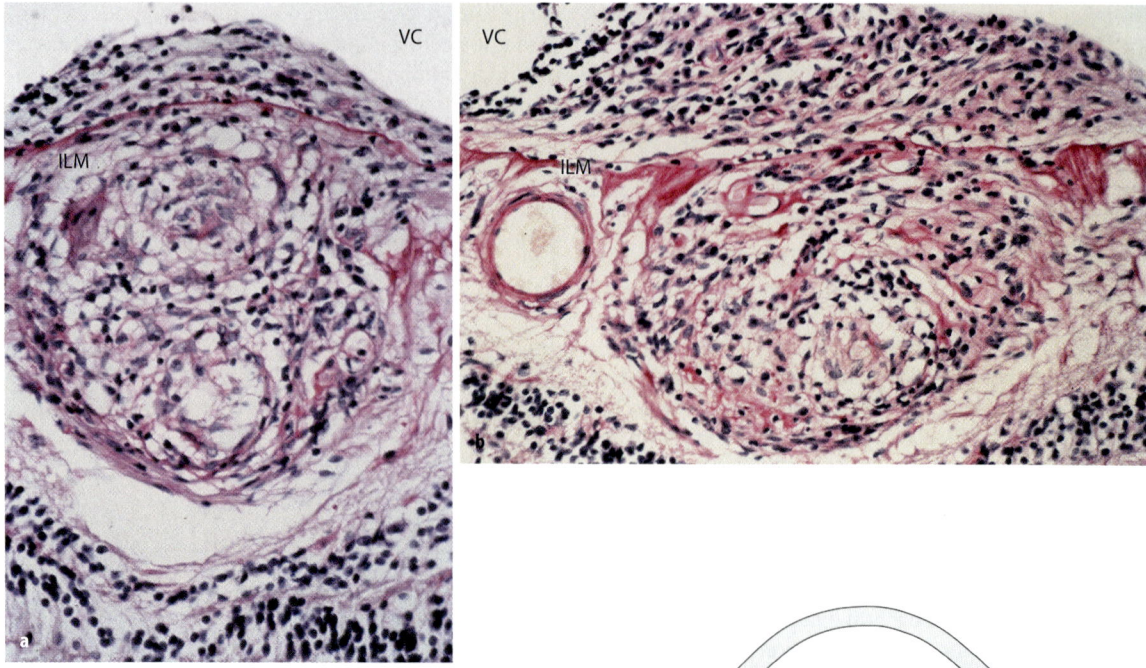

Fig. 5.6.33a, b. Sarcoidosis: granulomatous vasculitis of retina. Internal limiting membrane (*ILM*) vitreous cavity (*VC*) (PAS)

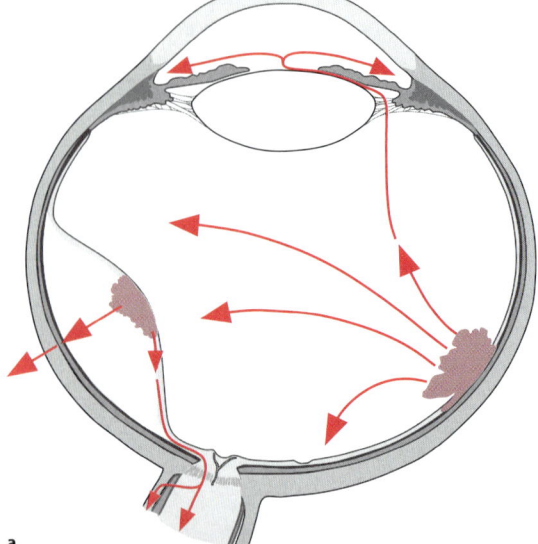

Fig. 5.6.34. Retinoblastoma, growth pattern: exophytic (**b1**) and endophytic (**b2**) tumor growth

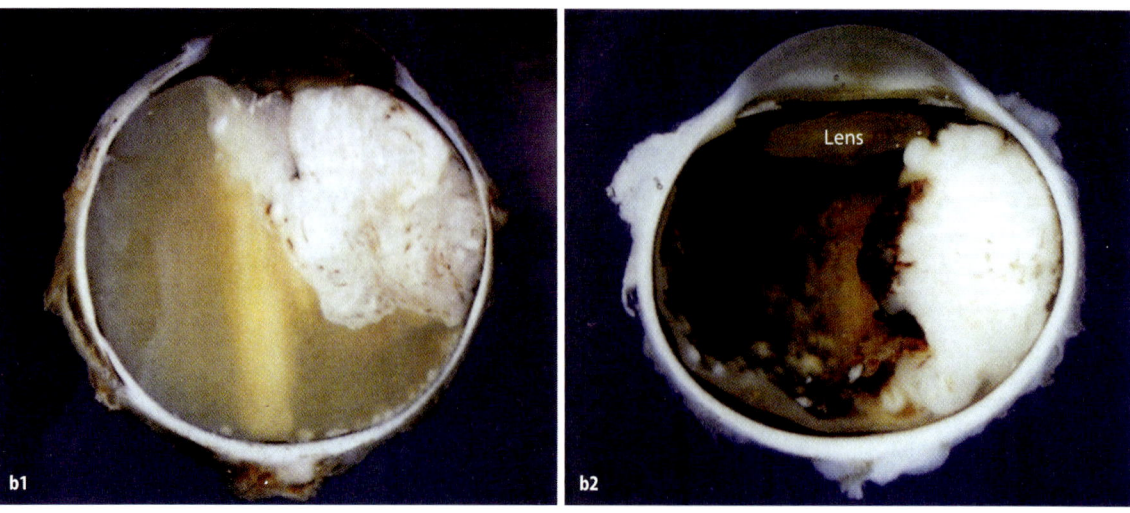

"black box" is important to choose the most suitable plane of section including disc and pupil. Cutting of the globe should be performed so that the principal histological section will pass through the center of the tumor. Further, the vortex veins should be dissected and excised, and examined for extraocular spread before the eye is opened. *Vortex vein spread* is more likely to occur if the base of the center of the tumor is located over the internal orifice of the vein, i.e., in the supero-/inferonasal and temporal quadrants. Similarly, *transcleral* spread can be found at any (Fig. 5.6.31). The sclera adjacent to the lamina cribrosa of the optic disc is less than half of the thickness elsewhere. Juxtapapillary malignant melanomas are less than 250 µm from the subdural space. Lymphocytic infiltration in the wall of a vortex vein is frequently seen on routine examination, while tumor cells are seen as clumps, partially or totally occluding the lumen or the wall of the vein.

The *microscopic evaluation* of the tumor distinguishes spindle cell type variants, epithelioid cell types, and mixed forms (McLean et al., 1978, 1983).

Spindle A cells are closely packed and have elongated oval nuclei with a longitudinal fold in the nuclear membrane. *Spindle B* cells are larger and have a rounder nucleus in which the nucleolus is prominent. Spindle cells are arranged in "fascicles," resembling the pattern seen in schwannomas, or demonstrate a perivascular fascicular arrangement. Mitotic figures are not usually seen.

Epithelioid cells are larger than spindle cells and the cytoplasmic rim is larger and more eosinophilic. The boundaries of these cells are more distinct and the cells appear to be separated by an intercellular space. There is a higher nuclear pleomorphism associated with epithelioid tumors, and they are associated with a poorer prognosis. These tumors have a higher *mitotic count* as determined per 10–40 high power fields on conventionally stained section. No consensus has been reached regarding which *proportion of epithelioid* cells qualifies a uveal melanoma as being of mixed and epithelioid type, respectively. Uveal melanoma cells stain usually (but with variability) for the melanocytic immunohistochemical markers, HMB-45, MelanA and S-100P.

Cells of macrophagic type, as identified by anti-CD68 staining, are often present within the uveal melanomas, sometimes as multinucleate cells. *Balloon cells* (degenerate melanoma cells) or lipid-laden macrophages may also be present within a tumor (Khalil 1983; Grossniklaus et al. 1997). Tumor melanin is not regarded as a significant prognostic marker. Tumor melanin is seen as fine light brown pigment granules, and contrasts the coarser and darker secondary melanophagosomes observed in perivenular macrophages. These are activated by tumor cell apoptosis and focal necrosis with melanin release.

In relation to the histological cell type, the *5-year survival rate* for patients with spindle cell melanomas is 80%, and for those with epithelioid cell melanomas it is 20% although epithelioid tumors at first appear to be more radiosensitive (Lommatzsch; Jensen et al. 1982). The peak mortality from metastatic disease, which usually involves the liver, occurs within 2 years of diagnosis or the date of enucleation (Jensen et al. 1982; McLean et al. 1982). While the presence of VEGF expression does not correlate with prognosis (Sheidow et al. 2000), a vascular network pattern and a closed loop pattern of the vasculature indicate a worse prognosis (Sakamoto et al. 1996; Folberg et al. 1997; McLean et al. 1997).

Other *prognostic factors* include indices of cell proliferation, ploidy analysis and the assessment of genetic abnormalities. Monosomy 3 and defined abnormalities of chromosomes 6 and 8, as determined using fluorescence in-situ hybridisaton (FISH), have consistently been associated with metastatic death in choroidal and ciliary body melanoma (Scholes et al., 1999–2003; Damato et al., 2007; Sisley et al., 1998; White et al., 1998). The strongest single predictor of prognosis is loss of heterozygosity detected in chromosome 3; because of the possibility of isochromosome, some of these patients falsely appear to be disomic e.g. in FISH analysis. Other molecular biological techniques, including gene expression profiling analysis (Tschentscher et al., 2003; Worley et al., 2007), may be more accurate ways than karyotyping ot differentiate uveal melanoma patients with favorable and adverse prognoses.

In addition to cell type, mitotic count, mean diameter of the ten largest nucleoli (measured e.g. from silver-stained sections), presence of defined extravascular matrix patterns (e.g. closed loops and networks detected with periodic acid-Schiff staining or clinically with confocal angiography), microvascular density (determined from areas of dense vascularization ofter staining with antibodies to vascular endothelial cells), as well as high numbers of tumor-infiltrating lymphocytes and macrophages have been shown to be independent predictors of subsequent survival in more than one study (Mäkitie et al., 1999, 2001). Determinants of cell proliferation, such as Ki67/MIB-1 or proliferating cell nuclear antigen (PCNA; also known as PC-10), have been investigated and found to be of value as prognostic indicators (Mooy and de Jong 1996; Seregard et al. 1998).

Tumor recurrence and metastases have been shown to correlate with the distribution of the amount of DNA in a tumor population using ploidy analyses on fixed tissue (Coleman et al. 1993). Others disagree (Elavathil et al. 1995). Several studies have shown that monosomy of chromosome 3 is by far the most important risk factor for metastasis. There are DNA probes available for detecting monosomy 3 in biopsies of tumors (Sisley 1992, 1997; Prescher 1990, 1992, 1996).

Choroidal metastases of extraocular solid tumors are most commonly of breast origin (about 70%) and bronchial carcinomas (Shields et al. 1997). Rare entities include metastasis of cutaneous melanoma, metastases from thyroid carcinoma (Ainsworth et al. 1991), hemangiosarcoma of the breast (Sach et al. 1998), endometrial carcinoma (Capeans et al. 1998) and others (Ferry and Font 1974). Bilateral involvement is not uncommon. Metastases are, however, also found rarely in patients with unknown systemic disease, presenting with unusual choroidal tumors. In cases of doubt, biopsies of these tumors can be considered in order to determine type and biologic dignity. Metastatic bronchial or breast carcinoma can be diagnosed clinically.

Very unusual *primary choroidal tumors* which have been misdiagnosed as amelanotic choroidal melanomas include primary choroidal lymphomas (Coupland et al. 2002, 2005), leiomyomas, neural tumors, alveolar osteomas and soft part sarcomas (von Domarus 1978; Warwar 1998; Shields 2005).

Intraocular lymphomas represent an heterogeneous group: Primary intraocular lymphoma (*PIOL*) is a relatively uncommon high-grade malignant non-Hodgkin lymphoma (NHL), involving predominantly the *retina* and the *vitreous* (Qualman 1983; Whitcup 1993) (Fig. 5.6.32). It may occur *independently, prior or subsequent to a primary central nervous system lymphoma* (PCNSL). "PIOL" frequently masquerades as a chronic, relapsing and steroid-resistant uveitis and vitritis: retino-vitreal lymphoma. As it simulates other conditions ("*masquerade syndrome*"), delays in the diagnosis of "PIOL" are common. If lymphoma involves the vasculature, this may lead to ischemic infarction of the retina and optic nerve (Guyer et al. 1990). Most "PIOLs" are of B-cell origin (B-PIOL) (Char 1988; Coupland 2005; Davis 1974; Nathwani 1978) and can be classified as diffuse large cell B-cell lymphomas (DLBCLs), according to the updated World Health Organization (WHO) Lymphoma Classification (Jaffe 2000).

Primary choroidal lymphomas are rare, with only 65 cases being reported (Coupland 2005). Primary choroidal and iridal lymphomas are the rarest of the three forms of lymphomatous manifestations occurring intraocularly. These lymphomas are considered to be *primary* tumors arising in the choroid, due to the absence of systemic lymphoma at the time of diagnosis, and to their *unilaterality* in the majority of patients (Jakobiec 1987). They usually occur in men in the 5th decade (Ben-Ezra 1989; Cockerham 2000; Coupland 2002). Typical presenting symptoms of *primary choroidal lymphoma* include recurrent episodes of blurred, painless loss of vision as well as metamorphopsia due to secondary serous detachment of the macula. There can be an initial response to steroid therapy, subconjunctival or episcleral extension may occur.

Table 5.6.11. Intraocular lymphomas

Lymphomatous manifestations can essentially be divided into three major groups:
1. *Primary intraocular lymphoma* (PIOL) in vitreous and the retina: high-grade malignant B-cell non-Hodgkin lymphomas (NHL) can be associated with primary central nervous system lymphomas (PCNSL)
2. *Lymphomas arising primarily in the choroid*, which are commonly low-grade malignant B-cell lymphomas. (The iris is exceptionally rarely involved in primary and secondary manifestations of lymphoma)
3. *Mainly choroidal* involvement in systemic lymphoma

The demonstration of *monoclonality* within the infiltrating lymphocytes using immunohistochemistry and, later, using molecular biological investigations, including polymerase chain reaction (PCR) for immunoglobulin heavy chain (IgH) rearrangements, resulted in the majority of these tumors being *re-defined* from "reactive lymphoid hyperplasia" of the uvea to low-grade B-cell NHL (Jakobiec 1987; Ciulla 1997; Ben-Ezra 1989; Grossniklaus 1998; Cockerham 2000).

They are more accurately subtyped as "*extranodal marginal zone B-cell lymphomas*" (EMZLs) of MALT type, according to the REAL lymphoma classification, as they demonstrate morphological, immunophenotypic and clinical features similar to EMZLs in other locations (Coupland 2002). The majority of uveal EMZLs have been diagnosed on eyes enucleated due to difficulties in differentiating the uveal lymphoproliferative lesion from a malignant uveal melanoma, or to painful secondary glaucoma.

Secondary intraocular lymphomas occur with systemic visceral lymphomas.

The clinical diagnosis of a *choroidal cavernous and retinal capillary hemangioma* can be made by fluorescein angiography. Exudation in larger tumors leads to retinal detachment and untreatable blind eyes (Shields 1992b). The rare cavernous hemangioma of the retina shows characteristic sedimentation (Messmer et al. 1984).

Choroidal osteoma is a rare entity. Generally, osteoma can be considered as benign static tumors occurring in the posterior choroid of female patients in the 2nd decade (Shields 1988). The tumor is easily recognized on clinical examination, particularly when ultrasound is used to enhance bone reflectivity. There is no treatment available. *Sclerochoroidal calcification* concerns the outer layer of the choroid, is of unknown origin and significance, and may be differentiated by echography.

Retinoblastoma is a malignant tumor originating from embryonal retinal cells, growing unilaterally or bilaterally, the latter often with *asymmetry* in size (Shields et al. 2001). The natural course can still be seen in developmental countries with tumor proliferation along the optic nerve to the intracranial meninges. Perforation of the corneoscleral envelope leads to intraorbital spread and death is the result of blood-borne visceral and skeletal metastases (Char et al. 1989). Nevertheless, with modern forms of management in specialized centers, cure rates in excess of 90% are the rule.

Retinoblastoma inheritance patterns have been thoroughly examined in recent decades (Bunin et al. 1989; De Luca et al. 1996; Yilmaz et al. 1998; Whitcup et al. 1999; Lohmann and Gallie 2004). Retinoblastoma is a monogenic disease, which occurs when both alleles of the *RB-1* gene are defective or not functional. Of note, patients with a germline mutation carry a risk of developing a *second malignancy* such as a pinealoblastoma (trilateral retinoblastoma) (Dudgeon and Lee 1984; Pesin and Shileds 1989; Kivela 1999).

Clinically, leucocoria is a key symptom as well as a squint in cases where central vision is affected. When in *exophytic growth* of the tumor, viable tumor cells may reach the uvea and later the anterior chamber presenting as pseudohypopyon. Retinoblastoma with extension into the vitreous (*endophytic growth*) may be differentiated from a retinal detachment due to subretinal tumor proliferation and exudation (exophytic growth) (Fig. 5.6.34).

For molecular genetic workup it is *essential to harvest viable tumor tissue* immediately after enucleation and *before* fixation. This is of the utmost importance in unilateral cases. Thus, first the *optic nerve is dissected from the globe* and *processed separately*. If the optic nerve is cut after opening the globe, loose tumor tissue may be smeared into the optic nerve and may cause serious confusion in the interpretation. Slides of the optic nerve are started at the *posterior resection* line and the blade wiped between each cut. After harvesting of tumor cells as described above, the globe is fixed in buffer formalin. Similarly, blocks should be taken through the calottes in an attempt to detect choroidal invasion. If significant choroidal invasion (i.e., leading to choroidal thickening) is demonstrated in combination with neovascular glaucoma, there is an increased risk of metastatic death (Shields et al. 1993). – An important parameter is pre- or postlaminar growth, infiltration of the optic nerve and choroidal invasion.

Microscopy in most cases demonstrates a tumor formed by uniform small round cells with a high mitotic rate and a tendency to individual cell necrosis. The nuclei are round with a fine granular nuclear chromatin. Tumor cells stain positive with anti-S-100 protein, anti-neuron-specific enolase (NSE), and anti-GFAP antibodies (Perentes et al. 1987). Anti-S antibody reacts against photoreceptor soluble retinal antigen (Nork et al. 1996) in the differentiated form. Survival of tumor cells is dependent on blood supply as manifested by rings (200–300 μm in diameter) of viable cells around widely spaced blood vessels ("pseudo-rosettes"). Endothelial budding can be found in tumor blood vessels indicating endothelial activation. Larger tumors often show wide areas of necrotic eosinophilic amorphous material with *calcifications*. Decalcification with a citric acid solution can be helpful in reducing cutting artefacts during sectioning.

While the tumor originates from undifferentiated retinoblasts (Tso 1980), in some tumors there is neuroglial differentiation (Messmer et al. 1985) and groups of cells can adopt some of the morphlogical characteristics of photoreceptor cells (Tso 1980). "*Fleurettes*" are circular or oval groups of cells in which cytoplasmic processes have the ultrastructural characteristics of inner segments of photoreceptors. In "*Flexner-Wintersteiner rosettes*," the cells are located in a circle which is limited internally by a continuous membrane, the lumen of which contains acid mucopolysaccharides (sialomucin resistant to hyaluronidase). Cells are united in these circles by adherent junctions. "*Homer-Wright rosettes*" are multilayered circles of nuclei surrounding eosinophilic fibrillar material.

5.6.2.10
Dyes, Vitreous Substitutes and Infusion Fluids (Fig. 5.6.35)

5.6.2.10.1
Dyes for Intravitreal Use

The introduction of intravitreal dyes was a breakthrough for vitreoretinal surgeons that largely *facilitated the challenging technique of ILM peeling* by allowing

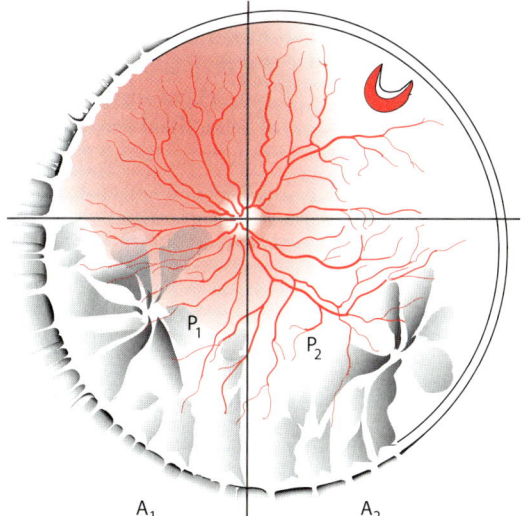

Fig. 5.6.35. The "Cologne" classification of proliferating vitreoretinopathy (PVR). In each quadrant PVR is determined to be either at the vitreous base (anterior, *A*) or at the posterior pole (posterior, *P*). In this sample the proper classification is A2/P2: anterior traction in two quadrants and posterior traction in two quadrants (modified from Heimann and Kirchhof)

a fast, more complete, and precise and less traumatic removal. *Indocyanine green* (ICG) was used initially followed by trypan blue. Even though the use of dyes is allowed for intraoperative visualization of previously invisible interface relationships, there is still considerable discussion about the potential toxicity of these dyes.

Indocyanine green is a tricarbocyanine dye with a long history of safety after intravenous administration for angiography (Hope-Ross et al. 1994). ICG binds quickly to proteins, particularly to serum albumin, but does not penetrate intact cell membranes. When used for *staining of the anterior capsule for "chromorhexis,"* no adverse effects have been reported in the anterior segment (Holley et al. 2002; Horiguchi et al. 1998). The initial use for improvement of macular hole surgery was quickly taken up by surgeons (Burk et al. 2000; Kadonoso et al. 2000). Interestingly, ICG stains vitreous collagen and the ILM selectively, but *not* epiretinal membranes. The current information on ICG toxicity is difficult to evaluate as different preparations with varying concentrations from 0.05% to 0.5% and exposure times are in use. To achieve experimentally pathologic damage, prolonged exposure times of >5 min and high concentrations (>0.5%) were necessary. It may be relevant to maintain pH neutrality and use iso-osmolar solutions (Kwok et al. 2003; Rivett et al. 2004) and to avoid direct contact with RPE cells as well as prolonged endoillumination (Haritoglou et al. 2004).

Trypan blue 0.3% has been used to examine endothelial cell viability of *organ-cultured corneas prior to transplantation* without signs of toxicity. Trypan blue gives a dose dependent staining of epiretinal membranes without morphological or functional alterations as investigated in a rabbit model 4 weeks after intravitreal injection of 0.06% trypan blue (Stalmanns 2003; Veckeneer et al. 2001). In retinal surgery this dye is applied onto the macula of an air filled eye. The staining of the epiretinal membrane is far better compared to staining of the ILM or vitreous and may be dependent on the composition of the epiretinal membrane (Feron et al. 2002). Clinically trypan blue has been used for peeling of macular pucker, PVR membranes and macular hole surgery (Feron et al. 2002; Perrier et al. 2003). Although there is *no apparent toxicity seen in histological studies* (Li et al. 2004), in vitro functional assays report some delay in the electroretinography (ERG) responses (Luke et al. 2005).

Triamcinolone acetonide is increasingly used as an intravitreal anti-inflammatory drug. Besides, *triamcinolone crystals can be useful in visualizing the transparent vitreous*. This is important in patients in whom a posterior vitreous detachment cannot be achieved by the usual suction maneuvers such as in high myopes and diabetic patients (Peyman et al. 2000). Triamcinolone assisted vitrectomy was also used to visualize the posterior hyaloid and cortical remnants and to outline peeled areas in cases of macular pucker, macular holes and PVR (Sakamoto 2002; Furino et al. 2003; Kimura et al. 2004). No adverse effects have been reported so far. In contrast, a reduction in the postoperative blood-retinal barrier breakdown and a reduced inflammatory response was noted (Sakamoto 2002). There are no reports of histological alterations by triamcinolone in the vitreous.

Studies of subconjunctival triamcinolone crystalline depots removed after prolonged induced ocular hypertension showed macrophages and a granulomatous reaction to the depot (Naumann 1972, unpublished observation).

5.6.2.10.2
Vitreous Substitutes and Tamponades

Internal tamponade holds a reattached retina in place until the scars formed by the laser or the cryoprobe have healed. In current practice, silicone oil, gas, e.g., "sulfur hexafluoride," or heavier-than-water liquids (perfluoro-octane or perfluoro-perhydrophenenthrene) are available to replace the vitreous substance which was removed by vitrectomy (Table 5.6.11).

Silicone oil is of low specific gravity and the physiochemical characteristics are such that an intact transparent bubble of oil will gently press against the region in the superior retina to be sealed. The oil has not always been of consistent purity and this may have been a factor in the emulsification, which is an unwelcome complication (Nakamura et al. 1990).

The characteristics of oil in a pathological specimen include *interference with lens metabolisms*, which induces lens opacities or exacerbates a preexisting cataract. Often the cataract is characterized by *posterior migration of epithelial cells* which are surrounded by a prominent PAS-positive basement membrane, but this feature may not necessarily be due to the silicone oil. A breakdown of the bubble leads to emulsification and escape of emulsified oil into the anterior chamber. The superior part of the outflow system is blocked by small globules of free oil and by macrophages laden with oil. The emulsified oil damages the corneal endothelium, which causes decompensation and edema. These changes may be seen in a corneal graft in which silicone oil spaces occur in the endothelium and the corneal stroma (Foulks et al. 1991; Azuara-Blanco 1999). And lastly angle closure glaucoma due to papillary block occurs in an aphakic eye due to the oil bubble pressing on the pupil when the patient is supine.

Despite all the possible adverse effects of silicone oil, it has experienced a triumphant advance through the world, allowing eyes to be saved which were lost due to failure of surgery without a long-term tamponading option.

Silicone oil with a viscosity of 5,000 cSt is now used in many surgical centers as the standard tamponade and appears to be less prone to emulsification; however, no difference in final outcome is found if 5,000 cSt silicone oil is compared to silicone oil of 1,000 cSt viscosity (Scott et al. 2005).

While in the initial years of silicone oil surgery the pathologist received more specimens after enucleation, today with improved surgical techniques the rate of enucleations has dropped. In samples investigated, it is possible that the surgeon will have removed the oil some time before enucleation. The oil vanishes from paraffin-embedded or plastic-embedded sections and the sole indication of its presence in emulsified form is the presence of circular spaces within tissue or within macrophages. The oil becomes resistant to lipid solvents if a short fixation time is followed by exposure to osmium tetroxide solution: oil red O may then stain the silicone oil droplets red in some cases. Evidence for the presence of oil in routine paraffin sections is provided by clusters of macrophages with large circular intracytoplasmatic spaces (Eckardt et al. 1992; Kirchhof et al. 1986). The cells may be seen in the posterior chamber, within the retina, in the vitreous and in membranes on the inner surface of the retina. Or the oil penetrates the retina and may be found in the subretinal space if the retina is detached and a retinal hole is not sealed and can be seen in RPE cells. Oil may pass from the prelaminar into the retrolaminar space if acute secondary glaucomas have caused ischemic infarction of optic nerve head analogous to cavernous atrophy (Schnabel's "cavernous silicophagic optic atrophy"). Similarly silicone has been found between the optic nerve fibers secondary to Schnabel's optic atrophy up to the osseous canal (Knorr et al. 1996; Wenkel 1999). In one remarkable case report there was migration of silicone oil into the lateral ventricles of the brain (Eller et al. 2000).

Sulfur hexafluoride (SF6) is a gas which *absorbs nitrogen*. Thus a gas bubble in the vitreous will expand and tamponade the retina. If the gas is too concentrated (>20%), expansion leads to a high intraocular pressure and occlusion of blood supply so that the retina is severely damaged by ischemia. This pathology has only been documented in the experimental literature. There is no distinctive feature in histopathology related to the use of intravitreal gas tamponade as the gas has usually vanished before histology is taken. Another gas with more long-standing properties is C3F8. All long-standing gases are at risk of causing *tractional retinal holes* in the inferior periphery, possibly due to massaging the remaining vitreous gel with extensions attached to the inferior peripheral retina. Secondary acute glaucomas leading to cavernous silicophagic optic atrophy must be avoided.

Perfluorocarbon liquids (PFCLs) are "*heavier than water liquids*," which have been used in preliminary studies for the treatment of retinal detachment or proliferative vitreoretinopathy. The high specific gravity of perfluorocarbon liquids allows the intraoperative hydrokinetic manipulation of the retina in eyes with severe proliferative vitreoretinopathy or trauma (see Sect. 5.6.4.2).

Retinal damage after short-term as well as extended vitreous substitution with heavy liquids has been demonstrated experimentally (Bryan et al. 1994; Chang et al. 1987, 1991; Eckardt et al. 1991; Flores-Aguilar 1995; Velikay et al. 1993). Impurities of perfluocarbon preparation (Meinert 1994; Velikay et al. 1995) may be among the limiting factors for long-term tolerance as well as dispersion of the liquids, foam cell (macrophagic) reaction, photoreceptor toxicity and preretinal membrane formation and tractional retinal detachment. Retinal gliosis has been demonstrated after a 1-month tamponade with perfluoroether (Miyamoto 1984). Similarly, hypertrophy of Müller cells with bump-like protrusions into the photoreceptor interspaces was observed after only 6 days tamponade with perfluoro-octane and perfluoropolyether (Eckardt 1991). Admixtures of vitreous and liquid perfluorocarbon bubbles or F6H8 may result in *whitish precipitates in the vitreous cavity* and behind the lens and are considered to represent condensed collagen without inflammatory alterations (Ekkardt 1991; Zeana 1999).

There is still controversy regarding the *damage seen with perfluorocarbon liquids*.

In contrast to the above observations, an unchanged retinal anatomy was found after tamponade with perfluorophenanthrene (Nahib et al. 1989) or after perfluoro-octylbromide tamponade of up to 6 months (Flores-Aguilar 1995).

Similarly, there was no tamponade related structural damage of the retina after a 3 months tamponade with F6H8, perfluorodecaline, and a mixture thereof in a rabbit model (Mackiewicz et al., submitted for publication).

Retinal damage has been at least partially attributed to inflammatory responses (Miyamoto 1984; Chang 1991; Eckardt 1991; Doi 1994). Nevertheless, in vivo, the presence of CD45 positive leukocytes was not associated with intraretinal damage and emulsification and foam cell formation was restricted to preretinal vitreous remnants in the inferior globe (Mackiewicz et al., submitted for publication). The macrophagic response by comparison with emulsified silicone or F6H8 differed with regard to the cytoplasmic features, which comprised a red-brown eosinophilic staining with very fine intracytoplasmic granules.

A prerequisite for emulsification is the combination of a vesicle shape of the tamponades with specific stabilizing or modifying surfactants (Kociok et al. 2005).

5.6.2.10.3
Infusion Fluids

To maintain a stable intraocular pressure during pars plana vitrectomy, the vitreous cavity is constantly irrigated with irrigation solution. The proper temperature needs to be maintained. Hypothermic infusion fluid (room temperature) may reduce the risk of blue light damage to the retina from the intraocular fiberoptic probe during vitreous surgery. *While retinal and RPE damage is present after the body temperature exposure, no damage was detected after infusion fluid of room temperature exposure in in-vivo studies.* Vitreoretinal surgeons should *avoid* warming intraocular infusion fluids to levels above room temperature! (Rinkhoff et al. 1986).

Adjunctive agents to prevent PVR or recurrence thereof have been investigated in clinical studies. The efficacy of the *antiproliferative agent daunomycin* in established PVR has been investigated in a prospective randomized controlled clinical trial (Wiedemann et al. 1998). While no significance with respect to the rate of attachment without additional surgery was achieved, the *reduction in the number of reoperations was statistically significant*, thus demonstrating that PVR was amenable to pharmacological treatment of limited duration. With a similar goal, a combination of the antiproliferative agent 5-fluorouracil (200 µg/ml) and low-molecular weight heparin (5 IU/ml) has been used. The development of postoperative PVR was lessened in the treatment group (Asaria et al. 2001). There are *no* reports of histological alterations caused by either of the treatments.

Intraoperative irrigation with aminoglycosides in the treatment and prophylaxis of endophthalmitis has become controversial because the *toxicity of 0.4 mg of gentamicin sulfate is well documented*. To reduce the risk of macular infarction amikacin sulfate or low-dose gentamicin is used. Nevertheless, a toxic reaction can occur even at low doses (Campochiaro et al. 1994). A *localized* increase in concentration in dependent areas of the retina may play a role in aminoglycoside toxicity. If some of the perifoveal capillaries are spared, retention of some central vision is possible.

5.6.3
Principal Indications

5.6.3.1
Closure of Defects

The photoreceptor layer of the retina can survive separation from the RPE only for a short period of time, and only if the layers are quickly reapposed will function be preserved after rhegmtogenous detachment (Barr 1990). TUNEL staining confirmed evidence that there is *apoptosis photoreceptor death* in the outer nuclear layer after traumatic detachment and this process becomes more extensive the longer the retina is detached (Chang et al. 1995; Luthert and Chong 1998). It is also of interest that the *blue cones* are lost selectively after retinal detachment (Nork et al. 1995).

Today surgery for retinal detachment is a routine but emergency procedure. Good anatomical and visual results are expected. Thus it becomes important to evaluate the causes of surgical failure and the side effects of new forms of treatment on the ocular tissues. The modern vitreoretinal surgeon has a variety of techniques available for reattachment of the retina and the pathologist must be aware of the spectrum of procedures in order to understand the changes which may be encountered in an eye in which the vitreoretinal surgery has been anatomically successful, but enucleation is required for secondary pathology in the anterior segment. Histological studies on successfully treated eyes are obviously a rarity, but when suitable material has become available the histology of the reattached retina has approached normal (Barr 1990). In other cases there has been a photoreceptor atrophy where the retina is reattached. This explains the poor visual outcome in addition to postoperative cystoid macular edema (intraretinal) and in some instances fluid accumulation subretinally in the foveolar cleft (see above).

Since rhegmatogenous detachment is due to a retinal break (hole, tear or dialysis), the purpose of treatment is to provide a firm adhesion between the retina and RPE, and choroid around the retinal hole to prevent further movement of fluid into the subretinal space.

In principle, a retinal hole can be sealed either from "*outside,*" by indentation of the sclera and choroid so that the retinal hole is reapposed to the choroid; or a sealing from "*inside*" is achieved by replacement of the vitreous with a bubble of inert gas, e.g., sulfur hexafluoride (SF6) gas or silicone oil, if a long-standing tamponade is required. The vitreous may also be replaced with compounds referred to as "*heavy liquids*" and "*heavy silicone oils*" which maintain mechanical adhesion in the inferior part of the retina. The current literature concentrates on the merits and demerits of the several compounds now available (see Sect. 5.6.2.8).

In general, both procedures, from "inside" or "outside," hold the neural retina against the RPE and allow the surgeon to form adherent RPE-glial scars between the retina and choroid. Chorioretinal fusion is established by cryotherapy or laser photocoagulation, which consists of a band of gliotic outer retinal tissue attached to Bruch's membrane. Cryotherapy induces glial replacement of outer retinal tissue. This glial tissue fuses with metaplastic RPE. While cryotherapy may be associated with a more prominent fibrous reaction, the application from outside allows the far periphery to be treated and does not require a completely attached retina as does laser photocoagulation. Laser photocoagulation destroys the "oven" of the pigment epithelium and outer retina, so that the gliotic retina fuses with Bruch's membrane. Both techniques result in a mechanically stable scar only after 5–8 days (see Sects. 5.6.2.1, 5.6.2.2).

5.6.3.1.1
Buckling or Scleral Indentation

Scleral indentation or buckling is used to approximate RPE choroids to sensory retina in the region of the hole after subretinal fluid has been drained, although the fluid may undergo spontaneous resorption – if the retinal defect is closed. The sclera can be indented with plumbs, buckles or silicone "tyres," which are held in place by matrix sutures in order to approximate the edges of the retinal hole to the pigment epithelium and Bruch's membrane. The scleral tissue reaction to nonabsorbable bands or buckles is minimal in most cases, but hydrogel implants may induce a granulomatous reaction (D'Hermies 1999). Aside of this, multilayered sutures cause a typical foreign body giant cell reaction.

The choice of material and approach (e.g., encircling band, radial buckle, or buckle parallel to the limbus) is detailed in the respective literature.

In *single retinal holes* in phakic eyes there is no doubt that buckling surgery is the method of choice. However, in "unclear hole situations" it is usually necessary to perform a detailed search for breaks and review the treatment of choice. If postoperatively subretinal fluid is still present, this might be because of either unclosed breaks with residual detachment, which hopefully is absorbed spontaneously, or overlooked breaks which need additional treatment. "Blind" encirclements may or may not work. Problems associated with external drainage include *choroidal hemorrhage, retinal incarceration, retinal perforation*, as well as that of *scleral perforation* during suturing of the explant. *Choroidal detachments* are found in 24–44% of eyes following scleral buckling surgery (Ambati 2000; Roider et al. 2001; see Chapters 2, 4).

Infections, intrusions and extrusion of explants have been reported (reference list summarized in Table 5.6.13). Likewise, diplopia has not been mentioned. "Fish mouthing," persisting ocular hypotony, and difficult to place buckles may be further complications. Postoperative diplopia and changes in refraction should be considered preoperatively.

Thus, scleral buckling is a straightforward, highly successful procedure in simple cases with good visualization of the retinal situation. However, in more complicated situations of rhegmatogenous detachment, the surgical procedure becomes more challenging. Location and size of the retinal breaks, the presence of cataract and vitreous opacities, and the presence of PVR should be considered before a decision is made on the surgical approach and it is discussed with the patient.

5.6.3.1.2
Vitrectomy Procedure

Primary vitrectomy was introduced when scleral buckling methods had been routinely implemented (Klöti 1983). The term "primary vitrectomy" for rhegmatogenous retinal detachment implies that pars plana vitrectomy is the first surgical intervention in the treatment of this disease.

Primary vitrectomy is today commonly performed with the help of a wide-angle viewing system, attached to an operating microscope. The sequence of surgical steps is as follows:

- Placement of an encircling band at 13 mm distance from the limbus (preequatorial) to support the vitreous base
- Access to the vitreous cavity via three ports in the pars plana
- Removal of the posterior vitreous, including the hyaloid
- Injection of 1–2 cc of perfluorocarbon liquid to stabilize the central retina (Brazitikos et al. 2003)
- Tightening of the band to better present peripheral retina and vitreous base
- Removal of the flap of the retinal tear (if present), to reduce persistent vitreous traction on the break
- Internal drainage of subretinal fluid (fluid needle) through the retinal break
- Relaxing incisions in the retina, and, in extreme circumstances, excision of the peripheral retina, may be required in cases of retinal shortening
- Fluid-air exchange
- Retinopexy by endolaser- or cryo-coagulation
- Exchange of air to SF6 20% or C3F8
- Adjustment of the tightness of the encircling band
- Adjustment of the intraocular pressure – potential for pupillary (and ciliary) block in eyes with vitreous implant

The placement of an encircling band depends on the preference of the individual surgeon. A circumferential buckle can be used as an ancillary tool to create scleral indentation for removal of peripheral vitreous and for the support of equatorial or preequatorial breaks. Oshima et al. (1999a) have stated that if the vitreous is removed entirely, an encircling buckle is not necessary. Whether vitrectomy with encircling band is superior to vitrectomy without an encircling band in rhegmatogenous retinal detachment is still an open debate.

The most frequent intraoperative complications are *iatrogenic breaks* (6%) and lens damage in phakic eyes (3%, in the series of Table 5.6.1). Iatrogenic breaks will supposedly not significantly influence the outcome of the surgery, if recognized and treated. There are still considerable rates of PVR in 6% of all patients. Macular pucker was seen in 9% of patients in studies in which this complication was investigated. A postoperative increase in nuclear cataract was established in one-third of phakic patients. These complications not only cause a decrease in visual acuity and a myopic shift of postoperative refraction but will cause *loss of accommodation* in young patients and, sooner or later, lead to the necessity of additional surgery in most patients.

The disadvantage of the pseudophakic situation for ophthalmoscopy in scleral buckling becomes an advantage for vitrectomy. *Unclear hole situations* and small *breaks are more common in pseudophakia*. In the presence of an encircling band, intraocular manipulation, especially during removal of anterior vitreous, is easier than in phakic eyes and cannot result in lens opacification during or after surgery. The high success rate of 91% seems to be significantly superior compared to those of scleral buckling. Also visual results after vitrectomy tend to be better after 6 months and 1 year (Bartz-Schmidt et al. 1996; Schmidt et al. 2003). Removal of vitreous opacifications, a better primary retinal reattachment rate, and a lower rate of PVR, at least for the series of Bartz-Schmidt et al., may explain the favorable functional outcome.

Possible mechanisms for the development of *new breaks* are accidental touching of the retina, new tangential forces from scar formation, especially in the region of the sclerotomies, contraction forces of the remaining vitreous cortex, and/or continuing posterior vitreous separation.

The SPR Study Group reviewed the literature comparing primary vitrectomy versus scleral buckling, in situations that were considered to be at high risk of failure if treated conventionally (Table 5.6.12).

The results of a randomized multicenter trial investigating buckle surgery versus primary vitrectomy (SPR Study; Heimann et al. 2001) are available.

Histopathology is available for assessment from the early vitrectomy era. There will be three scars in the pars plana where the entry ports of the vitreous cutter, the illumination source, and the infusion tube have been located. The scar tissue which forms in the sclera can penetrate the pars plana and grow into the vitreous.

Table 5.6.12. Physical properties of PFD, F6H8, their mixture and silicone oil 1,000

	Molecular weight (g/mol)	Specific gravity (g/cm^3) (25°C)	Boiling point (°C)	Refractive index (20°C)	Surface tension against air (mN/m)	Interface tension against water (mN/m)	Viscosity (mPa) (25°C)
PFD	462	1.93	142	1.310	19.0	57.8	5.68
F6H8	432	1.33	223	1.343	19.7	45.3	3.44
Silicone oil 1,000	–	0.97	–	1.404	20.9	39.4	≈1,000

Table 5.6.13. SPR study comparing primary vitrectomy versus scleral buckling

Author	Year	Buckle	No.	Primary success	Final success	PVR	VA >0.33	VA >0.4	VA >0.5
Escoffery et al. (1985)	1985	0%	29	79%	79%	7%		76%	
van Effenterre et al. (1987)	1987	0%	60	86%	92%	0%		76%	
Hakin et al. (1993)	1993	79%	124	64%	82%		34%		
Gartry et al. (1993)	1993	65%	114	74%	92%	8%	35%		
Girard and Karpouzas (1995)	1995	81%	103	74%	85%	16%			40%
Hoing et al. (1995)	1995	0%	32	78%	94%	19%			44%
Bartz-Schmidt et al. (1996)	1996	100%	33	94%	100%	3%		79%	
Heimann et al. (1996)	1996	0%	53	64%	92%	6%		41%	
Yang (1997)	1997	100%	9	89%	100%	0%		0%	
el-Asrar (1997)	1997	100%	22	100%	100%	0%		32%	
Desai and Strassman (1997)	1997	100%	10	100%	100%	0%		70%	
Hoerauf et al. (1997)	1997	83%	37	87%		8%			
Sharma et al. (1998)	1998	100%	21	90%	90%	10%		19%	
Brazitikos et al. (1999)	1999	36%	14	100%	100%	0%		69%	
Campo et al. (1999)	1999	0%	275	88%	96%	6%		69%	
Devenyi et al. 1999	1999	100%	94	100%	100%	0%			
Newman and Burton (1999)	1999	48%	25	84%	96%	8%			48%
Oshima et al. (1999)	1999	51%	63	92%	100%	0%			
Brazitikos et al. (2000)	2000		103	93%	97%	4%			
Gastaud et al. (2000)	2000	58%	19	84%	100%	0%			
Pournaras et al. (2000)	2000	100%	23	92%	100%	4%		65%	
Speicher et al. (2000)	2000	0%	78	94%	96%	5%			
Miki (2001)	2000		87	92%	100%	1%			
Tanner et al. (2001)	2001	0%	9	89%	100%	0%		67%	

PVR proliferative vitreoretinopathy, *VA* visual acuity

Delay in reattachment may be recognized in a histological preparation, when the retina is in situ, because there will be extensive photoreceptor atrophy without an obvious explanation, such as disease of the choriocapillaris, choroidal vascular sclerosis or disease of the posterior ciliary arteries.

Study of vitrectomy specimens has expanded our knowledge concerning preretinal, epiretinal and subretinal membranes (Hiscott et al. 2000). In PVR, the use of immunohistochemistry has established that RPE cells (cytokeratin+), glial cells (GFAP+), fibroblasts (vimentin+), lymphocytes (Charteris et al. 1992; Grierson et al. 1996) and macrophages (ACT+) are present in the collagenous tissue, which contains type I collagen, as distinct from the type II collagen usually present in the vitreous. It is important to look for the periodic acid–Schiff (PAS) positive ILM in these specimens (see Sect. 5.6.3.3). The presence of the membrane may indicate that the scaffold for epiretinal membrane proliferation has been taken away.

5.6.3.2
Release of Vitreous Traction

While both buckling procedures and vitrectomy may successfully release vitreous traction intraoperatively (see Sect. 5.6.3.1), it has emerged that postoperatively the formation of epiretinal membranes contributes significantly to the failure to reattach the retina. Hemorrhage, infection, secondary glaucomas or phthisis bulbi remain occasional indications for enucleation (see Chapter 3).

Traction leading to retinal detachment is seen in proliferative vitreoretinopathy (see Sect. 5.6.4.2) and in vasoproliferative disorders.

Membranes can be formed by glial cells derived from Müller cells or perivascular astrocytes, or metaplastic spindle-shaped RPE cells which have migrated through retinal holes (or possibly through the retina). If the retina is ischemic, blood vessels and fibroblasts migrate onto the retinal surface. The contractile properties of glial cells and metaplastic retinal pigment epithelial cells within a scaffold on the inner limiting membrane are responsible for wrinkling of the inner retina and distortion of the outer retina, a process referred to as *proliferative vitreoretinopathy* (PVR) (Hui et al. 1988; Morino et al. 1990; Nork et al. 1990; Ohira and de Juan 1990; Hiscott et al. 1994). Paradoxically, PVR can be a complication of surgical intervention as well as the primary indication for vitrectomy and/or membrane stripping (see Sect. 5.6.4.2).

Removal of membranes originating in vasoproliferative retinopathy, e.g., in diabetes or the retinopathy of prematurity, can lead to the reattachment of the retina. Vasoproliferative membranes contain small blood vessels which are populated by normal endothelial cells and pericytes in most specimens, but acellularity with ghost vessels may be a feature. *Endothelial cells* can be identified with *factor VIII* markers. Histological specimens of vasoproliferative retinopathy and immunohistochemical markers reveal fibroblastic growth factor and vascular endothelial growth factor (Frank et al. 1996; Chen et al. 1997; Boulton et al. 1998).

Vitrectomy and epiretinal membrane peeling and cutting are now standard procedures. The specimens obtained allow study of the cellular proliferations which may cause contraction of the inner surface of the retina and *"primary retinal traction detachment."*

Pars plana vitrectomy for vitreous hemorrhage without retinal detachment often provides striking visual improvement. However, the functional results in cases of complicated tractional detachment are disappointing in spite of satisfactory anatomical results. Complex surgery is performed in advanced sight-threatening disease; the modest aim is to preserve navigational vision, e.g., in severe proliferative diabetic retinopathy or hemoglobinopathies.

Helbig and coworkers report an overall intraoperative reattachment rate of 86% in patients with diabetic tractional detachment with persistent reattachment of 82% within 6 months postoperatively (Helbig 2002a, b). In contrast, complete tractional detachment was cured only in 9 out of 16 cases (56%), which is supported by recent reports (La Heij 2004). In general, longstanding detachments including the macula region signal a poor visual prognosis. Helbig and coworkers demonstrated a 13-fold higher risk for unfavorable outcome (VA <20/400) with preexisting macular detachment (Helbig 1996). This confirms previous results and supports the concept of *"early vitrectomy."* The improved recent results are likely to be attributable to a better visualization of the periphery, intraoperative photocoagulation and vitreous tamponade.

Besides macular detachment, risk factors for a reduced functional outcome are preoperative rubeosis iridis and subsequent neovascular glaucoma (Oldendoerp 1989), or as Helbig (1996) and coworkers describe, preexisting secondary glaucoma. Tractive macular detachment and a preoperative visual acuity of hand movement or less, allow only 87% to achieve a postoperative visual acuity of >20/400. Eyes with rubeosis iridis and complete retinal detachment with a duration of more than 6 months have a chance of only 2% for a final visual acuity of >20/400.

Furthermore, ischemic alterations of the macula as well as vitreopapillary traction damaging the anterior optic nerve and resulting in ischemic optic neuropathy are considered at risk for a poor outcome (La Heij 2004). Similarly, in eyes with a preoperative vitreous hemorrhage as well as those lacking preoperative photocoagulation a poor prognosis is expected (Rice 1983).

Nevertheless, in our opinion, vitrectomy is recommended even in eyes with active neovascularization and long-standing macular detachment to preserve the eye. Treatment should be performed according to the guidelines for antineovascular therapy (Bartz-Schmidt 1999) and aims to prevent phthisis or secondary glaucoma.

Different considerations apply to tractional retinal detachments *outside* the macula: Visual prognosis is far better. A defined peripheral detachment without active proliferation may be observed without surgical intervention. The risk of a severe visual loss in macular-sparing tractional detachment is reported as 14% per year (DRVS 1985; Charles 1979). Nevertheless, these cases require a close follow-up to prevent progression of the ischemic disease including rubeosis and related negative consequences.

5.6.3.3
Removal of Internal Limiting Membrane

The inner limiting membrane (ILM) is localized between the innermost layer of the retina and the outer boundary of the vitreous, thereby forming a structural barrier between the vitreous cavity and the retina. The ILM stains intensely with PAS and shows the typical ultrastructural characteristics of a basal lamina, in close contact with the foot processes of Müller cells, and containing proteins that are typically found in basal laminae such as collagen type IV and laminin (Bron 1997). With ageing – like other basement membranes – the ILM increases in thickness and attains a thickness of 0.5–2.0 µm at the posterior pole (Heegaard 1994). Striated collagen fibrils of the vitreous cortex insert into the inner portion of the ILM (Hogan 1971), which has been called the hyaloid membrane of the vitreous. Detachment of the posterior hyaloid membrane with ageing or pathology results in a *condensation of the posterior vitreous surface* (membrana hyaloidea posterior). Pathological adherence in the macular area may lead to hole formation in the macula (see Sect. 5.6.2.5). Ultrastructural studies in the eyes from individuals *aged 21 years or older* show that dissection of the retina off the vitreous results in complete cleavage between the vitreous cortex and the ILM. In contrast, if the same procedure is performed in children and young adults, the ILM can remain attached to the vitreous cortex. In addition, Müller cell foot processes become separated from their main cell body and remain connected to the posterior aspect of the ILM. These results suggest that, in youth, there is adhesion between the vitreous cortex and the ILM that is stronger than Müller's cells themselves (Sebag et al. 1991).

In general, basal laminae are specialized extracellular matrices, which underlay basically all epithelia and endothelia. They also surround several mesenchymal cell types such as smooth or striated muscles, as well as Schwann cells in the peripheral nervous system. Basal laminae do not just simply separate tissues, but may also have important functional roles such as directing axonal guidance, neuronal migration, neuronal survival or synapse formation (Libby et al 1999). Such functional roles may be mediated by the direct action of specific basal lamina compounds upon cellular receptors. Basal laminae do also function as a *reservoir for many growth factors,* in particular of the fibroblast growth factor (FGF) and transforming growth factor (TGF)β families (Lonai et al. 2003). All basal laminae are formed by members of three ubiquitous protein families, namely *laminins, nidogens, collagen type IV* and by the *proteoglycan perlecan.*

Of those matrix proteins only laminin is well studied in the retina (Libby et al. 2002). Laminin is not only found in the ILM or in other well organized basal laminae such as those of retinal vessels, but also in the extracellular matrix surrounding photoreceptors and in the first synaptic layer where photoreceptors synapse with retinal interneurons. The laminin β2 chain, present in laminins 14 and 15, appears to be particularly important for vision as it is vital for proper photoreceptor development in the mouse (Libby et al. 1999).

Laminin and fibronectin appear to play a role in the attachment of the vitreous to the ILM and that of the ILM to the cell membrane of Müller cell processes. A *double-laminated pattern* of fluorescence for both glycoproteins was frequently found at the ILM of the posterior retina only in aged eyes, which could predispose the eye to posterior vitreous detachment (Kohno et al. 1997). Recent work investigating the expression of ILM components demonstrated that ILM and vitreous body are synthesized during embryogenesis, but are maintained from early postnatal life onward with a very low turnover (Halfter et al. 2005). *Experimental removal of the ILM at early embryonic stages leads to a series of abnormalities* such as retinal dysplasia, retinal ectopias and massive loss of ganglion cells (Halfter 1998; Halfter et al. 2005b).

The embryonic origin of the ILM, which can be demonstrated as early as 4 weeks after gestation in the human eye, has been the subject of controversy (Rhodes et al. 1979; Spira et al. 1973). Traditionally, the ILM is considered to be synthesized by Müller cells. This concept has been challenged recently by research on the expression of collagen type IV during development of the mouse eye (Sarthy et al. 1993). Because collagen IV is an integral component of all basal laminae, the detection of its mRNA can be used to identify cellular sources of basal lamina production. By in situ hybridization at embryonic day 12 (E12), no or sparse mRNA for collagen type IV was found in the retina, while strong labeling was seen in and around the lens, especially in hyaloid vessels in the tunica vasculosa lentis. In contrast, collagen type IV itself could be readily detected in the ILM by immunohistochemistry. Thus ILM collagen type IV is very likely *not* produced in the retina itself, but rather in lens and tunica vasculosa lentis. From there it is apparently deposited on the inner retinal surface to form the ILM.

Also other ILM proteins such as perlecan, laminin-1, nidogen and collagen XVIII are expressed predominantly in lens and ciliary body, but are *not* detected in the retina (Halfter et al. 2005). Taken together, ILM proteins appear to originate largely from lens and ciliary body, although a contribution of retinal glial cells in ILM synthesis cannot be excluded.

The question arises as to why ILM synthesis is restricted to embryonic stages of development. Deposition of basal lamina compounds synthesized in lens and ciliary body onto the retinal surface may become too difficult as the eye grows in size. In addition, the tunica vasculosa lentis, an important source of collagen type IV production during embryogenesis, disappears later in fetal life. While the ILM is essential during embryonic development, it may very likely be dispensable later in life (Halfter et al. 2005). At least, ILM removal later in adult life does not cause those retinal abnormalities seen in animal models after ILM removal during embryogenesis. Still, the foot processes of Müller cells, which adhere to the ILM, may be damaged by traumatic peeling of the ILM off the retinal surface.

ILM peeling is the technique of choice for macular holes, macular edema, and for improved pucker surgery (see Sects. 5.6.2.5, 5.6.2.6). After pars plana vitrectomy, ILM is dissected from the retinal surface. *Staining* with ICG or other dyes can be used to facilitate visualization (Sect. 5.6.2.8). The ILM can be peeled with a microforceps and usually can be torn like the anterior lens capsule in patients with macular hole. However, it can be more fragile and adhesive in patients with diabetic cystoid maculopathy. The risks of retinal breaks and consecutive retinal detachment (about 5–8%), cataract (up to 63%), and endophthalmitis in any vitreous surgery are discussed below (Sect. 5.6.3.4).

Histological studies demonstrated cellular elements resembling the plasma membrane of Müller cells and other undetermined retinal structures adherent to the retinal side of the ILM (Haritoglou et al. 2002). It is unknown how this affects the role of Müller cells as living optical fibers (see Chapter 4; Reichenbach et al.).

There is an ongoing discussion as to whether the use of ICG and toxicity thereof leads to a more traumatic removal of the membrane compared to ILM peeling without staining. Arguments for the use of ICG are the better control of manipulation and the lower risk of iatrogenic damage. In general, the use of ICG allows surgery to be performed at an earlier stage and with better initial visual acuity.

As indicated above, ILM behaves differently during surgery depending on the respective diagnosis.

Gandorfer et al. describe a continuous layer of native vitreous collagen covering the ILM and a thickened premacular vitreous in *diabetic* patients (Gandorfer 2005). In these patients, peeling of the ILM is difficult, but may be rewarding, as it is thought to release macular edema by improving fluid movement between retina and vitreous.

In contrast to diabetic patients, ILM appears to be pathologically fragile after *blunt trauma*. This may be due to apoptosis of Müller cells, subsequent reorganization of neuronal cells and replacement by scar tissue.

Peeling of the ILM during macular pucker surgery may not have deleterious effects, but can even be beneficial by improving diffusion of fluid and by preventing regrowth of the pucker membrane.

It is important to keep in mind that it is not necessary to treat every *epiretinal membrane* (see Sect. 5.6.2.6), but only those associated with significant *visual loss* and/or, more importantly, with disturbing *metamorphopsia* (Michels et al. 1982; Magherio et al. 1985). Recurrence of the membrane has to be expected in 4–8% of cases. It is likely that the recurrence rate after prior ILM peeling is reduced, as the scaffold for regrowth of membranes has been removed (Park et al. 2003). Assuming that pucker formation needs ILM, then ILM peeling should be done together with the pucker. As indicated above, it is important to note for the discussion that ILM is a product of the primary vitreous and is not built by the Müller cells.

ILM peeling for *retinal detachment* was proposed recently (Bopp 2005). Obvious pucker formation occurs in 4–8% of cases after surgery for retinal detachment but a much larger percentage is found upon careful ophthalmoscopy. Preliminary studies demonstrated that after ILM peeling visual recovery was achieved more rapidly. ILM peeling may further reduce the rate of postsurgical cystoid macular edema and pucker formation, but randomized studies and long-term follow-up are needed.

5.6.3.4
Removal of Vitreous Opacities

Removal of vitreous opacities comprises a variety of indications and management options. Vitreous opacities can be allocated to three general groups: vitreous floaters and condensed vitreous collagen, vitreous hemorrhages and remaining blood cells, and as a third group inflammatory cells and cellular deposits. While the necessity for vitrectomy is obvious in some cases, the beneficial effect of removal of the opacities has to be judged against the risks and consequences of the treatment itself.

Vitreous floaters are areas of condensed vitreous collagen which are present more after posterior vitreous detachment.

- Precipitation of cholesterol crystals ("*synchisis scintillans*") may cause yellowish dots in the vitreous. Usually unilateral, they are a consequence of previous vitreous hemorrhages. Visual acuity may be affected.
- "*Asteroid hyalosis*" (or "synchisis nivea") results from Ca^{2+} soap deposits attached to the vitreous collagen, often bilateral.

The safety and effectiveness of pars plana vitrectomy as the primary treatment for visually disturbing vitreous floaters is established (Hoerauf et al. 2003; Roth et al. 2005; Schiff et al. 2000). Pre- and postoperative visual acuity mostly remains the same. In spite of the small number of patients suffering lowered postoperative visual acuity, which in the most severe cases amounted to a reduction of VA from 1.0 to 0.6 due to a nuclear sclerosis of the lens, the patients were satisfied overall. Selected patients experience after vitrectomy improved subjective vision even in eyes with full objective VA. As vitreoretinal complications including retinal detachment cannot be ruled out, a critical patient selection and a careful preoperative assessment of specific risks of vitrectomy are mandatory.

Retinal breaks and consecutive retinal detachment occur in about 5–8% of patients after vitrectomy for macular disease. Nuclear sclerosis and significant cataract develop in up to 63%, only rarely endophthalmitis (Michels 1984; Rice et al. 1968; de Bustros 1988a, b); we would recommend vitrectomy for "asteroid hyalosis and for synchisis nivea, only if other pathologies for visual deterioration have been excluded and the patient insists on surgery.

Vitreous hemorrhage is most likely a consequence of ruptured newly formed vessels at the vitreoretinal interface secondary to a (usually partial) posterior vitreous detachment. Vitreous hemorrhage was a major risk factor for a severe visual loss in the Early Treatment Diabetic Retinopathy Study (ETDRS) (Flynn 1992; Fong 1999).

The Diabetic Retinopathy Vitrectomy Study (DRVS) demonstrated the efficacy of vitrectomy in a randomized, prospective study; 616 eyes with severe diabetic vitreous hemorrhage (VA < 1/50) were randomized to either immediate vitrectomy or a postponed treatment after 1 year. At the 2-year follow-up visit, 25% of the patients receiving early vitrectomy demonstrated a visual acuity of 10/20 or better in comparison to only 15% of the late vitrectomy group ($p<0.01$) (DRVS 1985a, b). Later investigations, which included an intraoperative panretinal photocoagulation, confirmed this trend (Chaudhry 1995). A retrospective analysis of eyes with vitreous hemorrhage demonstrated a final visual acuity of 20/60 in one-third of the patients treated (Helbig et al. 1998a).

Accordingly, *early* vitrectomy should be considered in eyes with vitreous hemorrhage, precluding laser application, not resolving within 4–8 weeks. The general aim of the treatment is an *early adequate panretinal photocoagulation* (including the outer retinal periphery). As described above, it is advantageous to perform the panretinal photocoagulation intraoperatively using an illuminated laser probe and scleral indentation to complete the treatment to the peripheral retina.

If the hemorrhage is dense, a preoperative ultrasound examination (B-scan) is advisable to assess the retinal macula. If retinal detachment is about to extend the macula, or if the macula detached only recently, then vitrectomy should be performed soon. Early vitrectomy is further advisable in eyes lacking previous panretinal photocoagulation. Severe progressive proliferation of the fellow eye is another reason to perform vitrectomy instantly (DRVS 1990; Smiddy 1995). Surgical removal of vitreous hemorrhage may help to prevent progression to a tractional retinal detachment. Similarly, in any case of associated anterior segment neovascularization (either rubeosis iridis and/or manifest neovascular glaucoma), vitreous hemorrhage is an indication for early surgical intervention. Only instant vitrectomy and complete panretinal photocoagulation are able to inhibit progression of the neovascular process and to prevent occlusion of the chamber angle (Ho 1992).

Subhyaloidal hemorrhage develops if neovascular bridges tear between the retina and the posterior hyaloid surface. Spontaneous reabsorption can be awaited in most cases. However, long-standing subhyaloidal hemorrhage can serve as a scaffold for fibrovascular proliferation between ILM and the posterior vitreous surface. Then vitrectomy is advisable.

Vitreous hemorrhage requires *early* intervention in diabetic patients in the following situation: iris neovascularization, sonographic traction of the macula, and proliferative retinopathy in the fellow eye of patients with type I diabetes. Patients presenting with their first vitreous hemorrhage and type II diabetes or after previous panretinal photocoagulation should be considered less urgent for vitrectomy.

Similarly, vitreous hemorrhages after a known central retinal vein occlusion are less prone to traction, and vitrectomy may be delayed if panretinal laser photocoagulation seems possible after clearing of the vitreous blood.

Vitreous hemorrhages in elderly patients with sonographic evidence of a subretinal process mostly turn out to be a consequence of subretinal hemorrhage due to a (possibly peripheral) AMD that have penetrated the retina into the vitreous. Nevertheless, if a malignancy cannot be ruled out by non-invasive diagnostic methods, a pars plana vitrectomy and even a biopsy of the subretinal mass is maybe indicated.

Inflammatory, infiltrative or infectious disorders of the posterior segment of the eye may require vitreous surgery to diagnose or treat. Modern vitreoretinal surgical techniques have expanded the spectrum for intervention in various forms of uveitis. Removal of optically relevant vitreous opacities, improvement of secondary macular edema, delamination of epiretinal membranes, release of traction in the presence of abnormal vitreoretinal adhesions, and rhegmatogenous detachment represent indications for vitreoretinal procedures in uveitis patients (Table 1.3.4; Becker et al. 2003). Rhegmatogenous and tractional detachment and cystoid macula edema are discussed in other chapters. As a complication of intermediate uveitis not only vitreous cells can be present, but also vitreous hemorrhage (Potter 2001). Similarly, retinal vasculitis can produce ischemia and a neovascular response associated with vitreous infiltration and hemorrhage. Pars plana vitrectomy can relieve traction and clear the visual axis; however, panretinal photocoagulation may not be required in these patients (see Sect. 5.6.3.5).

The vitreous becomes opaque because of cellular deposits, proteinaceous infiltration and degeneration of the gel structure. In Caucasians the most frequent causes are *intermediate uveitis* and juvenile rheumatoid arthritis.

These entities often cannot be cured by anti-inflammatory treatment, but the surgical removal of the vitreous gel can restore vision in these patients – modified by the extent of cystoid macular edema. Pars plana vitrectomy and lentectomy in a patient with uveitis was first described in 1978 (Diamond and Kaplan). Pars plana vitrectomy is hoped to reduce the activity of inflammation that does not respond to immunosuppression. Removal of the gel is supposed to reduce the ability of the vitreous to retain inflammatory mediators and thereby reduces the recurrence of inflammation. Evidence for this remains uncertain and it could be argued that improvement following surgery is a result of the removal of the vitreous opacities rather than any influence on the inflammatory processes (Mieler 1988).

Furthermore, removal of the vitreous may have a positive effect on *macular edema* via elimination of inflammatory mediators and tractional forces and could improve penetration of anti-inflammatory medication to the retina (Heiligenhaus 1996).

Nevertheless, many of the patients affected are young and have an attached posterior hyaloid membrane which will require removal but is difficult to detach in the presence of vitreoretinal adhesions.

Becker and Davis have reviewed a total of 44 interventional case series on vitrectomy in patients with uveitis published between 1981 and 2005 that included 1,575 patients (1,762 eyes) (Becker et al. 2005). Intermediate uveitis was present in 841 eyes. Cystoid macular edema and cataract were commonly associated, and there were large numbers of additional surgical procedures. Visual outcomes in 39 articles were stated as improved in 708 eyes (68%), unchanged in 202 eyes (20%), and worsened in 124 eyes (12%). Reduction in systemic medication following PPV was reported in 25 out of 44 studies. This indicates that pars plana vitrectomy is possibly relevant to the outcomes of improving vision and reducing inflammation and cystoid macular edema. Still, inconsistent data exist regarding prognostic determinants and the role of perioperative immunosuppression as evident from the literature.

Randomized, controlled, collaborative trials or hypothesis-based case series with precise outcome measures that incorporate control group are required.

Uveitic syndromes may occasionally be difficult to discriminate from other causes of posterior infiltration such as infection and neoplasm. Thus, during vitrectomy, retinal and choroidal biopsies may be obtained if the precise etiology is unknown. This in turn offers the opportunity to better target pharmacological interventions. Recent developments in molecular biology allow novel diagnostic approaches in intraocular inflammation. Genetic markers as well as species-specific sequences are used for the diagnostics of infection or masquerade syndromes (Becker et al. 2003b).

For diagnosis of *lymphoma* a vitreous biopsy requires rapid processing of the sample because the lymphoma cells are fragile and barely viable using micropore-filter techniques (Williamson 2004). It is often difficult because of the tiny volume of the available tissue. Differentiation from inflammation can be a challenge and immunotyping to identify monoclonal cell lines is useful (Davids 1997). Ocular lymphoma should always be considered in a patient with steroid resistant posterior uveitis. If lymphoma cannot be ruled out by vitreous biopsy, it is advisable to consider chorioretinal biopsy to increase the chances of establishing an unequivocal diagnosis.

Table 5.6.14. Indications for pars plana vitrectomy in uveitis patients (adapted from Becker et al. 2003)

Absolute indications	If systemic steroid and immunosuppression fails
	Fuchs' uveitis syndrome with prominent vitreous infiltration
	Other forms of uveitis associated with heavy vitreous infiltration
	Epiretinal gliosis
	Tractional macular edema
	Peripheral traction in intermediate uveitis
	Detachment
Relative indications	Vitreous infiltration with intermediate uveitis
Questionable indications	Chronic uveitis in childhood (refractive to steroids, but responsive to immunosuppression)
	Anterior uveitis with vitreous affection without immunosuppression
Not recommended (contraindications)	Posterior uveitis without vitreous infiltrates (e.g., Behçet's disease, multifocal chorioretinitis, intermediate uveitis without affection of the macula)
	Any uveitis without vitreous infiltrates

5.6.3.5
Retinal Hypoxia

Retinal hypoxia is the number one reason for neoangiogenesis with end stages as neovascular glaucoma. Thus the major task is to reduce retinal hypoxia.

As early as 1956, Wise suggested that retinal hypoxia stimulated retinal neovascularization in the ischemic proliferative retinopathies (Steffanson 2001). Although not directly proven, this theory is strongly supported by a wealth of circumstantial information.

Little is known about the ocular oxygen consumption rate in retinal ischemia. Recently, vitreoperfusion was suggested to measure oxygen consumption during vitrectomy in retinal disease (Blair et al. 2004). Similarly, an MRI-based technique to measure the retinal oxygen response (ROR) as a change in vitreal oxygen level from room air breathing to a new hyperoxic condition (DeltaPO2) has been applied to human proliferative disease and can even be used as a surrogate marker of drug treatment efficacy (Berkowitz et al. 2000, 2005; Trick et al. 2005; Ito et al. 2001). Although these techniques may improve clinical judgement in the future, the area of *capillary non-perfusion* remains the current clinical indicator for retinal ischemia and thus a prognostic risk factor for retinal neovascularization in retinal occlusive diseases or diabetes (capillary occlusion).

VEGF mRNA was found to be elevated in the peripheral, avascular retina in eyes with retinopathy of prematurity (ROP), consistent with the hypothesis that retinal hypoxia *stimulates VEGF expression* (Young et al. 1997). Similarly, VEGF expression in the diabetic retina is associated with upregulation of *hypoxia inducible factor* (HiF-1a). While we are beginning to understand better the pathogenesis of hypoxia and hypoxic signaling (Poulaki et al. 2002), there is still no specific pharmacological inhibitor of ischemia available. Two *treatment modalities, vitrectomy and panretinal photocoagulation*, have been shown to be effective against retinal neovascularization in diabetics and other entities. Both of these treatment modalities improve retinal oxygenation, and supposedly that is the mechanism through which they halt retinal neovascularization (Steffanson 1990).

The physiologic mechanism of photocoagulation can been seen as evidenced in light and electron microscopy in cats in the following steps: The physical light energy is absorbed in the melanin granules of the RPE (the "oven" of Fankhauser). The adjacent photoreceptors are destroyed and are replaced by a glial scar and the oxygen consumption of the outer retina is reduced. Oxygen that normally diffuses from the choriocapillaris into the retina can now diffuse through the laser scars at the level of the former photoreceptor layer without being consumed in the mitochondria of the photoreceptors. This oxygen flux reaches the inner retina to relieve inner retinal hypoxia and raise the oxygen tension. As a result, the retinal arteries constrict and the bloodflow decreases. Hypoxia relief reduces production of growth factors such as VEGF and neovascularization is inhibited or stopped. Vasoconstriction increases arteriolar resistance, decreases hydrostatic pressure in capillaries and venules and reduces edema formation according to Starling's law (Steffanson 1986, 1990).

It is important to note that reduction of neovascularization in proliferative retinal disease cannot be achieved by direct coagulation of the proliferating vessels but by *indirect* effects of disseminated photoculation and reduction of the retinal hypoxia. Areas of ischemia should be coagulated, specifically the peripheral ischemic retina in diabetes or branch vein occlusion. In eyes with recurrent ROP but diode laser treatment of the peripheral avascular retina, VEGF mRNA was *not* detected in the photocoagulated areas of retina but was increased between laser scars (Young et al. 1990). This finding confirms the importance of laser photocoagulation and indicates that in the significant ischemia of the peripheral retina in the avascular zone of ROP, a very dense or even confluent photocoagulation may be required.

Vitrectomy on its own improves retinal oxygenation by allowing oxygen and other nutrients to be transported in *water currents* in the vitreous cavity from well oxygenated to ischemic areas of the retina. Vitrectomy and retinal photocoagulation both improve retinal oxygenation and both reduce diabetic macular edema and retinal neovascularization as well as hypoxia in branch vein occlusion (Steffanson 1990a, b). The major aim of vitrectomy after vitreous hemorrhage following diabetic retinopathy or central retinal vein occlusion is to have an adequate fundus view to complete photocoagulation and thus to quickly reduce ischemia. Only rarely does neovascularization not regress despite supposedly complete panretinal coagulation. If there is any doubt about a sufficient photocoagulation, it is advisable to further increase the number of laser spots per area. If panretinal photocoagulation is complete, then vitrectomy plus silicone oil tamponade aims at regression/prevention of rubeosis and ciliary body neovascularization, and at remedying preretinal neovascularization. Preretinal treelike neovascularization requires the presence of hyaloid scaffold (Wong et al. 1989).

Another important cause of retinal ischemia is *persistent peripheral retinal detachment*. A peripheral retinal detachment of the outer retina causes sufficient ischemia to result in a rubeosis iridis. In 38 patients with essentially reattached retinas after vitrectomy and silicone oil for PVR presenting with rubeosis, peripheral residual retinal detachment coexisted with rubeosis. *Removal of this peripheral detached retina* was statistically significantly associated with disappearance of rubeosis, which suggests that the peripheral detachment was a causative factor (van Meurs et al. 1996). Peripheral retinal hypoxia was similarly described to be associated with rubeosis in patients with juvenile retinoschisis (Pearson 1989; Hung et al. 1980).

5.6.3.6
Choroidal Neovascularization and Atrophy

Laser treatment of extrafoveal membranes, photodynamic therapy with verteporfin, and pharmacological approaches using steroids or antiangiogenic substances are described elsewhere.

Microsurgical extraction of the choroidal neovascularization (CNV) is technically feasible (Thomas et al. 1992; Adelberg et al. 1995; Hudson et al. 1995; Scheider et. al. 1999). In contrast to non-surgical treatment, approaches involving surgical removal of the neovascular membrane have been reported to improve visual function.

Submacular membrane extraction as performed in the Submacular Surgery Trial did *not* improve or preserve visual acuity for 24 months (SST Report No. 11). Besides simple removal of the neovascular membrane, which *inevitably injures the RPE, Bruch's membrane and the choriocapillaris*, more recent approaches attempt to retain a functional RPE layer (Berger and Kaplan 1992; Eckardt 1996; Lambert et al. 1992; Thomas et al. 1993; Thomas et al. 1994; Lappas 2000; Thumann 2000).

Preliminary data on *macular translocation* indicate that stabilization and even improvement of the visual acuity can be achieved (Wolf et al. 1999; Eckardt et al. 1999). Macular translocation is a tedious vitreoretinal technique, which bears the risk of retinal detachment, macular pucker or other forms of PVR and late macular edema (Ninomiya et al. 1996; Wolf et al. 1997).

Replacement of diseased or missing submacular RPE in AMD by *heterologous fetal RPE* was first performed by Algvere (RPE transplantation) (Algvere et al. 1994, 1997). Unfortunately all eyes developed macular edema, most likely due to host-graft rejection. Visual acuity declined and foveal fixation was lost in all patients. Peyman at al. (1991) suggested *autologous RPE translocation* to avoid immune reactions. This isolated RPE layer, however, is difficult to obtain under the retina. Iris-PE translocation remains easier for accessibility. However, its functionality remains to be shown. Whereas the short term results have been promising, there was *no proven benefit* in the long-term observations and the subretinally injected cells did *not* form a stable monolayer, but remained in cell clumps (Lappas 2000, 2004). This led to the assumption that the transplantation of a *stable monolayer* is required for the function of the transplant.

Peyman (1991) was the first to suggest a *translocation of the peripheral choroids and RPE*. van Meurs demonstrated the clinical feasibility of the new technique translocating a patch for peripheral choroids with the intact overlying RPE (van Meurs 2004).

The translocation of a *full-thickness patch* with autologous peripheral RPE to the macula after choroidal neovascular membrane extraction may theoretically result in a vital and functioning graft (Patch). Patients with unstable and/or extrafoveal fixation could achieve central fixation after surgery. Stable fixation prior to surgery could be maintained after Patch in most cases. As quality of fixation prior to surgery correlated to that afterwards, it is unlikely for patients with extrafoveal and unstable fixation to gain significantly better fixation through Patch unless compared to loss of fixation (Joussen et al. 2006, 2007). Long-term follow-up has to determine risks for subsequent graft fibrosis and long-term survival of the graft and recurrent CNV.

5.6.3.7
Chorioretinal Biopsy

Chorioretinal biopsy may provide useful information for determining the diagnosis and guiding the subsequent management of patients with progressive chorioretinal processes of unknown etiology.

After a complete pars plana vitrectomy, an area of choroid of about four to six disc areas in size is demarcated using long-lasting laser pulses to coagulate the choroid. It is important to choose an affected area with a *"fresh" lesion*. Burned-out scars are unlikely to give the information needed. The retina and the underlying choroid are then cut inside the laser demarcation and freed from the underlying sclera avoiding excessive manipulation and squeezing of the tissue. Importantly, the sclerotomy via which the specimen is taken out should be large enough to allow for atraumatic removal of the tissue. Depending on the suspected condition, the tissue should be immediately fixated or natively sent out for examination. On the basis of clinical indications, the specimens can be processed for light microscopy, electron microscopy, immunohistochemical staining, in situ DNA hybridization, and polymerase chain reaction including virology and microbiology.

The chorioretinal defect created by biopsy is secured by laser coagulation. A permanent tamponade with sil-

Table 5.6.15. Risk factors for age-related macular degeneration (AMD), from the literature

1.	Age	8.3×↑
2.	Sunlight exposure	2.1×↑
3.	Smoking	2.5×↑
4.	Diet	2.2×↑
5.	Pseudophakia	5.7×↑
6.	Female	2×↑
7.	"Blue" iris	1.3×↑
8.	Family history	4.5×↑

icone oil is *not* always necessary. Although the risk of PVR is evident, the chance of gaining diagnostic information can be relevant for the patient's life. *Indications for biopsy* in patients with progressive chorioretinal lesions of unknown etiology include: (1) macular-threatening lesions unresponsive to therapy, (2) suspicion of malignancy, or (3) suspicion of an infectious etiology. In all cases, it should be reasonably expected that the results would *alter therapy* or other aspects of clinical care (Rutzen et al. 1995; Martin et al. 1993). For example, chorioretinal biopsy was used to diagnose reactive lymphoid hyperplasia of the uvea (Cheung et al. 1994). The authors believe though that the indication for chorioretinal biopsy should be rather generous. Chorioretinal biopsy or fine needle biopsy should be avoided in any child *with suspected retinoblastoma* in order to prevent seeding of malignant cell along the tract of incision.

5.6.3.8
General Concepts in the Treatment of Tumors of Choroid and Retina

In general three possible methods of treating malignomas are in use, comprising *surgical excision, irradiation and systemic chemotherapy*. While detailed treatment protocols can be found in the specific literature, the following is meant to give an overview about possible approaches.

5.6.3.8.1
Controversies in the Management of Malignant Melanomas

With the known peak in the metastasis rate at 3 years after enucleation (Zimmerman et al. 1978), it was discussed whether surgical manipulation required during *enucleation* might promote metastatic spread by tumor cell penetration of blood vessels, resulting in an *"observation without intervention"* approach. This has been strongly opposed on the grounds that enucleation at a very early stage is most likely to prevent metastases (Manschot and van Peperzeel 1980; Zimmerman 1980). Nevertheless, there is no evidence that any form of intervention has a greater adverse effect than enucleation on the metastatic death rate! The availability of conservative treatment is particularly advantageous for a patient with a small melanoma in the only seeing eye. *Diagnostic biopsy* of the choroid (see Sect. 5.6.3.7) allows for a definite judgement about the presence or absence of a tumor (Gunduz et al. 1999).

A transscleral local excision of posterior uveal melanomas is technically feasible and follows a standardized technique (Damato et al. 1996a, b). A half-thickness scleral flap is raised over the base of the tumor. After diathermia of the choroid, the tumor is then excised with a surrounding flap of choroid and a *histological*

Table 5.6.16. Therapeutic options in malignant melanomas of choroid

Treatment modality	Indication
Brachytherapy with beta-ray plaques	Tumors < 6 mm thickness
Brachytherapy with gamma-ray plaques	Tumors 5–9 mm thickness
Transpupillary thermotherapy with infrared lasers	Only as ancillary treatment after brachytherapy or external beam radiation
External beam radiation: charged particles	Small to medium size tumors at the posterior pole not underlying the macula and not touching the optic disc
Transscleral resection	Large tumors of the peripheral choroid and the ciliary body not extending 15 mm in largest tumor diameter – followed by brachytherapy
Transretinal endoresection	"Experimental" in choroidal tumors exceeding 9 mm thickness and a basal diameter of 10–12 mm

examination proceeded with. The scleral flap is then sutured to the edges of the excision. This is followed by a pars plana vitrectomy to reattach the retina. In addition to tumor recurrence and cataract formation, the procedure itself holds the risk of expulsive bleeding and should be limited to experienced surgeons.

Evaluation of the *pathology* after transscleral excision of a melanoma requires specific attention as to whether or not residual tissue masses are recurrent tumor or reactive proliferations. Pigmented or white nodules at the periphery of the resection site may be due to reactive proliferation and fibrous metaplasia of the RPE. As histologically serial sections are impossible, the risk of residual tumors in the preserved scleral lamella cannot be ruled out. Therefore *Ru-brachytherapy of the area appears reasonable*. Scleral ectasia is even more frequently seen after external beam irradiation of the excision site.

Endoresection uses the advances of pars plana vitrectomy to remove the tumor from inside the eye. Access to the tumor can be gained either by a 180° retinotomy and subsequent surgery in the subretinal space, or by transretinal sacrifice of the retina overlying the tumor. Using the vitreous cutter the tumor is completely removed and the tumor fragments are collected for pathology. The best technique for dealing with the samples is to spin the fixed tissue in a micropore filter until a pellet can be processed for routine paraffin histology.

Carried out in order to avoid spread of viable tumor cells, endoresection under air did not improve the high rate of early metastasis (Hadden et al. 2004). The current approach of the authors is to irradiate the tumor by teletherapy and then in a second step perform the endoresection within the first 2 weeks to avoid reactions to irradiation induced tumor necrosis (Bornfeld 2002).

Brachytherapy

Using ionizing radiation, high tumoricidal doses are required: 90–100 Gy to the apex and 120–180 Gy to the base are necessary. Both in vitro and in vivo studies emphasize the radioresistant properties of uveal melanomas (Logani et al. 1995; Soulieres et al. 1995; Quivey et al. 1996). Irradiated tumors decrease slowly in size over a period of 1–2 years after treatment. This effect is likely to be due to a combination of *tumoricidal* radiotherapy and radiation *vasculopathy* (Schilling 1997; Shields 1990).

Survival studies after irradiation of melanomas have shown that pre-enucleation irradiation does not adversely affect the overall survival rate (COMS 1998; Augsburger et al. 1998). Brachytherapy, e.g., with ^{109}Ru plaques sutured to the sclera, is effective without causing scleral necrosis (Lommatzsch et al. 1986; Shields et al. 1990; Finger et al. 1999). Nevertheless, if the plaque is inaccurately located or separated from the globe by soft tissue or hemorrhage, tumor will *recur behind the irradiated area*. Appearances of the residual tumor vary from obvious and apparently unaffected proliferation to a pattern in which isolated bizarre cells with recognizable tumor morphology are located within fibrous tissue with scattered inflammatory cells of melanomacrophagic and lymphocytic type. Irradiation vasculopathy is rare after ^{109}Ru plaques. A plaque placed too close to the optic nerve will result in radiation endarteriopathy of the posterior ciliary vessels and an ischemic infarction of the optic nerve.

Teletherapy uses high energy charged particles such as protons or helium ions which are focused as a collimated beam from a distant source onto a tumor with sparing of the adjacent tissue (Gragoudas et al. 1987; Castro et al. 1997; Char et al. 1998). A major problem of this treatment approach is the possibility of focal necrosis within the tumor followed by the risk of remaining viable tumor tissue at the posterior limit of the treated area. *Even in the most advanced forms of radiation therapy, some 16% of patients will develop complications* (tumor recurrence or neovascular glaucoma), which will require *secondary enucleation* (Saornil et al. 1992; Finger et al. 1997; Jampol et al. 2002).

In contrast to radiation therapy, *photocoagulation* can only destroy the very superficial layers of tumors (Vogel 1972). Similarly, *transpupillary thermotherapy* (TTT), which has been proposed for primary treatment of small melanomas, did not meet the expectations in the long-term follow-up and is associated with a high incidence of recurrence. In TTT a diode laser beam is passed through the pupil to heat the tumor up to 45–60 °C for 1 min in order to achieve superficial tumor necrosis up to 4 mm in depth (Oosterhuis et al. 1998).

Treatment of *hemangiomas of the choroid* has been reported by external beam irradiation (Schilling et al. 1997a), radioactive plaque (Zografos et al. 1996) or PDT (Michels et al. 2005; Jurklies et al. 2003).

Retinoblastoma treatment has considerably changed within the past decade. In bilateral cases the worst eye was usually enucleated and the eye containing the smaller tumor was irradiated (40–50 Gy). Ortho- and mega voltage, ^{60}Co plaque and ^{109}Ru plaques (Kindy-Degman et al. 1989; Marcus et al. 1990; Shields et al. 1993) have been used. Macroscopically, a successful irradiation leaves small calcified egg-shaped structures within oval foci of complete depigmentation. Partial eradication with recurrence will show similar foci of calcification within web-like tissue where tumor tissue has been obliterated and typical gray/pink viable tumor tissue where the tumor has survived and continues to grow. Irradiation induced quiescence in a tumor appears as a thickened gray area within the retina.

Histologically, initially successful treatment followed by recurrence will be manifest as typical *well-differentiated retinoblastoma with fleurettes* and *Flexner-Winterstenier rosettes* – indicating radioresistance – adjacent to loosely spaced glial tissue. Pepper and salt depigmentation of the RPE and waxy intraretinal exudates are presumed to be due to radiation-induced damage to the vascular endothelium.

Unilateral retinoblastoma of small size can be treated by cryotherapy or photocoagulation (Shields et al. 1990a, b). *Systemic chemotherapy* is confined to advanced cases. Recent protocols using a regimen of vincristine 0.05 mg/kg, cyclophosphamide 40 mg/kg, carboplatin 10 mg/kg, and etoposide 15 mg/kg were unable to prove a curative effect of chemotherapy alone (Gallie et al. 1996; Murphree et al. 1996; Schüler et al. 2003). The ocular and systemic complications of retinoblastoma chemotherapy have been reviewed (Imperia et al. 1989; Nahum et al. 2001) and *histological studies* have revealed total tumor necrosis in some specimens and surviving tumor cells in others (Bechrakis et al. 1998; Dithmar et al. 2000). Nevertheless, a *combination of chemotherapy cycles* to reduce the tumor size in *combination with a subsequent local irradiation* seems to be efficient and is suggested for larger tumors outside the vascular arcades. Similarly, *thermochemotherapy* is a chemotherapy combined with laser photocoagulation which has been suggested for small multiloculated tumors. *Histologic* examination after enucleation is a relevant prerequisite to treatment decisions in patients with known retinoblastoma. Tumor spread into the optic nerve parenchyma or within the meninges will require irradiation of the orbit either alone or in combination with a pulsed chemotherapy. Invasion into the choroid is a striking sign for poor prognosis.

Trilateral Retinoblastoma

In this care condition both eyes and the corpus pineale are involved.

5.6.4
Wound Healing and Complications of Therapy

5.6.4.1
Retinal Pigment Epithelium Scars (Fig. 5.6.36)

Retinal pigment epithelium scars occur after trauma or in association with diseases affecting the choroid, sensory retina and RPE such as after retinochoroiditis, chorioretinitis or in age related macular degeneration.

Retinal pigment epithelium scarring has been extensively studied after *tears of the RPE* due to age related macular degeneration. In the majority of cases a plaque of fibrous tissue can be found in the bed of the tear. In a few eyes the inner surface of Bruch's membrane remains relatively unaltered or the process is covered by pigmented tissue resembling normal RPE. Alteration of the morphology occurred more quickly with extensive scarring, and in those with new vessels or significant blood in the subretinal space, when compared with those without such features (Chuang 1988). It has been discussed whether RPE cells in age related macular degeneration can also transdifferentiate to macrophages, e.g., in the case of soft drusen, or are only taking some of their function. The distinctive pathology associated with the changes of Bruch's membrane and RPE in age related macular degeneration is discussed in Sect. 5.6.2.8.

Following choroidal inflammation, RPE hypertrophy and scarring with RPE clumping is apparent as seen, e.g., in presumed ocular histoplasmosis choroiditis syndrome or after toxoplasmosis retinochoroiditis. The scar tissue is more prone to the development of choroidal neovascularization, probably due to secondary changes in Bruch's membrane allowing choroidal neovascularization to grow underneath the retina.

Interestingly, following detachment of the neural retina, the RPE monolayer is stimulated to proliferate and adopt the function of macrophages. However, a mitotic figure has never been demonstrated in the *monolayer* in routine histopathological preparations. Most commonly the cells become rounded and phagocytose lipoprotein (lipofuscin) so that the cytoplasm becomes foamy. In some specimens, plasma proteins are phagocytosed (endocytosed) and the RPE cells incorporate hyaline inclusions which are PAS positive (orange pigment lipofuscin). The most surprising property of the RPE is that the cells undergo fibrous pseudometaplasia to form large fibrous masses and nodules ("*Ringschwiele*") at the detached retinal periphery. More posteriorly this or thick bands of varying size may form beneath the retina and indent it and these may be identified on macroscopic examination when they appear as *subretinal cords*. Cutting of the subretinal cords by surgical maneuvers does not prevent the tenting of the retina. Migration into the vitreous or subhyaloidal space via a retinal hole induces spindle cell metaplasia in the RPE. The cells remaining in situ are also stimulated to form giant drusen. The choroid, optic nerve and posterior ocular structures are little affected by retinal detachment per se.

5.6.4.2
Proliferative Vitreoretinopathy

Proliferative vitreoretinopathy (PVR) is a complication of rhegmatogenous retinal detachment and of severe trauma to the posterior segment of the eye (intraocular foreign bodies, penetration, perforation, rupture, contusion). PVR is clinically characterized by the formation of *contractile periretinal membranes* on one or both faces of the retina. The membranes cause (tractional) retinal detachment or redetachment (see Sect. 5.6.3.2).

The PVR process is considered an "undesired" form of wound healing (Weller et al. 1990). The vitreous is "inflamed" or "changed" by blood ocular barrier breakdown (rhegmatogenous retinal detachment) or by whole blood (trauma), plus the presence of respon-

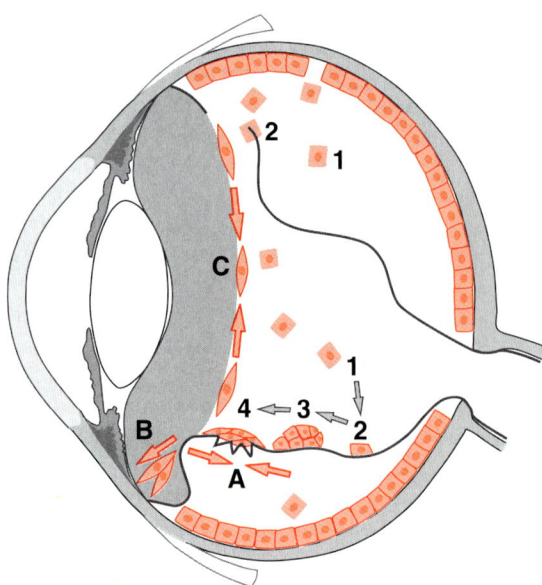

Fig. 5.6.36. Appearance of retinal pigment epithelium (RPE) in PVR. *1* RPE cells floating in the vitreous and subretinal space; *2* adhesion to free surfaces; *3* proliferation; *4* fibrous pseudometaplasia; *red arrows* vitreoretinal traction. (modified from Kirchhof)

sive fibroblastic cells. Fibroblastic cells in PVR are postulated to originate from the RPE, from retinal glia, and from fibrocytes. Interestingly, the *two preconditions of wound healing* – inflammation *and* responsive cells – need to be present at the same time. Blood ocular barrier breakdown alone, like in uveitis, is usually *not* complicated by PVR. Similarly, retinal tears in attached retina exposing RPE to a normal vitreous environment are generally *not* complicated by PVR.

It is accepted that PVR is *cell mediated* and stimulated by *serum* as well as cell-derived growth factors typical of wound healing since Robert Machemer investigated a primate PVR model (Machemer et al. 1968) and since the discovery of the myofibroblast (Gabbiani and Badonnel 1976). The individual cell functions considered to be crucial to the formation of periretinal contractile cell membranes are: attachment, migration, proliferation and deposition of extracellular matrix. Most cell types require cell attachment to extracellular matrix substratum to survive and to function (Meredith, Jr. et al. 1993).

In PVR as a complication of rhegmatogenous retinal detachment such membranes appear predominantly in the inferior circumference of the retina (Koerner et al. 1988). In PVR as a complication of ocular trauma, membranes typically grow from the site of the retinal and choroidal wound. PVR is a persistent clinical problem following *severe ocular trauma*, with rates of 10% up to more than 40%, depending on the type of trauma (Cardillo et al. 1997). The risk of PVR is especially present in children who are known to generate a fierce wound healing response (Karel et al. 1997; Scott et al. 1999). The relationship with "endophthalmitis hemogranulomatosa" – a granulomatous reaction to intraocular coagulated blood clots – is still unclear (Naumann and Völcker 1977).

Although with improved vitreoretinal techniques PVR has become less prevalent during the past few years, its incidence is increasing again with the introduction of new vitreoretinal surgical techniques, such as macular translocation in age related macular degeneration (Wolf et al. 1999; Abdel-Meguid et al. 2003; Aisenbrey et al. 2002; Wong et al. 2004) and retinectomy as an intraocular pressure lowering procedure (Joussen et al. 2003).

Removal of the vitreous collagen, which may act as the substratum to cell attachment, and the posterior hyaloid surface acting as a scaffold, has improved the prognosis of PVR (Abrams et al. 1997). Wide-angle viewing systems, heavy liquids (Brazitikos et al. 1999), and application of dyes aim at a more thorough and a less traumatic mode of removal of vitreous and periretinal membranes (see Sect. 5.6.2.8).

"*Early vitrectomy*" aims to reduce PVR by elimination of the wound healing environment prior to the establishment of contractile membranes.

"*Primary vitrectomy*" signifies vitrectomy instead of only buckling, and aims at prevention of PVR in complicated cases of rhegmatogenous retinal detachment.

Surgery for PVR should aim to *release all traction*. After complete peeling of all epiretinal membranes, subretinal membranes which prevent attachment should be excised. This can usually be done via a small retinotomy in the periphery. *Relaxing retinotomies* are always required when retinal shortening is present. It is important to make sure that the retina is attached without tension. Filling with perfluorcarbons and pressing the retina flat may result in a false impression.

Nevertheless, even the most meticulous vitrectomy technique cannot prevent cell adhesion on the residual collagen of the vitreous base (*anterior-posterior traction*) and cell adhesion on the inner retinal membrane (*star folds*).

Pharmacotherapy as an adjunct to vitrectomy to modulate the complex wound healing process was first proposed by Heimann and coworkers (Weller et al. 1990).

Daunorubicin, a cytostatic drug which acts independently to the cell cycle, was demonstrated to reduce the number of reoperations, but *not* to influence functional outcome in clinical trials (Wiedemann and Heimann 1986). This finding was later confirmed through trials using different drugs, or radiation: 5-fluorouracil (5-FU) and heparin (Allinson 2002), retinoic acid, *dexamethasone* (Machemer et al. 1979), colchicine (Lemor et al. 1986), Taxol (van Bockxmeer et al. 1985), heparin (Williams et al. 1996), and radiation (Binder et al. 1994). From the gathered experience, it was concluded that visual recovery is compromised by secondary retinal changes. Pharmacological therapy should therefore address the *prevention of PVR*, rather than already established PVR.

A heavier than water tamponade displaces the wound healing environment to the superior retinal circumference where the retina should be intact and where there should be no reactive fibroblastic cells. The hypothesis is that physically separating the PVR stimulating environment from the effector cell – the fibroblast or RPE cell – should inhibit the fibroblastic response. To clarify whether a heavier than water tamponade is indeed a useful tool to reduce the risk of PVR is the subject of an ongoing randomized multicenter trial investigating heavy silicone oil against standard oil (HSO Study, Cologne, Germany).

The standard anti-inflammatory drug, corticosteroid, is disputed as a choice for PVR, for its biphasic effect. Dexamethasone was found to stimulate cell growth in low concentrations and to inhibit PVR only in high concentrations (Wu et al. 2002). Nevertheless there is a need for anti-inflammatory drugs with a wider therapeutic range compared to the present cancer medication. Whether gene therapy is justified at this stage is questionable.

The analogy of PVR and wound healing makes it worthwhile to take advantage of progress in research on scarring in general. Presently, it seems to be *impossible to avoid scar formation completely*. But a reduction of experimental scarring is being achieved by antagonizing TGFβ1, by application of TGFβ3, by neutralizing platelet derived growth factor (PDFG) (Shah et al. 1992), and by application of hyaluronic acid (Longaker et al. 1989). These recent investigations were stimulated by an earlier observation that *fetal wounds heal without a scar* (Rowlatt 1979). Additional differences between fetal and adult wound healing, e.g., different gene expression, may also apply (Stelnicki et al. 1998). The problem of scarring in the eye is complicated by the *general lack of regeneration of central nerve system tissue*, and by the likeliness that lesions of retina and optic nerve are associated with permanent functional loss.

5.6.4.3
Active Cell Populations

Formation of scar tissue in PVR requires activated RPE cells and hyalocytes (see Sect. 5.6.4.2). Similarly, the angiogenic process in retinal and choroidal neovascularization requires activated endothelial cells and macrophages.

5.6.4.3.1
Retinal Pigment Epithelial Cells

Retinal pigment epithelial cells are hexanocuboidal cells and are described as a polarized epithelium. The RPE has both barrier and phagocytic functions in addition to the metabolic support given to the photoreceptor cells. The inner, apical parts of the RPE cells are joined by junctional complexes which comprise two types of junctions – zonula occludens (inner) and zonula adherens (outer). They form the Verhoeff membrane, one of the outer components of the blood-retinal barrier (see Chapter 4). Lateral cell membranes of the RPE cells have gap junctions which are responsible for transfer of ions and electrical impulses between the adjacent cells. Melanin granules are present in the apical part of the cell and these melanosomes migrate into the microvilli in bright light and thereby protect from damage by free radicals. One important function of the RPE cell is to control movements of water which pass from the vitreous across the retina to the choroid. The water transport is required for close structural interaction of the retina with its supportive tissues in establishment of an adhesive force between RPE and the retina. In one direction, the RPE transports electrolytes and water from the subretinal space to the choroid, and in the other direction, the RPE transports glucose and other nutrients from the blood to the photoreceptors.

Photoreceptors contain high amounts of photosensitive molecules and photoreceptor outer segments (POS) undergo a constant renewal process. Shed POS are phagocytosed by the RPE. In the RPE, shed POS are digested, and important molecules, such as retinol or docosahexaenoic acid, are redelivered to photoreceptors in a manner comparable to the visual cycle. For recycling, docosahexaenoic acid is removed from phospholipids and redelivered to photoreceptors as a fatty acid (for review, see Strauss 2005; Remé et al. 1991).

Furthermore, the RPE is known to produce and to secrete a variety of *growth factors* as well as factors that are essential for *maintenance of the structural integrity* of retina and choriocapillaris, e.g., different types of tissue inhibitor of matrix metalloprotease (TIMP). The RPE is able to secrete fibroblast growth factors (FGF-1, FGF-2, and FGF-5), transforming growth factor-β (TGF-β), insulin-like growth factor-I (IGF-I), ciliary neurotrophic factor (CNTF), platelet-derived growth factor (PDGF), members of the interleukin family, and pigment epithelium-derived factor (PEDF). In the healthy eye, the RPE secretes PEDF, which helps to maintain the retinal as well as the choriocapillaris structure in two ways. PEDF was described as a neuroprotective factor because it appeared to *protect* neurons against glutamate-induced or hypoxia-induced apoptosis. In addition, PEDF was shown to function as an *antiangiogenic* factor that inhibits endothelial cell proliferation and stabilizes the endothelium of the choriocapillaris (Strauss 2005).

Another vasoactive factor made in the RPE is vascular endothelial growth factor (VEGF), which is secreted in low concentrations by the RPE in the healthy eye, where it *prevents endothelial cell apoptosis* and is essential for an intact endothelium of the choriocapillaris. VEGF also acts as a permeability factor stabilizing the fenestrations of the endothelium. In a healthy eye, PEDF and VEGF are secreted at opposite sides of the RPE: PEDF to the apical side where it acts on neurons and photoreceptors, and the majority of VEGF is secreted to the basal side where it acts on the choroidal endothelium (Blauweegers et al. 1999). Growth factor secretion changes in response to damage or injury, which stimulates the RPE to also secrete neuroprotective factors including *bFGF* or *CNTF*. This is thought to protect photoreceptors from light-induced damage. The group of Remé and coworkers have demonstrated that following a range of intensified light exposures photoreceptors started to show signs of apoptosis that were fully reversible. This may be due to increased secretion and de novo synthesis of different neuroprotective factors by the RPE such as PEDF, CNTF, and bFGF, which are known to be protective against light damage.

The RPE closely interacts with photoreceptors in the maintenance of visual function. Mutations in genes that are expressed in the RPE can lead to photoreceptor degeneration. On the other hand, mutations in genes expressed in photoreceptors can lead to degenerations of the RPE. Thus both tissues can be regarded as a functional unit where both interacting partners depend on each other.

5.6.4.3.2
Hyalocytes

The embryonic development of the cell population of the mammalian vitreous has been traced to *two sources:* the undifferentiated *mesenchymal* cells of the eye primordium and the primitive reticular cells of the *bone marrow.* Undifferentiated mesenchymal cells invade the future vitreous space in two ways: through the annular opening between the rim of the optic cup and the lens primordium, and through the open embryonic fissure. They differentiate into prevascular cells, hemangioblasts, and fibrocytes located in the area of the optic nerve head. From the very beginning of fetal development, another ameboid-type cell of mesenchymal origin makes its entrance into the vitreous through the hyaloid vessels; these *monocyte-like cells differentiate into hyalocytes* and populate a well-defined area of the cortical vitreous close to the retina and to the ora serrata. Balacz and coworkers demonstrated in animal models that gamma-irradiation (600 rads) decreases the number of migrating amebocytes in their vitreous; 24 h later, however, they are replaced by monocytes from the hyaloid vessels (Balazs et al. 1980). There is further experimental evidence that hyalocytes are *bone marrow derived* (Quiao et al. 2005). If bone marrow cells are labeled and transplanted in a rodent model, the hyalocytes are not labeled if investigated right after bone marrow transplantation in the chimeric mouse. Interestingly, more than 60% of hyalocytes are replaced by labeled cells within 4 months and approximately 90% within 7 months after bone marrow transplantation. The rodent hyalocytes were shown to express tissue macrophage marker and were derived from bone marrow. Their turnover rate in the animal model is 7 months (Quiao et al. 2005).

In the adult organism, hyalocytes are distributed predominantly in the vitreous cortex and have an irregular shape with a spherical granule. Interestingly, hyalocytes maintain macrophage-like characteristics (Noda et al. 2004). They may have both physiologic and pathologic roles, such as the maintenance of vitreous transparency through fibrinolytic activity and the pathogenesis of proliferative-vitreoretinal diseases through cellular proliferation and vitreous hypercontraction (Noda et al. 2004). Hyalocytes have a contractile property in the presence of PDGF-BB and TGF-beta2. Whereas PDGF-BB initiates collagen gel contraction by transient activation of the Rho-kinase pathway, sustained activation of the Rho-kinase pathway and myofibroblast-like transdifferentiation appears to be involved in the TGF-beta2-dependent contractile properties of hyalocytes (Hirayama et al. 2004). The vitreous of normal human eyes usually contains very few cells. Therefore some skepticism is warranted as to whether translation of findings in experimental animals to humans is totally justified.

5.6.4.3.3
Müller Cells and Their Functions

Müller (radial glial) cells span the entire thickness of the retina, and contact and ensheathe every type of neuronal cell body and process (see Sect. 5.6.1.1). This morphological relationship is reflected by a multitude of functional interactions between retinal neurons and Müller cells, including extracellular ion homeostasis and glutamate recycling by Müller cells. Müller cells are the principal glial cells of the retina, assuming many of the functions carried out by astrocytes, oligodendrocytes and ependymal cells in other CNS regions (Newman 1996). Most diseases of the retina are associated with a *reactive Müller cell gliosis*. Massive reactive gliosis may mimic retinal tumors and even fill the entire vitreous cavity (Yanhoff and Zimmerman 1971; see Chapter 4). Müller cell gliosis may either support the survival of retinal neurons or accelerate the progress of neuronal degeneration (Bringmann 2001). Müller cells express numerous voltage-gated channels and neurotransmitter receptors, which recognize a variety of neuronal signals and trigger cell depolarization and intracellular Ca^{2+} waves. In turn, Müller cells modulate neuronal activity by regulating the extracellular concentration of neuroactive substances. The two-way communication between Müller cells and retinal neurons indicates that Müller cells play an active role in retinal function (Newman et al. 1996).

Winter and coworkers were able to demonstrate that Müller cells can only function with a small water film between retina and tamponading agent, allowing the potassium siphoning pump to work (Winter et al. 2000). The pathological changes observed after vitreous tamponade may be caused by excitotoxicity from potassium ion accumulation.

Müller cells are key mediators of nerve cell protection, especially via release of basic fibroblast growth factor, via uptake and degradation of the excitotoxin glutamate, and via secretion of the antioxidant glutathione. Neovascularization during hypoxic conditions is mediated by Müller cells via release of vascular endothelial growth factor and transforming growth factor beta or via direct contact to endothelial cells.

Primary Müller cell insufficiency has been suggested to be the cause of different cases of retinal degeneration including hepatic and methanol-induced retinopathy and glaucoma. It is conceivable that, in the future, new therapeutic strategies may utilize Müller cells for, e.g., somatic gene therapy or transdifferentiation of retinal neurons from dedifferentiated Müller cells (Bringmann et al. 2001).

5.6.4.3.4
Endothelial Cells, Astrocytes and Vascular Development (Fig. 5.6.37)

During development, the first vessels originate at the primitive optic nerve head and spread over the *inner surface of the retina*, forming a dense network (Hughes 2000). The inner vasculature of the retina develops as a spreading network, which is preceded by spindle-shaped cells. These cells are alleged to be vascular precursor cells (angioblasts). However, in the mouse retina the spindle-shaped cells preceding the forming vasculature are immature retinal astrocytes and not vascular precursor cells (Fruttinger et al. 2002). Thus, the primary vascular network in the retina develops by angiogenesis (budding from existing vessels) and not vasculogenesis (assembly of dispersed angioblasts).

The *network of astrocytes* that precedes the growths of vessels also spreads from the optic nerve head (Stone et al. 1987; Ling et al. 1989). Initially, retinal vessels seem to follow this network of retinal astrocytes (Jiang 1995). Retinal neurons release platelet-derived growth factor (PDGFA) to stimulate proliferation of astrocytes, which in turn stimulate blood vessel growth by secreting vascular VEGF (West et al. 2005). There is evidence that the developing vessels provide feedback signals that trigger astrocyte differentiation – marked by cessation of cell division, upregulation of glial fibrillary acidic protein (GFAP) and downregulation of VEGF (West 2005).

After the vascular network has spread across the entire retina, vessels start to sprout *downward,* into the inner plexiform layer, where they establish a *second* vascular network parallel to the first (Engermann 1965; Conolly 1988). The second vascular network is *not* associated with retinal astrocytes.

In adult proliferative disease endothelial activation is regulated by a complicated mechanism. The principal mediators involved in activation of endothelial cells include the regulators of embryogenic development as discussed, but are strongly dependent on interactions between blood cells and endothelial cells. This includes a low-grade inflammation based on neutrophil-leukocyte interaction which has been demonstrated to be a major component of a variety of postnatal angiogenic diseases (Joussen et al. 2003, 2004; Hirata 2005) (see Sect. 5.6.2.7).

5.6.4.4
Distant Defects
5.6.4.4.1
Nuclear Cataracts After Vitrectomy

The SPR study (scleral buckle versus vitrectomy in rhegmatogenous retinal detachment) demonstrated that the only differences in functional outcome were re-

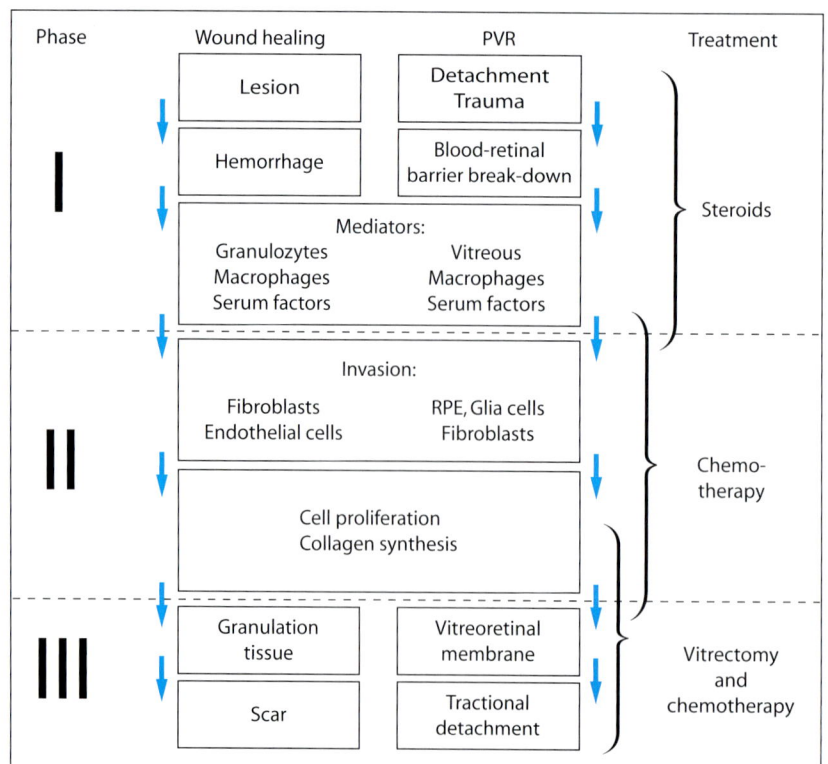

Fig. 5.6.37. Comparison of wound-healing reactions: PVR, including stage related therapy

lated to the higher rate of cataract formation after vitrectomy (SPR Study 2005, unpublished). Similarly, vitrectomy for epiretinal membranes has been shown to be safe in eyes with relatively good preoperative visual acuities, but cataract surgery is necessary in phakic eyes to achieve long-term visual acuity improvement (Thompson 2005).

In general, vitrectomy procedures may cause progression of nuclear sclerotic cataracts, and although some lenticular opacities clear spontaneously, others result in cataracts that impair vision (Blankenship 1982, 1985).

Cataract formation was attributed to intraoperative *osmotic* shifts caused by differences in glucose concentration between the infusion fluid and lens (Faulborn 1978; Green 1994), but is also likely to result from *inadvertent damage by surgical instruments* or from intraocular *gas bubble contact* (Blankenship 1979; Fineberg 1975; Norton 1976; Schachat 1983). While the rosette like structures which are frequently visible in gas filled eyes usually resolve after evaporation of the gas, nuclear cataracts develop usually years after surgery. Intravitreal gas bubbles are associated with a nuclear sclerosis increase of approximately 60% compared with eyes without use of a gas bubble (Thompson 2004). Similarly, contact with *silicone* oil results in cataract formation, which is even more clinically prominent as the duration of tamponade is usually longer and silicone oil in contact with the posterior capsule may result in a sealing phenomenon preventing diffusion of nutrients.

The association between duration of vitrectomy, as well as other risk factors, and the progression of nuclear sclerosis and posterior subcapsular cataract was investigated in the Vitrectomy for Macular Hole Study. *No* significant differences were found when eyes that experienced 45 min or less surgical duration were compared with eyes that endured more than 75 min surgical duration (Cheng 2001).

Patient related factors that dispose to cataract formation are controversial: age, blood pressure, and refractive power were not found to be predictors for nuclear sclerosis and posterior subcapsular cataract progression in a study by Freemann and coworkers (Cheng 2001). In contrast, Thompson (2004) demonstrated that patients older than 50 years of age had a rate approximately sixfold greater than in patients younger than 50 years of age. This observation is in congruence with the clinical observations of the authors.

The retinal disease itself can increase the risk of cataract formation. It was suggested that retinal detachment disturbs the function of the lens, and secondary swelling in the lens fibers and migration of the epithelium to the posterior pole lead to opacification (posterior subcapsular cataract) (Lee 2002).

Similarly, diabetic patients do frequently demonstrate a posterior subcapsular cataract even at an early age probably due to osmotic alterations caused by the underlying disease. Also, the rate of cataract extraction after vitrectomy in patients with diabetes was lower than in patients without diabetes (Smiddy 2004). Several studies have demonstrated that permanent visually significant cataracts occur in 17–37% of diabetic eyes undergoing vitrectomy (Brucker et al. 1978; Hutton et al. 1987; Novak et al. 1984). These eyes can be successfully managed with cataract extraction. A delay of at least 6 months after a vitrectomy procedure can be considered (Hutton et al. 1987; McDermott et al. 1997; Smiddy et al. 1987), keeping in mind that the postoperative cataract results in diabetic patients are inferior to those in patients without diabetes. Worsening or development of a macular edema is the main reason for visual deterioration after cataract surgery. Vice versa a potential postoperative worsening of macular edema is no argument against cataract surgery. Improvement of visual acuity after cataract surgery is achieved in spite of severe non-proliferative diabetic retinopathy in 55% of patients (Chew 1999).

It is of note that for macula diseases, a pars plana vitrectomy combined with cataract surgery compared to a consecutive two-step procedure is not associated with disadvantages regarding the functional outcome or macular edema formation (Staudt et al. 2003).

Regardless of the underlying condition, cataract surgery in combination with vitrectomy and in general cataract surgery in patients with retinal disease requires special precautions: Without any doubt phacoemulsification with implantation of a posterior chamber lens into the capsular bag remains the method of choice for combined vitreoretinal and cataract surgery. However, any type of extracapsular cataract surgery is associated with an increased risk of retinal detachment ($\times 4$) and AMD ($\times 3$) (see Chapter 5.5).

In order to facilitate later panretinal photocoagulation or vitrectomy, a *large* capsulorrhexis is required as well as an intraocular lens (IOL) with a large optic. Acryl is the recommended lens material, as these IOLs can be folded and implanted in small incision surgery. Furthermore, the risk of unfavorable interactions with silicone oil, which could become necessary in subsequent vitreous surgery, is reduced if acryl is used as lens impact material compared to silicone. A silicone lens may develop condensation on its posterior surface during fluid-air exchange, and it may bind to silicone oil as a tamponading agent requiring complicated wash-out procedures (Apple 1996; Eaton et al. 1995; Khawly et al. 1998).

5.6.4.4.2
Angle Closure Glaucoma After Vitreoretinal Surgery

In difficult vitreoretinal surgery several factors can contribute to angle closure in secondary glaucoma:

1. Overfilling of the vitreous cavity after vitrectomy may induce ciliary and/or papillary block and lead to irreversible angle closure.
2. The encircling band may induce an hourglass configuration of the equatorial region of the globe and also induce angle closure.
3. Combination of both potentially poses a risk of anterior segment ischemia.

References

Aaberg TM, Blair CJ, Gass JD. Macular holes. Am J Ophthalmol. 1970; 69: 555–562

Abdelsalam A, Del Priore L, Zarbin MA. Drusen in age-related macular degeneration: pathogenesis, natural course, and laser photocoagulation-induced regression. Surv Ophthalmol. 1999; 44: 1–29

Abdel-Meguid A, Lappas A, Hartmann K, Auer F, Schrage N, Thumann G and Kirchhof B. One year follow up of macular translocation with 360 degree retinotomy in patients with age related macular degeneration. Br J Ophthalmol 2003; 87: 615–621

Abrams GW, Azen SP, McCuen BW, Flynn HW, Jr., Lai MY and Ryan SJ. Vitrectomy with silicone oil or long-acting gas in eyes with severe proliferative vitreoretinopathy: results of additional and long-term follow-up. Silicone Study report 11. Arch Ophthalmol 1997; 115: 335–344

Adelberg DA, del Priore LV, Kaplan HJ. Surgery for subfoveal membranes in myopia, angioid streaks, and other disorders. Retina. 1995; 15: 198–205

Aiello LP, Northrup JM, Keyt BA, Takagi H, Iwamoto MA. Hypoxic regulation of vascular endothelial growth factor in retinal cells. Arch Ophthalmol. 1995; 113: 1538–1544

Ainsworth JR, Damato BE, Lee WR, Alexander WD. Follicular thyroid carcinoma metastatic to the iris: a solitary lesion treated with iridocyclectomy. Arch Ophthalmol. 1992; 110: 19–20

Aisenbrey S, Lafaut BA, Szurman P, Grisanti S, Luke C, Krott R, Thumann G, Fricke J, Neugebauer A, Hilgers RD, Esser P, Walter P and Bartz-Schmidt KU. Macular translocation with 360 degrees retinotomy for exudative age-related macular degeneration. Arch Ophthalmol 2002; 120: 451–459

Al-Abdulla NA, Thompson JT, Sjaarda RN. Results of macular hole surgery with and without epiretinal dissection or internal limiting membrane removal. Ophthalmology. 2004; 111: 142–149

Algvere PV, Berglin L, Gouras P, Sheng Y. Transplantation of fetal retinal pigment epithelium in age-related macular degeneration with subfoveal neovascularization. Graefes Arch Clin Exp Ophthalmol. 1994; 232: 707–716

Allinson RW. Adjuvant 5-FU and heparin prevent PVR. Ophthalmology 2002; 109: 829–830

Ambati J, Arroyo JG. Postoperative complications of scleral buckling surgery. Int. Ophthalmol. Clin. 2000; 40:175–185

Andersen SR, Warburg M. Norrie's disease: congenital bilateral pseudotumor of the retina with recessive X-chromosomal inheritance; preliminary report. Arch Ophthalmol. 1961; 66: 614–618

An International Classification of Retinopathy of Prematurity. II. The classification of retinal detachment. The International Committee for the Classification of the Late Stages of Retinopathy of Prematurity. Arch Ophthalmol. 1987; 105: 906–912

An International Classification of ROP revisited. The International Committee for the Classification of the Late Stages of Retinopathy of Prematurity. Arch Ophthalmol 2005; 123; 991–999

An International Classification of ROP. The International Committee for the Classification of the Late Stages of Retinopathy of Prematurity. Arch Ophthalmol 1984; 102: 1130–1134

Apple DJ, Federman JL, Krolicki TJ, Sims JC, Kent DG, Hamburger HA, Smiddy WE, Cox MS Jr, Hassan TS, Compton SM, Thomas SG. Irreversible silicone oil adhesion to silicone intraocular lenses. A clinicopathologic analysis. Ophthalmology. 1996; 103: 1555–1561

Apushkin MA, Fishman GA, Rajagopalan AS. Fundus findings and longitudinal study of visual acuity loss in patients with X-linked retinoschisis. Retina. 2005; 25: 612–618

Apushkin MA, Fishman GA, Janowicz MJ. Correlation of optical coherence tomography findings with visual acuity and macular lesions in patients with X-linked retinoschisis. Ophthalmology. 2005;113: 495–501

Archer DB. Bowman Lecture 1998. Diabetic retinopathy: some cellular, molecular and therapeutic considerations. Eye. 1999 Aug; 13: 497–523

Archer DB. Doyne Lecture. Responses of retinal and choroidal vessels to ionising radiation. Eye. 1993; 7: 1–13

Asaria RHY, Kon CH, Bunce C, Charteris DG, Wong D, Khaw PT, Aylward GW. Adjuvant 5-fluorouracil and heparin prevents proliferative vitreoretinopathy: results from a randomized, double-blind, controlled clinical trial. Ophthalmology 2001; 108: 1179–1183

Ashton, N. Oxygen and the growth and development of retinal vessels: In vivo and in vitro studies. Am J Ophthalmol 1966; 62: 412–435

Augsburger JJ, Correa ZM, Freire J, Brady LW. Long-term survival in choroidal and ciliary body melanoma after enucleation versus plaque radiation therapy. Ophthalmology. 1998; 105: 1670–1678

Azuara-Blanco A, Dua HS, Pillai CT. Pseudo-endothelial dystrophy associated with emulsified silicone oil. Cornea. 1999; 18: 493–494

Balazs EA, Toth LZ, Ozanics V. Cytological studies on the developing vitreous as related to the hyaloid vessel system. Albrecht Von Graefes Arch Klin Exp Ophthalmol. 1980; 213: 71–85

Barbazetto I, Burdan A, Bressler NM, Bressler SB, Haynes L, Kapetanios AD, Lukas J, Olsen K, Potter M, Reaves A, Rosenfeld P, Schachat AP, Strong HA, Wenkenstern A. Treatment of Age-Related Macular Degeneration with Photodynamic Therapy Study Group; Verteporfin in Photodynamic Therapy Study Group. Photodynamic therapy of subfoveal choroidal neovascularization with verteporfin: fluorescein angiographic guidelines for evaluation and treatment – TAP and VIP report No. 2. Arch Ophthalmol. 2003; 121: 1253–1268

Barr CC. The histopathology of successful retinal reattachment. Retina. 1990; 10:189–194

Bartels M. Über die Entstehung von Netzhautablösungen. Klin Monatsbl Augenheilkd 1933; 91: 437–450

Bartz-Schmidt KU, Thumann G, Psichias A, Krieglstein GK, Heimann K. Pars plana vitrectomy, endolaser coagulation of the retina and the ciliary body combined with silicone oil endotamponade in the treatment of uncontrolled neovascular glaucoma. Graefes Arch Clin Exp Ophthalmol. 1999; 237: 969–975

Bartz-Schmidt KU, Kirchhof B, Heimann K. Primary vitrectomy for pseudophakic retinal detachment. Br J Ophthalmol 1996; 80: 346–349

Bechrakis NE, Bornfeld N, Schueler A, Coupland SE, Henze G, Foerster MH. Clinicopathologic features of retinoblastoma after primary chemoreduction. Arch Ophthalmol. 1998; 116: 887–893

Becker MD, Bodaghi B, Holz FG, Harsch N, Hoang PL. Diagnostische Vitrektomie bei Uveitis: Möglichkeiten der Molekularbiologie. Ophthalmologe. 2003; 100: 796–801

Becker MD, Davis J: Vitrectomy in the treatment of uveitis. Am J Ophthalmol, 2005; in press

Becker MD, Harsch N, Zierhut M, Davis JL, Holz FG. Therapeutische Vitrectomie bei Uveitis: Aktueller Stand und Empfehlungen. Ophthalmologe. 2003; 100: 787–795

Bek T. Capillary closure secondary to retinal vein occlusion. A morphological, histopathological, and immunohistochemical study. Acta Ophthalmol Scand. 1998; 76: 643–648

Bek T. Glial cell involvement in vascular occlusion of diabetic retinopathy. Acta Ophthalmol Scand. 1997; 75: 239–243

Bek T. Immunohistochemical characterization of retinal glial cell changes in areas of vascular occlusion secondary to diabetic retinopathy. Acta Ophthalmol Scand. 1997; 75: 388–392

Bellhorn MB, Friedman AH, Wise GN, Henkind P. Ultrastructure and clinicopathologic correlation of idiopathic preretinal macular fibrosis. Am J Ophthalmol 1975; 79: 366–373

Ben-Ezra D, Sahel JA, Harris NL, Hemo I, Albert DM. Uveal lymphoid infiltrates: immunohistochemical evidence for a lymphoid neoplasia. Br J Ophthalmol. 1989; 73: 846–851

Berkowitz BA, Roberts R, Luan H, Peysakhov J, Knoerzer DL, Connor JR, Hohman TC. Drug intervention can correct subnormal retinal oxygenation response in experimental diabetic retinopathy. Invest Ophthalmol Vis Sci. 2005; 46: 2954–2960

Berkowitz BA, Zhang W. Significant reduction of the panretinal oxygenation response after 28% supplemental oxygen recovery in experimental ROP. Invest Ophthalmol Vis Sci. 2000; 41: 1925–1931

Berger AS, Kaplan HJ. Clinical experience with the surgical removal of subfoveal neovascular membranes. Ophthalmology. 1992; 99: 969–975

Beyer NE. Peripheral retinal lesions related to rhegmatogenous retinal detachment. In: Guyer DR, Yannuzzi LA, Chang S, Shields JA, Green WR: Retina Vitreous Macula, WB Saunders, Philadelphia 1999, p 1219–1223

Bidwell AE, Jampol LM, Goldberg MF. Macular holes and excellent visual acuity. Case report. Arch Ophthalmol. 1988; 106: 1350–1351

Binder S, Bonnet M, Velikay M, Gerard JP, Stolba U, Wedrich A and Hohenberg H (1994) Radiation therapy in proliferative vitreoretinopathy. A prospective randomized study. Graefes Arch Clin Exp Ophthalmol 232: 211–214

Blaauwgeers HG, Holtkamp GM, Rutten H, Witmer AN, Koolwijk P, Partanen TA, Alitalo K, Kroon ME, Kijlstra A, van Hinsbergh VW, Schlingemann RO. Polarized vascular endothelial growth factor secretion by human retinal pigment epithelium and localization of vascular endothelial growth factor receptors on the inner choriocapillaris. Evidence for a trophic paracrine relation. Am J Pathol. 1999; 155: 421–428

Blair NP, Liu T, Warren KA, Glaser DA, Kennedy M, Tran H, Larson CA, Atluri P, Saidel MA, Blair MP. Ocular oxygen consumption: estimates using vitreoperfusion in the cat. Retina. 2004; 24: 120–131

Blankenship G, Cortez R, Machemer R: The lens and pars plana vitrectomy for diabetic retinopathy complications, Arch Ophthalmol 1979; 97: 1263–1267

Blankenship GW, Machemer R. Long-term diabetic vitrectomy results: report of 10-year follow-up. Ophthalmology 1985; 92: 503–506

Blankenship GW. Preoperative prognostic factors in diabetic pars plana vitrectomy. Ophthalmology 1982; 89: 1246–1249

Boldrey EE, Egbert P, Gass JD, Friberg T (1985) The histopathology of familial exudative vitreoretinopathy: a report of two cases. Arch Ophthalmol 103:238–241

Bonnet M. Bielveltz B, Noel et al. Fluorescein angiography after retinal detachment microsurgery. Graefes Arch Clin Exp Ophthalmol 1983; 221: 35–40

Bopp S. Is there room for improvement in pucker surgery? In: Kirchhof B, Wong D (eds.) Essentials in Ophthalmology: Vitreo-retinal surgery. Springer, Heidelberg 2005; p 37–62

Bornfeld N, Talies S, Anastassiou G, Schilling H, Schuler A, Horstmann GA. Endoresektion maligner Melanome der Uvea nach präoperativer stereotaktischer Einzeldosis-Konvergenzbestrahlung mit dem Leksell-Gamma-knife. Ophthalmologe 2002; 99: 338–344

Boulton M, Foreman D, Williams G, McLeod D. VEGF localisation in diabetic retinopathy. Br J Ophthalmol 1998; 82: 561–568

Brazitikos PD. The expanding role of primary pars plana vitrectomy in the treatment of rhegmatogenous noncomplicated retinal detachment. Semin Ophthalmol 2000; 15: 65–77

Brazitikos PD, Androudi S, D'Amico DJ, Papadopoulos N, Dimitrakos SA, Dereklis DL, Alexandridis A, Lake S, Stangos NT. Perfluorocarbon liquid utilization in primary vitrectomy repair of retinal detachment with multiple breaks. Retina 2003; 23: 615–621

Brazitikos PD, D'Amico DJ, Tsinopoulos IT and Stangos NT (1999) Primary vitrectomy with perfluoro-n-octane use in the treatment of pseudophakic retinal detachment with undetected retinal breaks. Retina 19: 103–109

Bringmann A, Reichenbach A. Role of Muller cells in retinal degenerations. Front Biosci. 2001; 6: E 72–92

Brockhurst RJ, Albert DM (1981) Pathologic findings in familial exudative vitreoretinopathy. Arch Ophthalmol 99:2134–2146

Bron AJ, Tripathi RC, Tripathi BJ. The inner limiting membrane, Chapter 14, Wolff's anatomy of the eye, Chapman & Hall 1997; p 488

Brown SM, Jampol LM, Cantrill HL. Intraocular lymphoma presenting as retinal vasculitis. Surv Ophthalmol. 1994; 39: 133–140

Brucker AJ, Michels RG, Green WR. Pars plana vitrectomy in the management of blood-induced glaucoma with vitreous hemorrhage. Ann Ophthalmol 1978; 10: 1427–1437

Bryan JS, Friedman SM, Mames RN, Margo CE. Experimental vitreous replacement with Perfluorotri-n-Propylamine. Arch Ophthalmol 1994; 112: 1098–1102

Bunin GR, Emanuel BS, Meadows AT, Buckley JD, Woods WG, Hammond GD. Frequency of 13q abnormalities among 203 patients with retinoblastoma. J Natl Cancer Inst. 1989; 81: 370–374

Burk SE, da Mata AP, Snyder ME; Rosa RH, Foster RE. Indocyanine-green assisted peeling of the retinal internal limiting membrane. Ophthalmology 2000; 107: 2010–2014

Byer NE. Long-term natural history of lattice degeneration of the retina. Ophthalmology 1989; 96: 1396–1342

Byer NE. The long-term natural history of senile retinoschisis with implications for management. Ophthalmology 1986; 93: 1127–1137

Byer NE. Cystic retinal tufts and their relationship to retinal detachment. Arch Ophthalmol 1981; 99: 1788–1790

Byer NE. Lattice degeneration of the retina. Surv Ophthalmol 1979; 23: 213

Byer NE. Clinical study of senile retinoschisis. Arch Ophthalmol 1968; 79:36–44

Campochiaro PA, Lim JI. Aminoglycoside toxicity in the treatment of endophthalmitis. The Aminoglycoside Toxicity Study Group. Arch Ophthalmol. 1994 Jan;112(1):48–53.

Campo RV, Sipperley JO, Sneed SR, Park DW, Dugel PU, Jacobsen J, Flindall RJ. Pars plana vitrectomy without scleral buckle for pseudophakic retinal detachments. Ophthalmology 1999; 106:1811–1815

Campochiaro PA, Van Niel E, Vinores SA. Immunocytochemical labeling of cells in cortical vitreous from patients with premacular hole lesions. Arch Ophthalmol 1992; 110: 371–377

Canny CLB, Oliver GL (1976) Fluorescein angiographic findings in familial exudative vitreoretinopathy. Arch Ophthalmol 74:1114–1120

Capeans C, Santos L, Sanchez-Salorio M, Forteza J. Iris metastasis from endometrial carcinoma. Am J Ophthalmol. 1998; 125:729–730

Cardillo JA, Stout JT, LaBree L, Azen SP, Omphroy L, Cui JZ, Kimura H, Hinton DR and Ryan SJ (1997) Post-traumatic proliferative vitreoretinopathy. The epidemiologic profile, onset, risk factors, and visual outcome. Ophthalmology 104: 1166–1173.

Carpineto P, Ciancaglini M, Aharrh-Gnama A, Agnifili L, Cerulli AM, Cirone D, Mastropasqua L. Optical coherence tomography and fundus microperimetry imaging of spontaneous closure of traumatic macular hole: a case report. Eur J Ophthalmol. 2005; 15:165–169

Castro JR, Char DH, Petti PL, Daftari IK, Quivey JM, Singh RP, Blakely EA, Phillips TL. 15 years experience with helium ion radiotherapy for uveal melanoma. Int J Radiat Oncol Biol Phys. 1997; 39: 989–996

Chang A, Zimmerman NJ, Iwamoto T, Ortiz R, Faris D. Experimental vitreous replacement with Perfluorotributylamine. Am J Ophthalmol 1987; 103: 29–37

Chang CJ, Lai WW, Edward DP, Tso MO. Apoptotic photoreceptor cell death after traumatic retinal detachment in humans. Arch Ophthalmol. 1995; 113: 880–886

Chang S, Sparrow JR, Iwamoto T, Gershbein A, Ross R, Ortiz R. Experimental studies of tolerance to intravitreal Perfluoro-n-octane. Retina 1991; 11: 367–374

Char D, Kaleta-Michaels S, Engman E. Metastatic retinoblastoma. Case report. Arch Ophthalmol. 1989; 107: 1570–1571

Char DH, Ljung BM, Deschenes J, Miller TR. Intraocular lymphoma: immunological and cytological analysis. Br J Ophthalmol. 1988 Dec; 72: 905–911

Char DH, Kroll SM, Castro J. Long-term follow-up after uveal melanoma charged particle therapy. Trans Am Ophthalmol Soc. 1997; 95: 171–187 discussion 187–91

Charles S. Flinn CE: The natural history of diabetic extramacular traction detachment. Arch Ophthalmol 1979; 97: 1268–1272

Chaudhry NA, Lim ES, Saito Y, Mieler WF, Liggett PE, Filatov V: Early vitrectomy and endolaser photocoagulation in patients with type I diabetes with severe vitreous hemorrhage. Ophthalmology 1995; 102: 1164–1169

Cheng L, Azen SP, El-Bradey MH, Scholz BM, Chaidhawangul S, Toyoguchi M, Freeman WR. Duration of vitrectomy and postoperative cataract in the vitrectomy for macular hole study. Am J Ophthalmol. 2001; 132: 881–887

Chuang EL, Bird AC. Repair after tears of the retinal pigment epithelium. Eye. 1988; 2:106–113

Chen YS, Hackett SF, Schoenfeld CL, Vinores MA, Vinores SA, Campochiaro PA. Localisation of vascular endothelial growth factor and its receptors to cells of vascular and avascular epiretinal membranes. Br J Ophthalmol. 1997; 81: 919–926

Cheung MK, Martin DF, Chan CC, Callanan DG, Cowan CL, Nussenblatt RB. Diagnosis of reactive lymphoid hyperplasia by chorioretinal biopsy. Am J Ophthalmol. 1994; 118: 457–462

Chew EY, Benson WE, Remaley NA, Lindley AA, Burton TC, Csaky K, Williams GA, Ferris Fl 3rd (1999) Results after lens extraction in patients with diabetic retinopathy. The Early Treatment Diabetic Retinopathy Study Report number 25. Arch Ophthalmol 117: 1600–1606

Ciulla TA, Pesavento RD, Yoo S. Subretinal aspiration biopsy of ocular lymphoma. Am J Ophthalmol. 1997; 123: 420–422

Clarkson JG, Green WR, Massof D. A histopathologic review of 168 cases of preretinal membrane. Am J Ophthalmol 1977; 84: 1–7

Cockerham GC, Hidayat AA, Bijwaard KE, Sheng ZM. Re-evaluation of "reactive lymphoid hyperplasia of the uvea": an immunohistochemical and molecular analysis of 10 cases. Ophthalmology. 2000; 107: 151–158

Cogan DG, Kuwabara T. Comparison of retinal and cerebral vasculature in trypsin digest preparations. Br J Ophthalmol 1984; 68(1):10–2

Coleman K, Baak JP, Dorman A, Mullaney J, Curran B, Tiernan D, Farrell M, Fenton M, Leader M. Deoxyribonucleic acid ploidy studies in choroidal melanomas. Am J Ophthalmol. 1993; 115: 376–383

Collins ET. Unusual changes to the macular region. Trans Ophthalmol Soc UK 1900; 20: 196–197

Condon GP, Brownstein S, Wang NS, Kearns JA, Ewing CC. Congenital hereditary (juvenile X-linked) retinoschisis. Histopathologic and ultrastructural findings in three eyes. Arch Ophthalmol. 1986;104:576–583

Connolly SE, Hores TA, Smith LE, D'Amore PA. Characterization of vascular development in the mouse retina. Microvasc Res 1988; 36: 275–290

Coupland SE, Anastassiou G, Bornfeld N, Hummel M, Stein H. Primary intraocular lymphoma of T-cell type: report of a case and review of the literature. Graefes Arch Clin Exp Ophthalmol. 2005; 243: 189–197

Coupland SE, Hummel M, Muller HH, Stein H. Molecular analysis of immunoglobulin genes in primary intraocular lymphoma. Invest Ophthalmol Vis Sci. 2005; 46: 3507–3514

Coupland SE, Loddenkemper C, Smith JR, Braziel RM, Charlotte F, Anagnostopoulos I, Stein H. Expression of immunoglobulin transcription factors in primary intraocular lymphoma and primary central nervous system lymphoma. Invest Ophthalmol Vis Sci. 2005;46: 3957–3964

Coupland SE, Bechrakis NE, Anastassiou G, Foerster AM, Heiligenhaus A, Pleyer U, Hummel M, Stein H. Evaluation of vitrectomy specimens and chorioretinal biopsies in the diagnosis of primary intraocular lymphoma in patients with Masquerade syndrome. Graefes Arch Clin Exp Ophthalmol. 2003; 241: 860–870

Coupland SE, Foss HD, Hidayat AA, Cockerham GC, Hummel M, Stein H. Extranodal marginal zone B cell lymphomas of the uvea: an analysis of 13 cases. J Pathol. 2002; 197: 333–340

Couvillion SS, Smiddy WE, Flynn HW Jr, Eifrig CW, Gregori G. Outcomes of surgery for idiopathic macular hole: a case-control study comparing silicone oil with gas tamponade. Ophthalmic Surg Lasers Imaging. 2005; 36: 365–371

Cramer T, Johnson RS. A novel role for the hypoxia inducible transcription factor HIF-1alpha: critical regulation of inflammatory cell function. Cell Cycle. 2003; 2:192–193

Cramer T, Yamanishi Y, Clausen BE, Forster I, Pawlinski R, Mackman N, Haase VH, Jaenisch R, Corr M, Nizet V, Firestein GS, Gerber HP, Ferrara N, Johnson RS. HIF-1alpha is essential for myeloid cell-mediated inflammation. Cell. 2003; 112: 645–657

Criswick VG, Schepens CL (1969) Familial exudative vitreoretinopathy. Am J Ophthalmol 68:578–594

Cursiefen C, Holbach LM, Schlötzer-Schrehardt U, Naumann GOH. Persisting retinal ganglion cell axons in blind atrophic human eyes. Graefe's Arch Clin Exp Ophthalmol 2001; 239: 158–164

Da Mata AP, Burk SE, Foster RE, Riemann CD, Petersen MR, Nehemy MB, Augsburger JJ. Long-term follow-up of indocyanine green-assisted peeling of the retinal internal limiting membrane during vitrectomy surgery for idiopathic macular hole repair. Ophthalmology. 2004; 111: 2246–2253

Damato B, Duke C, Coupland SE, Hiscott P, Smith PA, Campbell I, Douglas A, Howard P. Clinical cytogenetics in uveal melanoma: seven years experience. Ophthalmology, 2007 Oct; 114(10): 1925–1931

Damato B, Foulds WS. Indications for trans-scleral local resection of uveal melanoma. Br J Ophthalmol. 1996; 80: 1029–1030

Damato BE, Paul J, Foulds WS. Risk factors for metastatic uveal melanoma after trans-scleral local resection. Br J Ophthalmol. 1996; 80: 109–116

Das T, Biswas J, Kumar A, Nagpal PN, Namperumalsamy P, Patnaik B, Tewari HK. Eales' disease. Indian J Ophthalmol 1994 Mar;42(1):3–18

Davis JL, Viciana AL, Ruiz P. Diagnosis of intraocular lymphoma by flow cytometry. Am J Ophthalmol. 1997; 124: 362–372

Davids JL, Hummer J, Feuer WJ. Laser photocoagulation for retinal detachments and retinal tears in cytomegalovirus retinitis. Ophthalmology 1997; 104: 2053–2060

Davis MD, Segal PP and McCormick A. The natural course followed by the fellow eye in patients with rhegmatogenous retinal detachment. In: Pruett RC and Regan CDJ (eds): Retinal Congress, New York 1974, Appleton-Century-Crofts, 643–648

de Bustros S. Vitrectomy for prevention of macular holes. Results of a randomized multicenter clinical trial. Vitrectomy for Prevention of Macular Hole Study Group. Ophthalmology. 1994;101:1055–1059

de Bustros S, Thompson JT, Michels RG, Rice TA, Glaser BM. Vitrectomy for idiopathic epiretinal membranes causing macular pucker. Br J Ophthalmol. 1988; 72: 692–695

de Bustros S, Thompson JT, Michels RG, Enger C, Rice TA, Glaser BM. Nuclear sclerosis after vitrectomy for idiopathic epiretinal membranes. Am J Ophthalmol. 1988; 105: 160–164

de Juan E, Lambert HM (1985) Recurrent proliferations in macular pucker, diabetic retinopathy, and retrolental fibroplasias-like disease after vitrectomy. Graefes Arch Clin Exp Ophthalmol 223:174–183

De Luca A, Esposito V, Baldi A, Giordano A. The retinoblastoma gene family and its role in proliferation, differentiation and development. Histol Histopathol. 1996; 11: 1029–1034

Delaney WV Jr, Torrisi PF, Hampton GR, Seigart CR, Hay PB. Hemorrhagic peripheral pigment epithelial disease. Arch Ophthalmol. 1988; 106: 646–650

Desai UR, Strassman IB (1997) Combined pars plana vitrectomy and scleral buckling for pseudophakic and aphakic retinal detachments in which a break is not seen preoperatively. Ophthalmic Surg. Lasers 28:718–722

Devenyi RG, de Carvalho NH. Combined scleral buckle and pars plana vitrectomy as a primary procedure for pseudophakic retinal detachments. Ophthalmic Surg. Lasers 1999; 30: 615–618

D'Hermies F, Korobelnik JF. Histological evidence of hydrogel fragmentation. Arch Ophthalmol. 1999; 117: 1449

D'Hermies F, Korobelnik JF, Chauvaud D, Pouliquen Y, Parel JM, Renard G. Scleral and episcleral histological changes related to encircling explants in 20 eyes. Acta Ophthalmol Scand. 1999; 77: 279–285

Diabetic Retinopathy Vitrectomy Study Research Group. Early vitrectomy for severe vitreous hemorrhage in diabetic retinopathy. Four-year results of a randomized trial: Diabetic Retinopathy Vitrectomy Study Report 5. Arch Ophthalmol. 1990; 108: 958–964

Diabetic Retinopathy Vitrectomy Study Research Group. Two-year course of visual acuity in severe proliferative diabetic retinopathy with conventional management. Diabetic Retinopathy Vitrectomy Study (DRVS) report #1. Ophthalmology. 1985; 92: 492–502

Diabetic Retinopathy Vitrectomy Study Research Group. Two-year results of a randomized trial. Diabetic Retinopathy Vitrectomy Study report 2. Arch Ophthalmol. 1985; 103: 1644–1652

Diamond J, Kaplan H. Uveitis: effect of vitrectomy combined with lensectomy. Ophthalmology 1978; 86:1320–1329

Dithmar S, Aabert TM Jr, Grossniklaus HE. Histopathologic changes in retinoblastoma after chemoreduction. Retina. 2000; 20: 33–36

Doi M, Refojo MF. Histopathology of rabbit eyes with intravitreous silicone-fluorosilicone copolymer oil. Exp Eye Res 1994; 59: 737–746

Donders PC. Malignant melanoma of the choroid. Trans Ophthalmol Soc U K 1973; 93(0):745–51

Dudgeon J, Lee WR. The trilateral retinoblastoma syndrome. Trans Ophthalmol Soc U K. 1983; 103 (Pt 5): 523–529

Duke Elder S: System of Ophthalmology Vol III, pp 294–308, St Louis: CV Mosby Co 1968

Dumas J and Schepens CL. Chorioretinal lesions predisposing to retinal breaks. Am J Ophthalmol 1966; 61: 620–630

Dunn WJ, Lambert HM, Kincaid MC, Dieckert JP, Shore JW. Choroidal malignant melanoma with early vitreous seeding. Retina. 1988; 8: 188–192

Eaton AM, Jaffe GL, McCuen BW II, Mincey GJ. Condensation on the posterior surface of silicone intraocular lenses during fluid-air exchange. Ophthalmology 1995; 102: 733–736

Eckardt C, Eckardt U, Conrad HJ. Macular rotation with and without counter-rotation of the globe in patients with age-related macular degeneration. Graefe's Arch Clin Exp Ophthalmol. 1999; 237: 313–325

Eckardt C. Chirurgische Entfernung von submakulären Neovaskularisationsmembranen. Ophthalmologe. 1996; 93: 688–693

Eckardt C, Nicolai U, Czank M, Schmidt D. Identification of silicone oil in the retina after intravitreal injection. Retina. 1992; 12: S17–22

Eckard C, Nicolai U, Winter M, Knop E. Experimental intraocular tolerance to liquid Perfluorooctane and Perfluoropolyether. Retina 1991; 11: 375–384

Eisner G. Autoptische Spaltlampenuntersuchung des Glaskörpers. I–III. Graefes Arch Clin Exp Ophthalmol 1971; 182: 1–40

el-Asrar AM. Primary vitrectomy for bullous rhegmatogenous retinal detachments due to complex breaks. Eur J Ophthalmol. 1997 Oct–Dec;7(4):322–6

Elavathil LJ, LeRiche J, Rootman J, Gallagher RP, Phillips D. Prognostic value of DNA ploidy as assessed with flow cytometry in uveal melanoma. Can J Ophthalmol. 1995; 30: 360–365

Eller AW, Friberg TR, Mah F. Migration of silicone oil into the brain: a complication of intraocular silicone oil for retinal tamponade. Am J Ophthalmol. 2000; 129: 685–688

Engerman, RL, Meyer, RK. Development of retinal vasculature in rats Am J Ophthalmol 1965; 60: 628–641

Escoffery RF, Olk RJ, Grand MG, Boniuk I. Vitrectomy without scleral buckling for primary rhegmatogenous retinal detachment. Am. J. Ophthalmol. 1985; 99:275–281

Ezra E, Fariss RN, Possin DE, Aylward WG, Gregor ZJ, Luthert PJ, Milam AH. Immunocytochemical characterization of macular hole opercula. Arch Ophthalmol. 2001; 119:223–231

Ezra E, Gregor ZJ; Morfields Macular Hole Study Group Report No. 1. Surgery for idiopathic full-thickness macular hole: two-year results of a randomized clinical trial comparing natural history, vitrectomy, and vitrectomy plus autologous serum: Moorfields Macular Hole Study Group Report no. 1. Arch Ophthalmol. 2004; 122: 224–236

Ezra E, Munro PMG, Charteris DG, et al. Macular hole opercula. Arch Ophthalmol 1997; 115: 1381–1387

Ezra E. Idiopathic full thickness macular hole: natural history and pathogenesis. Br J Ophthalmol. 2001; 85:102–128

Faude F, Reichenbach A, Wiedemann P. Zur Geschichte der Hypothese einer Mitwirkung der Müllerzellen bei der Entwicklung des idiopathischen Makulaforamens. Klin Monatsbl Augenheilkd. 2004; 221: 519–520

Faude F, Francke M, Makarov F, Schuck J, Gartner U, Reichelt W, Wiedemann P, Wolburg H, Reichenbach A. Experimental retinal detachment causes widespread and multilayered degeneration in rabbit retina. J Neurocytol. 2001; 30: 379–390

Faulborn J, Ardjomand N. Tractional retinoschisis in proliferative diabetic retinopathy: a histopathological study. Graefes Arch Clin Exp Ophthalmol. 2000; 238: 40–44

Faulborn J, Conway BP, Machemer R. Surgical complications of pars plana vitreous surgery. Ophthalmology, 1978; 85: 116–125

Feron EJ, Veckeneer M, Parys-Van Ginderdeuren R, Van Lommel A, Melles GRJ, Stalmans P. Trypan blue staining of epiretinal membranes in proliferative vitreoretinopathy. Arch Ophthalmol 2002; 120: 141–144

Ferry AP, Font RL. Carcinoma metastatic to the eye and orbit. I. A clinicopathologic study of 227 cases. Arch Ophthalmol. 1974; 92: 276–286

Fineberg E, Machemer R, Sullivan P, Norton EWD, Hamasaki D, Anderson D. Sulfur hexafluoride in owl monkey vitreous cavity. Am J Ophthalmol 1975; 79: 67–76

Finger PT, Berson A, Szechter A. Palladium-103 plaque radiotherapy for choroidal melanoma: results of a 7-year study. Ophthalmology. 1999; 106: 606–613

Finger PT. Radiation therapy for choroidal melanoma. Surv Ophthalmol. 1997; 42: 215–232

Flores Aquilar M, Munguia D, Loeb E, Crapotta JA, Vuong C, Shakiba S. Intraocular tolerance of Perfluoro-octylbromide (Perflubrom). Retina 1995; 15: 3–13

Flynn HW Jr, Chew EY, Simons BD, Barton FB, Remaley NA, Ferris FL 3rd. Pars plana vitrectomy in the Early Treatment Diabetic Retinopathy Study. ETDRS report number 17. The Early Treatment Diabetic Retinopathy Study Research Group. Ophthalmology. 1992; 99: 1351–1357

Folberg R, Mehaffey M, Gardner LM, Meyer M, Rummelt V, Pe'er J. The microcirculation of choroidal and ciliary body melanomas. Eye. 1997; 11 (Pt 2): 227–238

Folk JC, Arrindell EL and Klugman NR. The fellow eye of patients with phakic lattice retinal detachment. Ophthalmology 1989; 96: 72–79

Fong DS, Ferris FL 3rd, Davis MD, Chew EY. Causes of severe visual loss in the early treatment diabetic retinopathy study. ETDRS report number 24: Early Treatment Diabetic Retinopathy Study Research Group. Am J Ophthalmol 1999, 127: 137–141

Font RL, Croxatto JO, RAO NA. Armed Forces Institute of Pathology atlas of tumors of the eyes and ocular adnexa. Series 4 ed. Washington: AFIP Press, 2006. Pages 56–59

Font RL, Naumann GOH. Ocular histopathology of pulseless disease. Arch Ophthalmol 1969; 82: 784–788

Foos RY. Ultrastructural features of posterior vitreous detachment. Graefes Arch Clin Exp Ophthalmol 1974; 196: 103–111

Foos RY. Vitreous base, retinal tufts and retinal tears: Pathogenic relationships. In: Pruett RC, Regan CDJ (Eds): Retinal Congress. Chapter 20, New York, 1974, Apple-Century-Crofts, Page 259

Foos RY. Post oral peripheral retinal tears. Ann Ophthalmol 1974; 6: 679–689

Foos RY. Vitreoretinal juncture – simple epiretinal membranes. Graefes Arch Clin Exp Ophthalmol 1973; 189: 231–250

Foos RY. Zonular traction tufts of the peripheral retina in cadaver eyes. Arch Ophthalmol 1969; 82: 620–632

Foos RY, Allen RA. Retinal tears and lesser lesions of the peripheral retina in autopsy eyes. Am J Ophthalmol 1967; 64: 643–655

Foulks GN, Hatchell DL, Proia AD, Klintworth GK. Histopathology of silicone oil keratopathy in humans. Cornea. 1991; 10: 29–37

Foulds WS, Lee WR, Taylor WO. Clinical and pathological aspects of choroidal ischaemia. Trans Ophthalmol Soc U K. 1971;91:323–41

Frank RN, Amin RH, Eliott D, Puklin JE, Abrams GW. Basic fibroblast growth factor and vascular endothelial growth factor are present in epiretinal and choroidal neovascular membranes. Am J Ophthalmol. 1996; 122: 393–403

Francke M, Faude F, Pannicke T, Uckermann O, Weick M, Wolburg H, Wiedemann P, Reichenbach A, Uhlmann S, Bringmann A. Glial cell-mediated spread of retinal degeneration during detachment: a hypothesis based upon studies in rabbits. Vision Res. 2005; 45: 2256–2267

Fraser-Bell S, Guzowski M, Rotchina E, Wang JJ, Mitchell P. Five-year cumulative incidence and progression of epiretinal membranes. The Blue Mountains Eye Study. Ophthalmology 2003; 110: 34–40

Freeman WR, Azen SP, Kim JW, el-Haig W, Mishell DR 3rd, Bailey I. Vitrectomy for the treatment of full-thickness stage 3 or 4 macular holes. Results of a multicentered randomized clinical trial The Vitrectomy for Treatment of Macular Hole Study Group. Arch Ophthalmol. 1997; 115: 11–21

Freeman WR. Vitrectomy surgery for full-thickness macular holes. Am J Ophthalmol. 1993; 116: 233–235

Fruttiger M. Development of the mouse retinal vasculature: angiogenesis versus vasculogenesis. Invest Ophthalmol Vis Sci. 2002; 43: 522–557

Furino C, Micelli Ferrari T, Boscia F, Cardascia N, Recchimurzo N, Sborgia C. Triamcinolone-assisted pars plana vitrectomy for proliferative vitreoretinopathy. Retina 2003; 23: 771–776

Gabbiani G and Badonnel MC (1976) Contractile events during inflammation. Agents Actions 6: 277–280

Gallie BL, Budning A, DeBoer G, Thiessen JJ, Koren G, Verjee Z, Ling V, Chan HS. Chemotherapy with focal therapy can cure intraocular retinoblastoma without radiotherapy. Arch Ophthalmol. 1996; 114: 1321–1328

Gandorfer A, Rohleder M, Grosselfinger S, Haritoglou C, Ulbig M, Kampik A. Epiretinal pathology of diffuse diabetic macular edema associated with vitreomacular traction. Am J Ophthalmol. 2005; 139: 638–652

Gariano RF, Iruela-Arispe ML, Sage EH, Hendrickson AE. Immunohistochemical characterization of developing and mature primate retinal blood vessels. Invest Ophthalmol Vis Sci. 1996; 37: 93–103.

Gariano RF, Sage EH, Kaplan HJ, Hendrickson AE. Development of astrocytes and their relation to blood vessels in fetal monkey retina. Invest Ophthalmol Vis Sci. 1996; 37: 2367–2375

Gartry DS, Chignell AH, Franks WA, Wong D. Pars plana vitrectomy for the treatment of rhegmatogenous retinal detachment uncomplicated by advanced proliferative vitreoretinopathy. Br J Ophthalmol 1993; 77: 199–203

Gass JDM. Bullous retinal detachment. An unusual manifestation of idiopathic central serous choroidopathy. Am J Ophthalmol 1973; 75(5):810–21

Gass JDM. Muller cell cone, an overlooked part of the anatomy of the fovea centralis. Hypotheses concerning its role in the pathogenesis of macular hole and foveomacular retinoschisis. Arch Ophthalmol 1999; 117: 821–823

Gass JDM. Reappraisal of biomicroscopic classification of stages of development of a macular hole. Am J Ophthalmol 1995; 119: 752–759

Gass JD. Biomicroscopic and histopathologic considerations regarding the feasibility of surgical excision of subfoveal neovascular membranes. Am J Ophthalmol. 1994; 118: 285–298

Gass JDM. Idiopathic senile macular hole: its early stages and development. Arch Ophthalmol 1988; 106: 629–639

Gastaud P, Rouhette H, Negre F, Leguay JM, Dorafourg F. Place de la "vitrectomie exploratrice" dans le traitement du décollement de rétine sans prolifération vitréo-rétinienne. J Fr Ophtalmol 2000; 23: 482–487

George ND, Yates JR, Moore AT. Clinical features in affected males with X-linked retinoschisis. Arch Ophthalmol. 1996; 114:274–280

Gibran SK, Alwitry A, Cleary PE. Foveal detachment after successful retinal reattachment for macula on rhegmatogeneous retinal detachment: an ocular coherence tomography evaluation. Eye. 2005 Sep 30

Gieser AS, Murphy RP: Eales disease. Retina 1994; 2: 1503–1507

Girard P, Karpouzas I. Vitrectomie dans le traitement du décollement de rétine simplement. J Fr Ophtalmol 1995; 18: 188–193

Glazer LC, Maguire A, Blumenkranz MS, Trese MT, Green WR. Improved surgical treatment of familial exudative vitreoretinopathy in children. Am J Ophthalmol 1995; 120:471–479

Glaser BM, Michels RG, Kupperman BD, Sjaarda RN, Pena RA. The effects of pars plana vitrectomy and transforming growth factor-beta 2 for the treatment of full-thickness macular holes: a prospective randomized study. Ophthalmology 1992; 99: 1162–1173

Gloor B. Zur Entwicklung des Glaskörpers und der Zonula. V. Zur Entwicklung der Netzhautgefäße des Kaninchens. von Graefes Arch Clin Exp Ophthalmol 1973; 187: 147

Gloor B.P. Zur Entwicklung des Glaskörpers und der Zonula. I. Überblick und chronologischer Ablauf der Glaskörper- und Zonulaentwicklung bei Kaninchen und Maus. Graefes Arch Clin Exp Ophthalmol 1973; 186: 299

Goldberg MF. Retinal vaso-occlusion in sickling hemoglobinopathies. Birth Defects Orig Artic Ser 1976; 12(3):475–515. Review

Gonin J. Pathogenie et anatomie pathologique des decollemends retiniens. Bull Mem Soc d'Ophtalmol 1920; 33:1–8

Gow J, Oliver GL (1971) Familial exudative vitreoretinopathy: an expanded view. Arch Ophthalmol 86:150–155

Gragoudas ES, Seddon JM, Egan K, Glynn R, Munzenrider J, Austin-Seymour M, Goitein M, Verhey L, Urie M, Koehler A. Long-term results of proton beam irradiated uveal melanomas. Ophthalmology. 1987; 94: 349–353

Green RL, Byrne SF. Diagnostic ophthalmic ultrasound. Ryan SJ, et. Retina, et 2, St. Louis, 1994; Mosby

Grossniklaus HE, Martin DF, Avery R, Shields JA, Shields CL, Kuo IC, Green RL, Rao NA. Uveal lymphoid infiltration. Report of four cases and clinicopathologic review. Ophthalmology. 1998; 105(7): 1265–1273

Grossniklaus HE, Gass JD. Clinicopathologic correlations of surgically excised type 1 and type 2 submacular choroidal neovascular membranes. Am J Ophthalmol. 1998; 126: 59–69

Grossniklaus HE, Albert DM, Green WR, Conway BP, Hovland KR. Clear cell differentiation in choroidal melanoma. COMS report no. 8. Collaborative Ocular Melanoma Study Group. Arch Ophthalmol. 1997; 115: 894–898

Gunduz K, Shields JA, Shields CL, Eagle RC Jr, Diniz W, Mercado G, Chang W. Transscleral choroidal biopsy in the diagnosis of choroidal lymphoma. Surv Ophthalmol. 1999; 43: 551–555

Guyer DR, Green WR, de Bustros S, Fine SL. Histopathologic features of idiopathic macular holes and cysts. 1990. Retina. 2005; 25: 1045–1051

Guyer DR, Green WR, Schachat AP, Bastacky S, Miller NR. Bilateral ischemic optic neuropathy and retinal vascular occlusions associated with lymphoma and sepsis. Clinicopathologic correlation. Ophthalmology. 1990; 97: 882–888

Guyer DR, Green WR, de Bustros S, Fine SL. Histopathologic features of idiopathic macular holes and cysts. Ophthalmology. 1990; 97: 1045–1051

Hadden PW, Hiscott PS, Damato BE. Histopathology of eyes enucleated after endoresection of choroidal melanoma. Ophthalmology. 2004; 111: 154–160

Haimann MH, Burton TC, Brown CK. Epidemiology of retinal detachment. Arch Ophthalmol 1982; 100: 289–292

Hagimura N, Iida T, Suto K, Kishi S. Persistent foveal retinal detachment after successful rhegmatogenous retinal detachment surgery. Am J Ophthalmol. 2002; 133: 516–520

Hakin KN, Lavin MJ, Laever PK. Primary vitrectomy for rhegmatogenous retinal detachment. Graefes Arch Clin Exp Ophthalmol 1993; 231: 344–346

Halfter W, Dong S, Schurer B, Ring C, Cole GJ, Eller A. Embryonic synthesis of the inner limiting membrane and vitreous body. Invest Ophthalmol Vis Sci. 2005; 46: 2202–2209

Halfter W, Willem M, Mayer U. Basement membrane-dependent survival of retinal ganglion cells. Invest Ophthalmol Vis Sci 2005; 46: 1000–1009

Halfter W. Disruption of the retinal basal lamina during early embryonic development leads to a retraction of vitreal endfeet, and increased number of ganglion cells, and aberrant axon outgrowth. J Comp Neurol 1998; 397: 89–104

Haritoglou C, Gandorfer A, Gass CA, Kampik A. Histology of the vitreoretinal interface after staining of the internal limiting membrane using 5% diluted indocyanine and infracyanine green. Am J Ophthalmol 2004; 137: 345–348

Haritoglou C, Gandorfer A, Gass CA, Schaumberger M, Ulbig MW, Kampik A. Indocyanine green-assisted peeling of the internal limiting membrane in macular hole surgery affects visual outcome: a clinicopathologic correlation. Am J Ophthalmol. 2002; 134: 836–841

Heiligenhaus A, Bornfeld N, Wessing A. Longterm results of pars plana vitrectomy in the management of intermediate uveitis. Curr Opin Ophthalmol 1996; 7:77–79

Helbig H: Diabetische Traktionsablatio. Klin Monatsbl Augenheilkd 2002; 219: 186–190

Helbig H, Kellner U, Bornfeld N, Foerster MH: Vitrektomie bei diabetischer Retinopathie: Ergebnisse, Risikofaktoren, Komplikationen. Klin Monatsbl Augenheilkd 1998; 212: 339–342

Helbig H, Kellner U, Bornfeld N, Foerster MH: Rubeosis iridis after vitrectomy for diabetic retinopathy. Graefes Arch Clin Exp Ophthalmol 1998; 236: 730–733

Helbig H, Kellner U, Bornfeld N, Foerster MH: Grenzen und Möglichkeiten der Glaskörperchirurgie bei diabetischer Retinopathie 1996; 93: 647–654

Heimann H, Bornfeld N, Friedrichs W, Helbig H, Kellner U, Korra A, Foerster MH. Primary vitrectomy without scleral buckling for rhegmatogenous retinal detachment. Graefes Arch Clin Exp Ophthalmol 1996; 234: 561–568

Heimann H, Hellmich M, Bornfeld N, Bartz-Schmidt KU, Hilgers RD, Foerster MH. Scleral buckling versus primary vitrectomy in rhegmatogenous retinal detachment (SPR Study): design issues and implications. SPR Study report no. 1. Graefes Arch Clin Exp Ophthalmol 2001; 239:567–574

Hirata F, Yoshida M, Ogura Y. High glucose exacerbates neutrophil adhesion to human retinal endothelial cells. Exp Eye Res. 2005 Sep 29 online

Hirayama K, Hata Y, Noda Y, Miura M, Yamanaka I, Shimokawa H, Ishibashi T. The involvement of the rho-kinase pathway and its regulation in cytokine-induced collagen gel contraction by hyalocytes. Invest Ophthalmol Vis Sci. 2004; 45: 3896–3903

Hiscott P. Macrophages in the pathobiology of epiretinal membranes: multifunctional cells for a multistage process. Br J Ophthalmol 1993;77: 686–687

Ho AC, Guyer DR, Fine SL. Macular hole. Surv Ophthalmol. 1998;42: 393–416

Ho T, Smiddy WE, Flynn HWJ: Vitrectomy in the management of diabetic eye disease. Surv Ophthalmol 1992; 37: 190–202

Hoerauf H, Müller M, Laqua H. Mouches volantes und Vitrektomie bei vollem Visus? Ophthalmologe. 2003; 100: 639–643

Hoerauf H, Roider J, Herboth T, Hager A, Laqua H. Ergebnisse der Vitrektomie bei rhegmatogener Amotio und dichten Glaskörpertrübungen. Klin. Monatsbl. Augenheilkd. 1997; 211:369–374

Hofman P, van Blijswijk BC, Gaillard PJ, Vrensen GF, Schlingemann RO. Endothelial cell hypertrophy induced by vascular endothelial growth factor in the retina: new insights into the pathogenesis of capillary nonperfusion. Arch Ophthalmol. 2001; 119: 861–866

Hogan MJ, Alvarado JA, Weddell JE. Histology of the human eye. An atlas and textbook. Philadelphia: WB Saunders, 1971; 492–497

Hogan MJ, Alvarado JA, Weddell JE (eds): Histology of the human eye. Philadelphia: WB Saunders, CA; 1971, p 607–637

Hogan MJ, Alvarado JA, Weddell J.E. Retina. In: Histology of the Human Eye, W.B. Saunders Company 1971, pp. 393–522

Hoing C, Heidenkummer HP and Kampik A. Primäre Vitrektomie bei der rhegmatogenen Netzhautablösung. Ophthalmologe 1995; 92:668–671

Hoing C, Kampik A, Heidenkummer HP. Pars plana Vitrektomie mit intraokularer SF6 Tamponade bei komplizierter Netzhautablösung. Ophthalmologe 1994; 91:312–318

Hollenberg MJ, Spira AW. Human retinal development: ultrastructure of the outer retina. Am J Anat. 1973; 137: 357–385

Holey GP, Alam A, Kiri A, Edelhauser HF. Effect of indocyanine green intraocular stain on human and rabbit corneal endothelial structure and viability. An in vitro study. J Cat Refr Surg 2002; 28: 1027–1033

Hope-Ross M, Yannuzzi LA, Gragoudas ES, Guyer DR, Slakter JS, Sorenson JA, Krupsky S, Orlock DA, Puliafito CA. Adverse reactions due to indocyanine green. Ophthalmology. 1994; 101: 529–533

Horiguchi M, Miyake K, Ohta IN, Ito Y. Staining of the lens capsule for circular continuous capsulorrhexis in eyes with white cataracts. Arch Ophthalmol 1998; 116: 535–537

Hovlang KR. Vitreous findings in fellow eyes of aphakic retinal detachment. Am J Ophthalmol 1978; 86: 350–353

Hudson HL, Frambach DA, Lopez PF. Relation of the functional and structural fundus changes after submacular surgery for neovascular age-related macular degeneration. Br J Ophthalmol. 1995; 79: 417–423

Hughes S, Yang H, Chan-Ling T. Vascularization of the human fetal retina: roles of vasculogenesis and angiogenesis. Invest Ophthalmol Vis Sci 2000; 41: 1217–1228

Hui YN, Goodnight R, Zhang XJ, Sorgente N, Ryan SJ. Glial epiretinal membranes and contraction. Immunohistochemical and morphological studies. Arch Ophthalmol. 1988; 106: 1280–1285

Hung JY, Hilton GF. Neovascular glaucoma in a patient with X-linked juvenile retinoschisis. Ann Ophthalmol. 1980; 12: 1054–1055

Hutton WL, Pesicka GA, Fuller DG. Cataract extraction in the diabetic eye after vitrectomy. Am J Ophthalmol 1987; 104: 1–4

Imperia PS, Lazarus HM, Lass JH. Ocular complications of systemic cancer chemotherapy. Surv Ophthalmol. 1989; 34: 209–230

Ishida S, Yamazaki K, Shinoda K, Kawashima S, Oguchi Y. Macular hole retinal detachment in highly myopic eyes: ultrastructure of surgically removed epiretinal membrane and clinicopathologic correlation. Retina. 2000; 20: 176–183

Ito Y, Berkowitz BA. MR studies of retinal oxygenation. Vision Res. 2001; 41: 1307–1311

Jaffe ES, Sander CA, Flaig MJ. Cutaneous lymphomas: a proposal for a unified approach to classification using the R.E.A.L./WHO Classification. Ann Oncol. 2000; 11: 17–21

Jakobiec FA, Sacks E, Kronish JW, Weiss T, Smith M. Multifocal static creamy choroidal infiltrates. An early sign of lymphoid neoplasia. Ophthalmology. 1987; 94: 397–406

James M, Fenman SS. Macular holes. Graefes Arch Klin Exp Ophthalmol 1980; 215: 59–63

Jampol LM, Moy CS, Murray TG, Reynolds SM, Albert DM, Schachat AP, Diddie KR, Engstrom RE Jr, Finger PT, Hovland KR, Joffe L, Olsen KR, Wells CG; Collaborative Ocular Melanoma Study Group (COMS Group). The COMS randomized trial of iodine 125 brachytherapy for choroidal melanoma: IV. Local treatment failure and enucleation in the first 5 years after brachytherapy. COMS report no. 19. Ophthalmology. 2002;109: 2197–206

Jensen OA. Malignant melanomas of the human uvea: 25-year follow-up of cases in Denmark, 1943–1952. Acta Ophthalmol (Copenh). 1982; 60: 161–182

Jiang B, Bezhadian MA, Caldwell RB. Astrocytes modulate retinal vasculogenesis: effects on endothelial cell differentiation Glia 1995; 15: 1–10

Johnson RN, Gass JDM. Idiopathic macular holes. Observations, stages of formation and implications for surgical intervention. Ophthalmology 1988; 95: 917–924

Jonas JB, Schneider U, Naumann GOH. Count and density of human retinal photoreceptors. Graefes Archiv Clin Exp Ophthalmol 1992; 230: 505–519

Joussen AM, Heussen FMA, Joeres S, Llacer H, Prinz B, Rohrschneider K, Maaijwee KJM, van Meurs J, Kirchhof B. Autologous translocation of the choroid and RPE in age related macular degeneration. Am J Ophthalmol 2006; Jul;142(1):17–30

Joussen AM, Poulaki V, Le ML, Koizumi K, Esser C, Janicki H, Schraermeyer U, Kociok N, Fauser S, Kirchhof B, Kern TS, Adamis AP. A central role for inflammation in the pathogenesis of diabetic retinopathy. FASEB J. 2004; 18: 1450–1452

Joussen AM, Poulaki V, Mitsiades N, Cai WY, Suzuma I, Pak J, Ju ST, Rook SL, Esser P, Mitsiades CS, Kirchhof B, Adamis AP, Aiello LP. Suppression of Fas-FasL-induced endothelial cell apoptosis prevents diabetic blood-retinal barrier breakdown in a model of streptozotocin-induced diabetes. FASEB J. 2003; 17: 76–78

Joussen AM, Walter P, Jonescu-Cuypers CP, Koizumi K, Poulaki V, Bartz-Schmidt KU, Krieglstein GK and Kirchhof B (2003) Retinectomy for treatment of intractable glaucoma: long term results. Br J Ophthalmol 87: 1094–1102

Joussen AM, Poulaki V, Qin W, Kirchhof B, Mitsiades N, Wiegand SJ, Rudge J, Yancopoulos GD, Adamis AP. Retinal vascular endothelial growth factor induces intercellular adhesion molecule-1 and endothelial nitric oxide synthase expression and initiates early diabetic retinal leukocyte adhesion in vivo. Am J Pathol 2002; 160: 501–509

Joussen AM, Murata T, Tsujikawa A, Kirchhof B, Bursell SE, Adamis AP. Leukocyte-mediated endothelial cell injury and death in the diabetic retina. Am J Pathol. 2001; 158: 147–152

Joussen AM, Joeres S, Fawzy N, Heussen FM, Llacer H, van Meurs JC, Kirchhof B. Autologous translocation of the choroid and retinal pigment epithelium in patients with geographic atrophy. Ophthalmology. 2007 Mar;114(3):551–60

Jurklies B, Anastassiou G, Ortmans S, Schuler A, Schilling H, Schmidt-Erfurth U, Bornfeld N. Photodynamic therapy using verteporfin in circumscribed choroidal haemangioma. Br J Ophthalmol. 2003; 87: 84–89

Kadonoso K, Itoh N, Uchio E, Makamura S, Ohno S. Staining of internal limiting membrane in macular hole surgery. Arch Ophthalmol 2000; 118: 1116–1118

Karel I, Michalickova M and Kuthan P (1997) [Long-term results of pars plana vitrectomy and silicone oil in large retinal tears in children]. Cesk Slov Oftalmol 53: 147–154

Kelly NE, Wendel RT. Vitreous surgery for idiopathic macular holes: results of a pilot study. Arch Ophthalmol 1991; 190: 654–659

Khalil MK. Balloon cell malignant melanoma of the choroid: ultrastructural studies. Br J Ophthalmol. 1983; 67: 579–584

Khawly JA, Lambert RJ, Jaffe GJ. Intraocular lens changes after short- and long-term exposure to intraocular silicone oil. An in vivo study. Ophthalmology. 1998; 105: 1227–1233

Kim JW, Freeman WR, Azen SP, el-Haig W, Klein DJ, Bailey IL. Prospective randomized trial of vitrectomy or observation for stage 2 macular holes. Vitrectomy for Macular Hole Study Group. Am J Ophthalmol. 1996; 121: 605–614

Kimura H, Kuroda S, Nagata M. Triamcinolone acetonide-assisted peeling of the internal limiting membrane. Am J Ophthalmol 2004; 137: 172–173

Kindy-Degnan NA, Char DH, Castro JR, Kroll S, Stone RD, Quivey JM, Phillips TL, Irvine AR. Effect of various doses of radiation for uveal melanoma on regression, visual acuity, complications, and survival. Am J Ophthalmol. 1989; 107: 114–120

Kirchhof B, Tavakolian U, Paulmann H, Heimann K. Histopathological findings in eyes after silicone oil injection. Graefes Arch Clin Exp Ophthalmol. 1986; 224: 34–37

Kishi S, Shimizi K: Posterior precortical vitreous pocket. Arch Ophthalmol 1990; 108: 979–982

Kivela T. Trilateral retinoblastoma: a meta-analysis of hereditary retinoblastoma associated with primary ectopic intracranial retinoblastoma. J Clin Oncol. 1999; 17(6): 1829–1837

Klöti R. Amotio-Chirurgie ohne Skleraeindellung. Primäre Vitrektomie. Klin Monatsbl Augenheilkd 1983; 182, 474–478

Knorr HL, Seltsam A, Holbach L, Naumann GO. [Intraocular silicone oil tamponade. A clinico-pathologic study of 36 enucleated eyes]. Ophthalmologe. 1996 Apr;93(2):130–8

Kociok N, Gavranic C, Kirchhof B, Joussen AM. Influence on membrane-mediated cell activation by vesicles of silicone oil or perfluorohexyloctane. Graefes Arch Clin Exp Ophthalmol. 2005; 243: 345–358

Kohno T, Sorgente N, Ishibashi T, Goodnight R, Ryan SJ. Immunofluorescent studies of fibronectin and laminin in the human eye. Invest Ophthalmol Vis Sci. 1987; 28: 506–514

Kokame GT, de Bustros S, The Vitrectomy for Prevention of Macular Hole Study Group. Visual acuity as a prognostic indicator in stage 1 macular holes. Am J Ophthalmol 1995; 119: 112–114

Koniszewski G, Lang GK, Naumann GOH, Knorr HLJ. Prophylaktische YAG-Iridotomie zur Vermeidung des sekundären Winkelblock-Glaukoms nach Pars-Plana-Vitrektomie und Silikon in phaken Augen. Fortschr Ophthalmol 1988; 85: 462–463

Küchle M, Nguyen NX, Naumann GOH. Aqueous flare in eyes with choroidal malignant melanoma. Am J Ophthalmol 1992; 113: 207–208

Kurihara T, Noda K, Ishida S, Inoue M. Pars plana vitrectomy with internal limiting membrane removal for macular hole associated with proliferative diabetic retinopathy. Graefes Arch Clin Exp Ophthalmol. 2005; 243: 724–726

Kwok AK, Lai TY, Yuen KS, Tam BS, Wong VW. Macular hole surgery with or without indocyanine green stained internal limiting membrane peeling. Clin Exp Ophthalmol 2003; 31: 470–475

Lafaut BA, Aisenbrey S, Van den Broecke C, Bartz-Schmidt KU, Heimann K. Polypoidal choroidal vasculopathy pattern in age-related macular degeneration: a clinicopathologic correlation. Retina. 2000; 20: 650–654

La Heij EC, Tecim S, Kessels AG, Liem AT, Japing WJ, Hendrikse F: Clinical variables and their relation to visual outcome after vitrectomy in eyes with diabetic retinal traction detachment. Graefes Arch Clin Exp Ophthalmol 2004; 242(3): 210–217.

Lai JC, Stinnett SS, McCuen BW. Comparison of silicone oil versus gas tamponade in the treatment of idiopathic full-thickness macular hole. Ophthalmology. 2003; 110: 1170–1174

Lambert HM, Capone AJ, Aaberg TM, Strenberg PJ, Mandell BA, Lopez PF. Surgical excision of subfoveal neovascular membranes in age-related macular degeneration. Am J Ophthalmol. 1992; 113: 257–262

Lang GE: Differential diagnosis vitreoretin. Klin Monatsbl Augenheilkde 1990

Lang GK, FJ Daumann: The Peripheral Retina and Choroid in Healthy Eyes (3125 Airplane Pilots). Klin. Mbl. Augenheilk. 181 (1982) 493–495

Lang GE, B Laudi, RA Pfeiffer: Autosomal dominant vitreoretinal dystrophy with skeletal dysplasia in one generation. Klin. Mbl. Augenhk. 198 (1991) 207–214

Lang GE, Lang GK, Naumann GOH. Akzidentelle bilaterale asymmetrische Rubin-Laser-Makulopathie. Klin Monatsbl Augenheilkd 1985; 186:366–370

Lang GE, Maumanee I. KMO

Lang Glaskörper, Daumann FJ. Periphere Fundusveränderungen bei "Augengesunden" (Piloten). Klin Monatsbl Augenheilkd 1982; 181: 493–495

Lansing MB, Glaser BM, Liss H, et al. The effect of pars plana vitrectomy and transforming growth factor-beta 2 without epiretinal membrane peeling on full-thickness macular holes. Ophthalmology 1993; 100: 868–871

Lappas A, Foerster AM, Weinberger AW, Coburger S, Schrage NF, Kirchhof B. Translocation of iris pigment epithelium in patients with exudative age-related macular degeneration: long-term results. Graefes Arch Clin Exp Ophthalmol. 2004; 242: 638–647

Lappas A, Weinberger AWA, Foerster AMH, Kube Th, Kirchhof B. Iris pigment epithelium translocation in age related macular degeneration, Graefes Arch Exp Clin Ophthalmol. 2000; 238: 631–641

Laqua H (1980) Familial exudative vitreoretinopathy. Graefes Arch Clin Exp Ophthalmol 213:121–133

Lee WR (Ed.), Ophthalmic histopathology, Chapter 7: Treatment of retinal detachment, Springer Heidelberg 2002; p 217–235

Lemor M, Yeo JH and Glaser BM (1986) Oral colchicine for the treatment of experimental traction retinal detachment. Arch Ophthalmol 104: 1226–1229

Lewis GP, Fisher SK. Muller cell outgrowth after retinal detachment: association with cone photoreceptors. Invest Ophthalmol Vis Sci. 2000; 41(6): 1542–1545

Lewis GP, Matsumoto B, Fisher SK. Changes in the organization and expression of cytoskeletal proteins during retinal degeneration induced by retinal detachment. Invest Ophthalmol Vis Sci. 1995; 36: 2404–2416

Lewis H. Peripheral retinal degenerations and the risk of retinal detachment. Am J Ophthalmol. 2003; 136: 155–160

Lewis H, Cowan GM, Straatsma BR. Apparent disappearance of a macular hole associated with development of an epiretinal membrane. Am J Ophthalmol. 1986; 102: 172–175

Li K, Wong D, Hiscott P, Stanga P, Groenwald C, McGalliard J. Trypan blue staining of the internal limiting membrane and epiretinal membrane during vitrectomy: visual results and histopathological findings. Br J Ophthalmol 2003; 87: 216–219

Ling TL, Mitrofanis J, Stone J. Origin of retinal astrocytes in the rat: evidence from migration from the optic nerve J Comp Neurol 1989; 286: 345–352

Loeffler KU, Lee WR. Terminology of sub-RPE deposits: do we

all speak the same language? Br J Ophthalmol. 1998; 82: 1104–1105

Logani S, Cho AS, Ali BH, Withers HR, McBride WH, Kozlov KL, Hall MO, Lee DA, Straatsma BR. Single-dose compared with fractionated-dose radiation of the OM431 choroidal melanoma cell line. Am J Ophthalmol. 1995; 120: 506–510

Lohmann DR, Gallie BL. Retinoblastoma: revisiting the model prototype of inherited cancer. Am J Med Genet C Semin Med Genet. 2004 Aug 15;129(1):23–8. Review

Lommatzsch PK. Results after beta-irradiation (106Ru/106Rh) of choroidal melanomas: 20 years experience. Br J Ophthalmol 1986; 70: 844–851

Longaker MT, Chiu ES, Harrison MR, Crombleholme TM, Langer JC, Duncan BW, Adzick NS, Verrier ED and Stern R (1989) Studies in fetal wound healing. IV. Hyaluronic acid-stimulating activity distinguishes fetal wound fluid from adult wound fluid. Ann Surg 210: 667–672

Luke C, Luke M, Dietlein TS, Hueber A, Jordan J, Sickel W, Kirchhof B. Retinal tolerance to dyes. Br J Ophthalmol. 2005; 89: 1188–1191

Luthert PJ, Chong NH. Photoreceptor rescue. Eye 1998; 12: 591–596

Machemer R, Sugita G and Tano Y. Treatment of intraocular proliferations with intravitreal steroids. Trans Am Ophthalmol 1979; Soc 77: 171–180

Machemer R (1968) Experimental retinal detachment in the owl monkey. II. Histology of retina and pigment epithelium. Am J Ophthalmol 66: 396–410.

Machemer R. Experimental retinal detachment in the owl monkey. IV. The reattached retina. Am J Ophthalmol 1968; 66: 1075–1091

Madreperla SA, McCuen BW II, Hickingbotham D, et al. Clinicopathologic correlation of surgically removed macular hole opercula. Am J Ophthalmol 1995; 120: 197–207

Mäkitie T, Summanen P, Tarkkanen A, Kivelä T. Microvascular density in predicting survival of patients with choroidal and ciliary body melanoma. Invest Ophthalmol Vis Sci 1999; 40:2471–2480

Mäkitie T, Summanen P, Tarkkanen A, Kivelä T. Microvascular loops and networks as prognostic indicators in choroidal and ciliary body melanomas. J Natl Cancer Inst 1999; 91:359–367

Mäkitie T, Summanen P, Tarkkanen A, Kivelä T. Tumor-infiltrating macrophages (CD68(+) cells) and prognosis in malignant uveal melanoma. Invest Ophthalmol Vis Sci 2001; 42:1414–1421

Manschot WA, Van Peperzeel HA. Uveal melanoma: location, size, cell type, and enucleation as risk factors in metastasis. Hum Pathol. 1982; 13: 1147–1148

Marcus DM, Craft JL, Albert DM. Histopathologic verification of Verhoeff's 1918 irradiation cure of retinoblastoma. Ophthalmology. 1990; 97: 221–224

Margherio RR, Cox MS Jr, Trese MT, Murphy PL, Johnson J, Minor LA. Removal of epimacular membranes. Ophthalmology. 1985; 92: 1075–1083

Marmor MF. Control of subretinal fluid: experimental and clinical studies. Eye. 1990; 4 (Pt 2): 340–344

Martegiani F: Novae Observationes de oculo humano, Neapoli: Typis Cajetani Eboli 1814; pp 16–24

Martin DF, Chan CC, de Smet MD, Palestine AG, Davis JL, Whitcup SM, Burnier MN Jr, Nussenblatt RB. The role of chorioretinal biopsy in the management of posterior uveitis. Ophthalmology. 1993;100: 705–714

Matsumura N, Ikuno Y, Tano Y. Posterior vitreous detachment and macular hole formation in myopic foveoschisis. Am J Ophthalmol. 2004; 138: 1071–1073

Mazzuca DE, Benson WE. Central serous retinopathy: variants. Surv Ophthalmol. 1986; 31:170–174

McDermott HR, Puklin JE, Abrams GW, Eliott D: Phacoemulsification for cataract following pars plana vitrectomy. Ophthalmic Surg Lasers 1997; 28: 558–564

McDonnell PJ, Fine SL, Hillis AI. Clinical features of idiopathic macular cysts and holes. Am J Ophthalmol 1982; 93: 777–786

McLean IW, Foster WD, Zimmerman LE. Uveal melanoma: location, size, cell type, and enucleation as risk factors in metastasis. Hum Pathol. 1982; 13: 123–132

McLean IW, Foster WD, Zimmerman LE, Gamel JW. Modifications of Callender's classification of uveal melanoma of the Armed Forces Institute of Pathology. Am J Ophthalmol 1983; 96:502–509

McLean IW, Keefe KS, Burnier MN. Uveal melanoma. Comparison of the prognostic value of fibrovascular loops, mean of the ten largest nucleoli, cell type, and tumor size. Ophthalmology. 1997; 104: 777–780

McLean IW, Zimmerman LE, Evans RM. Reappraisal of Callender's spindle a type of malignant melanoma of choroid and ciliary body. Am J Ophthalmol 1978; 86:557–564

McLeod DS, Merges C, Fukushima A, Goldberg MF, Lutty GA. Histopathologic features of neovascularization in sickle cell retinopathy. Am J Ophthalmol. 1997 Oct; 124: 455–472

McPherson A, O'Malley R and Beltangady SS. Management of the fellow eyes of patients with rhegmatogenous retinal detachment. Ophthalmology 1981; 88: 922–934

McPherson A. (ed.) "New and Controversial Aspects of Retinal Detachment", Hoeber Pub. New York, 1968

Meinert H, Knoblich A. The use of semifluorinated alkanes in blood-substitutes. Biomater Artif Cells Immobilization Biotechnol. 1993; 21: 583–595

Meredith JE Jr, Fazeli B, Schwartz MA. The extracellular matrix as a cell survival factor. Mol Biol Cell 1993; 4: 953–961

Messmer EM, Heidenkummer HP, Kampik A. Ultrastructure of epiretinal membranes associated with macular holes. Graefes Arch Clin Exp Ophthalmol. 1998; 236: 248–254

Messmer EP, Font RL, Kirkpatrick JB, Hopping W. Immunohistochemical demonstration of neuronal and astrocytic differentiation in retinoblastoma. Ophthalmology. 1985; 92: 167–173

Messmer EP, Laqua H, Wessing A et al. Nine cases of cavernous hemangioma of the retina. Am J Ophthalmol 1983; 95: 383–390

Messmer EP, Font RL, Laqua H, Höppng W, Naumann GOH. Cavernous hemangioma of the retina. Immunohistochemical and ultrastructural observations. Arch Ophthalmol 1984; 102: 413–418

Meyer-Schwickerath G, Lund OE, Wessing A, von Barsewisch B. Classification and terminology of ophthalmological changes in the retinal periphery. Mod Probl Ophthalmol 1975; 15: 50–52

Michaelides M, Luthert PJ, Cooling R, Firth H, Moore AT. Norrie disease and peripheral venous insufficiency. Br J Ophthalmol. 2004; 88: 1475

Michels RG. Vitrectomy for macular pucker. Ophthalmology 1984; 91: 1364–1388

Michels RG. A clinical and histopathological study of epiretinal membranes affecting the macula and removed by vitreous surgery. Trans Am Ophthalmol Soc 1982; 80: 580–656

Michels S, Michels R, Simader C, Schmidt-Erfurth U. Verteporfin therapy for choroidal hemangioma: a long-term follow-up. Retina. 2005; 25: 697–703

Mieler WF, Will BR, Lewis H, Aaberg TM. Vitrectomy in the management of peripheral uveitis. Ophthalmology 1988; 95: 859–864

Miki D, Hida T, Hotta K, Shinoda K, Hirakata A. Comparison of scleral buckling and vitrectomy for retinal detachment resulting from flap tears in superior quadrants. Jpn J Ophthalmol 2001; 45:187–191

Miyamoto K, Khosrof S, Bursell SE, Rohan R, Murata T, Clermont AC, Aiello LP, Ogura Y, Adamis AP. Prevention of leukostasis and vascular leakage in streptozotocin-induced diabetic retinopathy via intercellular adhesion molecule-1 inhibition. Proc Natl Acad Sci U S A. 1999; 96: 10836–10841

Miyamoto K, Refolo MF, Tolentino FI, Fournier GA, Albert DM. Perfluoroether liquid as a long-term vitreous substitute. An experimental study. Retina 1984; 4: 264–268

Montero JA, Ruiz-Moreno JM. Optical coherence tomography characterisation of idiopathic central serous chorioretinopathy. Br J Ophthalmol. 2005; 89:562–564

Mooy CM, De Jong PT. Prognostic parameters in uveal melanoma: a review. Surv Ophthalmol. 1996; 41: 215–228

Morino I, Hiscott P, McKechnie N, Grierson I. Variation in epiretinal membrane components with clinical duration of the proliferative tissue. Br J Ophthalmol. 1990; 74: 393–399

Murakami-Nagasako F, Ohba N. Phakic retinal detachment associated with cystic retinal tuft. Graefes Arch Clin Exp Ophthalmol. 1982; 219:188–192

Murphree AL, Villablanca JG, Deegan WF 3rd, Sato JK, Malogolowkin M, Fisher A, Parker R, Reed E, Gomer CJ. Chemotherapy plus local treatment in the management of intraocular retinoblastoma. Arch Ophthalmol. 1996; 114; 1348–1356

Nahib, M, Peyman GA, Clark LC, Hoffmann RE, Miceli M, Abou-Steit M. Experimental evaluation of perfluoro-phenanthrene as a high specific gravity vitreous substitute: a preliminary report. Ophthalmic Surg 1989; 20: 289–293

Nahum MP, Gdal-On M, Kuten A, Herzl G, Horovitz Y, Weyl Ben Arush M. Long-term follow-up of children with retinoblastoma. Pediatr Hematol Oncol. 2001; 18: 173–179

Nakamura K, Refojo MF, Crabtree DV. Factors contributing to the emulsification of intraocular silicone and fluorosilicone oils. Invest Ophthalmol Vis Sci. 1990; 31: 647–656

Nathwani BN, Kim H, Rappaport H, Solomon J, Fox M. Non-Hodgkin's lymphomas: a clinicopathologic study comparing two classifications. Cancer. 1978; 41: 303–325

Naumann G, Hellner KA, Naumann LR. Pigmented Nevi of the Choroid. Clinical Study of Secondary Changes in the Overlying Tissue. Trans Am Acad Ophthalmol 1971; 75: 110–123

Naumann G, Yanoff M, Zimmerman LE. Histogenesis of Malignant Melanomas of the Uvea. I. Histopathologic Characteristics of Nevi of the Choroid and Ciliary Body. Arch Ophthalmol 1966; 76: 784–796

Naumann GOH, Seibel, W. Surgical Revision of Vitreous and Iris-Incarceration in Persisting Cystoid Maculopathy (Hruby-Irvine-Gass Syndrome) – report on 27 eyes. Dev Ophthalmol 1985; 11: 181–187

Naumann GOH and Völcker HE. Endophthalmitis haemogranulomatosa (eine spezielle Reaktion auf intraokulare Blutungen). Klin Mbl Augenheilkd 1977; 171: 352–359

Newman DK, Burton RL. Primary vitrectomy for pseudophakic and aphakic retinal detachments. Eye 1999; 13 (Pt 5):635–639

Newman E, Reichenbach A. The Muller cell: a functional element of the retina. Trends Neurosci. 1996; 19: 307–312

Nicholson DH, Galvis V (1984) Criswick-Schepens syndromes (familial exudative vitreoretinopathy): a study of a Colombian kindred. Arch Ophthalmol 102:1519–1522

Ninomiya Y, Lewis JM, Hasegawa T, Tanoi Y. Retinotomy and foveal translocation for surgical management of subfoveal choroidal neovascular membranes. Am J Ophthalmol. 1996; 122: 613–621

Noda Y, Hata Y, Hisatomi T, Nakamura Y, Hirayama K, Miura M, Nakao S, Fujisawa K, Sakamoto T, Ishibashi T. Functional properties of hyalocytes under PDGF-rich conditions. Invest Ophthalmol Vis Sci. 2004; 45: 2107–2114

Nork TM, Millecchia LL, de Venecia GB, Myers FL, Vogel KA. Immunocytochemical features of retinoblastoma in an adult. Arch Ophthalmol. 1996; 114: 1402–1406

Nork TM, Millecchia LL, Strickland BD, Linberg JV, Chao GM. Selective loss of blue cones and rods in human retinal detachment. Arch Ophthalmol. 1995; 113: 1066–1073

Nork TM, Wallow IH, Sramek SJ, Stevens TS, De Venecia G. Immunocytochemical study of an eye with proliferative vitreoretinopathy and retinal tacks. Retina. 1990; 10: 78–85

Norton EWD, Fuller DG. The use of intraocular sulphur hexafluoride in vitrectomy. In Irvine AR, O'Malley C eds.: Advances in vitreous surgery, Springfield, III, 1976; Charles C Thomas Lecture

Novak MA, Rice TA, Michels RG, Auer C. The crystalline lens after vitrectomy for diabetic retinopathy. Ophthalmology. 1984; 91: 1480–1484

Noyes HD. Detachment of the macula with laceration of the macula lutea. Trans Am Ophthalmol Soc 1971; 1:128–134

Ohlmann A, Scholz M, Goldwich A, Chauhan BK, Hudl K, Ohlmann AV, Zrenner E, Berger W, Cvekl A, Seeliger MW, Tamm ER. Ectopic norrin induces growth of ocular capillaries and restores normal retinal angiogenesis in Norrie disease mutant mice. J Neurosci. 2005; 25:1701–1710

Ohira A, de Juan E Jr. Characterization of glial involvement in proliferative diabetic retinopathy. Ophthalmologica. 1990; 201: 187–195

Ohlmann AV, Adamek E, Ohlmann A, Lutjen-Drecoll E. Norrie gene product is necessary for regression of hyaloid vessels. Invest Ophthalmol Vis Sci. 2004; 45: 2384–2390

Oldendoerp J, Spitznas M: Factors influencing the results of vitreous surgery in diabetic retinopathy. I. Iris rubeosis and/or active neovascularization at the fundus. Graefes Arch Clin Exp Ophthalmol 1989; 227: 1–8

O'Malley PF, Allen RA. Peripheral cystoid degeneration of the retina. Incidence and distribution in 1,000 autopsy eyes. Arch Ophthalmol. 1967; 77: 769–776

Oosterhuis JA, Journee-de Korver HG, Keunen JE. Transpupillary thermotherapy: results in 50 patients with choroidal melanoma. Arch Ophthalmol. 1998; 116: 157–162

Orrellana J, Lieberman RM. Stage III macular hole surgery. Br J Ophthalmol 1993; 77: 555–558

Oshima Y, Emi K, Motokura M, Yamanishi S. Survey of surgical indications and results of primary pars plana vitrectomy for rhegmatogenous retinal detachments. Jpn J Ophthalmol 1999; 43:120–126.

Oshima Y, Emi K, Motokura M, Yamanishi S. [A comparative study of visual outcomes following primary vitrectomy and scleral buckling procedures to manage macular off rhegmatogenous retinal detachments]. Nippon Ganka Gakkai Zasshi 1999; 103:215–222

Paques M, Chastang C, Mathis A, Sahel J, Massin P, Dosquet C, Korobelnik JF, Le Gargasson JF, Gaudric A. Effect of autologous platelet concentrate in surgery for idiopathic macular hole: results of a multicenter, double-masked, randomized trial. Platelets in Macular Hole Surgery Group. Ophthalmology. 1999; 106: 932–938

Park DW, Dugel PU, Garda J, Sipperley JO, Thach A, Sneed SR, Blaisdell J. Macular pucker removal with and without internal limiting membrane peeling: pilot study. Ophthalmology. 2003; 110: 62–64

Pearlstone AD. The incidence of idiopathic preretinal macular gliosis. Am Ophthalmol 1985; 17: 378–380

Pearson R, Jagger J. Sex linked juvenile retinoschisis with optic disc and peripheral retinal neovascularisation. Br J Ophthalmol. 1989; 73: 311–313

Pe'er J, Neufeld M, Baras M, Gnessin H, Itin A, Keshet E. Rubeosis iridis in retinoblastoma. Histologic findings and the possible role of vascular endothelial growth factor in its induction. Ophthalmology. 1997; 104: 1251–1258

Perentes E, Herbort CP, Rubinstein LJ, Herman MM, Uffer S, Donoso LA, Collins VP. Immunohistochemical characterization of human retinoblastomas in situ with multiple markers. Am J Ophthalmol. 1987; 103: 647–658

Perrier M, Sebag M. Epiretinal membrane surgery assisted by trypan blue. Am J Ophthalmol 2003; 135: 909–911

Pesin SR, Shields JA. Seven cases of trilateral retinoblastoma. Am J Ophthalmol. 1989; 107: 121–126

Peyman GA, Blinder KJ, Paris CJ, Alturki W, Nelson NC, Desai U. A technique for retinal pigment epithelium transplantation for age-related macular degeneration secondary to extensive subfoveal scarring. Ophthalmic Surg. 1991; 22: 102

Peyman GA, Cheema R, Conway MD, Fang T. Triamcinolone acetonide as an aid to visualization of the vitreous and the posterior hyaloid during pars plana vitrectomy. Retina 2000; 20: 554–555

Piccolino FC, de la Longrais RR, Ravera G, Eandi CM, Ventre L, Abdollahi A, Manea M. The foveal photoreceptor layer and visual acuity loss in central serous chorioretinopathy. Am J Ophthalmol. 2005; 139: 87–99

Potter MJ, Myckatyn SO, Maberley AL, Lee AS. Vitrectomy for pars planitis complicated by vitreous hemorrhage: visual outcome and long-term follow-up. Am J Ophthalmol, 2001; 131: 514–515

Poulaki V, Qin W, Joussen AM, Hurlbut P, Wiegand SJ, Rudge J, Yancopoulos GD, Adamis AP. Acute intensive insulin therapy exacerbates diabetic blood-retinal barrier breakdown via hypoxia-inducible factor-1alpha and VEGF. J Clin Invest. 2002; 109: 805–815

Pournaras CJ, Donati G, Sekkat L, Kapetanios AD. Décollement de rétine du pseudophake. Traitement par vitrectomie et cerclage. Étude pilote. J. Fr. Ophtalmol. 2000; 23:1006–1011

Prescher G, Bornfeld N, Becher R. Nonrandom chromosomal abnormalities in primary uveal melanoma. J Natl Cancer Inst. 1990; 82: 1765–1769

Prescher G, Bornfeld N, Horsthemke B, Becher R. Chromosomal aberrations defining uveal melanoma of poor prognosis. Lancet. 1993; 339: 691–692

Prescher G, Bornfeld N, Becher R. Two subclones in a case of uveal melanoma. Relevance of monosomy 3 and multiplication of chromosome 8q. Cancer Genet Cytogenet. 1994 Oct 15;77(2):144–6

Prescher G, Bornfeld N, Hirche H, Horsthemke B, Jockel KH, Becher R. Prognostic implications of monosomy 3 in uveal melanoma. Lancet. 1996 May 4;347(9010):1222–5

Qiao H, Hisatomi T, Sonoda KH, Kura S, Sassa Y, Kinoshita S, Nakamura T, Sakamoto T, Ishibashi T. The characterisation of hyalocytes: the origin, phenotype, and turnover. Br J Ophthalmol. 2005; 89: 513–517

Qualman SJ, Mendelsohn G, Mann RB, Green WR. Intraocular lymphomas. Natural history based on a clinicopathologic study of eight cases and review of the literature. Cancer. 1983; 52: 878–886

Quinn RH, Quong JN, Miller SS. Adrenergic receptor activated ion transport in human fetal retinal pigment epithelium. Invest Ophthalmol Vis Sci. 2001; 42: 255–264

Quivey JM, Augsburger J, Snelling L, Brady LW. 125I plaque therapy for uveal melanoma. Analysis of the impact of time and dose factors on local control. Cancer. 1996; 77: 2356–2362

Rehm HL, Gutierrez-Espeleta GA, Garcia R, Jimenez G, Khetarpal U, Priest JM, Sims KB, Keats BJ, Morton CC. Norrie disease gene mutation in a large Costa Rican kindred with a novel phenotype including venous insufficiency. Hum Mutat 1997; 9: 402–408

Rehm HL, Zhang DS, Brown MC, Burgess B, Halpin C, Berger W, Morton CC, Corey DP, Chen ZY. Vascular defects and sensorineural deafness in a mouse model of Norrie disease. J Neurosci 2002; 22: 4286–4292

Reese AB, Jones IS, Cooper WC. Macular changes secondary to vitreous traction. Am J Ophthalmol. 1967; 64: 544–549

Remé CE, Braschler UF, Roberts JE, Dillon J. Light damage in the rat retina: Effect of radioprotective agent (WR77913) on acute rod outer segment disk disruptions. Photochem Photobiol 1991; 54: 137–142

Rhodes RH. A light microscopic study of the developing human neural retina. Am J Anat. 1979; 154: 195–209

Ricci A. Classification des degenerescences vitreo-retiniennes et chorio-retiniennes en relation avec le decollement de retine. Bibl Ophthalmol. 1969; 79:183–205

Rice TA, de Bustros S, Michels RG, et al. Prognostic factors in vitrectomy for epiretinal membranes of the macula. Ophthalmology 1986; 93: 602–610

Rice TA, Michels RG, Rice EF: Vitrectomy for diabetic traction retinal detachment involving the macula. Am J Ophthalmol 1983, 95: 22–33

Richter M, Gottanka J, May CA, Welge-Lussen U, Berger W, Lutjen-Drecoll E. Retinal vasculature changes in Norrie disease mice. Invest Ophthalmol Vis Sci 1998; 39: 2450–2457

Rinkoff J, Machemer R, Hida T, Chandler D. Temperature-dependent light damage to the retina. Am J Ophthalmol. 1986; 102: 452–462

Rivett K, Kruger L, Radloff S. Infracyanine green-assisted internal limiting membrane peeling in macular hole surgery: does it make a difference? Graefes Arch Clin Exp Ophthalmol 2004; 242: 393–396

Roider J, Hoerauf H, Hager A, Hoerboth T, Laqua H. Konventionelle Ablatiochirurgie oder primäre Vitrektomie bei komplizierten Lochsituationen Ophthalmologe 2001; 98: 887–891

Romayanada N, Goldberg MF, Green WR. Histopathology of sickle cell retinopathy. Trans Am Acad Ophthalmol Otolaryngol. 1973; 77: OP 642–676

Rosen PH, Wong HC, McLeod D. Indentation microsurgery: internal searching for retinal breaks. Eye 1989; 3 (Pt 3): 277–281

Rosengren B, Osterlin S. Hydrodynamic events in the vitreous space accompanying eye movements. Significance for the pathogenesis of retinal detachment. Ophthalmologica 1976: 173: 513–517.

Roth AM, Foos RY. Surface wrinkling retinopathy in eyes enucleated at autopsy. Trans Am Acad Ophthalmol Otolaryngol 1971; 75: 824–829

Roth M, Trittibach P, Koerner F, Sarra G. Pars-plana-Vitrektomie bei idiopathischen Glaskörpertrübungen. Klin Monatsbl Augenheilkd. 2005; 222: 728–732

Rowlatt U. Intrauterine wound healing in a 20 week human fetus. Virchows Arch A Pathol Anat Histol 381: 1979; 353–361

Ruby AJ, Williams DF, Grand MG, et al. Pars plana vitrectomy for treatment of stage 2 macular holes. Arch Ophthalmol 1994; 112: 359–364

Rutzen AR, Ortega-Larrocea G, Dugel PU, Chong LP, Lopez PF, Smith RE, Rao NA. Clinicopathologic study of retinal and choroidal biopsies in intraocular inflammation. Am J Ophthalmol. 1995;119: 597–611

Ryan EH, Gilbert HD. Results of surgical treatment of recent onset full-thickness idiopathic macular holes. Arch Ophthalmol 1994; 112: 1545–1553

Ryan SJ. The development of an experimental model of subretinal neovascularization in disciform macular degeneration. Trans Am Ophthalmol Soc. 1979; 77: 707–745

Sach J, Krepelkova J, Kuchynka P. Haemangiosarcoma of the breast, metastatic to the ciliary body and iris. Br J Ophthalmol. 1998; 82:709–711

Sakamoto T, Miyazaki M, Hisatomi T, Nakamura T, Ueno A,

Itaya K, Ishibashi T. Triamcinolone-assisted pars plana vitrectomy improves the surgical procedures and decreases the postoperative blood-ocular barrier breakdown. Graefes Arch Clin Exp Ophthalmol 2002; 240: 423–429

Sakamoto T, Sakamoto M, Yoshikawa H, Hata Y, Ishibashi T, Ohnishi Y, Inomata H. Histologic findings and prognosis of uveal malignant melanoma in Japanese patients. Am J Ophthalmol. 1996;121: 276–283

Saornil MA, Egan KM, Gragoudas ES, Seddon JM, Walsh SM, Albert DM. Histopathology of proton beam-irradiated vs enucleated uveal melanomas. Arch Ophthalmol. 1992; 110: 1112–1118

Sarks JP, Sarks SH, Killingsworth MC. Evolution of geographic atrophy of the retinal pigment epithelium. Eye. 1988; 2: 552–577

Sarks JP, Sarks SH, Killingsworth MC. Evolution of soft drusen in age-related macular degeneration. Eye. 1994; 8: 269–283

Sarks SH. Ageing and degeneration in the macular region: a clinico-pathological study. Br J Ophthalmol. 1976; 60: 324–341

Sarthy V. Collagen IV mRNA expression during development of the mouse retina: an in situ hybridization study. Invest Ophthalmol Vis Sci. 1993; 34: 145–152

Sato H, Kawasaki R, Yamashita H. Observation of idiopathic full-thickness macular hole closure in early postoperative period as evaluated by optical coherence tomography. Am J Ophthalmol. 2003; 136: 185–187

Sautter H, Lüllwitz W, Naumann G. Die Infrarot-Photographie in der Differential-Diagnose pigmentierter, tumorverdächtiger Fundusveränderungen. Klin Monatsbl Augenheilkd 1974; 164: 597–602

Schachat AP, Oyakawa RT, Michels RG, Rice TA. Complications of vitreous surgery for diabetic retinopathy. II. Postoperative complications. Ophthalmology. 1983; 90: 522–530

Schatz H, McDonald HR. Atrophic macular degeneration. Rate of spread of geographic atrophy and visual loss. Ophthalmology. 1989; 96: 1541–1551

Scheider A, Gündisch O, Kampik A. Surgical extraction of subfoveal choroidal new vessels and submacular haemorrhage in age-related macular degeneration: results of a prospective study. Graefe's Arch Clin Exp Ophthalmol. 1999; 237: 10–15

Schepens CL. Diagnostic and prognostic factors as found in preoperative examination. Trans Am Acad Ophthalmol Otolaryngol 1952; 56: 398–418

Schiff WM, Chang S, Mandava N, Barile GR. Pars plana vitrectomy for persistent, visually significant vitreous opacities. Retina. 2000; 20: 591–596

Schilling H, Sauerwein W, Lommatzsch A, Friedrichs W, Brylak S, Bornfeld N, Wessing A. Long-term results after low dose ocular irradiation for choroidal haemangiomas. Br J Ophthalmol. 1997; 81: 267–273

Schilling H, Sehu KW, Lee WR. A histologic study (including DNA quantification and Ki-67 labeling index) in uveal melanomas after brachytherapy with ruthenium plaques. Invest Ophthalmol Vis Sci. 1997; 38: 2081–2092

Schlötzer-Schrehardt U, Viestenz Arne, Naumann GOH, Laqua H, Michels S, Schmidt-Erfurth U. Dose-related structural effects of photodynamic therapy on choroidal and retinal structures of human eyes. Graefes Arch Clin Exp Ophthalmol 2002; 240: 748–757

Schmidt-Erfurth U, Laqua H, Schlötzer-Schrehardt U, Viestenz A, Naumann GOH. Histopathological changes following photodynamic therapy in human eyes. Arch Ophthalmol 2002; 120: 835–844

Schmidt-Erfurth U, Schlötzer-Schrehardt U, Cursiefen C, Michels S, Beckendorf A, Naumann GOH. Influence of photodynamic therapy on expression of vascular endothelial growth factor (VEGF), VEGF receptor 3, and pigment epithelium-derived factor. Invest Ophthalmol Vis Sci 2003; 44: 4473–4480

Schmidt JC, Rodrigues EB, Hoerle S, Meyer CH, Kroll P. Primary vitrectomy in complicated rhegmatogenous retinal detachment – a survey of 205 eyes. Ophthalmologica 2003; 217:387–392

Scholes AG, et al. Monosomy 3 in uveal melanoma: correlation with clinical and histologic predictors of survival. Invest Ophthalmol Vis Sci, 2003. 44(3): p. 1008–1011

Scholes AG, et al. Allelic imbalance at tumour suppressor loci in uveal melanoma. Ophthalmic Research, 1999. 31 (Suppl. 1): p. 135

Scholes AG et al. Loss of heterozygosity on chromosomes 3, 9, 13 and 17, including the retinoblastoma locus, in uveal melanoma. Invest Ophthalmol Vis Sci, 2001. 42(11): p. 2472–2477

Schueler AO, Jurklies C, Heimann H, Wieland R, Havers W, Bornfeld N. Thermochemotherapy in hereditary retinoblastoma. Br J Ophthalmol. 2003;87: 90–95

Schultz GS, Grant MB. Neovascular growth factors. Eye. 1991; 5: 170–180

Scott IU, Flynn HW Jr, Murray TG, Smiddy WE, Davis JL, Feuer WJ. Outcomes of complex retinal detachment repair using 1000- vs 5000-centistoke silicone oil. Arch Ophthalmol. 2005; 123: 473–478

Scott IU, Flynn HW, Jr., Azen SP, Lai MY, Schwartz S and Trese MT. Silicone oil in the repair of pediatric complex retinal detachments: a prospective, observational, multicenter study. Ophthalmology 1999; 106: 1399–1407

Scott JD. Lens epithelial proliferation in retinal detachment. Trans Ophthalmol Soc U K. 1982; 102 Pt 3: 385–389

Sebag J. Classifying posterior vitreous detachment: a new way to look at the invisible. Br J Ophthalmol 1997; 81: 527–532

Sebag J. Age-related differences in the human vitreoretinal interface. Arch Ophthalmol 1991; 15: 100–107

Sebag J. Age-related differences in the human vitreoretinal interface. Arch Ophthalmol. 1991; 109: 966–971

Sebag J, Balazcs EA: Morphology and ultrastructure of human vitreous fibers. Invest Ophthalmol Vis Sci 1989; 30: 1867–1871

Sebag J. Balazs EA. Human vitreous fibres and vitreoretinal disease. Trans Ophthalmol Soc UK. 1985; 104: 123–128

Seregard S, Spangberg B, Juul C, Oskarsson M. Prognostic accuracy of the mean of the largest nucleoli, vascular patterns, and PC-10 in posterior uveal melanoma. Ophthalmology. 1998; 105: 485–491

Shah M, Foreman DM and Ferguson MW. Control of scarring in adult wounds by neutralising antibody to transforming growth factor beta. Lancet 1992; 339: 213–214

Sharma T, Gopa IL, Badrinath SS. Primary vitrectomy for rhegmatogenous retinal detachment associated with choroidal detachment. Ophthalmology 1998; 105:2282–2285

Shastry BS, Hiraoka M, Trese MT. Lack of association of the Norrie disease gene with retinoschisis phenotype. Jpn J Ophthalmol. 2000;44: 627–629

Sheidow TG, Hooper PL, Crukley C, Young J, Heathcote JG. Expression of vascular endothelial growth factor in uveal melanoma and its correlation with metastasis. Br J Ophthalmol. 2000; 84: 750–756

Shields CL, Sun H, Demirci H, Shields JA. Factors predictive of tumor growth, tumor decalcification, choroidal neovascularization, and visual outcome in 74 eyes with choroidal osteoma. Arch Ophthalmol. 2005; 123: 1658–1666

Shields CL, Shields JA, De Potter P, Quaranta M, Freire J, Brady LW, Barrett J. Plaque radiotherapy for the management of uveal metastasis. Arch Ophthalmol. 1997; 115: 203–209

Shields CL, Shields JA, Baez KA, Cater J, De Potter PV. Choroidal invasion of retinoblastoma: metastatic potential and clinical risk factors. Br J Ophthalmol. 1993; 77: 544–548

Shields CL, Shields JA, Minelli S, De Potter P, Hernandez C, Cater J, Brady L. Regression of retinoblastoma after plaque radiotherapy. Am J Ophthalmol. 1993; 115: 181–187

Shields CL, Shields JA, Karlsson U, Menduke H, Brady LW. Enucleation after plaque radiotherapy for posterior uveal melanoma. Histopathologic findings. Ophthalmology. 1990; 97: 1665–1670

Shields CL, Shields JA, Augsburger JJ. Choroidal osteoma. Surv Ophthalmol. 1988; 33: 17–27

Shields JA, Shields CL, Honavar SG, Demirci H. Clinical variations and complications of Coats disease in 150 cases: the 2000 Sanford Gifford Memorial Lecture. Am J Ophthalmol. 2001; 131: 561–571

Shields JA, Stephens RF, Eagle RC Jr, Shields CL, De Potter P. Progressive enlargement of a circumscribed choroidal hemangioma. A clinicopathologic correlation. Arch Ophthalmol. 1992; 110: 1276–1278

Shields JA, Shields CL, Parsons H, Giblin ME. The role of photocoagulation in the management of retinoblastoma. Arch Ophthalmol. 1990; 108: 205–208

Shields JA, Shields CL. Treatment of retinoblastoma with cryotherapy. Trans Pa Acad Ophthalmol Otolaryngol. 1990; 42: 977–980

Sisley K, et al. Abnormalities of chromosomes 3 and 8 in posterior uveal melanoma correlate with prognosis. Genes Chromosom Cancer, 1997. 19: p. 22–28

Sisley K, Cottam DW, Rennie IG, Parsons MA, Potter AM, Potter CW, Rees RC. Non-random abnormalities of chromosomes 3, 6, and 8 associated with posterior uveal melanoma. Genes Chromosomes Cancer. 1992; 5: 197–200

Sisley K, Rennie IG, Parsons MA, Jacques R, Hammond DW, Bell SM, Potter AM, Rees RC. Abnormalities of chromosomes 3 and 8 in posterior uveal melanoma correlate with prognosis. Genes Chromosomes Cancer. 1997; 19: 22–28

Smiddy WE, Feuer W. Incidence of cataract extraction after diabetic vitrectomy. Retina. 2004; 24: 574–81

Smiddy WE, Michels RG, Gilbert HD, Green WR. Clinicopathologic study of idiopathic macular pucker in children and young adults. Retina. 1992; 12: 232–236

Smiddy WE, Flynn HW Jr, Nicholson DH, Clarkson JG, Gass JD, Olsen KR, Feuer W. Results and complications in treated retinal breaks. Am J Ophthalmol 1991; 112:623–631

Smiddy WE, Michels RG, Green WR. Morphology, pathology, and surgery of idiopathic vitreoretinal macular disorders. Retina 1990; 10: 288–296

Smiddy WE, Michels RG, de Bustros S, et al. Histopathology of tissue removed during vitrectomy for impending idiopathic macular holes. Am J Ophthalmol 1989; 108: 360–364

Smiddy WE, Stark WJ, Michels RG, Maumenee AE, Terry AC, Glaser BM. Cataract extraction after vitrectomy. Ophthalmology 1987; 94: 483–487

Smiddy WE. Contusion in monkeys, Kap. 11

Soulieres D, Rousseau A, Tardif M, Larochelle M, Tremblay M, Vaillancourt L, Pelletier G. The radiosensitivity of uveal melanoma cells and the cell survival curve. Graefes Arch Clin Exp Ophthalmol. 1995; 233: 85–89

Speicher MA, Fu AD, Martin JP, von Fricken MA. Primary vitrectomy alone for repair of retinal detachments following cataract surgery. Retina 2000; 20:459–464

Spira AW, Hollenberg MJ. Human retinal development: ultrastructure of the inner retinal layers. Dev Biol. 1973; 31: 1–21

Spitznas M, Meyer-Schwickerath G, Stephan B: The clinical picture of Eales' disease. Graefes Arch Clin Exp Ophthalmol 1975; 194(2): 73–85.

Spraul CW, Lang GE, Grossniklaus HE, Lang GK. Histologic and morphometric analysis of the choroid, Bruch's membrane, and retinal pigment epithelium in postmortem eyes with age-related macular degeneration and histologic examination of surgically excised choroidal neovascular membranes. Surv Ophthalmol. 1999; 44: S10–32

Stalmans P, Van Aken EH, Melles G, Veckeneer M, Feron EJ, Stalmans I. Trypan blue not toxic for retinal pigment epithelium in vitreo. Am J Ophthalmol 2003; 135: 234–236

Staudt S, Miller DW, Unnebrink K, Holz FG. Inzidenz und Ausprägung von postoperativem Makulaödem nach Makuloforamenoperation mit und ohne kombinierte Kataraktoperation. Ophthalmologe. 2003; 100: 702–707

Stefansson E, Hatchell DL, Fisher BL, Sutherland FS, Machemer R. Panretinal photocoagulation and retinal oxygenation in normal and diabetic cats. Am J Ophthalmol. 1986; 101 :657–664

Stefansson E, Novack RL, Hatchell DL. Vitrectomy prevents retinal hypoxia in branch retinal vein occlusion. Invest Ophthalmol Vis Sci. 1990; 31: 284–289

Stefansson E. Oxygen and diabetic eye disease. Graefes Arch Clin Exp Ophthalmol. 1990; 228: 120–123

Stefansson E. The therapeutic effects of retinal laser treatment and vitrectomy. A theory based on oxygen and vascular physiology. Acta Ophthalmol Scand. 2001; 79: 435–440

Stelnicki EJ, Arbeit J, Cass DL, Saner S, Harrison M and Largman C. Modulation of the human homeobox genes PRX-2 and HOXB13 in scarless fetal wounds. J Invest Dermatol 1998; 111: 57–63

Stone J, Chan-Ling T, Pe'er J, Itin A, Gnessin H, Keshet E. Roles of vascular endothelial growth factor and astrocyte degeneration in the genesis of retinopathy of prematurity. Invest Ophthalmol Vis Sci. 1996; 37: 290–299

Stone J, Dreher Z. Relationship between astrocytes, ganglion cells and vasculature of the retina. J Comp Neurol 1987; 255: 35–49

Straatsma BR, Foos RY, Feman SS (1986) Degenerative disease of the peripheral retina. In Duane DD (ed): Clinical ophthalmol. Vol.3, Chapter 26, Philadelphia, 1986, Harper & Row, 1–16

Straatsma BR, Foos RY and Feman SS. Degenerative disease of the peripheral retina. In: Duane DD (ed): Clinical Ophthalmol. Vol. 3, Chapter 26, Philadelphia, 1986, Harper & Row, 1–19

Straatsma BR, Foos RY. Typical and reticular retinoschisis. Am J Ophthalmol 1973; 75: 551–575

Straatsma BR, Zeegen, Foos RY, Feman SS, Shabo AL. Lattice degeneration of the retina. XXX Edward Jackson Memorial Lecture. Am J Ophthalmol 1974; 77: 619–649

Strahlman ER, Fine SL, Hillis A. The second eye of patients with senile macular degeneration. Arch Ophthalmol. 1983; 101: 1191–1193

Strauss O. The retinal pigment epithelium in visual function. Physiol Rev. 2005; 85: 845–881

Streilein JW, Ma N, Wenkel H, Ng TF, Zamiri P. Immunobiology and privilege of neuronal retina and pigment epithelium transplants. Vision Res. 2002; 42:487–495

Surgery Trial Research Group. Surgery for subfoveal choroidal neovascularization in age-related macular degeneration. Ophthalmic findings: SST Report No.11 Ophthalmology. 2004; 111: 1967–1980

Szurman P, Di Tizio FM, Lafaut B, Aisenbrey S, Grisanti S, Roters S, Bartz-Schmidt KU. Notwendigkeit der Kopftieflage nach Makuloforamenchirurgie: eine konsekutive Fall-Kontroll Studie. Klin Monatsbl Augenheilkd. 2000; 217: 351–355

Takada Y, Fariss RN, Tanikawa A, Zeng Y, Carper D, Bush R, Sieving PA. A retinal neuronal developmental wave of retinoschisin expression begins in ganglion cells during layer formation. Invest Ophthalmol Vis Sci. 2004; 45: 3302–3312

Takeuchi A, Kricorian G, Marmor MF. Albumin movement out of the subretinal space after experimental retinal detachment. Invest Ophthalmol Vis Sci. 1995; 36:1298–305

Tanner V, Minihan M, Williamson TH. Management of inferior retinal breaks during pars plana vitrectomy for retinal detachment. Br J Ophthalmol 2001; 85: 480–482

The Collaborative Ocular Melanoma Study (COMS) randomized trial of pre-enucleation radiation of large choroidal melanoma III: local complications and observations following enucleation COMS report no. 11. Am J Ophthalmol. 1998; 126: 362–372

The Collaborative Ocular Melanoma Study (COMS) randomized trial of pre-enucleation radiation of large choroidal melanoma II: initial mortality findings. COMS report no. 10. Am J Ophthalmol. 1998;125: 779–796

The Collaborative Ocular Melanoma Study (COMS) randomized trial of pre-enucleation radiation of large choroidal melanoma I: characteristics of patients enrolled and not enrolled. COMS report no. 9. Am J Ophthalmol. 1998; 125: 767–778

Theodossiadis PG, Georgalas IG, Emfietzoglou J, Kyriaki TE, Pantelia E, Gogas PS, Moschos MN, Theodossiadis GP. Optical coherence tomography findings in the macula after treatment of rhegmatogenous retinal detachments with spared macula preoperatively. Retina. 2003; 23:69–75

Thomas JW, Grossniklaus HE, Lambert HM, Aaberg TM, L'Hernault N. Ultrastructural features of surgically excised idiopathic subfoveal. Retina. 1993; 13: 93–98

Thomas MA, Dickinson JD, Melberg NS, Ibanez HE, Dhaliwal RS. Visual results after surgical removal of subfoveal choroidal membranes. Ophthalmology. 1994; 101: 1384–1396

Thomas MA, Grand MG, Williams DF, Lee CM, Pesin SR, Lowe MA. Surgical management of subfoveal choroidal neovascularization. Ophthalmology. 1992; 99: 952–968

Thompson JT. Epiretinal membrane removal in eyes with good visual acuities. Retina. 2005; 25: 875–882

Thompson JT. The role of patient age and intraocular gas use in cataract progression after vitrectomy for macular holes and epiretinal membranes. Am J Ophthalmol. 2004; 137: 250–257

Thumann G, Aisenbrey S, Schraermeyer U, et al. Transplantation of autologous iris pigment epithelium after removal of choroidal neovascular membranes. Arch Ophthalmol. 2000; 118: 1350–1355

Tielsch JN, Legro LW, Cassard SD. Risk factors for retinal detachment after cataract surgery. A population based case controlled study. Ophthalmology 1996; 103: 1537–1545

Tillery WV and Lucier LC. Round atrophic holes in lattice degeneration – an important cause of phakic retinal detachment. Trans Am Acad Ophthalmol Otolaryngol 1976; 81: 509–518

Tolentino F, Schepens CL and Freeman HN. Vitreoretinal disorders diagnosis and management, W.B. Saunders, Philadelphia 1976; p 340–349

Tolentino FI, Lapus JV, Novalis G, Trempe CL, Gutow GS, Ahmad A. Fluorescein angiography of degenerative lesions of the peripheral fundus and rhegmatogenous retinal detachment. Int Ophthalmol Clin. 1976; 16: 13–29

Trick GL, Berkowitz BA. Retinal oxygenation response and retinopathy. Prog Retin Eye Res. 2005; 24: 259–274

Tschentscher F, Husing J, Holter T, Kruse E, Dresen IG, Jockel KH, Anastassiou G, Schilling H, Bornfeld N, Horsthemke B, Lohmann DR, Zeschnigk M. Tumor classification based on gene expression profiling shows that uveal melanomas with and without monosomy 3 represent two distinct entities. Cancer Res 2003; 63:2578–2584

Tso MO. Clues to the cells of origin in retinoblastoma. Int Ophthalmol Clin. 1980; 20: 191–210

van Bockxmeer FM, Martin CE, Thompson DE and Constable IJ. Taxol for the treatment of proliferative vitreoretinopathy. Invest Ophthalmol Vis Sci 26: 1985; 1140–1147

van Effenterre G, Haut J, Larricart P, Abi-Rached J, Vachet JM. Gas tamponade as a single technique in the treatment of retinal detachment: is vitrectomy needed? A comparative study of 120 cases. Graefes Arch Clin Exp Ophthalmol 1987; 225: 254–258

Van Meurs JC, ter Averst E, Croxen R, Hofland L, van Hagen PM. Comparison of the growth potential of retinal pigment epithelial cells obtained during vitrectomy in patients with age-related macular degeneration or complex retinal detachment. Graefes Arch Clin Exp Ophthalmol 2004; 242: 442–443

van Meurs JC, Bolt BJ, Mertens DA, Peperkamp E, De Waard P. Rubeosis of the iris in proliferative vitreoretinopathy. Retina. 1996; 16: 292–295

van Meurs JC, Schwoerer J, Schwartz B, Mulder PG, Meiselmann HJ, Johnson CS. Retinal vessel autoregulation in sickle cell patients. Graefes Arch Clin Exp Ophthalmol. 1992; 230: 442–445.

van Meurs JC. Relationship between peripheral vascular closure and proliferative retinopathy in sickle cell disease. Graefes Arch Clin Exp Ophthalmol. 1991; 229: 543–538

van Nouhuys CE (1991) Signs, complications, and platelet aggregation in familial exudative vitreoretinopathy. Am J Ophthalmol 111:34–41

van Nouhuys CE (1989) Juvenile retinal detachment as a complication of familial exudative vitreoretinopathy. Fortschr Ophthalmol 86:221–223

van Nouhuys CE (1982) Dominant exudative vitreoretinopathy and other vascular developmental disorders of the peripheral retina. Doc Ophthalmol 54:1–414

van Nouhuys CE (1981) Congenital retinal fold as a sign of dominant exudative vitreoretinopathy. Graefes Arch Clin Exp Ophthalmol 217:55–67

van Velthoven ME, Verbraak FD, Garcia PM, Schlingemann RO, Rosen RB, de Smet MD. Evaluation of central serous retinopathy with en face optical coherence tomography. Br J Ophthalmol. 2005 Nov;89(11):1483–8.

Veckeneer M, van Overdam K, Monzer J, Kobuch K, van Marle W, Spekreijse H, van Meurs J. Ocular toxicity of trypan blue injected into the vitreous cavity of rabbit eyes. Graefes Arch Clin Exp Ophthalmol 2001; 239: 698–704

Velikay M, Stolba U, Wedrich A, Li Y, Datlinger P, Binder S. The effect of chemical stability and purification of perfluorocarbon liquids in experimental extended-term vitreous substitution. Graefes Arch Clin Exp Ophthalmol. 1995; 233: 26–30

Velikay M, Wedrich A, Stolba U, Datlinger P, Li Y, Binder S. Experimental long-term vitreous replacement with purified and non purified Perfluorodecaline. Am J Ophthalmol 1993; 116: 565–570

Vogel M. Treatment of malignant choroidal melanomas with photocoagulation. Evaluation of ten-year follow-up data. Am J Ophthalmol 1972; 74:1

Vogel M. Histopathologic observation of photocoagulated malignant melanomas of the choroid. Am J Ophthalmol 1972; 74: 468

Vogt A. Die Operative Therapie und Die Pathogenese der Netzhautablösung. Stuttgart Ferdinand Enke Verlag, 1936

von Domarus D, Mitschke H. Primäres alveolares Weichteilsarkom der Aderhaut. Ophthalmologie und Histiogenese. Ophthalmologica 1978; 177: 229–235

Warburg M, Hauge M, Sanger R. Norrie's disease and the XG blood group system: linkage data. Acta Genet Stat Med. 1965; 15:103–115

Warwar RE, Bullock JD, Shields JA, Eagle RC Jr. Coexistence of 3 tumors of neural crest origin: neurofibroma, meningioma, and uveal malignant melanoma. Arch Ophthalmol. 1998; 116: 1241–1243

Weinstock SJ, Morin JD. Traumatic macular hole. Can J Ophthalmol. 1976; 11: 249–251

Weller M, Wiedemann P and Heimann K. Proliferative vitreoretinopathy – is it anything more than wound healing at the wrong place? Int Ophthalmol 1990; 14: 105–117

Wells JA, Gregor ZJ. Surgical treatment of full-thickness macular holes using autologous serum. Eye 1996; 10: 593–599.

Wendel RT, Patel AC, Kelly NE, Salzano TC, Wells JW, Novack GD. Vitreous surgery for macular holes. Ophthalmology 1993; 100: 1671–1676

Wenkel H, Streilein JW. Evidence that retinal pigment epithelium functions as an immune-privileged tissue. Invest Ophthalmol Vis Sci. 2000; 41:3467–3473

Wenkel H, Streilein JW, Young MJ. Systemic immune deviation in the brain that does not depend on the integrity of the blood-brain barrier. J Immunol. 2000; 164:5125–5131

Wenkel H, Chen PW, Ksander BR, Streilein JW. Immune privilege is extended, then withdrawn, from allogeneic tumor cell grafts placed in the subretinal space. Invest Ophthalmol Vis Sci. 1999; 40:3202–3208

Wenkel H, Naumann GO. Retrolaminäre Infiltration des Sehnervenkopfes nach Silikonöltamponade. Klin Monatsbl Augenheilkd. 1999; 214: 120–122

Wenkel H, Streilein JW. Analysis of immune deviation elicited by antigens injected into the subretinal space. Invest Ophthalmol Vis Sci. 1998; 39:1823–1834

West H, Richardson WD, Fruttiger M. Stabilization of the retinal vascular network by reciprocal feedback between blood vessels and astrocytes. Development. 2005; 132: 1855–1862

Whitcup SM, de Smet MD, Rubin BI, Palestine AG, Martin DF, Burnier M Jr, Chan CC, Nussenblatt RB. Intraocular lymphoma. Clinical and histopathologic diagnosis. Ophthalmology. 1993; 100: 1399–1406

Whitcup SM, Park WS, Gasch AT, Eagle RC, Filie AC, Nussenblatt RB, Zhuang Z, Chan CC. Use of microdissection and molecular genetics in the pathologic diagnosis of retinoblastoma. Retina. 1999; 19: 318–324

White VA, et al. Correlation of cytogenetic abnormalities with the outcome of patients with uveal melanoma. Cancer, 1998. 83: p. 354–359

Wiedemann P, Hilgers RD, Bauer P, Heimann K. Adjunctive daunorubicin in the treatment of proliferative vitreoretinopathy: results of a multicenter clinical trial. Am J Ophthalmol 1998; 126: 550–559

Wiedemann P and Heimann K. Proliferative Vitreoretinopathie. Pathogenese und Möglichkeiten der Zytostatikatherapie. Klin Monatsbl Augenheilkd 1986; 188: 559–564

Wieger G. Über den Canalis petiti und ein Ligamentum hyaloideocapsulare (dissertation) Strassburg 1883

Wilkes SR, Beard CN, Kurland LT. The incidence of retinal detachment in Rochester, Minnesota, 1970–1978. Am J Ophthalmol 1982; 94: 670–673

Wilkinson CP. Evidence-based analysis of prophylactic treatment of asymptomatic retinal breaks and lattice degeneration. Ophthalmology 2000; 107:12–15

Williams RG, Chang S, Comaratta MR and Simoni G. Does the presence of heparin and dexamethasone in the vitrectomy infusate reduce reproliferation in proliferative vitreoretinopathy? Graefes Arch Clin Exp Ophthalmol 1996; 234: 496–503

Williamson TH. Vitreous surgery in uveitis and allied disorders. In: Kirchhof B, Wong D (eds): Vitreo-retinal surgery, Essentials in Ophthalmology Series, Springer, Berlin 2005, pp 163–174

Winter M, Eberhardt W, Scholz C, Reichenbach A. Failure of potassium siphoning by Muller cells: a new hypothesis of perfluorocarbon liquid-induced retinopathy. Invest Ophthalmol Vis Sci. 2000; 41: 256–261

Witschel H, Font RL. Hemangioma of the choroid. A clinicopathologic study of 71 cases and review of the literature. Surv Ophthalmol 1976; 20: 415–431

Wolf S, Lappas A, Weinberger AW, Kirchhof B. Macular translocation for surgical management of subfoveal choroidal neovascularizations in patients with AMD: first results. Graefes Arch Clin Exp Ophthalmol. 1999; 237: 51–57

Wolfensberger TJ. Foveal reattachment after macula-off retinal detachment occurs faster after vitrectomy than after buckle surgery. Ophthalmology. 2004;111:1340–1343

Wong D, Stanga P, Briggs M, Lenfestey P, Lancaster E, Li KK, Lim KS and Groenewald C. Case selection in macular relocation surgery for age related macular degeneration. Br J Ophthalmol 2004; 88: 186–190

Wong HC, Sehmi KS, McLeod D. Abortive neovascular outgrowths discovered during vitrectomy for diabetic vitreous haemorrhage. Graefes Arch Clin Exp Ophthalmol. 1989; 227: 237–240

Worley LA, Onken MD, Person E, Robirds D, Branson J, Char DH, Perry A, Harbour JW. Transcriptomic versus cromosomal prognostic markers and clinical outcome in uveal melanoma. Clin Cancer Res 2007; 13:1466–1471

Worst JGF: The bursa intravitrealis premacularis. New Developments in Ophthalmology. Nijmegen, Doc Ophthalmol Proc Ser 1975; 275–279

Worst JGF, Sebag J, Kishi S, Shimizi K: posterior vitreous pocket: Correspondence. Arch Ophthalmol 1991; 109: 1058–1060

Yamada E. Some structural features of the fovea centralis in the human retina. Arch Ophthalmol 1969; 82: 152–159

Yang CM, Pars plana vitrectomy in the treatment of combined rhegmatogenous retinal detachment and choroidal detachment in aphakic or pseudophakic patients. Ophthalmic Surg Lasers 1997; 28: 288–293

Yanoff M. Pseudogliomas: differential diagnosis of retinoblastoma: Ophthal. Dig. 1972; 34: 9

Yanhoff M and Zimmerman LE, Davis RL. Massive gliosis of the retina. Int Ophthalmol Clin 1971; 11: 211

Yanoff M, EK Rahn, LE Zimmerman: Histopathology of juvenile retinoschisis. Arch. Ophthalmol 79 (1968):49–53

Yaoeda H. Clinical observation on macular hole. Acta Soc Ophthalmol Jpn 1967; 71: 1723–1736

Yilmaz S, Horsthemke B, Lohmann DR. Twelve novel RB1 gene mutations in patients with hereditary retinoblastoma. Mutations in brief no. 206. Hum Mutat. 1998; 12: 434

Young TL, Anthony DC, Pierce E, Foley E, Smith LE. Histopathology and vascular endothelial growth factor in untreated and diode laser-treated retinopathy of prematurity. J AAPOS. 1997; 1:105–110

Zeana D, Becker J, Kuckelkorn R, Kirchhof B. Perfluorohexyloctane as a long-term vitreous tamponade in the experimental animal. International Ophthalmology 1999; 23: 17–24

Zimmerman LE, McLean IW, Foster WD. The Manschot–van Peperzeel concept of the growth and metastasis of uveal melanomas. Doc Ophthalmol. 1980; 50: 101–121

Zimmerman LE, McLean IW, Foster WD. Does enucleation of the eye containing a malignant melanoma prevent or accelerate the dissemination of tumour cells. Br J Ophthalmol. 1978; 62: 420–425

Zimmerman LE, Naumann GOH. Pathology of Retinoschisis in "New and Controversial Aspects of Retinal Detachment", McPherson A (ed), New York, Hoeber, 400–423, 1968

Zimmerman LE, Spencer WH. The pathologic anatomy of retinoschisis. Arch Ophthalmol 1960; 63: 10–19

Zografos L, Bercher L, Chamot L, Gailloud C, Raimondi S, Egger E. Cobalt-60 treatment of choroidal hemangiomas. Am J Ophthalmol. 1996; 121: 190–199

Optic Nerve and Elschnig's Scleral Ring

C.Y. Mardin, G.O.H. Naumann

5.7.1 Anatomy, Landmarks, Harmless and Other Anomalies, Age Related Changes, Juxtapapillary Coni

The optic nerve consists of intrascleral, orbital and canalicular portions and about 1.2 million axons. It is in the true sense of the word a fascicle of axons (nerve fibers). Histologically it loses about 5,000 nerve fibers per year – in an 80-year life span 400,000 axons or a third of the total equals (Jonas et al. 1992) a loss of neuroretinal rim area of 0.1%/year in vivo. This is important for the long-term follow-up of the neuroretinal rim in glaucomas, where in addition to axons astrocytes and oligodendrocytes are likely also lost although their reduction in number is more difficult to measure.

In principle, hereditary, inflammatory, compressive and ischemic processes result in loss of axons, initially leaving most of the astrocytes intact. The clinical picture of a glial and fibrous proliferation of the intermediate nerve tissue is called simple optic atrophy. We differentiate between an ascending and descending atrophy in the course of the disease (Table 5.7.1). While ascending optic atrophy results in simple disc atrophy after 2 weeks to 1 month, a descending atrophy may become visible at the disc after 6 weeks. In many cases of ascending disc atrophy vascular supply plays an important role (Fig. 5.7.2).

The optic disc is the place where loss of axons and astrocytes becomes obvious on ophthalmoscopy (Fig. 5.7.3). It is demarcated by Elschnig's scleral rim and can be divided into prelaminar, laminar and retrolaminar portions. The prelaminar portion consists of 64% axonal tissue, whereas the retrolaminar part is composed of 20% axons (Table 5.7.2, Fig. 5.7.4). This fact holds implications for in vivo measurements of the neuroretinal rim in various diseases. The retrolaminar nerve is characterized by the myelinization of the retrolaminar axons by the oligodendrocytes. Congenital myelinization of the visible retinal nerve fibers (RNF)

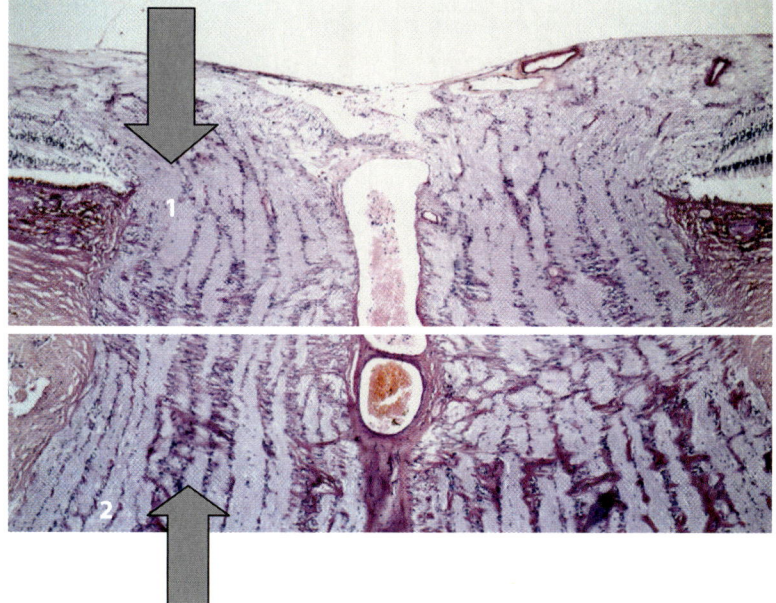

Fig. 5.7.1. Optic atrophy: ascending (after 2 weeks), descending (after 4–6 weeks). *1* intraocular axons, *2* retrobulbar axons with myelin sheaths (PAS)

5.7 Optic Nerve and Elschnig Scleral Ring

Table 5.7.1. Pathogenetic classification of optic atrophies

I. *Descending* optic atrophy (primary defect in retrolaminar optic nerve: intracranial or retrobulbar)
   1. Primary optic nerve processes, demyelinating, axial retrobulbar neuritis, tumors
   2. Secondary diseases outside the optic nerve
      – Intracranial and orbital tumors, e.g., pituitary tumors
      – Retrobulbar perineuritis
      – Elevated intracranial pressure
      – Trauma

II. *Ascending* optic atrophy (primary defect in the prelaminar optic disc or retina)
   1. After central artery occlusion
   2. Cerebromacular dystrophies
   3. Secondary after papilledema
   4. Secondary after papillitis due to intraocular inflammation
   5. Glaucomatous optic atrophy, chronic
   6. After ischemic disc processes: arteriosclerosis, AION, giant cell arteritis, acute glaucomas
   7. End stage of tapetoretinal degenerations
   8. In all diffuse retinal processes with loss of ganglion cells

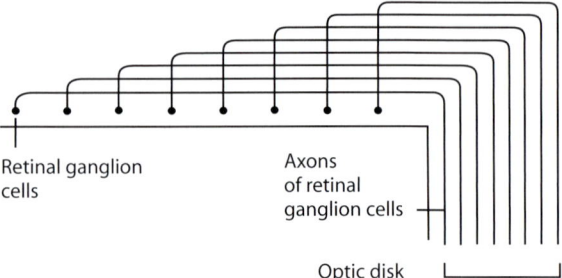

Fig. 5.7.3. Course of the retinal nerve fibers in the optic disc according to the position of their ganglion cells. Note: the greater the distance of the ganglion cell to the disc, the nearer it is to Elschnig's scleral rim at the optic disc, while the nearer the ganglion cell, the more it is to the center

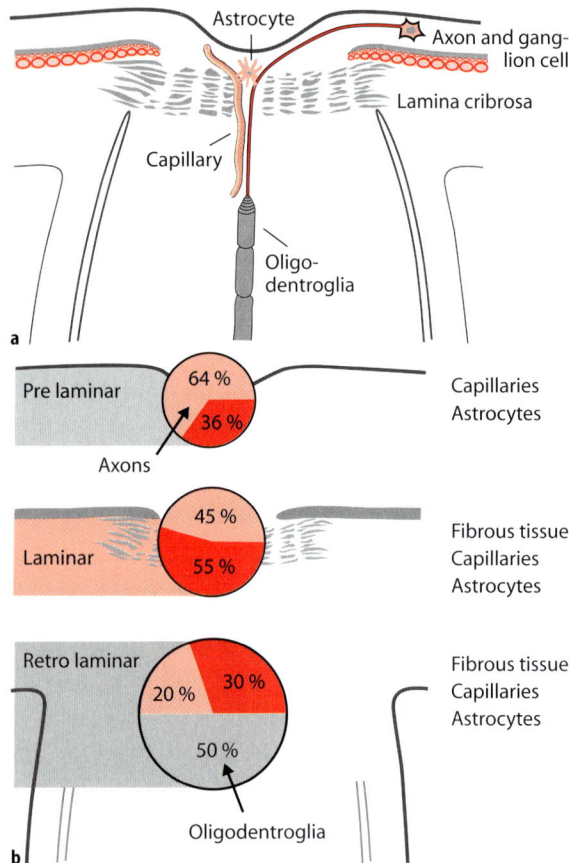

Fig. 5.7.4a, b. Cross section through the optic disc with its prelaminar, laminar and retrolaminar parts. Percentage of axons (*pink*) in relation to capillaries, astrocytes, fibrous tissue and oligodendroglia. For assumptions see Table 5.7.2

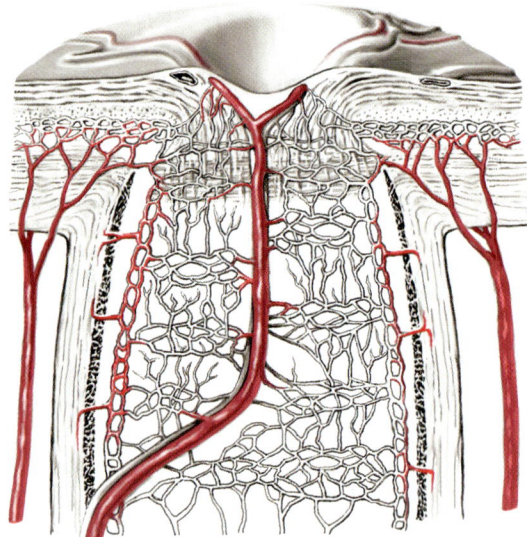

Fig. 5.7.2. Schematic drawing of the vascular supply of the anterior optic nerve. Retina, choroidea, lamina cribrosa, dura, arachnoidea, short posterior ciliary arteries, central retinal vessels (artery, vein), arachnoid vessels, Zinn-Haller circle, and anastomosis of the central retinal artery with the choroidal and arachnoidal vessels (see also 5.6.20)

results in a relative or absolute scotoma in the static perimetry and may be confused with RNF infarction (cotton-wool spots) if it is not in contact with the optic disc. Starting from the prelaminar surface towards the orbit, the relation of axons to glial and fibrovascular tissue is shifted from the axon to the surrounding tissue (Jonas et al. 1993) (Table 5.7.2, see also 5.2.7, 5.2.8). The thickness of the lamina cribrosa is measured histologically and has a mean value of 0.35 mm in the center and 0.39 mm in the periphery (Jonas et al. 2004) (Table 5.7.3). This is important for the discussion of whether the optic disc should be incised horizontally and nasally in central vein occlusion. The mean disc area measured with optic disc photographs is 2.7 mm^2 (Jonas et al. 1993) and 2.2 mm^2 with the Heidelberg Retina Tomograph (HRT II, Heidelberg Engineering, Dossenheim, Germany) (Burk et al. 2004). The vari-

5.7.2 Surgical Pathology and Indications for Microsurgery   341

Table 5.7.6. Critical details of glaucomatous disc atrophy in chronic glaucomas (after working groups Airaksinen et al. 1983; Jonas et al. 1989–1995; Quigley et al. 1979–1995; Spaeth et al. 1971; Burk, Kruse, Rohrschneider, Völcker 1989–1994)

I. Cupping: cup-disc ratio
  1. Disc size
     Pseudonormal micro cupping in small discs
     Pseudoglaucomatous macro cupping in macro discs
     Asymmetry: in relation to the de facto disc size
  2. Vertical configuration of the cup: glaucoma suspected
II. Neuroretinal rim zone
  1. Locally isolated loss temporal inferiorly or superiorly (notch)
  2. Diffuse thinning
  3. Paleness
	III. Lamina cribrosa
	  1. Pore visibility increased
	  2. Deformation to the posterior and compression
	  3. Slitlike pores
	IV. Retinal vessels
	  1. Nasal dislocation
	  2. Narrowing
	  3. Kinking at the scleral rim
	Stripped appearance in the disc zone

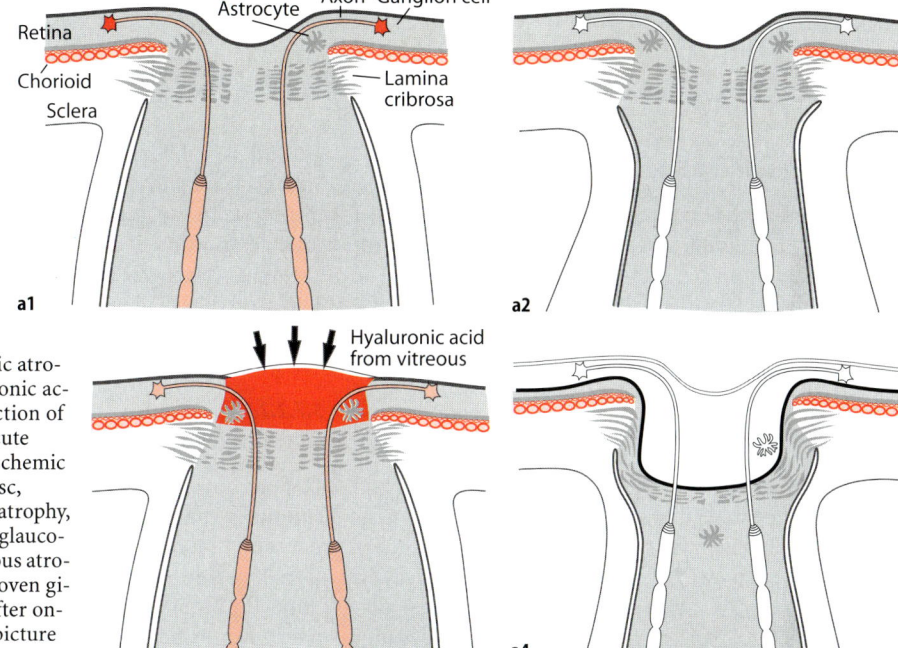

Fig. 5.7.11. Cavernous optic atrophy. Impression of hyaluronic acid into the ischemic infarction of the optic nerve head in acute glaucomas and anterior ischemic neuropathy. **a1** Normal disc, **a2** ascending/descending atrophy, **a3** Cavernous atrophy, **a4** glaucomatous atrophy **b** Cavernous atrophy of the optic disc in proven giant cell arteritis 18 days after onset of blindness. Clinical picture of pale edematous optic disc

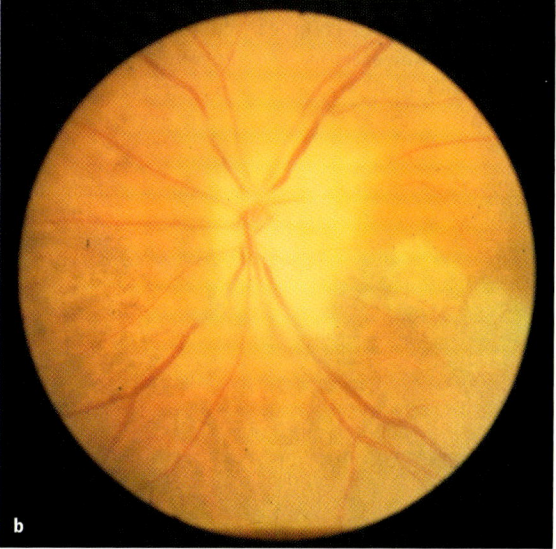

In contrast to the chronic glaucomatous changes, the disc in acute glaucomas with very high intraocular pressures shows a different pattern of atrophy. Initially a disc edema and not a cupping may appear as a result of hydropic swelling, ischemic necrosis of prelaminar tissue and later a ballooning of necrotic papillary tissue due to impression of hyaluronic acid from the vitreous (Fig. 5.7.11). Later cupping after the initial edema develops; this entity is called Schnabel's cavernous optic disc atrophy. Hyaluronidase sensitive mucopolysaccharide acids can be demonstrated also in the retrolaminar tissue. These changes can also be observed in eyes after arteritic and non-arteritic infarction of the disc. Similar changes are evident in eyes with silicone-filled vitreous cavity, suffering from high intraocular pressure (see below and Chapter 5.6).

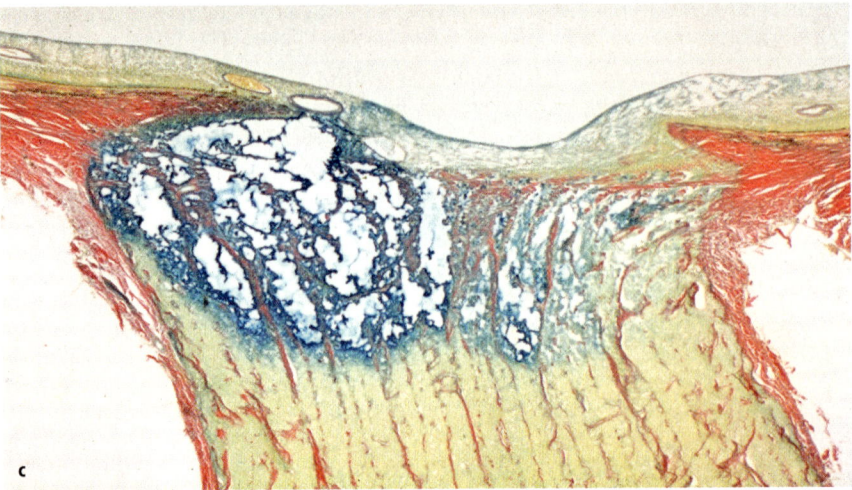

Fig. 5.7.11. c Cavernous optic atrophy: Hyaluronic acid (*blue*) in area of ischemic infarction in proven giant cell-arteriitis 3 weeks after onset (case reported by Hinzpeter and Naumann, 1976)

5.7.2.2
Giant Cell Arteritis and Biopsy of the Temporal Artery

Disc swelling with functional loss of central vision and visual field is among others (Table 5.7.7) a common sign and symptom for this generalized disease of the cranial arteries (Horton disease). Occlusion of the short, posterior ciliary arteries is the common cause both for non-arteritic and arteritic anterior ischemic neuropathy. The role of ultrasound biomicroscopy and Doppler flowmetry in confirming obstruction of the temporal artery needs to be established more definitely (Wenkel and Michelson 1996). The ischemic infarction of the optic nerve head in Horton's disease is an indication for surgical intervention; a biopsy of the branches of the temporal artery is done to confirm the clinical diagnosis. A negative biopsy does not rule out the disease. Immediate onset of near complete vision loss is accompanied by pale swelling of the disc with juxtapapillary hemorrhages, thin arterioles and dilated venules. In the course of 4 weeks simple (axon loss, glial cells unchanged) or complex (axon loss, proliferation of glial cells) or even pseudoglaucomatous (axon and glial cell loss) optic atrophy may occur. Hyaluronic acid is found in necrotic areas of the optic nerve on histology and is called cavernous Schnabel's atrophy (Fig. 5.7.11). It may even extend into the orbital portion of the nerve. In the ischemic necrosis of most of the disc a total destruction of all neuronal and connective tissues is found. Microglia may phagocytose necrotic tissue. The optic nerve also displays a fibrous and astrocytic optic atrophy.

5.7.2.2.1
Biopsy and Histology of the Temporal Artery

Doppler investigation of both *external carotid arteries* should be mandatory to rule out a stenosis and a compensatory, secondary shunt between internal and external carotid artery via the temporal artery. If this is done, the biopsy is a safe procedure and in our hands in over 700 biopsies no major complications were noticed. Histopathologic changes in the temporal artery are similar to those in the cranial and retrobulbar, ciliary arteries (Jacobs et al. 1994). Biopsy of branches of the temporal artery leads to a solid basis for the treatment of Horton's disease, *but does not exclude the disease if negative*. Knowledge of the exact anatomic location is mandatory for a successful biopsy. Prior to surgery a branch of the artery has to be localized and marked. The characteristic local finding is the palpable, thickened, pulseless, painful artery and erythema of the skin. A normal local finding does not rule out the disease, and 9–61% of the biopsies are reported to be negative. In bilateral biopsies only *10% were positive only for one side*. Therefore a bilateral biopsy is recommended. The excised arteries should be at least 20 mm long, and prepared in different step-sections, because in 7% of the specimens "skip lesions" are revealed. In histology a granulomatous reaction against smooth muscle cells and the lamina elastica interna usually, but not always, with giant cells can be observed. The lamina elastica is fragmented as it is phagocytosed by giant cells.

Table 5.7.7. Clinical manifestations of giant cell arteritis in the eye and visual system (modified after Jacobs and Foster 1994)

1. Ischemic infarction of the optic nerve: optic nerve head, retrobulbar
2. Occlusion of the central artery or its branches
3. Cerebral ischemic infarction
4. Disturbance of motility, intermittent paresis of nerves III, IV; and VI, internuclear ophthalmopathy
5. Horner's syndrome
6. Orbital pseudotumor with exophthalmus
7. Ischemic ophthalmopathy with ocular hypotony
8. Uveal infarctions: choroidal, iridal
9. Scleritis and episcleritis
10. Polymyalgia rheumatica

Muscle cells are degenerated and replaced by fibrous tissue. Adventitia and nourishing vessels of the artery show also an inflammatory infiltration. Initially the inflammation may start with the adventitia and continues into the muscularis media. Severity of histology in the temporal artery does not correlate with the degree of the clinical ocular manifestation. The biopsy is not an emergency procedure but should be performed preferably within 1 week. As soon as the clinical suspicion of Horton's disease arises high dose corticosteroid-therapy should be started immediately. Evans et al. (1994) even report proof for active inflammation after steroid medication for several weeks.

5.7.2.3
Optic Disc in Non-/Ischemic Central Retinal Vein Occlusion and Opticotomy

Optic disc swelling in the course of a central vein occlusion (CVO) demands consideration of the natural course of the disease, particularly as "opticotomy" at the level of the lamina cribrosa via pars plana vitrectomy (ppVy) recently has been recommended in the management of this disease without reliable clinically controlled studies.

5.7.2.3.1
Non-ischemic Central Vein Occlusion

Disc swelling, tortuous and dilated venules and a varying amount of retinal hemorrhages with or without cotton-wool spots describes the entity of "simple" central vein occlusion. This condition may occur in young patients, unilaterally in most cases with nearly unaffected visual acuity and enlarged blind spot. This disorder may be associated with coagulopathies like factor V Leyden defect, apolipoprotein C or antithrombin III defect. Some authors call this condition "papillophlebitis," but it presents a non-ischemic central vein occlusion. Non-ischemic CVOs are also associated with disc swelling. There are no signs of capillary occlusion, and turbulences at the level of the lamina cribrosa are described to be the site of origin. The deeper the place of obstruction the higher is the likelihood of the appearance of collateral vessels and the more positive the outcome.

An important differential diagnosis is *"venous stasis retinopathy,"* which may resemble CVO, but does not show disc edema and the retinal hemorrhages appear to be spot like and situated in the deep retina. An occlusion of the internal carotid artery causing an ischemic ophthalmopathy should be ruled out (DDx, Table 5.7.8 according to Kearns and Hollenhorst 1963).

5.7.2.3.2
Ischemic Central Vein Occlusion

Disc swelling in ischemic central vein occlusion is a condition diagnosed with fluorescein angiography (FLA) or visual field examination and is clinically characterized by a relative afferent pupillary defect or Marcus-Gunn pupillary sign and massive retinal hemorrhage. Most causes are reported to be situated at the level of the optic disc as in hyperviscosity syndrome, vasculitis, reduction of arterial perfusion pressure, intravasal turbulences due to vein compression of an atheromatous central artery (associated with systemic arterial hypertension, hyperlipidemia and smoking), massive drusinosis of the disc, congenital anomalies of the lamina cribrosa and venous outflow obstruction due to intracranial or intraocular rise of pressure (bottle height of infusion in ppVy in relation to systemic blood pressure) or compressive neoplasia. In a prospective study of 29 eyes with CVO (Green et al. 1981), only in 24.6% could an arterial insufficiency be demonstrated. Also, in animal models (monkey), a capillary occlusion appeared in eyes without arterial malperfusion.

Radial optic neurotomy (RONT) horizontally and nasally in ischemic CVO has been proposed to improve blood flow and visual acuity (Kim et al. 2005; Opremcak et al. 2006). The surgical dissection of the optic disc at the level of the lamina cribrosa is supposed to lower pressure in the axoplasmatic and venous flow or induce cilioretinal anastomoses. This anastomosis is thought to rise from the intact Zinn-Haller's circle, which gives branches tranversely to the prelaminar and laminar portion of the optic disc. Usually the circle is divided into two half circles, which provides altitudinal blood supply to the superior and inferior part of the disc. An infarction of the short posterior arteries may result in an altitudinal pattern of visual loss (Risco et al. 1981). The efficacy of RONT is very controversial and subject to considerable discussion. Case series of RONT after ppVy (Opremcak et al. 2006) demonstrated an improvement of visual acuity and decrease of central retinal thickness, measured with OCT. Opremcak et al. (2006) showed in 117 eyes that anatomical resolution of CVO occurred in 95% and visual acuity improved in 71% with no surgical complications and a rate of rubeosis of the iris of 6%.

On the other hand, Vogel et al. (2006) studied a surgi-

Table 5.7.8. Central retinal venous occlusion, variants, according to Kearns and Hollenhorst (1963)

	Non-ischemic central vein occlusion	Ischemic vein occlusion	Venous-stasis retinopathy
Age	Normal	Older adults	Older adults
Disc	Hyperemic, sometimes edematous	Disc edema	Pale disc, hemorrhages sharp border Disc neovascularization

cally enucleated eye after RONT and absolute secondary glaucoma due to rubeosis: RONT neither involved the adjacent sclera nor the retinal vessels. The authors could not find evidence for the above mentioned hypothetical mechanism of action. Horio et al. (2006) measured with video angiography and OCT the postoperative results after 1 week and 6 months in seven eyes with CVO and macular edema after RONT and ppVy. Dye dilution curves did not differ significantly in these seven eyes from the preoperative measurements, and chorioretinal anastomosis occurred in all eyes after 6 months. Kim et al. (2005) found no significant anatomical and functional differences between RONT and panretinal photocoagulation in 27 eyes. Wrede et al. (2006) concluded from histopathological studies and measurements that the cutting depth of RONT should at least be 1.45 mm, not taking into account the amount of papilledema in CVO. Randomized, controlled studies are surely needed to judge the value of this experimental intervention.

The desired surgical benefit is influenced by the amount of ischemia in the capillary bed and the amount of hemorrhage in the macula. Therefore an upstream relief by RONT in the area of the optic disc need not always result in an improvement in downstream perfusion and oxygenation in the perifoveal capillary bed. Finally, the juxtapapillary sclera – in front of the subarachnoidal space of the optic nerve – is less than half as thick as the rest of the sclera: theoretically an opening of the liquor-space may occur (Fig. 2.16c).

5.7.2.4
Congenital Pits of the Optic Nerve

Optic pits are associated with *large* optic discs and are found mostly temporally. Histology shows a defect in the lamina cribrosa, which is covered with collagen and dysplastic retina. Optic pits often lead to serous detachment of the macular retina and may be complicated by macular retinoschisis (*Kranenburg syndrome, KS*) (Fig. 5.7.12). The source of subretinal fluid is still a matter of debate. Direct flow from the arachnoidal space and failure of the retina-vessel barrier of the prelaminar capillaries in the dysplastic retina can be discussed. Postel, Johnson et al. (1998) provide clinical confirmation of a defect in tissue overlying cavitary optic disc anomalies and implied interconnections between the vitreous cavity, subarachnoid space, and subretinal space. They theorize that intermittent pressure gradi-

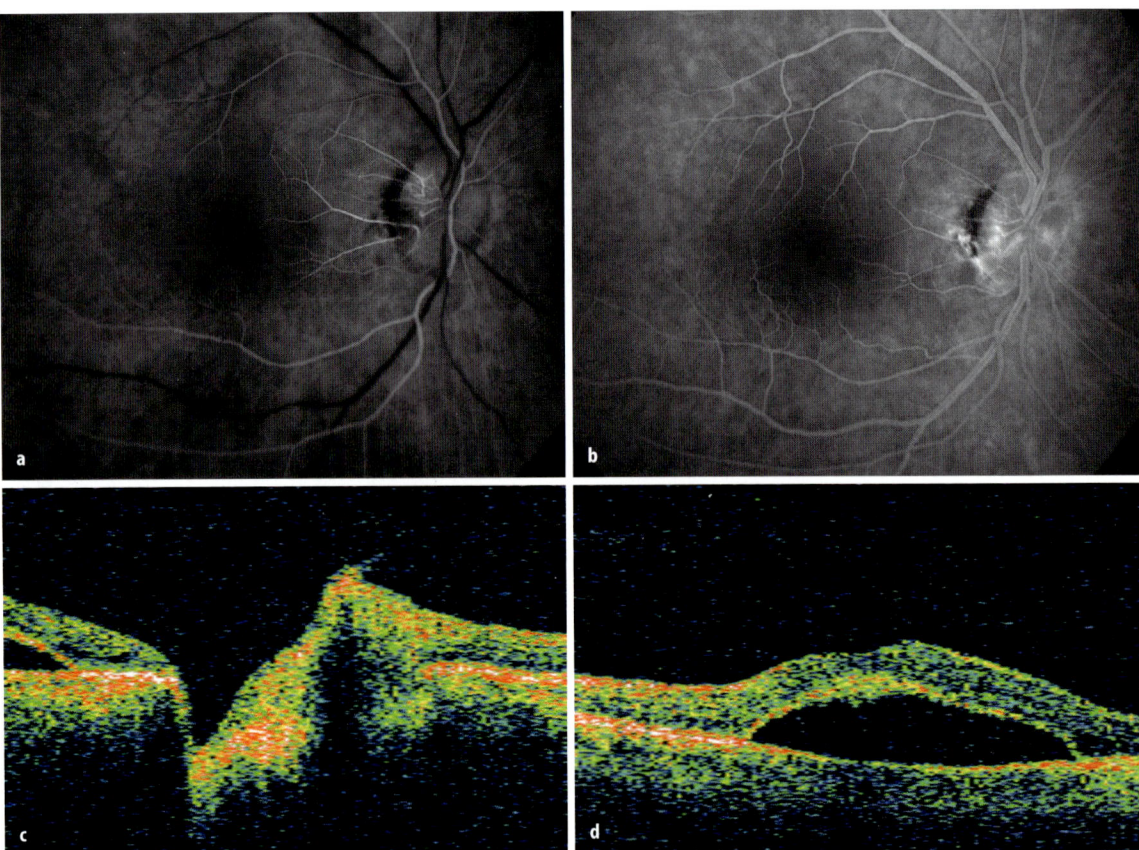

Fig. 5.7.12. Fluorescence angiography of a patient's fundus with Kranenburg's syndrome. Early (**a**) and late (**b**) phase showing the area of the pit (*dark*) and overlay of retinal, vascular anomaly and serous detachment of the retina. OCT showing a cross section through the optic disc (**c**): note the area of the pit and detached retina and detached fovea (**d**)

ents resulting from normal variations in intracranial pressure may play a critical role in the pathogenesis of retinopathy associated with cavitary disc anomalies (Fig. 5.7.12). The juxtapapillary sclera in front of the subarachnoidal space is very thin – loss of more than half of the scleral thickness elsewhere, approximately 200 µm (see above and Chapters 2 and 4).

5.7.2.4.1
Vitreoretinal Microsurgery

In optic pits and consecutive serous detachment of the retina (Annesley et al. 1987), ppVy can improve visual acuity by reattachment of the retina and avoid secondary, irreversible retinoschisis. ppVy includes posterior vitreous detachment, peeling of the internal limiting membrane and long acting gas tamponade (Hotta et al. 2004). By OCT imaging in optic disc pits, associated maculopathy tractional forces from the vitreous could be shown on the optic disc pit, and that vitrectomy with ILM peeling released this traction (Ishikawa et al. 2005; Konno et al. 2000). "Besides the exudative component of macular detachment, the vitreoretinal interface seems to play an underestimated role in the pathogenesis of maculopathy associated with optic pits. Tractional forces could explain the delay of macular detachment in young adulthood and the frequency of treatment failure after laser coagulation and gas tamponade. Pars plana vitrectomy with complete removal of all vitreoretinal adhesions should be a suitable technique in the treatment of macular detachment associated with optic pits" (Irvine et al. 1986; Gandorfer et al. 2000).

5.7.2.5
Tumors of the Optic Nerve

Tumors of the optic nerve (Table 5.7.9) may be primary or secondary, situated either prelaminar (intraocular) or retrobulbar and infiltrate the optic nerve head or the intraorbital nerve. Here loss of vision or visual field is not always a sign for malignancy (Fig. 5.7.13). The signs and symptoms may be a healthy disc and functional deficit (visual acuity and visual field, color vision), disc swelling with or without function loss and simple disc

Table 5.7.9. Tumors of the optic nerve

I. Prelaminar tumors (intraocular) of the disc
  1. Pigmented
      Melanocytoma
      Malignant melanoma of the choroid with overgrowth of the disc
      Pigment epithelial proliferation and neoplasia
  2. Non-pigmented
      Drusen (pseudotumors)
      Hamartoma, often associated with phakomatoses
      Real astrocytomas
      Retinoblastoma, invasive from neighboring retina
      Metastatic tumors and lymphomas of the disc
      Granulomatous inflammation, e.g., sarcoidosis

II. Retrobulbar tumors of the optic nerve
  1. Glioma (pilocytic astrocytoma)
  2. Meningioma
  3. Zimmerman choristoma
  4. Metastasis

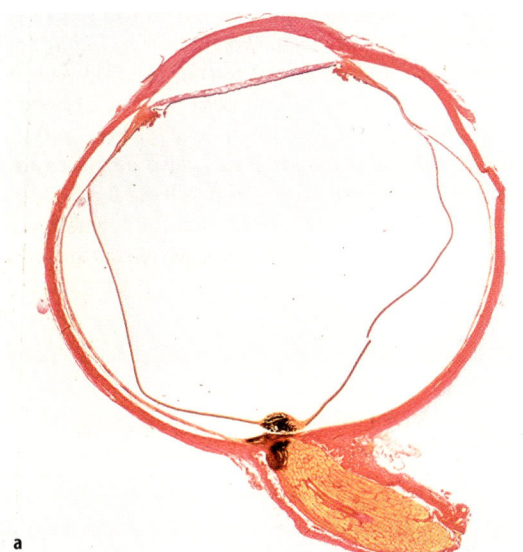
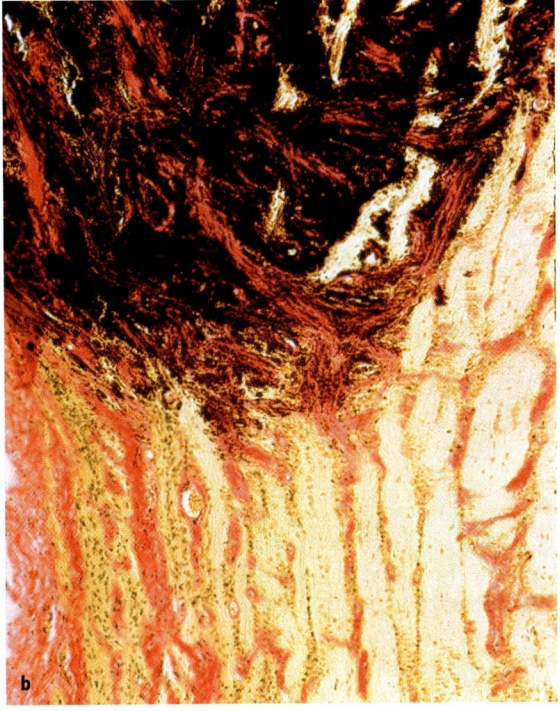

Fig. 5.7.13a, b. Melanocytoma of the optic disc within the optic nerve head. The eye was enucleated due to visual function – and field loss, mistaken for malignant melanoma of the optic disc. Histology reveals a densely pigmented melanocytoma consisting of benign tumor cells and corresponding focal optic nerve atrophy (case reported by Naumann, 1966)

Table 5.7.10. Clinical signs of the disc for optic nerve head involvement

Sign	Interpretation
Spontaneous venous pulse	Normal in 80% of population, pathologic if it disappears, when cranial pressure > 200 mm Hg
Asymmetric color of disc	Beginning of disc atrophy, one eyed pseudophakia
Hyperemic disc	Early sign for disc swelling
Nasally blurred disc margin	Early sign for disc swelling
Peripapillary hemorrhages	In the retinal nerve fiber layer, sign for disc swelling
Peripapillary cotton wool	In the retinal nerve fiber layer, among others in disc edema
Concentric lines around disc	Paton lines, sign for disc edema
Bilateral disc edema	Elevation of intracranial pressure, exclude drusen
Unilateral disc edema, and contralateral simple atrophy	Suspect Foster-Kennedy syndrome (frontal intracranial mass), exclude second eye with AION
Focal, juxtapapillary hemorrhage in retinal nerve fiber layer	Hemorrhagic microinfarct preceding sectorial RNF loss in early glaucoma

atrophy with loss of function (Table 5.7.10). *Pilocytic astrocytoma* (glioma) may even produce prominent optociliary shunt vessels due to chronic compression and venous outflow obstruction. Axial exophthalmus and secondary strabism due to sensory loss are extraocular signs. Very distal tumors may present late changes of the optic disc, such as swelling (elevation) or simple (descending) disc atrophy.

The main differential diagnoses for retrobulbar tumors in imaging (echography, MRI) are inflammatory, infiltrative processes, as in sarcoidosis, neuritis due to multiple sclerosis and infections with bacteria, viruses and fungi.

Tumors of the intraorbital optic nerve are managed together with neurosurgeons and demand differential diagnosis by the neuro-ophthalmologist and neuroradiologist.

Primary lesions infiltrating the optic disc are optic glioma (benign, malignant), ganglioglioma, hemangioma (capillary, cavernous), hemangioblastoma and rare others.

Secondary tumors are metastatic carcinoma, nasopharynx carcinoma, lymphoma (e.g., Burkitt) and leukemia. Echography, CT scan and MRI are mandatory prior to surgical management. Impending involvement of the optic chiasm is crucial to weigh indications for intervention in benign primary tumors.

5.7.2.6
Intracranial Hypertension: Acute and Chronic Variants Must Be Distinguished

5.7.2.6.1
Acute Intracranial Pressure Rise and Terson's Syndrome

Acute rise in intracranial pressure may develop with various rapidly expanding processes and lead earlier or later to disc edema (*Stauungspapille*). The most dramatic is Terson's syndrome in case of massive subarachnoidal hemorrhage.

The vitreoretinal surgeon is confronted with the problem of vitreous hemorrhage in *Terson's syndrome*. Here an *acute* rise of intracranial pressure as in subarachnoidal hemorrhage leads not only to uni- or bilateral intravitreal but also to subhyaloidal, subinternal limiting membrane hemorrhage (Friedmann et al. 1997). The pressure is also elevated in the subarachnoidal space of the optic nerve up to the sclera. Normally there is no anatomical connection between the subarachnoidal space and vitreous cavity. However, the juxtapapillary sclera behind Elschnig's spur is less than 250 µm thick (Fig. 2.16c). The intravitreal hemorrhage arises from the optic nerve head, probably by acute obstruction of the central retinal venous outflow. Bilateral hemorrhage presents a severe handicap for recovery in patient's with Terson's syndrome. Pars plana vitrectomy with removal of the hemorrhagic vitreous and internal limiting membrane of the retina may achieve fast visual rehabilitation (Kuhn et al. 1998) in persisting hemorrhages without spontaneous resorption. Later complications of this operation are cataract formation, retinal damage, endophthalmitis, and recurrence of hemorrhage. Formation of epiretinal membranes with secondary retinal traction was reported by Yokoi et al. (1997) and Tsai et al. (1995) if during ppVy a posterior vitreal detachment could not be achieved or was incomplete. It also appeared that multiple pathological processes involving the vitreoretinal interface were responsible for the formation of epiretinal membranes. These changes may also lead to a higher incidence of retinal ora tears during surgery (personal observations – C.M.).

5.7.2.6.2
Benign Intracranial Chronic Hypertension and Optic Disc Swelling (Pseudotumor Cerebri)

Optic disc swelling without loss of visual acuity and an enlarged blind spot are the clinical characteristics of optic disc involvement in benign intracranial hypertension, after localized expanding processes are ruled out. It must also be differentiated from disc edema due to neuritis and ischemic infarction (Table 5.7.11).

Table 5.7.11. Differential diagnosis of papilledema (*Stauungspapille*)

1. Expanding intracranial processes
2. Benign intracranial hypertension
3. Drusen of the optic disc
4. Terson's syndrome
5. Cavernous optic atrophy in acute glaucomas (Schnabel)-pseudocavernous optic atrophy in acute glaucomas due to silicone oil
6. Retinal vein occlusion
7. Papilledema due to myositis, borreliosis, encephalitis disseminata
8. Papilledema due to inflammation and orbital tumors

Fenestration of the Dural Sheath

The fenestration of the dural sheath of the optic nerve (ONSF) presents an alternative option to medical therapy to reduce pressure on the axonal tissue in patients with pseudotumor cerebri (PTC). By the performance of multiple slits in the dural sheath either by a nasal or temporal transconjunctival approach immediately behind the globe fluid of the arachnoidal space is directed into the orbit. A sudden relief of pressure of neuronal axons is achieved by creating a kind of filtration mechanism, leading to a resolution of papilledema and prevention of further vision loss. Even a unilateral ONSF was reported to relieve the contralateral side via the optic chiasm. Seiff et al. (1990) showed in an optic nerve model that when one nerve was fenestrated, fluid flow along the nerve was initiated and pressure in that nerve sheath dropped substantially. Pressure in the unfenestrated sheath dropped due to fluid communication across the chiasm. These lower intrasheath pressures were consistent with the bilateral resolution of papilledema after unilateral fenestration. As the underlying pathogenesis is not treated and wound healing of the dura sheaths may prevent long-term filtration, 80% of ONSF treated patients showed recurrent papilledema after 6 years (Seiff et al. 1990).

Tsai et al. (1995) showed in two autopsy eyes that "histopathological and ultrastructural examination of the tissue revealed fibroblasts localized to the sites of fenestration. Adipose tissue was also adherent to the optic nerve pia in areas of incised dura. *No patent fistula site was observed.*"

Corbett et al. (1989) showed that in patients suffering from visual field deterioration and PTC ventriculoperitoneal shunting was as effective as ONSF. Therefore weight reduction, oral treatment with carboanhydrase inhibitors and ventriculoperitoneal shunting provide a safe and efficient alternative. In ischemic optic neuropathy (AION) ONSF was shown to be not of any benefit. Glaser et al. (1994) showed no beneficial effect on visual morbidity in the common ischemic optic neuropathy. In the light of the pathogenesis of AION it seems logical that a relief of intraneural pressure will not show functional improvement, as it is caused by occlusion of the posterior short ciliary arteries and ischemic infarcts of the disc and not by elevated intracranial pressure.

5.7.3
Wound Healing and Complications

5.7.3.1
Pseudocavernous Optic Neuropathy

Pseudocavernous optic neuropathy in silicone oil filled eyes. Silicone oil filled eyes with acute glaucomas can develop an acute ischemic infarction of the optic nerve head: as the vitreous with hyaluronic acid has been removed silicone oil invades the necrotic disc and nerve. Thus one potential complication of ppVy with silicone oil is this pseudocavernous optic neuropathy. Here necrotic axonal tissues after ischemic infarction due to elevated intraocular pressures after surgery lead to a multiple silicone oil vacuoles or silicone oil filled macrophages in the prelaminar and retrolaminar optic nerve in analogy to Schnabel's optic neuropathy. Apoplexia of the optic nerve with arteritic or non-arteritic origin has been described to be the prerequisite. The course is an initial swelling of the optic nerve head, necrosis of axonal tissue and glaucomatous cupping. Silicone oil may even reach the cerebral ventricles. This case has been shown in an eye after ppVy due to retinal cytomegalo infection in HIV with highly elevated intraocular pressure (IOP) over months (Eller et al. 2000).

5.7.3.2
Radiation Opticoneuropathy

Radiation opticoneuropathy (RONP) may develop as a side effect of radiation therapy of intraocular and extraocular tumors. This may appear months or years after radiation therapy being the result of a radiation arteriopathy of the retrobulbar vessels (Fig. 5.7.14), leading to ischemic disorder of the optic nerve (Knorr, Heindl, data in publication). The total dose and fractionation of the radiation influences the risk of the delayed necrosis of nerve tissue. The risk of RONP seems to appear at doses of over 50 Gy and the tolerance level appears to be 50–55 Gy. RONP is seen in eyes with external beam or plaque radiation of intraocular tumors, orbital, sinus or brain tumors. The affected disc shows swelling, cotton-wool spots (microinfarction) and exudative retinopathy. Early recognition, treatment and follow-up may be facilitated by measuring the blood-ocular barrier breakdown by laser tyndallometry.

The surgical procedures by the ophthalmologist in the area of the optic disc and the orbital part of the optic nerve are limited. This has its reason mainly in the lack of regeneration of the highly differentiated axons.

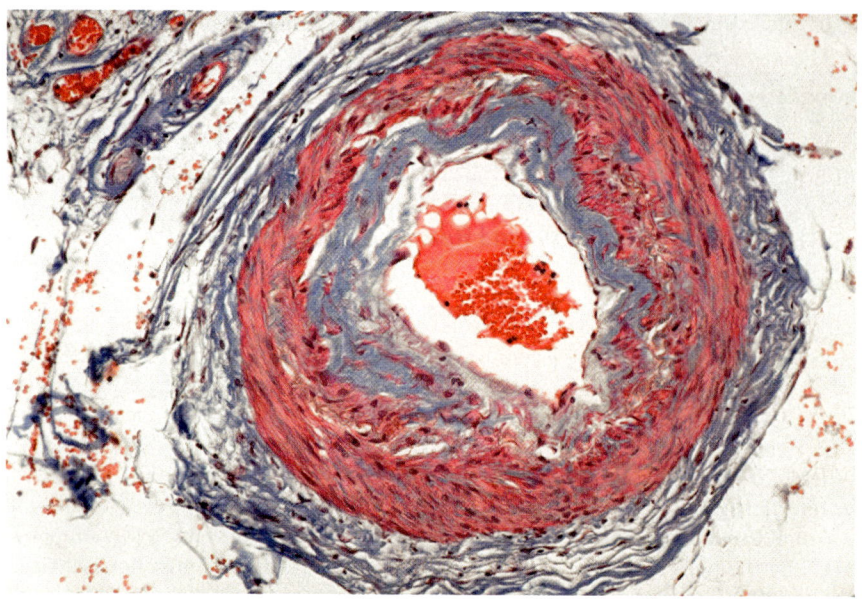

Fig. 5.7.14. Radiation arteriopathy: cross section through a posterior ciliary artery (Masson trichrome) 2 years after radiation of an ethmoidal and maxillary cell carcinoma, resulting in an ischemic ophthalmopathy. Note the irregular wall thickening, narrowed lumen with thrombosis, and concentric myointimal proliferation

Latest results of Heiduschka, Thanos and colleagues (2005) show that, at least in cats, under certain circumstances the regeneration of axons in a crash model of the optic nerve can be demonstrated.

We have tried to sketch the basic principles of anatomy and pathology of the optic nerve in the context of ocular and non-ocular diseases.

References (see also page 379)

Annesley W, Brown G, Bolling J, Goldberg R, Fisher D. Treatment of retinal detachment with congenital optic pit by krypton laser photocoagulation. Graefes Arch Clin Exp Ophthalmol 1987. 225;5: 311–314

Brodsky MC. Morning glory disc anomaly or optic disc coloboma? Arch Ophthalmol 1994. 112;2: 153

Burk RO, Rendon R. Clinical detection of optic nerve damage. Surv Ophthalmol 2004. 45;3: 297–303

Cohen AI. Is there a potential defect in the blood retinal barrier at the choroidal level of the optic nerve canal? Invest Ophthal 1973; 12: 513

Corbett JJ, Thompson HS. The rational management of idiopathic intracranial hypertension. Arch Neurol 1989. 46; 10: 1049–1051

Dichtl A, Jonas JB, Holbach L, Naumann GOH. Retinal nerve fiber layer thickness in human eyes. Graefes Arch Clin Exp Ophthalmol 1999. 237; 6: 474–479

Eller AW, Friberg TL, Mah F. Migration of silicone oil into the brain. Am J Ophthalmol 2002; 133: 429-438

Evans JM, Batts KP, Hunder GG. Persistent giant cell arteritis despite corticosteroid treatment. Mayo Clin Proc 1994. 69;11: 1060–1061

Friedmann SM, Margo CE. Bilateral subinternal limiting membrane hemorrhage with Terson syndrome. Am J Ophthalmol 1997. 124;6: 850–851

Gandorfer A, Kampik A. Role of vitreoretinal interface in the pathogenesis and therapy of macular disease associated with optic pits. Ophthalmologe 2000. 97; 4: 276–279

Glaser JS, Teimory M, Schatz NJ. Optic nerve sheath fenestration for progressive optic neuropathy. Results in second series consisting of 21 eyes. Arch Ophthalmol 1994. 112;8: 1047–1050

Green WR, Chan CC, Hutchins GM, Terry JM. Central vein occlusion: A prospective histopathologic study of 29 eyes in 28 cases. Retina 1981. 1;1: 27–55

Heiduschka P, Fischer D, Thanos S. Recovery of visual evoked potentials after regeneration of cut ganglion cell axons within the ascending visual pathway in rats. Restorative Neurology and Neuroscience 2005. 23; 5–6: 303–312

Hinzpeter EN, Naumann GOH. Ischemic papilledema in giant cell arteriitis. Mucopolysaccharide deposition with normal intraocular pressure. Arch Ophthalmol 1976; 94: 624–628

Horio N, Horiguchi M. Retinal blood flow and macular edema after radial optic neurotomy for central retinal vein occlusion. Am J Ophthalmol 2006. 141;1: 31–34

Hotta K. Unsuccessful vitrectomy without gas tamponade for macular retinal detachment and retinoschisis without optic disc pit. Ophthalmic Surg Lasers Imaging. 2004 Jul-Aug;35(4):328–31

Irvine AR, Crawford JB, Sullivan JH. The pathogenesis of retinal detachment with morning glory discs and pit. Retina 1986. 6; 3: 146–150

Ishikawa K, Terasaki H, Mori M, Sugita K, Miyake Y. OCT before and after vitrectomy with internal limiting membrane removal in a child with optic pit maculopathy. Jpn J Ophthalmol 2005. 49;5: 411–413

Jacobs DS, Foster CS. Temporal arteriitis. In: Alber DM, Jacobiec FA (eds) Principles and practice of ophthalmology, vol.5. Philadelphia: Saunders 1994; 2901–2908

Jonas JB, Berenshtein E, Holbach L. Lamina cribrosa thickness and spatial relationships between intraocular space and cerebrospinal fluid space in highly myopic eyes. Invest Ophthalmol Vis Sci 2004. 45;8: 2660–2665

Jonas JB, Naumann GOH. The optic nerve: Its embryology, histology and morphology. In: Varma R, Spaeth GL (eds) The optic nerve in glaucoma. Philadelphia: Lippincott 1993; pp 3–26

Jonas JB, Schmidt AM, Müller-Bergh JA, Schlötzer-Schrehardt UM, Naumann GOH. Human optic nerve fiber count and optic disc size. Invest Ophthalmol Vis Sci 1992. 33; 6: 2012–2018

Kearns TP, Hollenhorst RW. Venous stasis retinopathy of occlusive disease of the carotid artery. Majo Clinic Proc 1963;38:304

Kim TW, Lee SJ, Kim SD. Comparative evaluation of radial optic neurotomy and panretinal photo coagulation in the management of central vein occlusion. Korean J Ophthalmol 2005. 19;4: 269–274

Konno S, Akiba J, Sato E, Kuriyama S, Yoshida A. OCT in successful surgery of retinal detachment associated with optic nerve head pit. Ophthalmic Surg Lasers 2000. 31; 3: 236–239

Kubota T, Holbach L, Naumann GOH. Corpora amylacea in glaucomatous and non-glaucomatous optic nerve and retina. Graefes Arch Clin Exp Ophthalmol 1993. 231;1: 7–11

Kubota T, Jonas JB, Naumann GOH. Direct clinico-histological correlation of parapapillary chorioretinal atrophy. Br J Ophthalmol 1993. 77; 2: 103–106

Kuhn F, Morris R, Witherspoon CD, Mester V. Terson syndrome. Results of vitrectomy and the significance of vitreous hemorrhage in patients with subarachnoid hemorrhage. Ophthalmology 1998. 105;3: 472–477

Lippe von der I, Wuermeling MJ, Naumann GOH. Akute druckabhängige Veränderungen des neuroretinalen Randsaums in einer juvenilen Glaukompapille – Messungen mittels Laser Scanning Tomographie und planimetrischer Papillometrie. Klin Monatsbl Augenheilkd 1994; 204:126–130

Naumann GOH, Mardin CY, Bergua A. Bedeutung und Perspektive der Glaukom-Mikrozirkulationsforschung. Klin Monatsbl Augenheilkd 1993; 203: 286

Naumann GOH. Benign melanocytoma of the optic nerve papilla. Doc Ophthalmol. 1966;20: 468–483

Okinami S, Ohkuma M, Tsukahara I. Kuhnt intermediary tissue as a barrier between the optic nerve and retina. Albrecht v Graefes Arch klin exp Ophthal 1977; 201: 57

Opremcak EM, Rehmar AJ, Ridenour CD, Kurz DE. Radial optic neurotomy for central retinal vein occlusion: 117 consecutive cases. Retina 2006. 26;3: 297–305

Postel EA, Pulido JS, McNamara JA, Johnson MW. The etiology and treatment of macular detachment associated with optic nerve pits and related anomalies. Trans Am Ophthalmol Soc 1998; 96:73–88

Quigley HA. The pathogenesis of reversible cupping in congenital glaucoma. Am J Ophthalmol 1977;84:358

Richardson KT, Shaffer RN. Optic nerve cupping in congenital glaucoma. Am J Ophthalmol 1966;62:507

Risco JM, Grimson BS, Johnson PT. Angioarchitecture of the ciliary artery circulation of the posterior pole. Arch Ophthalmol 1981. 99; 5: 864–868

Seiff SR, Shah L. A model for the mechanism of optic nerve fenestration. Arch Ophthalmol 1990. 108; 9: 1326–1329

Sharma T, Gopal L, Biswas J, Shanmugam MP, Bhende PS, Agrawal R, Shetty NS, Sanduja N. Results of vitrectomy in Terson's syndrome. Ophthalmic Surg Lasers 2002. 33;3: 195–199

Traboulsi EI, O'Neill JF. The spectrum in the morphology of the so called morning glory disc anomaly. J Pediatr Ophthalmol Strabismus 1988. 25;2: 93–98

Tsai JC, Petrovich MS, Sadun AA. Histopathological and ultrastructural examination of optic nerve sheath decompression. Br J Ophthalmol 1995. 79;2: 182–185

Vogel A, Holz G, Loeffler KU. Histopathologic findings after radial optic neurotomy in central retinal vein occlusion. Am J Ophthalmol 2006. 141;1: 203–205

Wenkel H, Michelson G. Korrelation der Ultraschallbiomikroskopie mit histologischen Befunden in der Diagnostik der Riesenzellarteriitis. Klin Monatsbl Augenheilkd 1996; 210: 48–52

Wenkel H, Naumann GOH. Retrolaminäre Infiltration des Nervus opticus durch als intraokulare Tamponade verwendetes Silikonöl. Klin Monatsbl Augenheilkd 1999; 214: 120–122

Wietholter S, Steube D, Stotz HP. Terson syndrome: A frequently missed ophthalmologic complication in subarachnoid hemorrhage. Zentrabl Neurochir 1998. 59;3: 166–170

Wrede J, Varadi G, Volcker HE, Dithmar S. Radial optic neurotomy for central retinal vein occlusion – how deep should it be. Ophthalmologe 2006. 103; 4: 321–324

Yokoi M, Kase M, Hyodo T, Horimoto M, Kitagawa F, Nagata R. Epiretinal membrane formation in Terson's syndrome. Jpn J Ophthalmol 1997. 41;3: 168–173

6 Influence of Common Generalized Diseases on Intraocular Microsurgery

G.O.H. Naumann, U. Schlötzer-Schrehardt

Most generalized diseases lead to manifestations also in the ocular tissues. In this chapter we shall briefly review the intraocular consequences of the following common generalized diseases of relevance for ocular microsurgery: (1) diabetes mellitus, (2) arterial hypertension and "vis a tergo," (3) pseudoexfoliation syndrome (PEX) and its intraocular and systemic manifestations andcomplications, (4) infectious diseases, and (5) hematologic disorders. – The intraocular pathology of PEX shall be reviewed in more detail because of its significantly increased risks for intra- and postoperative complications.

In addition, neurologic diseases, e.g., multiple sclerosis and Parkinson's disease, and muscular problems like myotonic dystrophy and endocrine orbitopathy as manifestations of thyroid disease require the conscious cooperation of the entire surgical team, anesthesiologist and their consultants.

Diabetes Mellitus

G.O.H. Naumann

This very common metabolic disorder currently affects 170 million people and will concern an estimated 370 million people by 2030. Not only the population in the industrialized part of the world but particularly the inhabitants in the low- and middle-income countries are suffering from this "pandemic." More than 75% of those suffering from diabetes mellitus for over 20 years will have some sort of retinopathy. "Metabolic control matters!" Well controlled glucose and Hb1Ac levels are most important for the prevention or delayed onset of the late microangiopathy involving the sensory retina, kidney and peripheral nerves. Proper medical therapy can reduce the risk of blindness and moderate vision loss significantly, but does not totally prevent it.

The following manifestations are of particular significance for the ophthalmic microsurgeon.

6.1.1 Diabetic Retinopathy

Retinopathia diabetic simplex involves the capillaries of the sensory retina by formation of microaneurysms due to loss of pericytes and finally capillary occlusion. The resulting hypoxic and ischemic areas in the sensory retina induce release of vasoproliferative factors leading to preretinal proliferating retinopathy and to rubeosis iridis and cyclitic membrane (see Chapters 2, 5.6). Awareness of such neovascularization is necessary, particularly in open eye surgery.

6.1.2 Diabetic Iridopathy

Persisting glucose levels above 200 mg% lead to accumulation of glycogen in the pigment epithelium of the iris (Fig. 5.3.7). These ballooned cells are often an obstacle for satisfactory mydriasis for diagnostics and laser therapy. Glycogen deposits in the iris pigment epithelium make it friable and during iris movements cause rupture and induce *secondary melanin granule dispersion syndrome* (Tables 5.3.1, 5.3.3, 5.3.11) and melanin phagocytosis in the corneal and trabecular endothelium. The multifocal loss of melanin leads to the appearance of a "starry sky" on retroillumination. Ruptured cell bodies of the iris pigment epithelium pose a risk for posterior synechiae. Melanin granules are also phagocytized by the corneal endothelium, which may induce heat damage during laser coagulation of the retinal periphery or trabeculoplasty (see 5.2).

6.1.3 Recurrent Corneal Erosions

Markedly thickened basement membranes of the corneal epithelium and decreased corneal sensitivity from diabetic neuropathy loosen the hemidesmosomes of the corneal epithelium with an increased risk of recurrent erosions. This concerns not only patients wearing contact lenses but also all diagnostic or therapeutic manipulations of the corneal surface during microsurgery. In view of the risks of bacterial infections from blepharitis and increased bacterial contamination of the tear film, the risk of complicating bacterial ulcers of the cornea is a real threat (see Chapter 5.1).

6.1.4 Cataracts

Diabetic cataract in *juvenile* diabetes: They present the pathognomic "snowflake" phenotype (Fig. 5.5.20).

Earlier Manifestation of Age-Related Cataracts in Adult Onset Diabetes

The mechanisms of this common entity are poorly understood. Secondary cataract after extracapsular cataract extraction (ECCE) seems to be less frequent than, e.g., in pseudoexfoliation (PEX) syndrome (see Chapter 5.5; 6.3; Küchle et al., 1997).

6.1.5
Risk of Infection

Bacterial and mycotic colonization of the lid margins and accessory glands of the lid pose an increased risk of intra- and postoperative infection and endophthalmitis.

Arterial Hypertension and "Vis A Tergo"

G.O.H. Naumann

Intraoperative control of arterial blood pressure and choice of anesthesia are particularly relevant in wide open eye surgery (see Chapter 2 and 4).

Uncontrolled arterial hypertension is associated with an increased risk of spontaneous and intra-/postoperative hemorrhage in all organs. An important distinguishing feature of intraocular versus extraocular surgery includes the forward movement of the iris lens diaphragm by increased blood filling of the choroid – "*vis a tergo*" – with any opening of the eye as soon as the intraocular pressure falls. In its extreme expression as expulsive hemorrhage it may lead to loss of the eye (see Chapter 2). Prevention of such potential catastrophic complications is of the utmost importance: During the phase of the open eye the systemic arterial blood pressure should be well controlled and ideally should be around 100 mm Hg systolic in demanding and difficult intraocular surgery, e.g., block excision and penetrating corneal grafts (see Chapters 5.1, 5.4).

Preexisting arterial hypertension requires close cooperation with the internist and anesthesiology team to evaluate the individual situation.

6.3 Pseudoexfoliation Syndrome: Pathological Manifestations of Relevance to Intraocular Surgery

U. Schlötzer-Schrehardt, G.O.H. Naumann

6.3.1
Introduction

Pseudoexfoliation* (PEX) syndrome is a common age-related, although often overlooked disorder that predisposes to a number of conditions requiring intraocular surgery, most notably cataract and glaucomas but also corneal endothelial decompensation. It has been estimated that the number of people with PEX syndrome in the world varies between 60 and 100 million (Ritch and Schlötzer-Schrehardt 2001). With a rising mean age not only in western populations, PEX syndrome is increasing in prevalence, although it is not an integral part of ageing but represents a distinct clinical entity (Naumann et al. 1998). PEX syndrome is presently acknowledged as the most common identifiable cause of open-angle glaucoma, accounting for the majority of glaucoma in some countries and for about 25% of all open-angle glaucomas worldwide (Ritch 1994a). The condition is characterized by an abnormal turnover of extracellular matrix material resulting in the deposition of an abnormal fibrillar substance (PEX material) in virtually all tissues of the anterior segment of the eye (Naumann et al. 1998). Despite its clinical significance and extensive research, the precise etiology and pathogenesis of PEX syndrome remain unclear; however, there is evidence for a genetic basis of the disease (Damji et al. 1998; Orr et al. 2001).

Although concepts of PEX are often dominated by its association with chronic open-angle glaucoma and by the visible changes on the anterior lens capsule (Lindberg 1989) depicted by Vogt almost 100 years ago (Vogt 1925), lens capsule involvement is only one aspect of the various ocular manifestations of PEX syndrome (Naumann et al. 1998). There is also direct in situ involvement of the ciliary body and zonular apparatus, the juxtacanalicular and trabecular tissue, the corneal endothelium, and virtually all cell populations of the iris, predisposing to a number of intraocular complications including phacodonesis and lens subluxation, pupillary block angle-closure glaucoma, melanin dispersion, insufficient mydriasis, blood-aqueous barrier dysfunction and pseudouveitis, anterior segment hypoxia, posterior synechiae as well as corneal endothelial decompensation (Table 6.3.1) (Naumann et al. 1998; Ritch and Schlötzer-Schrehardt 2001).

The pathological changes also explain the spectrum of complications that occur in association with intraocular surgery on PEX patients (Table 6.3.1). At our institution, approximately 15% of patients undergoing cataract surgery and 40% of patients undergoing glaucoma filtering surgery have PEX. In relation to these procedures, numerous studies have reported a wide range of intra- and postoperative complications including zonular dehiscence, vitreous loss, posterior capsular rupture, intraocular hemorrhage, corneal endothelial failure, postoperative inflammation and intraocular pressure spikes, secondary cataract, and luxation of intraocular lens implants (Naumann et al. 1988; Küchle et al. 1997).

Moreover, recent evidence indicates that the ocular features of PEX syndrome are actually only one facet of a broader systemic process, since typical PEX material deposits have been identified in the skin and in connective tissue portions of various visceral organs including lungs, kidney, gallbladder, liver and heart (Schlötzer-Schrehardt et al. 1992; Streeten et al. 1992). Although the clinical consequences of these systemic deposits await further clarification, PEX syndrome has been repeatedly associated with cardiovascular and cerebrovascular disease, such as aneurysms of the abdominal aorta, transient ischemic attacks, and a history of angina pectoris, hypertension, myocardial infarction or stroke (Mitchell et al. 1997; Schumacher et al. 2001).

---

* The current terminology is very unsatisfactory. The term "exfoliation" implies a "minus" of tissue as it really occurs in "glassblowers' cataract" (infrared exposure lens capsule exfoliation). "Pseudoexfoliation" is the correct ophthalmopathologic description for the newly produced material (a "plus") deposited on the intact lens capsule and other structures of the anterior segment. However, to use the prefix "pseudo" for a serious and common entity may appear misleading. We suggest to use both terms to sustain awareness that details are important to understand the manifestations and complications. A new nomenclature will be suggested as soon as we better understand the etiology and pathogenesis of this puzzling entity.

Table 6.3.1. Diagnosis of early stages, and clinical and surgical complications of pseudoexfoliation (PEX) syndrome

Tissue involvement	Early clinical signs	Clinical complications	Surgical complications
Lens, ciliary body and zonules (phakopathy, cyclopathy, zonulopathy)	Diffuse precapsular layer Phacodonesis PEX deposits on zonules (UBM)	Cataract (nuclear) Zonular instability Phacodonesis Lens (sub)luxation Angle closure glaucoma due to pupillary and ciliary block	Zonular rupture/dialysis Vitreous loss Posterior capsule rupture Decentration of the lens implant Anterior capsule fibrosis Secondary cataract
Iris (iridopathy)	Peripupillary atrophy and iris sphincter region transillumination Melanin dispersion associated with pupillary dilation Poor mydriasis, asymmetric pupil sizes	Melanin dispersion Poor mydriasis Iris rigidity Capillary hemorrhage Blood-aqueous barrier defects, pseudouveitis Anterior chamber hypoxia Posterior synechiae	Miosis/poor surgical access Intra- and postoperative hyphema Postoperative inflammation Prolonged blood-aqueous barrier breakdown Posterior synechiae and pupillary block Postoperative IOP rise
Trabecular meshwork (trabeculopathy)	Pigment deposition Marked asymmetry of IOP Marked IOP rise after pupillary dilation	Intraocular hypertension Open-angle glaucoma	Postoperative IOP rise
Cornea (keratopathy)	Atypical cornea guttata	Reduced endothelial cell count Endothelial decompensation Endothelial migration/proliferation	Endothelial decompensation
Posterior segment		Central retinal vein occlusion	

IOP intraocular pressure, *UBM* ultrasound biomicroscopy

Hyperhomocysteinemia has been suggested as one possible cause for an increased vascular risk in PEX patients (Vessani et al. 2003; Bleich et al. 2004). However, the mortality rate appears not to be increased in PEX patients (Shrüm et al. 2000). Other investigators reported on an association of PEX syndrome and hearing loss or Alzheimer's disease.

6.3.2
Pathobiology of PEX Syndrome

The exact pathogenesis of PEX syndrome is still not known. However, the pathologic process is characterized by the progressive accumulation of an abnormal fibrillar matrix product, which is either the result of an excessive production and/or an insufficient breakdown, and which is regarded as pathognomonic for the disease based on its unique light microscopic and ultrastructural criteria (Fig. 6.3.1a–d) (Naumann et al. 1998; Ritch and Schlötzer-Schrehardt 2001). The characteristic fibrils, which are composed of microfibrillar subunits resembling elastic microfibrils (Fig. 6.3.1e), contain predominantly epitopes of elastic fibers, such as elastin, tropoelastin, amyloid P, vitronectin, and components of elastic microfibrils, such as fibrillin-1, microfibril-associated glycoprotein MAGP-1, and the latent TGF-β binding proteins LTBP-1 and LTPB-2 (Fig. 6.3.1f). These immunohistochemical and recent molecular biologic data, confirming an overexpression of fibrillin-1 and LTBP-1/2 mRNA in most cell types involved (Schlötzer-Schrehardt et al. 2001; Zenkel et al. 2005), give strong support to the elastic microfibril theory of pathogenesis, which explains PEX syndrome as a type of elastosis affecting elastic microfibrils (Streeten 1993). The PEX fibrils appear to be multifocally produced by various intra- and extraocular cell types including the preequatorial lens epithelium, nonpigmented ciliary epithelium, trabecular endothelium, corneal endothelium, vascular endothelial cells, and virtually all cell types in the iris, by active fibrillogenesis involving all anterior segment tissues (Figs. 6.3.1g, h, 6.3.2). This fibrillogenesis is accompanied by a destruction of the normal extracellular matrix of the cells, normally represented by their basement membrane, and is followed by a degeneration of the cells involved due to a disturbed cell-matrix interaction (degenerative fibrillopathy).

The currently acknowledged pathogenetic concept describes PEX syndrome as a specific type of a stress-induced elastosis, an elastic microfibrillopathy, associated with the excessive production of elastic microfibrils and their aggregation into typical PEX fibrils by a variety of potentially elastogenic cells in intra- and extraocular locations (Ritch and Schlötzer-Schrehardt 2001; Ritch et al. 2003; Schlötzer-Schrehardt and Nau-

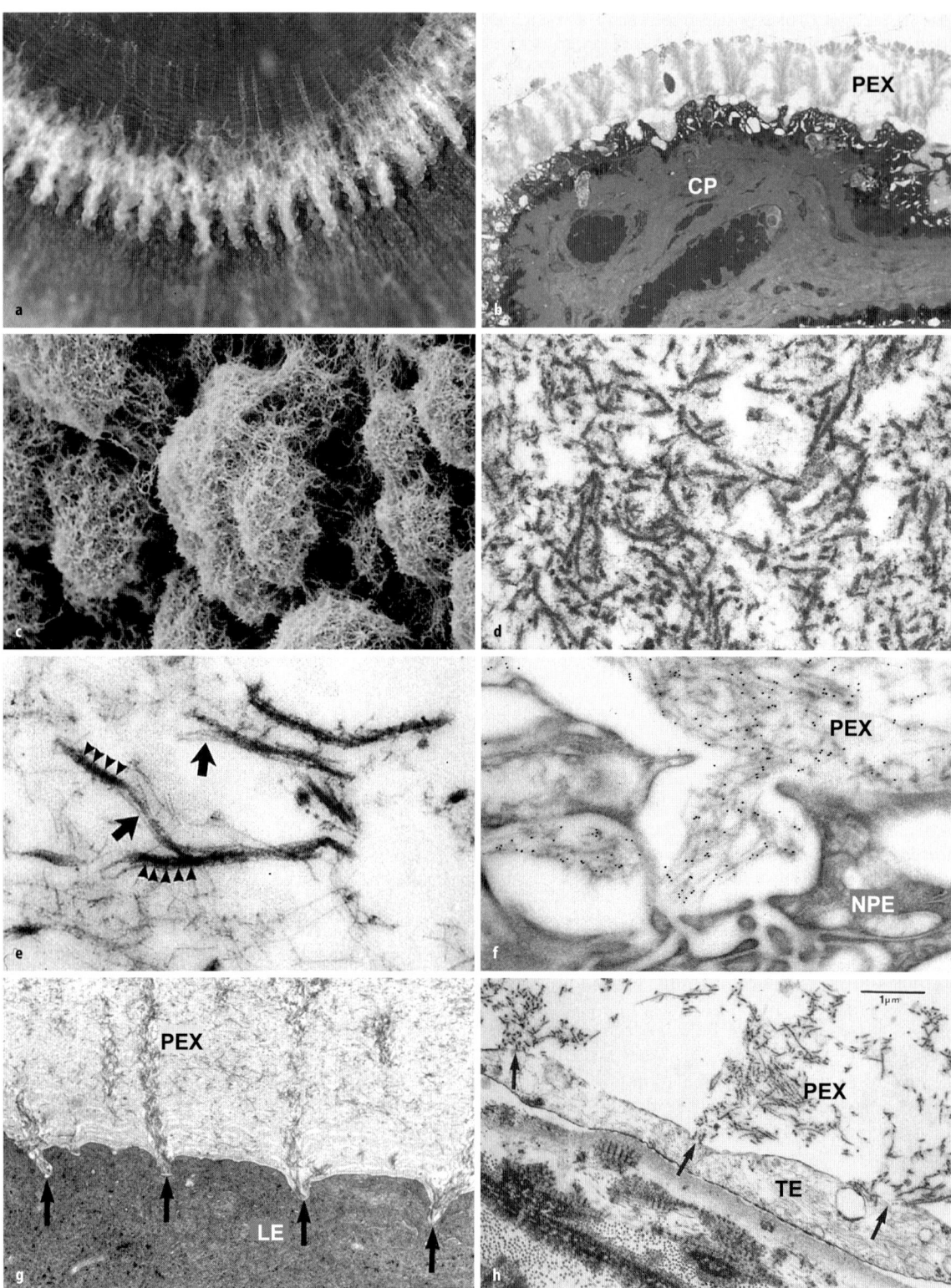

Fig. 6.3.1. Light and electron micrographs showing structure and origin of PEX material. **a** Macroscopic appearance of PEX deposits on ciliary processes and zonules. **b** Bush-like, feathery *PEX* deposits on ciliary process (*CP*) by light microscopy (toluidine blue, ×400). **c** Scanning electron micrograph of PEX deposits. **d** Ultrastructure of PEX fibrils. **e** Aggregation of microfibrils (*arrows*) into mature PEX fibrils showing cross-bands at 50 nm (*arrowheads*). **f** Immunogold labeling using antibodies against fibrillin-1 showing clear association of the gold marker with *PEX* fibrils emerging from a nonpigmented ciliary epithelial cell (*NPE*). **g** Intracapsular *PEX* fibrils emerging from pits (*arrows*) in the preequatorial lens epithelium (*LE*). **h** Apparent production of *PEX* fibrils (*arrows*) by a trabecular endothelial cell (*TE*)

mann 2006). Growth factors, particularly TGF-β1, increased cellular and oxidative stress, but also the stable aggregation of misfolded stressed proteins, appear to be involved in this fibrotic process. Due to an imbalance of matrix metalloproteinases (MMPs) and their inhibitors TIMPs and extensive cross-linking processes involved in PEX fiber formation, the newly formed material is not properly degraded but progressively accumulates within the tissues over time with potentially deleterious effects.

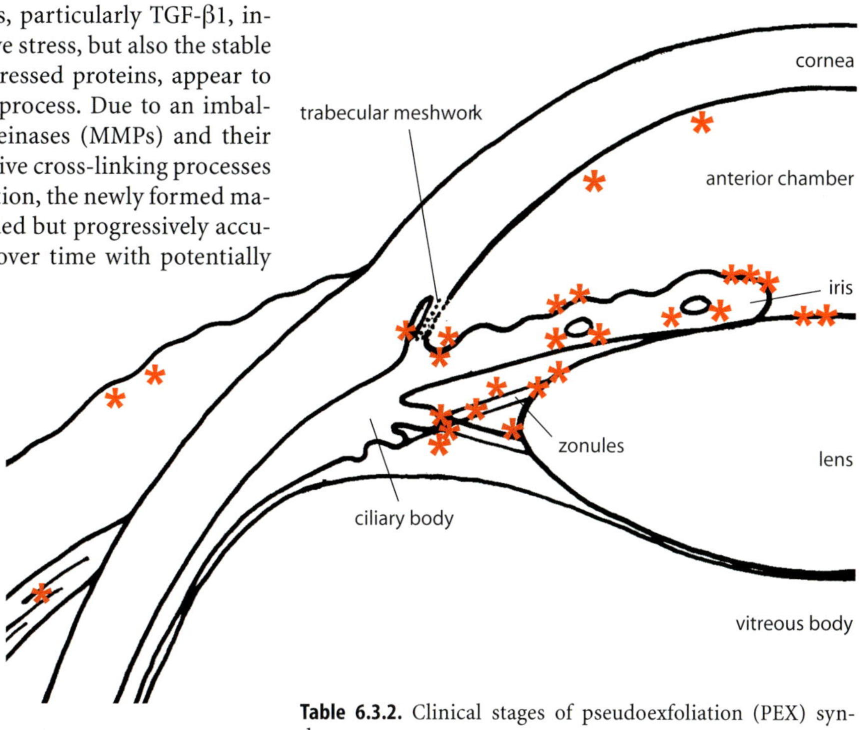

Fig. 6.3.2. Schematic representation of anterior segment tissues involved in active production and subsequent deposition of PEX material (*)

In a recent landmark study, polymorphisms in the lysyl oxidase-like 1 (*LOXL1*) gene located on chromosome 15q24 have been shown to be associated with PEX syndrome and PEX glaucoma in two Scandinavian populations (Thorleifsson et al., 2007). LOXL1 is a member of the lysyl oxidase familiy of enzymes that are necessary for the stabilizaton of elastic fibers by cross-linking tropoelastin molecules to mature elastin. These genetic variants may contribute to the elastotic process characteristic of PEX syndrome.

6.3.3
Clinical Diagnosis and Early Recognition

Several clinical stages of PEX syndrome can be recognized (Table 6.3.2, Fig. 6.3.3).

6.3.3.1
Manifest PEX Syndrome

The most important diagnostic criteria of PEX syndrome are the whitish flake-like deposits of PEX material on anterior segment structures, particularly on the anterior lens surface (Fig. 6.3.4a, b) and the pupillary margin (Fig. 6.3.4c, d), occasionally also on the posterior surface of the cornea (Fig. 6.3.4e), on the surface of intraocular lens implants, and on the anterior vitreous face in aphakic eyes. The characteristic target-shaped pattern on the lens, consisting of a rather homogeneous central disc, an intermediate clear zone, and a peripheral granular zone, can be only seen after pupillary dilation (Fig. 6.3.4a). In routine examinations without pupillary dilation, the diagnosis may be easily missed, because the central disc may be very subtle or even absent in 20–50% of cases (Fig. 6.3.4b). However, the ma-

Table 6.3.2. Clinical stages of pseudoexfoliation (PEX) syndrome

Suspect
Early PEX (precapsular diffuse dewy layer on anterior lens surface)
"Masked PEX" (posterior synechiae without other obvious cause)

Definite
"Mini-PEX" (focal defects in precapsular layer, mostly nasal superiorly)
Manifest PEX (characteristic target-like pattern of PEX material deposition)

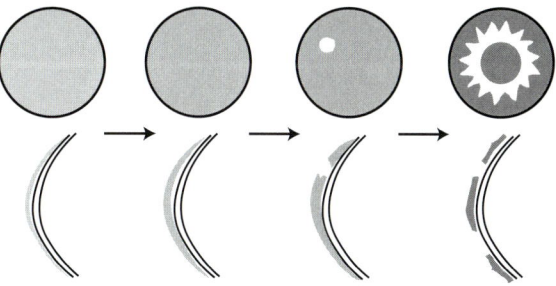

Preclinical stage (clinically invisible) | "Suspected PEX" (precapsular layer) | "Mini-PEX" (focal defect) | "Manifest PEX" (target pattern)

Fig. 6.3.3. Schematic representation of clinical classification of PEX syndrome based on morphologic alterations of the anterior lens surface

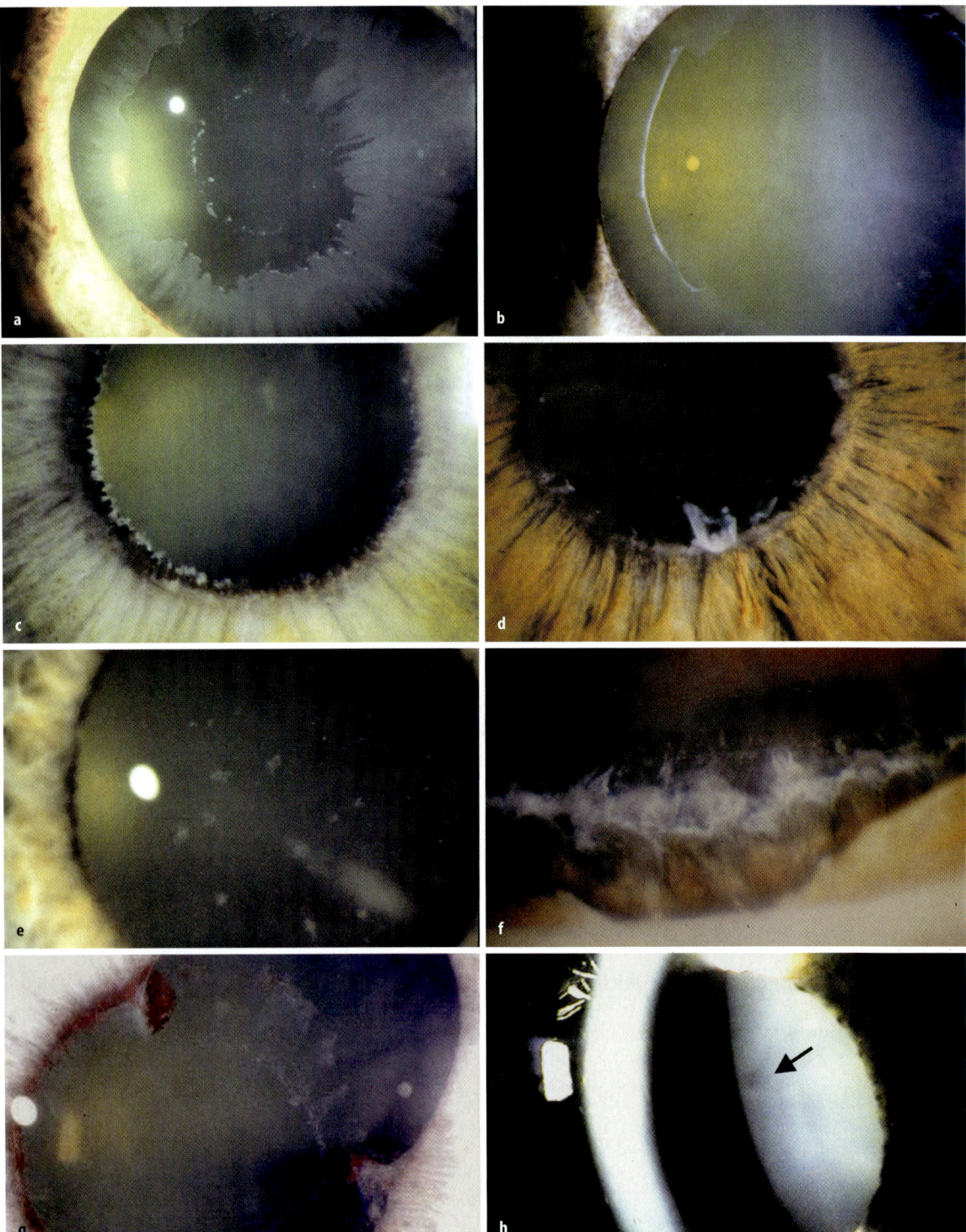

Fig. 6.3.4. Various clinical appearances of PEX material deposition in PEX syndrome. **a** Appearance of the classic "target" pattern with the central disc and peripheral zone separated by a clear intermediate zone; a few remaining bridges of PEX material span the clear zone. **b** The central disc may be absent; lenticular PEX deposits can only be seen after pupillary dilation. **c, d** PEX material deposition along the pupillary rim. **e** Retrocorneal PEX flakes. **f** PEX material deposits on ciliary processes and zonules as seen through an iris defect (surgical sector coloboma). **g** Appearance of "masked PEX"; the central disk is absent and the majority of the peripheral zone is obscured by circular posterior synechiae. Only in one segment, where the synechiae have broken down due to pharmacological dilatation, is the peripheral zone revealed. **h** Appearance of "mini-PEX" as an early stage of ocular PEX syndrome; an early rub-off defect (*arrow*) is seen in the superonasal midzone

Table 6.3.3. Aqueous flare values (photon counts/ms) in normal controls, pseudoexfoliation (PEX) with or without secondary open-angle glaucoma (SOAG) and primary open-angle glaucoma (POAG) (statistics: Mann-Whitney test) (from Küchle et al. 1995)

Group	Eyes (*n*)	Flare values (mean ± SD)	Range	Significance (*P*)
Normal controls	164	4.6 ± 1.1	2.0 – 7.2	} 0.1
POAG eyes	100	4.7 ± 1.6	2.0 – 7.4	
All PEX eyes	90	14.3 ± 9.2	6.0 – 43.2	< 0.0001
PEX with SOAG	40	14.5 ± 9.8	7.4 – 43.2	} 0.5
PEX without SOAG	50	14.1 ± 7.9	6.0 – 42.0	

jority of intraocular PEX deposits cannot be observed by direct biomicroscopy, and the accumulations on zonules, ciliary processes (Fig. 6.3.4f), and trabecular meshwork may be only detected on gonioscopy or cycloscopy or may be visualized by high resolution ultrasound biomicroscopy (Naumann et al. 1998; Inazumi et al. 2002).

In addition to deposits of PEX material, several other clinical signs aid in the diagnosis. Pigment loss from the peripupillary iris pigment epithelium and its deposition on anterior chamber structures is a hallmark of PEX syndrome. Further PEX-associated clinical signs that can alert the clinician to the presence of PEX include phacodonesis, iris stroma atrophy, iris hemorrhages after pupillary dilation, increased aqueous flare values, posterior synechiae, elevated intraocular pressure, and insufficient pupillary dilation, particularly if asymmetrically present. An atypical cornea guttata may precede the full clinical picture for decades. The differential diagnosis of PEX syndrome is presented in Table 6.3.3.

6.3.3.2
Masked PEX Syndrome

In cases of circular posterior synechiae, which frequently form in PEX eyes, particularly under miotic therapy, the evaluation of the anterior lens surface may be hindered and PEX deposits may be masked by the synechiae (Fig. 6.3.4g) (Mardin et al. 2001). In these cases, high resolution ultrasound biomicroscopy may be useful to reveal PEX deposits on the lens or zonules (Inazumi et al. 2002; Naumann et al. 1998). The presence of "spontaneous" posterior synechiae without any other obvious cause should alert the clinician to suspect PEX.

6.3.3.3
Early Stages of PEX Syndrome

The classical picture of lens deposits represents, however, a very late stage of the disease, which is preceded by a long, chronic, preclinical course. Early recognition is critical for reducing operative complications due to PEX. By thorough biomicroscopic examination, a diffuse-matte homogeneous film on the surface of the anterior lens capsule can be observed prior to the formation of obvious PEX deposits (Fig. 6.3.4h) (Naumann et al. 1998; Tetsumoto et al. 1992). To visualize these early changes at the slit lamp, it has been suggested to place the slit beam at 45 degrees to the axis of observation, reducing the light source, and focus temporally from the center of the lens to highlight the subtle deposits on the lens surface (Ritch and Schlötzer-Schrehardt 2001). Electron microscopy shows this surface film to consist of a layer of microfibrils, a precursor of PEX fibrils, diffusely deposited on the entire surface of the anterior lens capsule from the aqueous humor (Dark et al. 1990; Tetsumoto et al. 1992) (Fig. 6.3.5). As the precapsular layer becomes thicker, focal defects begin to form in the mid-peripheral zone by abrasive movements of the iris, often in the upper nasal quadrant ("*mini-PEX*") (Fig. 6.3.4h), which further enlarge and become confluent to form the classical picture of manifest PEX syndrome (Figs. 6.3.3, 6.3.5).

Additional clinical signs, which help alert the ophthalmologist to the presence of these early stages, comprise peripupillary atrophy of the iris pigment epithelium, melanin dispersion associated with pupillary dilation, increased trabecular pigmentation, and poor mydriasis (Table 6.3.1) (Prince et al. 1987; Tetsumoto et al. 1992). As PEX often is an asymmetric condition (see below), comparison with the fellow eye is diagnostically helpful in highlighting these early changes.

6.3.3.4
Asymmetry of Involvement

For unknown reasons, PEX patients can present clinically with either unilateral or bilateral involvement, which may be markedly asymmetric. Unilateral involvement is often regarded as a precursor to bilateral involvement. PEX syndrome manifests unilaterally in about 50 – 70 % of patients and the conversion rates from clinically unilateral to bilateral disease were found to vary from 15 % to 40 % within 5 years (Ritch and Schlötzer-Schrehardt 2001). Clinically, the involved eye often has a poorer visual acuity, more advanced lens opacity, higher intraocular pressure, a smaller pupil, and a more pronounced trabecular pigmentation than the noninvolved fellow eye.

However, in the majority of clinically unilateral cases, there are subtle histopathological and ultrastructural changes in the fellow eye suggesting that *all* cases are in fact asymmetric (Hammer et al. 2001; Kivelä et al. 1997). PEX material has been shown to be almost invariably present on electron microscopy in the conjunctiva (Prince et al. 1987) and in the iris, particularly in the dilator muscle and blood vessel walls, of the clini-

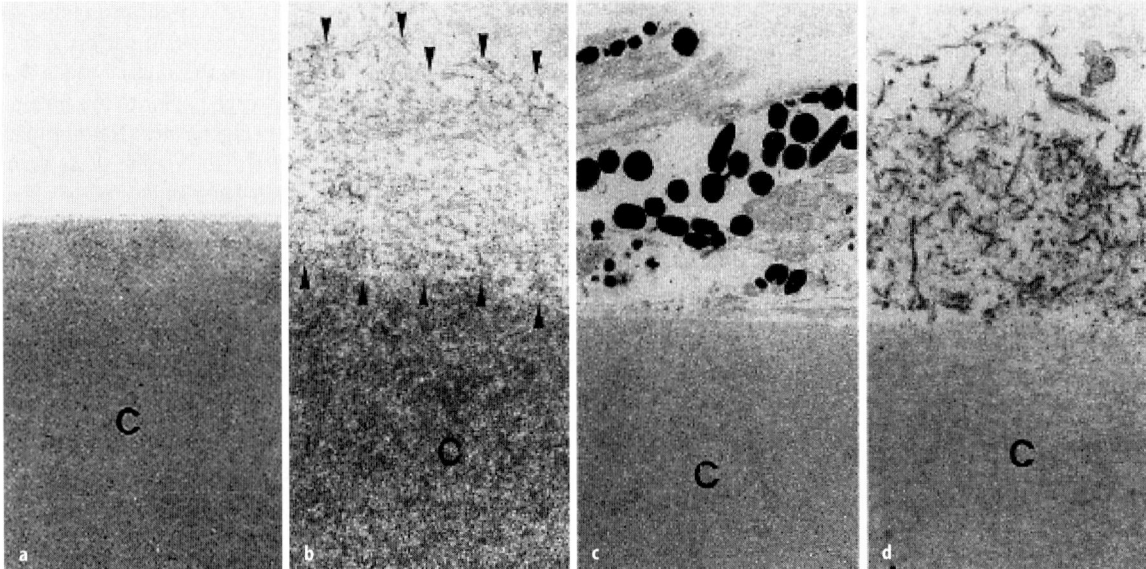

Fig. 6.3.5. Classification of PEX syndrome based on ultrastructural alterations of the anterior lens capsule (*C*) surface. **a** Normal capsule with smooth surface. **b** "Suspected PEX" with a precapsular layer of microfibrils (*arrowheads*). **c** "Masked PEX" with melanin granules derived from the iris pigment epithelium forming posterior synechiae adhering to the precapsular layer. **d** "Manifest PEX" with both microfibrils and typical mature PEX fibers in the area of the central disc

cally uninvolved fellow eye (Hammer et al. 2001; Kivelä et al. 1997). These early changes may account for the clinical signs characteristic of early stages, such as melanin dispersion, peripupillary atrophy, insufficient mydriasis, and blood-aqueous barrier defects leading to increased aqueous flare values measured by laser tyndallometry (Küchle et al. 1995). They further support the concept of PEX syndrome as a generalized, basically bilateral disorder with a clinically marked asymmetric presentation.

6.3.4
Surgical Pathology

6.3.4.1
Lens, Ciliary Body, and Zonular Apparatus

Lens opacification occurs in a high proportion of eyes with PEX syndrome and is the most common cause of PEX patients to require surgical intervention. An increased incidence of cataract, most commonly of a *nuclear type*, is known to be associated with PEX syndrome (Hietanen et al. 1992) and may be causally linked to the presence of ocular ischemia, anterior chamber hypoxia (Helbig et al. 1994), reduced protection against ultraviolet radiation by lower levels of ascorbic acid in the aqueous humor (Koliakos et al. 2003), and abnormal aqueous composition such as increased growth factor levels in the aqueous humor evident as "PEX hydropathy."

The *zonules* are affected early in the course of the PEX process (Fig. 6.3.6a). The zonular fibers may separate from their attachments to the ciliary body and lens and produce a characteristic phacodonesis or inferior displacement of the lens (Fig. 6.3.6b) (Bartholomew 1970; Freissler et al. 1995). The zonular fibers proper may be intact or partially fragmented; however, in cases associated with phacodonesis or lens subluxation, marked degenerative changes of the zonular fibers are observed. Weakening of the zonular support and subsequent laxity of the lens allows lens movement to occur. Especially in the prone position, anterior lens movement can occur resulting in pupillary or even ciliary block predisposing to angle-closure glaucoma, which is more common in eyes with PEX (Ritch 1994b; von der Lippe et al. 1993). Miotics may exacerbate forward movement of the iris-lens diaphragm and cause attacks of pupillary block angle-closure glaucoma. This pronounced instability of the zonular apparatus is easily understood by analyzing the underlying histopathologic alterations of the zonules and their attachments at the lens and ciliary body (see below).

Although the changes of the anterior lens capsule are important for diagnosis, they are relatively harmless. In the classic manifestation, a "target" pattern of deposited PEX material is recognizable with a dilated pupil (Figs. 6.3.4a, 6.3.7a) (Vogt 1925). It consists of a loosely attached central disc of fibrillar PEX material (Fig. 6.3.7b), which is separated from the peripheral zone with nodular PEX aggregates (Fig. 6.3.7c) by a 1- to 2-mm-wide clear intermediate zone produced by removal of the deposits by iris movements. The central disc, corresponding to the size of the pupil, appears to result from diffuse sedimentation of PEX material from

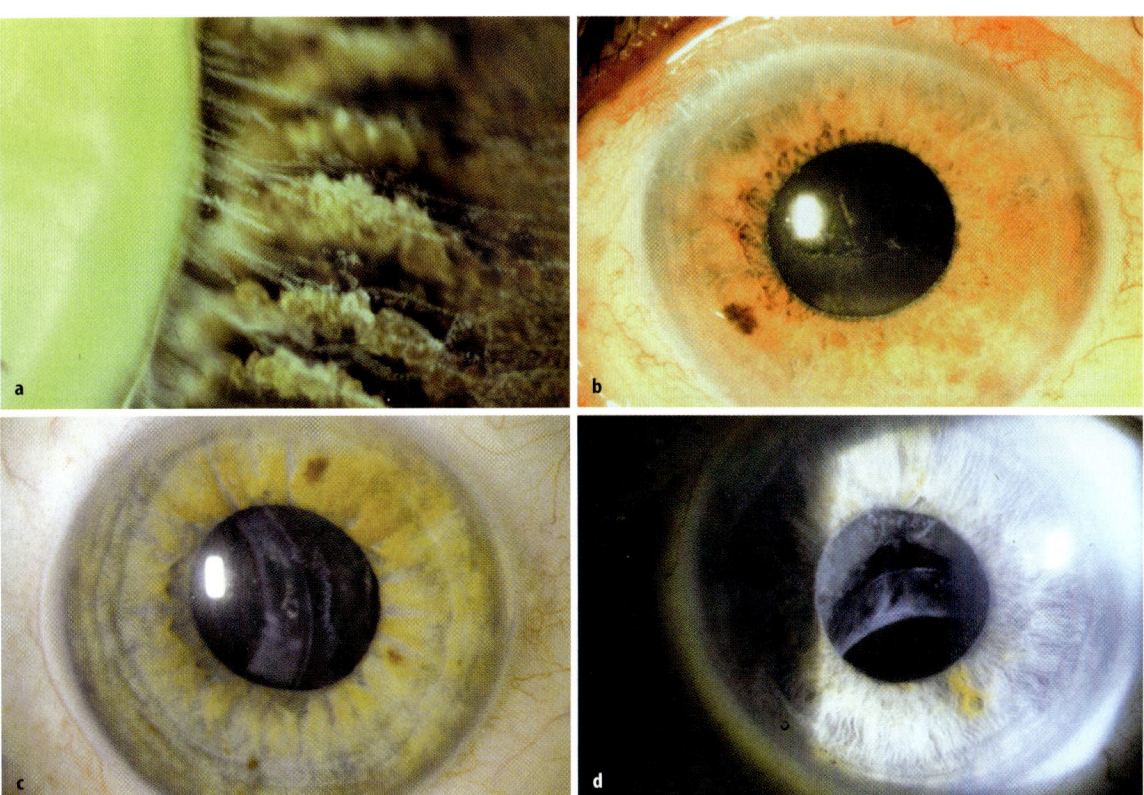

Fig. 6.3.6. Clinical involvement of the zonular apparatus in PEX syndrome. **a** Macroscopic view of ciliary processes and zonules encrusted with PEX material. **b** Luxated lens in an 87-year-old patient; note the superior equator and zonular fibers loaded with PEX material. **c, d** Postoperative decentration of the lens implant within the capsular bag

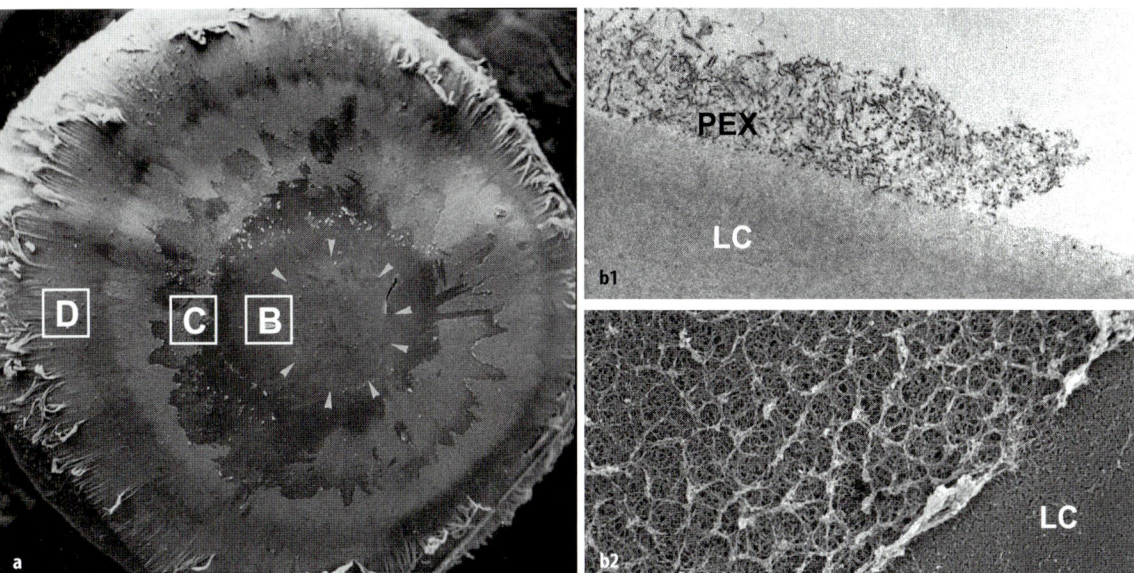

Fig. 6.3.7. Histopathologic involvement of the lens in PEX syndrome. **a** Scanning electron micrograph of the anterior lens surface showing signs of manifest PEX syndrome with a central disc (*arrowheads, B*), the peripheral granular zone (*C*), and the preequatorial zone of zonular insertion (*D*); the *boxed areas* are shown in higher magnification in **b–d**. **b** Scanning (*top*) and transmission (*bottom*) electron micrographs showing the fibrillar deposits of the loosely attached central disc

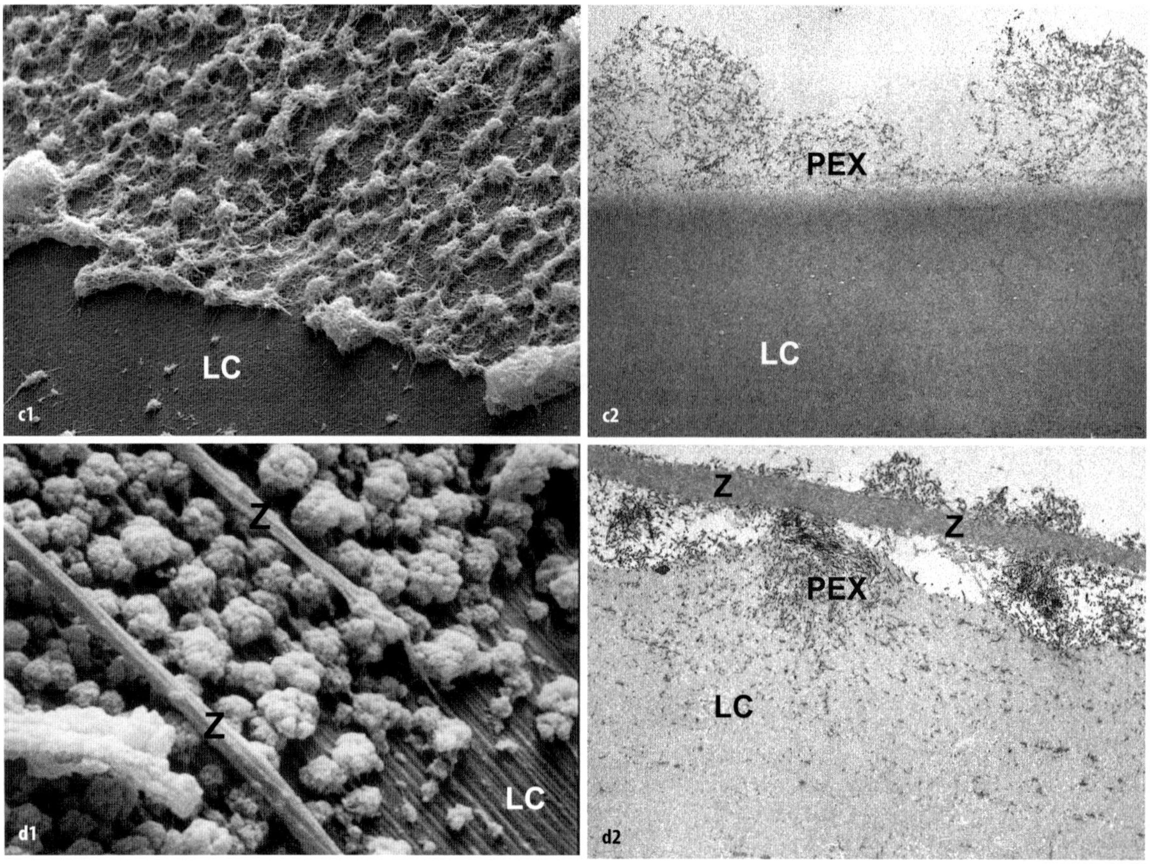

Fig. 6.3.7. c Scanning (*left*) and transmission (*right*) electron microscopic appearance of nodular PEX deposits in the peripheral granular zone. **d** Scanning (*left*) and transmission (*right*) electron micrographs of the preequatorial zone of the lens capsule showing nodular PEX aggregates separating the zonular lamella from the capsular surface (*LC* lens capsule, *Z* zonules)

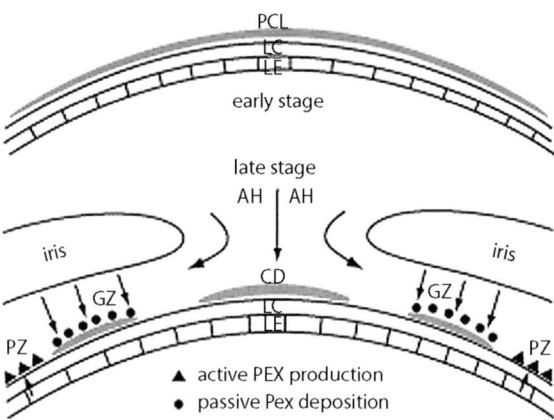

Fig. 6.3.8. Schematic representation of the presumed origin of lenticular PEX material (*AH* aqueous humor, *CD* central disc, *GZ* granular zone, *LC* lens capsule, *LE* lens epithelium, *PCL* precapsular layer, *PZ* preequatorial zone)

the aqueous, whereas the peripheral granular zone builds up by undisturbed accumulation of nodular PEX aggregates produced by the iris pigment epithelium; the intermediate clear zone is created by abrasive movements of the peripupillary iris during pupillary movement (Fig. 6.3.8) (Naumann et al. 1998).

The anterior and posterior lens capsules proper appear to be morphologically normal and have been reported to have a similar mean thickness and elasticity compared to control eyes. In contrast, the preequatorial capsule, corresponding to the proliferative zone of the lens epithelium and the zone of zonular anchorage, is associated with significant alterations and dangers for the intraocular surgeon. In this area, active production of PEX material occurs by the preequatorial lens epithelium. Exuberant bundles of PEX fibrils appear to originate from the adjacent lens epithelial cells, which disrupt the capsule proper and invade the zonular lamella, resulting in separation of the zonules from their insertion onto the capsule (Schlötzer-Schrehardt and Naumann 1994) (Figs. 6.3.7d, 6.3.9a, b). These alterations are usually not visible on clinical examination, being hidden behind the iris, but give rise to a marked instability of the zonular attachment to the lens (Fig. 6.3.10).

Similarly, at their origin and anchorage in the non-pigmented ciliary epithelium, the zonular bundles are separated from their connection to the disrupted epi-

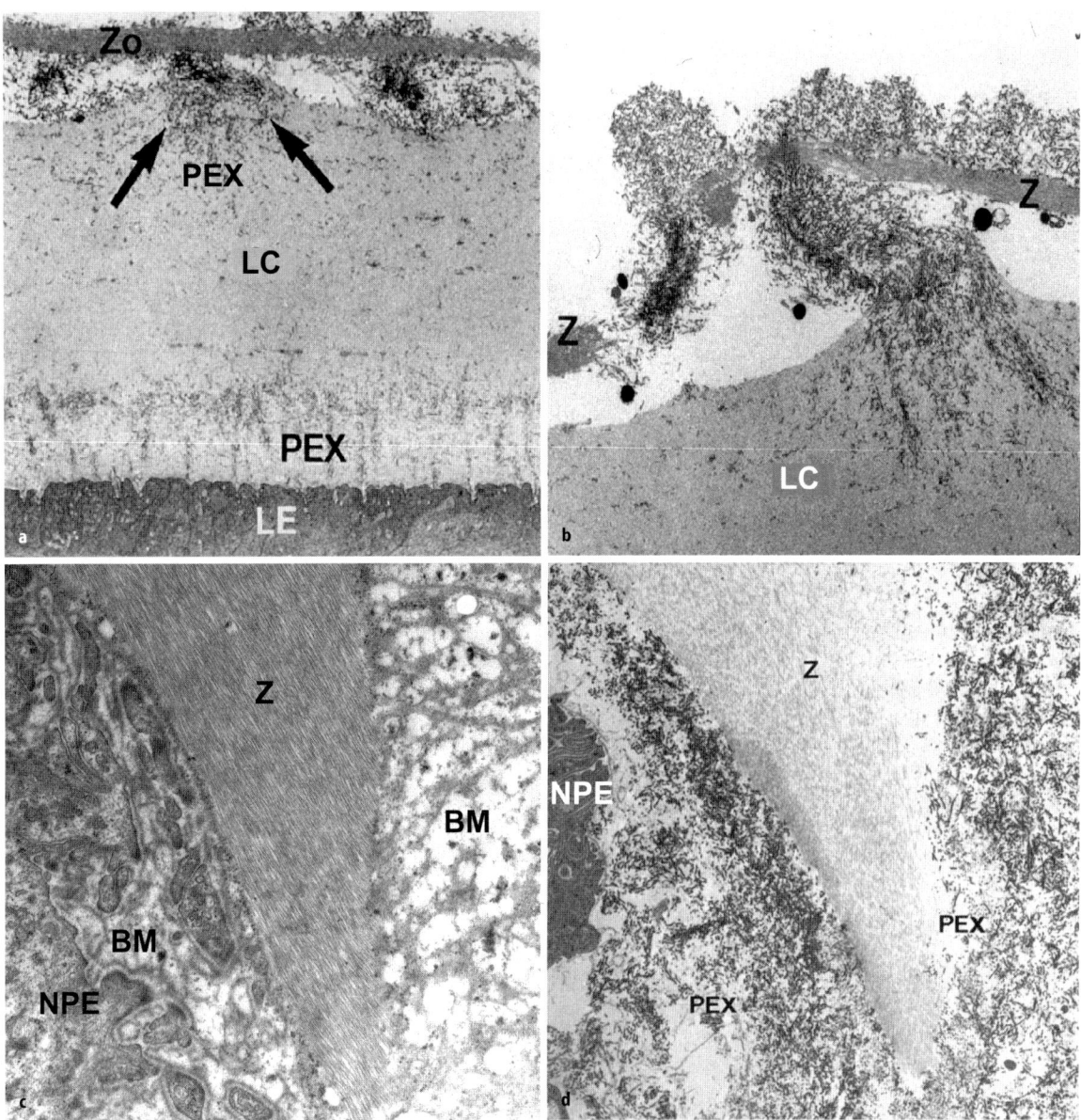

Fig. 6.3.9. Histopathologic involvement of the zonular apparatus in PEX syndrome. **a, b** In the preequatorial region of the lens, the zonular attachment (*Z*) to the anterior lens capsule (*LC*) is disrupted due to the exuberant production of *PEX* material by the underlying lens epithelial cells (*LE*). **c, d** Zonular bundles at their insertion into the ciliary epithelium. The zonular fibers (*Z*) are firmly attached to the basement membrane (*BM*) of the nonpigmented ciliary epithelium (*NPE*) in normal age-matched eyes (**c**), but are loosened due to complete destruction of the epithelial basement membrane by intercalating *PEX* material in PEX eyes (**d**)

thelial basement membrane by locally produced, intercalating PEX fibers (Fig. 6.3.9c, d) (Schlötzer-Schrehardt and Naumann 1994). Zonular disintegration may be further facilitated by degenerative changes of the freely suspended zonular fiber bundles between ciliary body and lens, which are focally infiltrated by PEX material containing proteolytic enzymes (Fig. 6.3.9e, f). Every ophthalmologist planning intraocular surgery in patients with PEX syndrome should recall these alterations of the zonular apparatus. As they are biomicroscopically not visible, they "must be kept in mind." They present a real risk particularly in advanced stages.

Production of PEX material by the remaining lens epithelial cells continues to occur after extracapsular cataract extraction and may cause late decentration or even subluxation of the lens implant within the capsular bag (Fig. 6.3.6c, d) (Auffahrt et al. 1996).

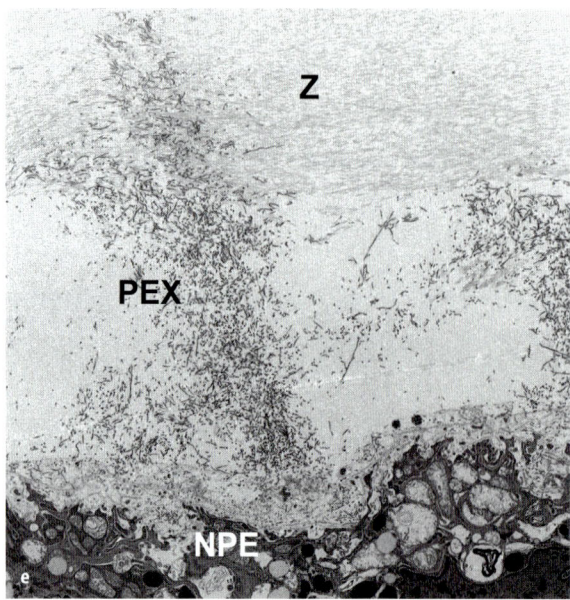
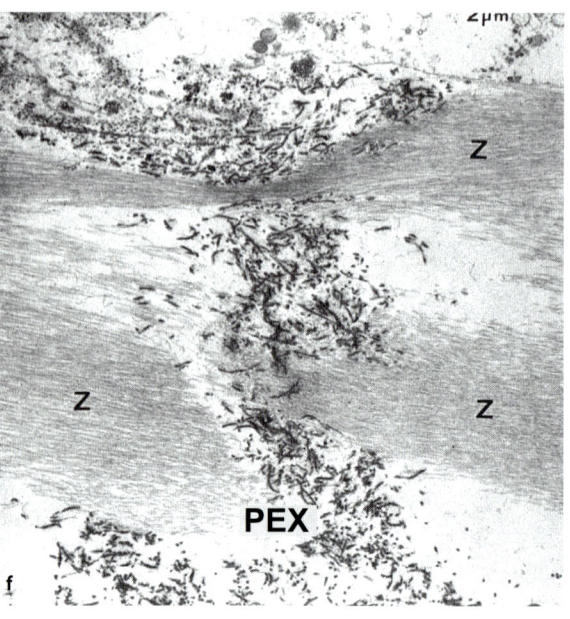

Fig. 6.3.9. e, f Freely suspended zonular bundles (*Z*) passing alongside the nonpigmented ciliary epithelium (*NPE*) are infiltrated (*E*) and disrupted (*F*) by *PEX* material

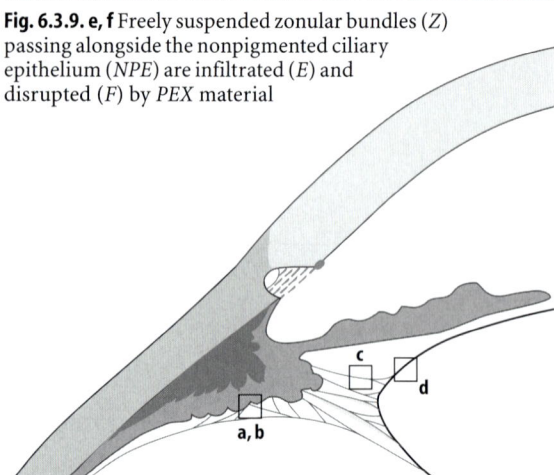
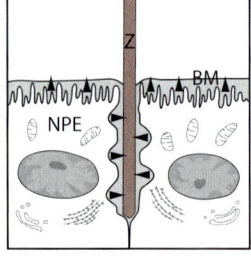
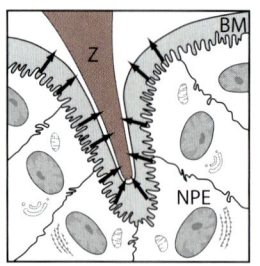
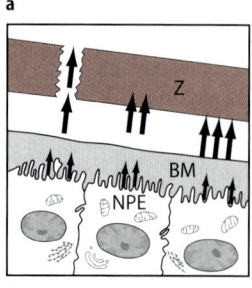
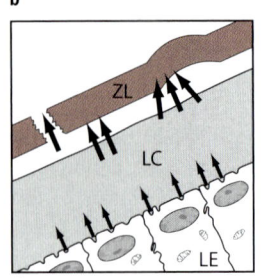

6.3.4.2
Iris

PEX syndrome has a multitude of effects on iris tissues with clinical importance. Numerous histopathologic studies have demonstrated that virtually all iris cell types (epithelial cells, fibrocytes, melanocytes, vascular endothelial cells, pericytes, and smooth muscle cells) are involved in PEX material production and deposition including the posterior pigment epithelium, dilator and sphincter muscles, anterior border layer, stromal fibroblasts and melanocytes, and blood vessels (Fig. 6.3.11) (Asano et al. 1995; Naumann et al. 1998). This abnormal metabolic activity disturbs their normal function and leads to progressive tissue damage.

Clinically, the PEX iris is characteristically rigid with *reduced dilating properties* (Carpel 1988), which has been attributed to a combination of PEX fiber deposition in the stroma and muscle tissues along with degenerative changes of sphincter and dilator muscles (Fig. 6.3.12a, c) (Asano et al. 1995).

Concomitantly, the pigment epithelial cells in the pupillary ruff and sphincter regions show marked degenerative changes with focal membrane ruptures and

Fig. 6.3.10. Schematic representation of the typical localizations of zonular alterations in PEX syndrome; PEX material production and zonular infiltration is indicated by *arrows* and *arrowheads*. **a** Origin of zonular fibers in the nonpigmented ciliary epithelium. **b** Zonular anchorage within the nonpigmented ciliary epithelium. **c** Freely suspended zonular bundles passing along the ciliary processes. **d** Zonular attachment to the anterior lens capsule (*BM* basement membrane, *LC* lens capsule, *LE* lens epithelium, *NPE* nonpigmented ciliary epithelium, *Z* zonular fibers, *ZL* zonular lamella)

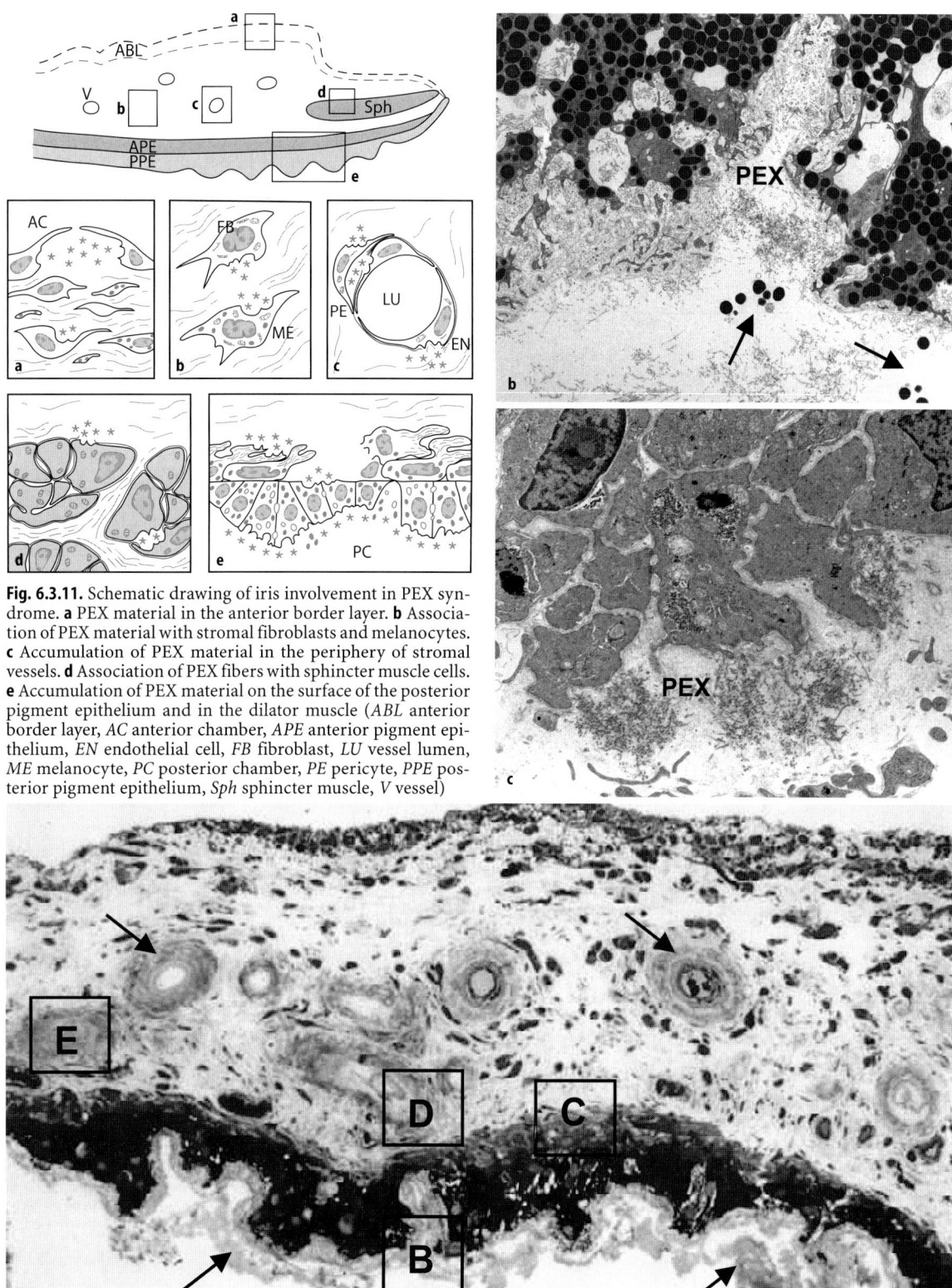

Fig. 6.3.11. Schematic drawing of iris involvement in PEX syndrome. **a** PEX material in the anterior border layer. **b** Association of PEX material with stromal fibroblasts and melanocytes. **c** Accumulation of PEX material in the periphery of stromal vessels. **d** Association of PEX fibers with sphincter muscle cells. **e** Accumulation of PEX material on the surface of the posterior pigment epithelium and in the dilator muscle (*ABL* anterior border layer, *AC* anterior chamber, *APE* anterior pigment epithelium, *EN* endothelial cell, *FB* fibroblast, *LU* vessel lumen, *ME* melanocyte, *PC* posterior chamber, *PE* pericyte, *PPE* posterior pigment epithelium, *Sph* sphincter muscle, *V* vessel)

Fig. 6.3.12. Histopathologic involvement of the iris in PEX syndrome. **a** Light microscopic appearance and PEX material deposits (*arrows*) on the surface of the posterior pigment epithelium and in the periphery of blood vessels (toluidine blue, ×250); the *boxed areas* are shown in higher magnification in **b–e**. **b** Transmission electron micrograph of iris pigment epithelial cells; the epithelial cells are involved by thick deposits of *PEX* material on their surface and display degenerative changes evidenced by the liberation of melanin granules (*arrows*). **c** Electron micrograph showing *PEX* aggregates between dilator muscle cells

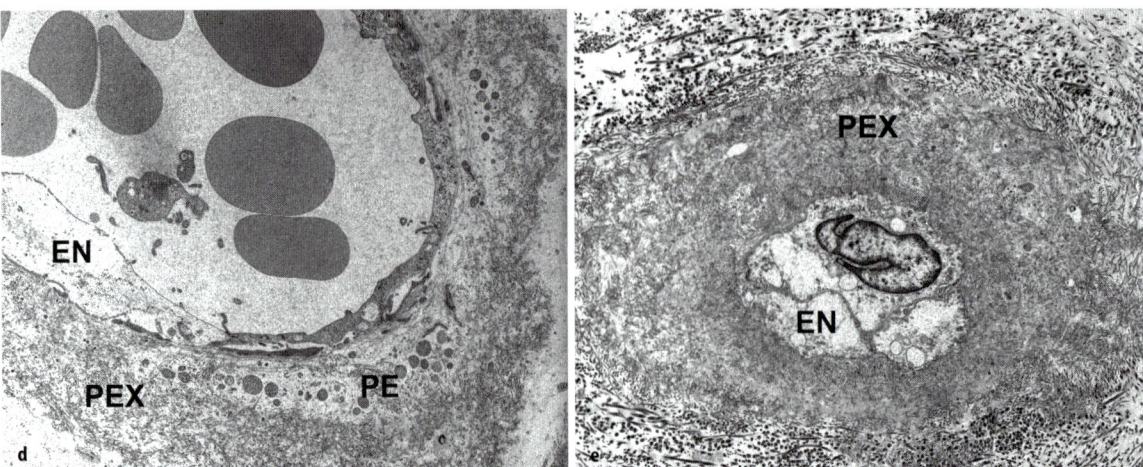

Fig. 6.3.12. d, e Electron micrographs of iris blood vessels; the vessel wall is thickened by *PEX* material accumulations, whereas the vascular wall cells (*EN* endothelial cells, *PE* pericytes) are largely degenerated (**d**) or swollen to obstruct the vessel lumen (**e**)

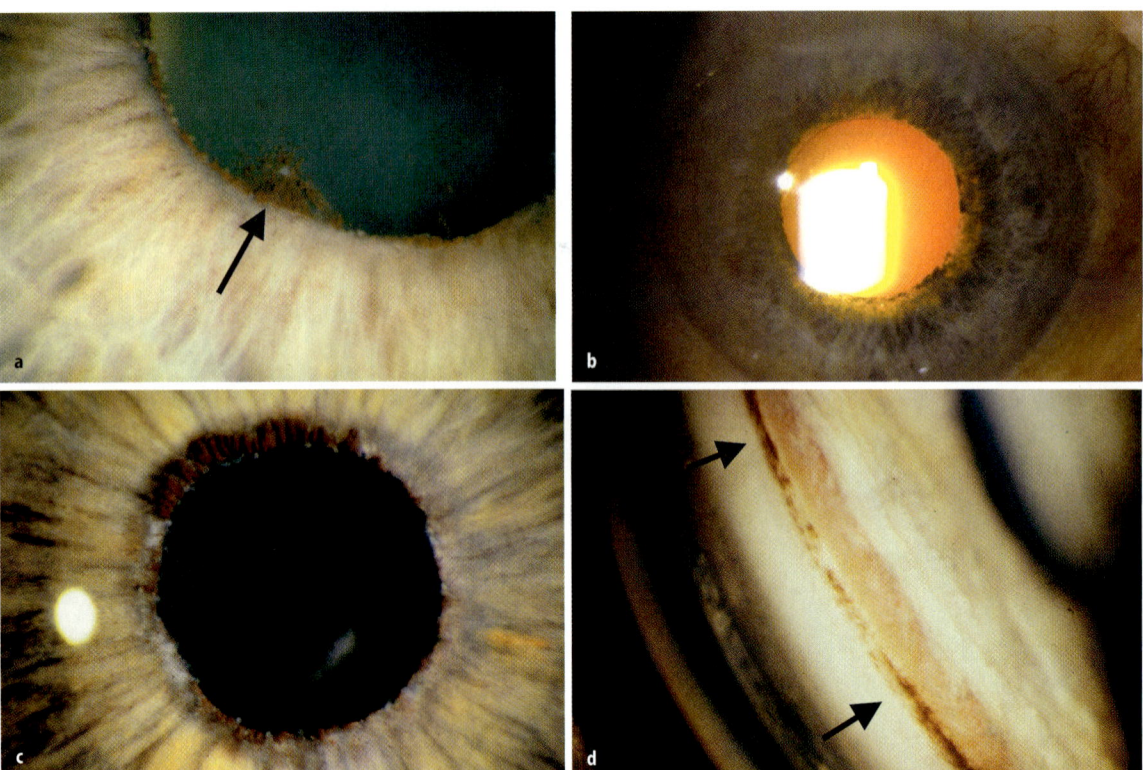

Fig. 6.3.13. Clinical appearance of the iris affected by PEX. The degenerative changes of the iris pigment epithelial cells result clinically in melanin dispersion (**a**), in atrophic degeneration and transillumination defects in the peripupillary region (**b**), in defects of the pupillary ruff (**c**), and in melanin deposition on the trabecular meshwork (**d**) and corneal endothelial surface (**e**); vascular damage leads to intrastromal hemorrhages (**f**). **g, h** Iris indocyanine green angiographies from PEX eyes illustrating regions of microvascular abnormalities including dye leakage (**g**) as well as hypoperfusion and complex plexuses of anastomotic vessels (**h**) (courtesy of Dr. M.B. Parodi, University of Trieste, Italy)

liberation of melanin granules (Fig. 6.3.12a, b) (Asano et al. 1995). These changes result in a diagnostically important peripupillary atrophy and characteristic "moth-eaten" transillumination defects in the peripupillary region (Fig. 6.3.13a–c) accompanied by a characteristic pattern of pigment deposition on the iris surface, trabecular meshwork, corneal endothelium, and other anterior segment structures (Fig. 6.3.13d, e) (Prince et al. 1987). Additionally, *dispersion of melanin granules* following pharmacological dilatation due to

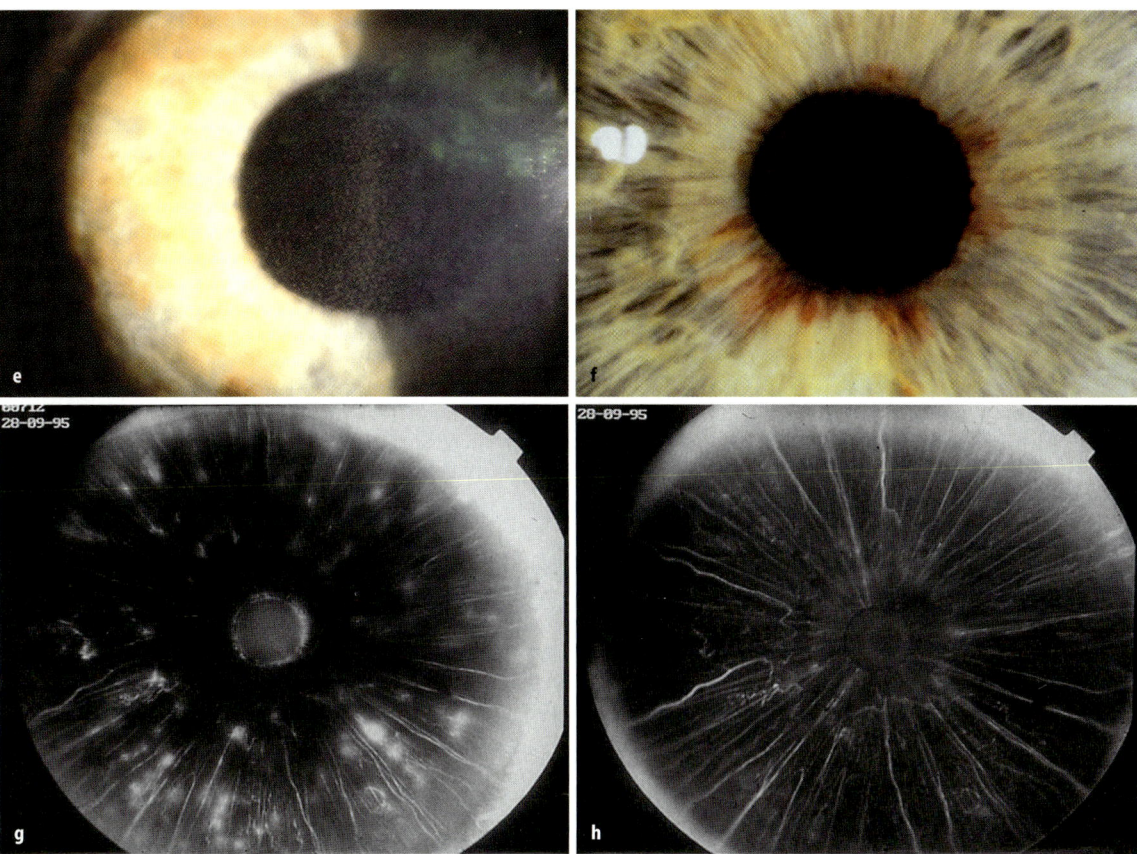

Fig. 6.3.13. (*Cont.*)

rupture of degenerative pigment epithelial cells may be marked and even result in an acute rise in intraocular pressure (Fig. 6.3.13a). In the absence of other causes for melanin dispersion, PEX should always be considered in the differential diagnosis of this phenomenon.

Involvement of the iris stromal vessels has major functional consequences. PEX fibers are deposited in the wall of iris vessels associated with degeneration of smooth muscle cells, pericytes, and endothelial cells up to complete destruction of the vessel wall (Fig. 6.3.12a, d) (Asano et al. 1995). In advanced stages, iris blood vessels may become obliterated (Fig. 6.3.12e) resulting in iris hypoperfusion and reduced partial pressure of oxygen in the anterior chamber (Helbig et al. 1994). On fluorescein or indocyanine green angiography, changes including iris vessel dropout and dye leakage may be seen (Fig. 6.3.13g, h) (Brooks and Gillies 1983; Parodi et al. 2000). Cataract formation and altered behavior of corneal endothelial cells (see below) have also been attributed to anterior chamber hypoxia in PEX eyes. *"Spontaneous" intrastromal hemorrhages* after mydriasis indicate significant vascular damage and friability and may be more common than appreciated, but overlooked particularly in brown irides (Fig. 6.3.13f) (Naumann et al. 1998) because the small hemorrhages are

Table 6.3.4. Differential diagnosis of pseudoexfoliation syndrome

True exfoliation of the lens capsule (infrared or "glassblowers" cataract)
Fibrin or inflammatory precipitates on anterior lens capsule
Melanin dispersion
Diabetes
"Senile"
Idiopathic "melanin dispersion syndrome," pigmentary glaucoma (both in young myopes)
Uveitis, Fuchs' heterochromia complicata
Trauma
Intraocular tumors
Segmental iris necrosis (e.g., chronic angle-closure glaucoma, pupillary block, herpes zoster)
Long-standing mydriasis
Senile iridoschisis
Marfan syndrome (homocystinuria)

hidden in iris stroma crypts. In lightly pigmented blue irides such hemorrhages are more easily recognized.

Another important consequence of the iris vasculopathy is a chronic breakdown of the blood-aqueous barrier in eyes with PEX syndrome (Küchle et al. 1995). Clinically this may manifest as a *pseudouveitis* with elevated aqueous flare and formation of posterior synechiae due to adherence of the posterior pigment epithelium to the PEX material-coated anterior lens capsule (Table 6.3.4). The inhibition of iris movement by miotic agents may enhance posterior synechiae formation. Furthermore, blood-aqueous barrier dysfunction is compromised to a greater extent in eyes with PEX compared to eyes without PEX following intraocular surgery including cataract surgery, trabeculectomy, and laser trabeculoplasty (Nguyen et al. 1999; Schumacher et al. 1999).

6.3.4.3
Trabecular Meshwork

Compared to primary open-angle glaucoma (POAG), PEX-associated secondary open-angle glaucoma represents a relatively severe and progressive type of glaucoma with a generally poor prognosis associated with higher mean intraocular pressure (IOP), increased frequency and severity of optic nerve damage, greater diurnal fluctuation in IOP, poorer response to medical therapy, and more frequent need for surgery (Konstas et al. 1997). PEX glaucoma further differs from POAG by a more frequent and pronounced asymmetry of manifestation, more intense chamber angle pigmentation, and acute pressure rises after mydriasis. A significant correlation between the IOP level at the time of diagnosis and the mean visual field defect could be only established in PEX glaucoma but not in POAG patients (Teus et al. 1998), suggesting that glaucomatous damage in patients with PEX glaucoma may be more directly related to IOP than in POAG patients.

The markedly raised IOP characteristic of PEX glaucoma is understood by observing the pathological changes in the trabecular meshwork. Although there may be deposits of PEX material throughout the trabecular meshwork, the focus of PEX material accumulation and pathological alterations is the juxtacanalicular tissue beneath the inner wall of Schlemm's canal, the site of greatest resistance to aqueous outflow. This critical area becomes thickened through gradual deposition of *locally* produced *endotrabecular* PEX material, whereas *exotrabecular* PEX material, passively washed in with the aqueous flow, adheres to the inner surface of the uveal meshwork (Fig. 6.3.14). The gradual build-up of PEX material in the juxtacanalicular tissue may be often associated with progressive degenerative changes of Schlemm's canal including narrowing, fragmentation and obstruction in advanced cases (Fig. 6.3.15a–c) (Gottanka et al. 1997; Schlötzer-Schrehardt and Naumann 1995). Ultrastructural indications suggest that the PEX fibrils are *locally* produced by the endothelial cells lining Schlemm's canal leading to a progressive accumulation of the pathologic matrix product in the subendothelial area, thus limiting access of aqueous humor to Schlemm's canal and resulting in degenerative alterations of the canal wall (Fig. 6.3.16a–d) (Schlötzer-Schrehardt and Naumann 1995). From these changes it can be appreciated that therapeutic efforts to improve outflow need to address the alterations in this area to obtain lasting intraocular pressure reduction. PEX material accumulations can be also found along the outer wall of Schlemm's canal and in the periphery of collector channels and scleral aqueous veins, occasionally leading to collapse of aqueous veins. Partly, PEX clumps may be also passively washed in with the aqueous flow after abrasion from the lens and pupillary margin and may become trapped in the uveal pores of the meshwork (Fig. 6.3.16e–f).

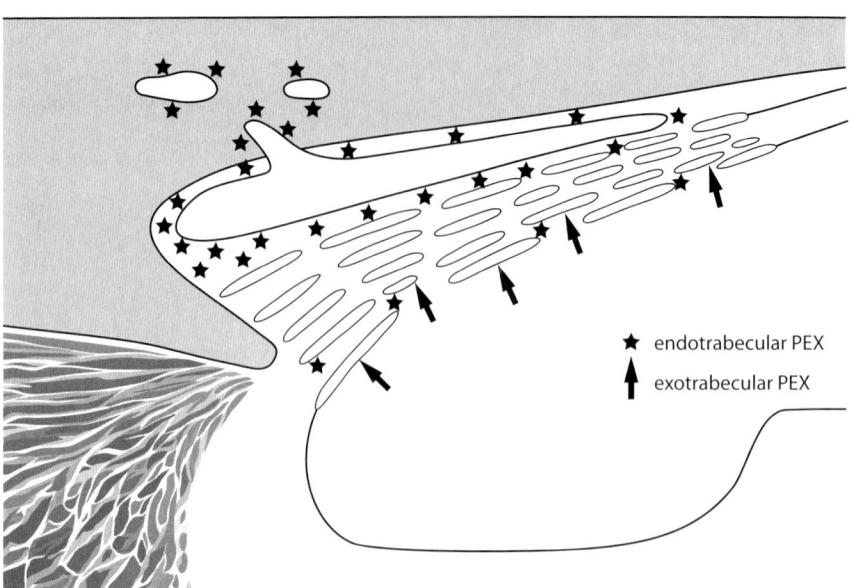

Fig. 6.3.14. Schematic representation of the trabecular meshwork in PEX syndrome showing the localization of PEX deposits of presumed endotrabecular (local production) and exotrabecular (passive inflow) origin

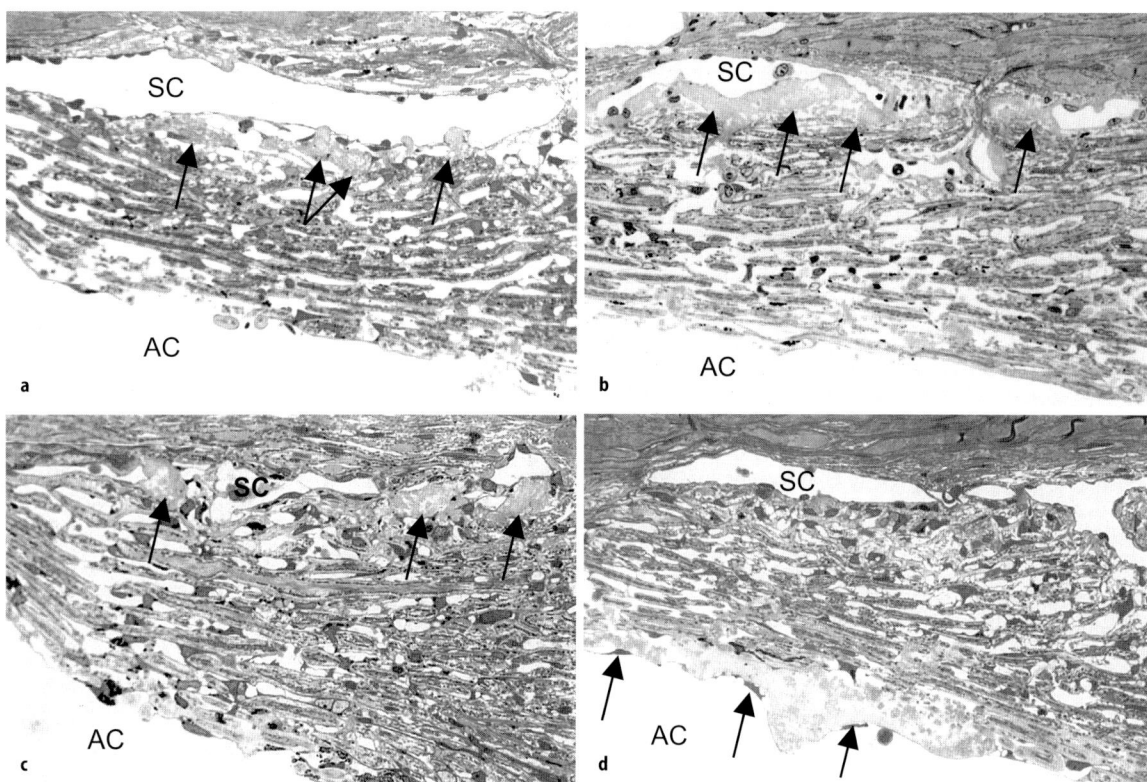

Fig. 6.3.15. Light microscopic semithin sections showing involvement of the trabecular meshwork and Schlemm's canal in PEX syndrome (toluidine blue, ×250) (*AC* anterior chamber, *SC* Schlemm's canal). **a** Accumulation of small deposits of PEX material (*arrows*) in the juxtacanalicular meshwork. **b** Accumulation of large masses of PEX material (*arrows*) in the juxtacanalicular tissue. **c** Disorganization of Schlemm's canal area by PEX material accumulation (*arrows*) in the juxtacanalicular tissue. **d** Pretrabecular deposits of PEX material overgrown by migrating corneal endothelial cells

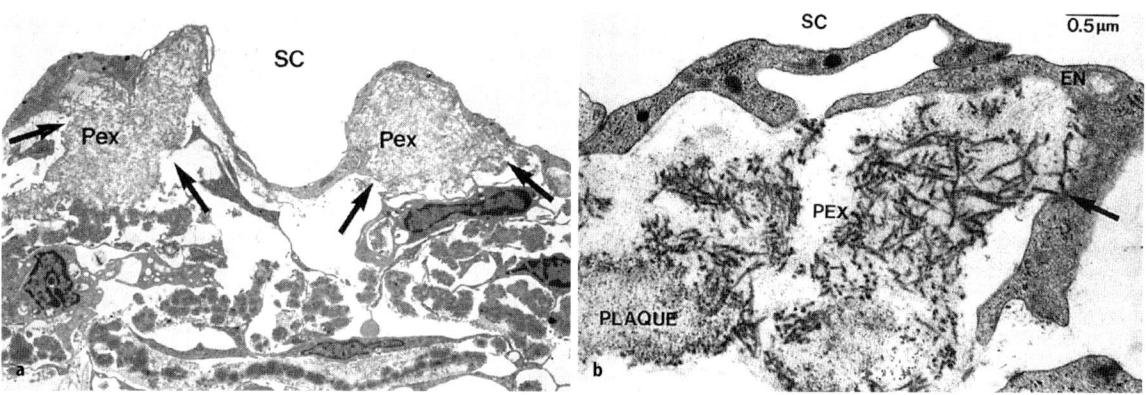

Fig. 6.3.16a–f. Electron micrographs showing involvement of the trabecular meshwork in PEX syndrome. **a** Accumulation of *PEX* material (*arrows*) in the subendothelial juxtacanalicular tissue along the inner wall of Schlemm's canal (*SC*). **b** Apparent production of *PEX* fibrils (*arrow*) by the inner wall endothelium (*EN*) of Schlemm's canal (*SC*)

The amount of PEX material within the juxtacanalicular region *correlated* with the presence of glaucoma, the average thickness of the juxtacanalicular tissue and the mean cross-sectional area of Schlemm's canal in one study (Schlötzer-Schrehardt and Naumann 1995) and also with the intraocular pressure level and the axon count in the optic nerve in another (Gottanka et al. 1997). These findings indicate a direct causative relationship between the buildup of PEX material in the meshwork and glaucoma development and progression.

Even though obstruction of the trabecular outflow channels by locally produced PEX material appears to be the major mechanism of increased outflow resistance and chronic pressure elevation, contributions due to pigment dispersion and increased aqueous pro-

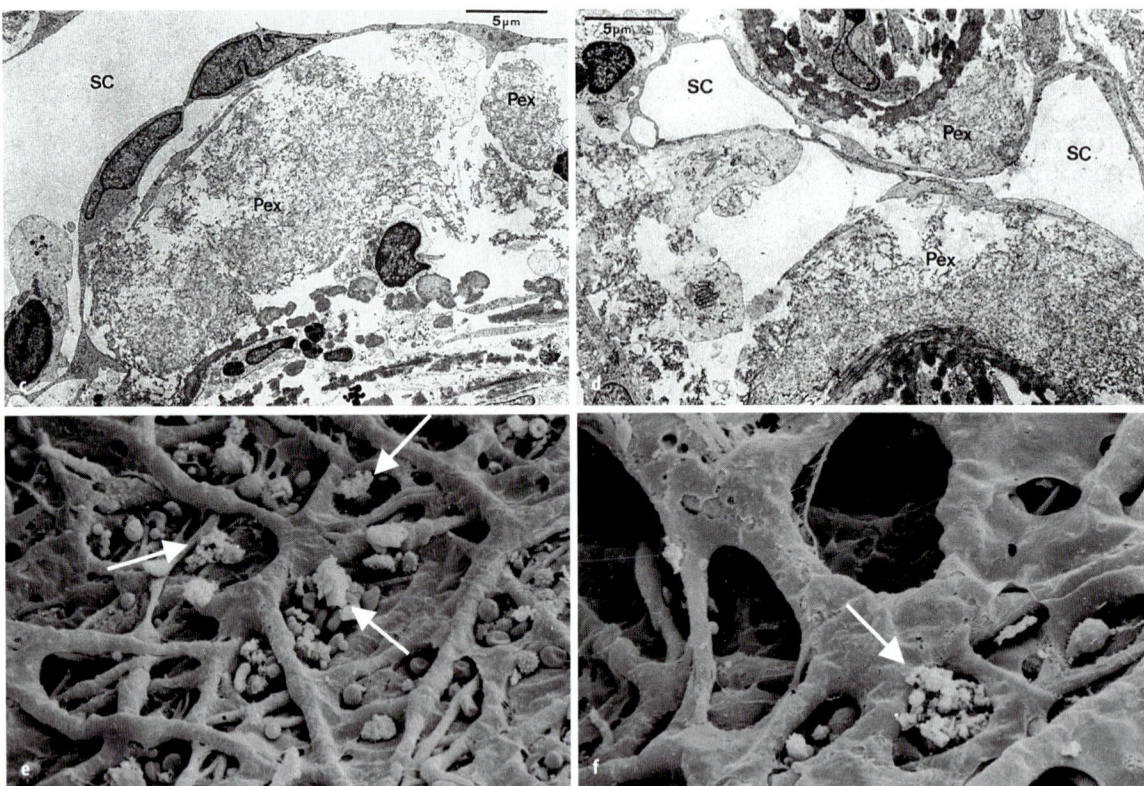

Fig. 6.3.16. c Thickening of the juxtacanalicular tissue and narrowing of Schlemm's canal lumen by massive accumulation of *PEX* material. **d** Focal collapse of Schlemm's canal (*SC*) with contact of inner and outer walls due to accumulating PEX masses. **e, f** Scanning electron micrographs of the inner surface of the trabecular meshwork showing PEX deposits (*arrows*) in the uveal pores

Table 6.3.5. Pathogenetic factors of ocular hypertension and glaucoma development in PEX syndrome

1. Ocular hypertension and open-angle glaucoma	Locally produced (endotrabecular) PEX material Passively deposited (exotrabecular) PEX material Melanin dispersion during mydriasis Increased aqueous protein concentrations Proliferation/migration of corneal endothelial cells
2. Angle closure glaucomas (pupillary/ciliary block)	Zonular instability and subtle lens subluxation Rigid iris and poor mydriasis Posterior synechiae Protein-rich aqueous humor Relative anterior microphthalmos

tein concentrations have also been proposed (Table 6.3.5). Increased trabecular meshwork pigmentation, particularly in the inferior half, is a prominent and early sign of PEX syndrome, sometimes associated with flecks of PEX material. Unlike that in primary melanin dispersion syndrome, the distribution of the pigment tends to be less dense and rather uneven or patchy (Fig. 6.3.13d). Pigment is also characteristically deposited on or anterior to Schwalbe's line (Sampaolesi's line). By electron microscopy, pigment granules are invariably present within trabecular endothelial cells, preferably in the innermost uveal portions of the meshwork (Sampaolesi et al. 1988; Schlötzer-Schrehardt and Naumann 1995). Another interesting observation has been the migration and proliferation of corneal endothelial cells beyond Schwalbe's line resulting in a pretrabecular layer of extracellular material including PEX fibrils produced by migrating/proliferating endothelial cells (Fig. 6.3.15d) (Schlötzer-Schrehardt and Naumann 1995; Schlötzer-Schrehardt et al. 1999). This may be a consequence of anterior chamber hypoxia in PEX eyes (Helbig et al. 1994), stimulating corneal endothelial cell proliferation (Zagorski et al. 1989). Such observations may partially explain why there is a variable response to medical therapy with some patients seeming to respond so poorly.

Dispersion of melanin granules and PEX material in the anterior chamber is common after diagnostic pupillary dilation (Fig. 6.3.13a) and may lead to marked rises in intraocular pressure, sometimes causing, together with an early corneal endothelial decompensation and diffuse corneal edema, the clinical picture of an acute glaucoma (Naumann et al. 1998). Such pressure peaks can even mimic an acute pupillary block with a red eye, corneal edema, and pressure rises over 50 mm Hg, in spite of an open angle. Krause et al. (1973) noted a positive correlation between the degree of pressure rise and the amount of pigment liberation, which both reach a maximum after 2 h following mydriasis and may go back to normal levels after 10–24 h. Postdilation intraocular pressure should be, therefore, checked in all patients receiving mydriatics.

Glaucoma in PEX syndrome usually occurs in the presence of an open chamber angle, but an association between PEX and angle-closure glaucoma is not rare either (Table 6.3.5) (Gross et al. 1994; Ritch 1994b). Because eyes with PEX syndrome often have narrowed chamber angles and smaller anterior chamber volumes (Gross et al. 1994; Wishart et al. 1985) in the presence of a weak zonular apparatus, a minimal anterior subluxation of the lens predisposes to the development of angle-closure glaucoma via a pupillary block mechanism. The decrease in anterior chamber depth between the supine and prone position was shown to be greater in eyes with PEX than in fellow eyes (Lanzl et al. 2000). Further features of PEX eyes that may predispose to the development of pupillary block angle-closure glaucoma include the formation of posterior synechiae, an increased iris rigidity and decreased iris motility, an impairment of the blood-aqueous barrier and increased protein concentrations of aqueous humor (Naumann et al. 1998). Miotics may aggravate both pupillary block and forward movement of the lens-iris diaphragm. In extreme and rather rare cases with marked zonular laxity, anterior displacement of the lens may be so pronounced that a ciliary block angle-closure glaucoma ("malignant glaucoma") is induced by contraction of the ciliary muscle (von der Lippe et al. 1993). A narrow angle associated with PEX syndrome may, therefore, represent an additional argument for prophylactic iridotomy.

Secondary angle-closure glaucoma following central retinal vein occlusion with rubeosis iridis ("neovascular glaucoma") may also occur in PEX eyes, because retinal vein occlusion appears to be more common in patients with PEX syndrome/glaucoma (Cursiefen et al. 1997; Gillies and Brooks 2002). In rare cases, the spontaneous luxation of the lens into the vitreous or of lens fragments in complicated cataract surgery may induce the development of an acute phakolytic glaucoma (Lim et al. 2001).

6.3.4.4
Cornea

In some eyes with PEX syndrome, focal retrocorneal flakes of PEX material can be clinically observed adhering to the corneal endothelium (Fig. 6.3.17a, b). Ultrastructural evidence suggests *focal in situ* production of PEX fibers by corneal endothelial cells, which finally degenerate and detach from Descemet's membrane (Fig. 6.3.18a–d). Subsequent reendothelialization of denuded areas by neighboring fibroblastic endothelial cells leads to incorporation of PEX aggregates into Descemet's membrane (Fig. 6.3.18e, f) (Schlötzer-Schrehardt et al. 1993). Associated with these changes, the corneal endothelium shows nonspecific ultrastructural alterations, focal degeneration, and abnormal extracellular material production. Together with a reduced endothelial cell density, a diffuse non-guttate-like thickening of Descemet's membrane, and marked endothelial phagocytosis of melanin granules, the active involvement of the corneal endothelium in the PEX process leads to the concept of a distinctive PEX-associated keratopathy (Naumann and Schlötzer-Schrehardt 2000). The changes at the corneal endothelial surface may be seen clinically by slit-lamp biomicroscopy as a corneal edema associated with a diffusely thickened Descemet's membrane with irregular excrescences, different from typical guttata, and diffuse melanin deposition on the corneal endothelium (Fig. 6.3.17c). Specular microscopy reveals pronounced polymorphism of corneal

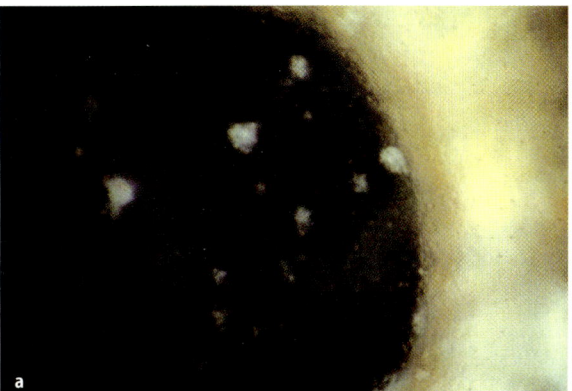
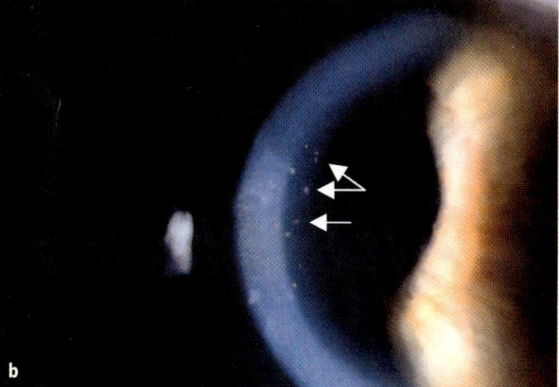

Fig. 6.3.17. Clinical appearance of corneal involvement in PEX syndrome (PEX keratopathy). **a, b** Retrocorneal deposits of PEX material (*arrows*)

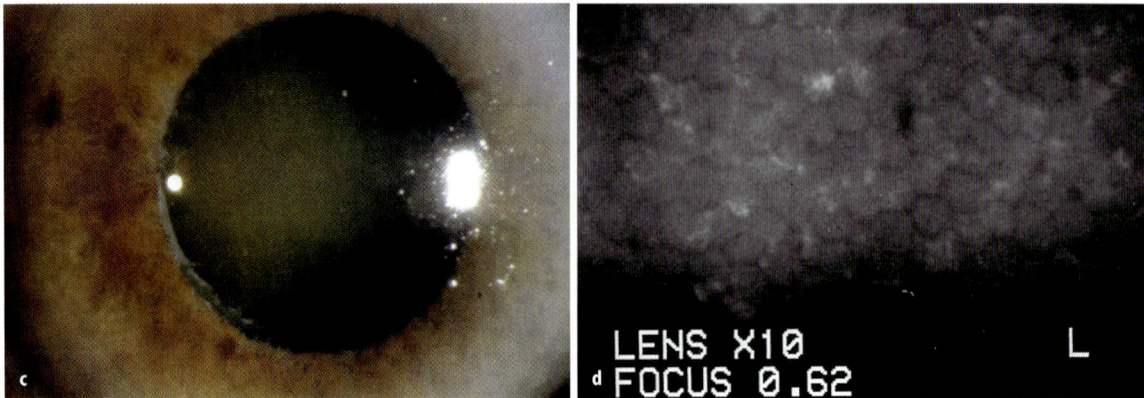

Fig. 6.3.17. c Diffuse corneal endothelial decompensation after diagnostic mydriasis. **d** Specular microscopy showing corneal endothelial pleomorphism and polymegathism and whitish PEX material deposits

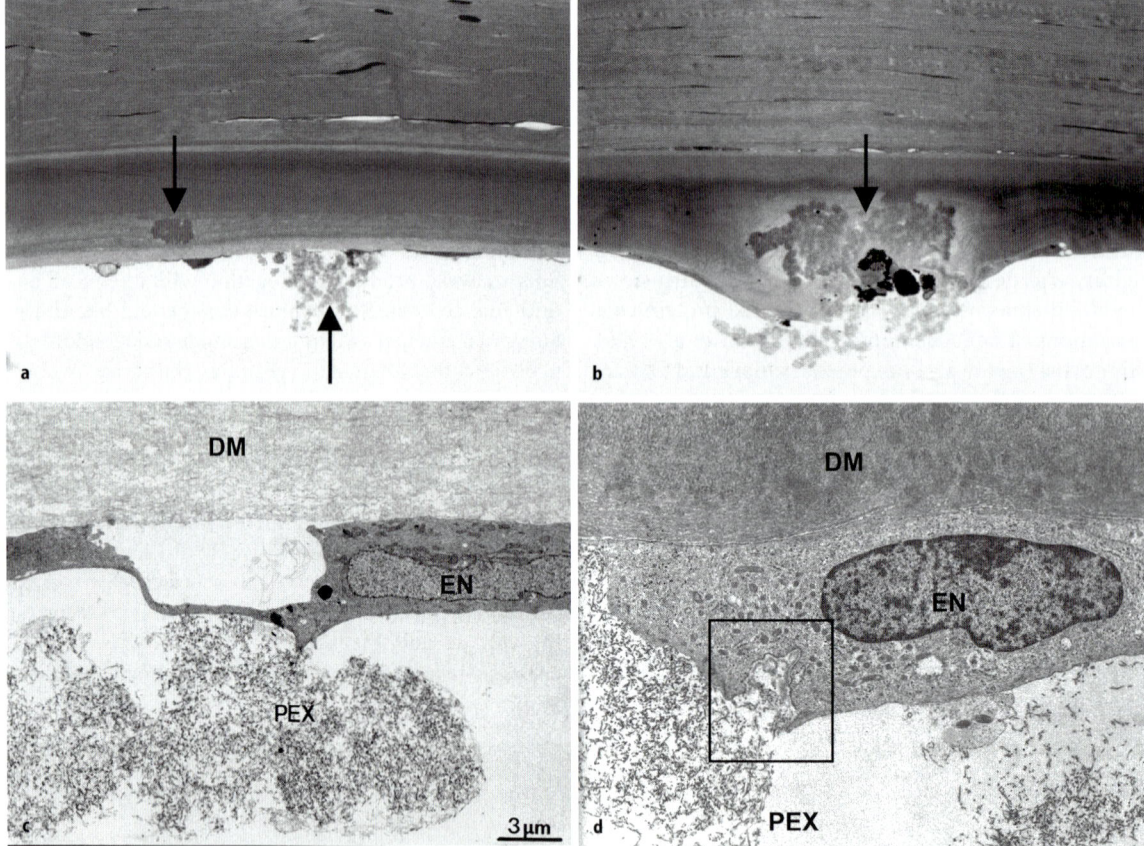

Fig. 6.3.18. Histopathologic features of PEX keratopathy. **a** Semithin section showing retrocorneal and intradescemetal deposits of PEX material (*arrows*). **b** Semithin section showing incorporation of PEX material (*arrow*) into the markedly thickened Descemet's membrane by overgrowing fibroblastic endothelial cells. **c** Transmission electron micrograph of the posterior corneal surface showing *PEX* fibers in association with an endothelial cell detaching from Descemet's membrane. **d** Electron micrograph showing *PEX* material in association with an endothelial cell; the *inset* shows PEX material intermingled with abnormal basement membrane material that appears to arise from an invagination of the corneal endothelial cell

endothelial cells and reduced cell counts of 800–1,500 cells/mm^2, occasionally also whitish PEX material deposits (Fig. 6.3.17d) (Knorr et al. 1991; Seitz et al. 1995).

This specific PEX keratopathy, which is independent of the presence of glaucoma and differs from Fuchs' endothelial dystrophy – approximately 10% patients clinically diagnosed as having Fuchs' dystrophy are in fact

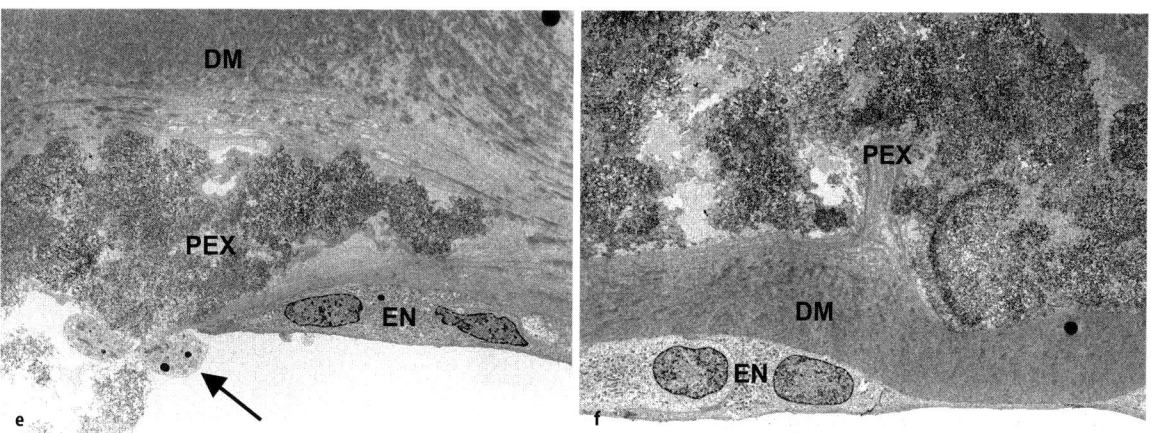

Fig. 6.3.18. e *PEX* clump incorporated into Descemet's membrane by overgrowing fibroblastic endothelial cells. **f** Massive incorporation of *PEX* material into posterior Descemet's membrane forming protrusions or warts (*DM* Descemet's membrane, *EN* endothelial cell)

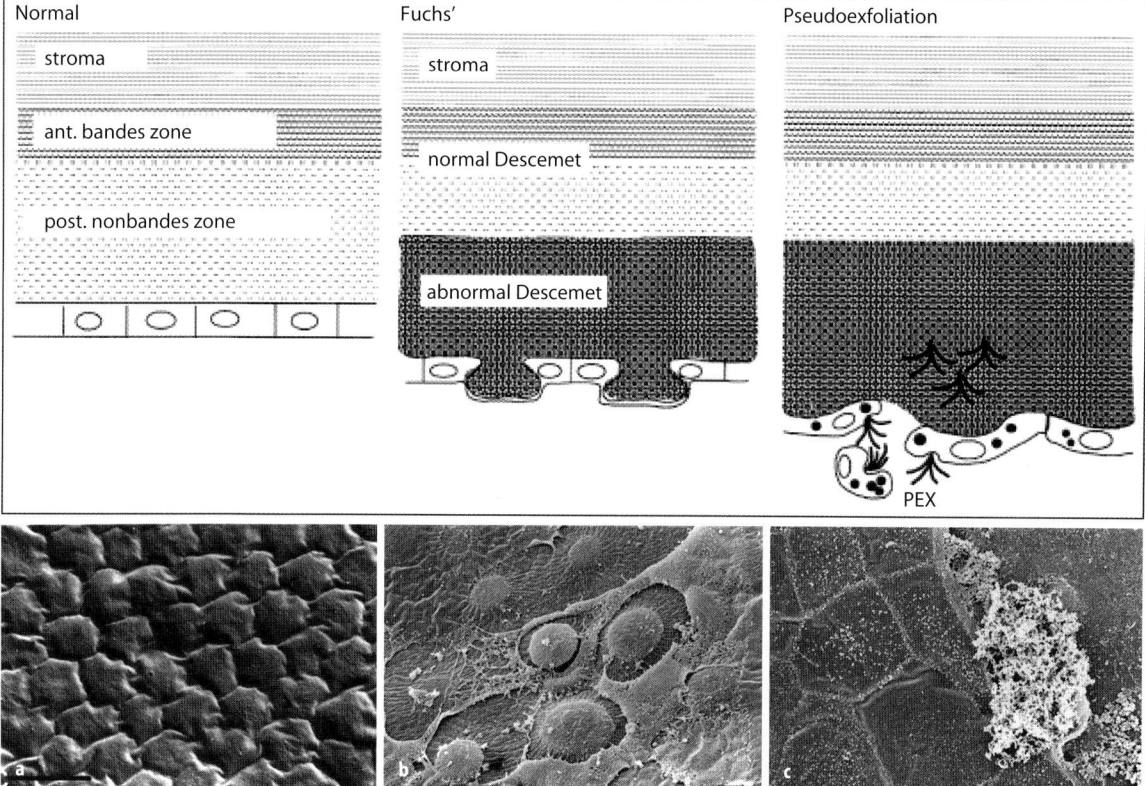

Fig. 6.3.19. Schematic representation of the posterior cornea and scanning electron micrographs of the corneal endothelium displaying the differential histopathologic diagnosis of PEX keratopathy (**c**) and Fuchs' endothelial dystrophy (**b**) compared with the normal structure of the posterior cornea (**a**)

suffering from PEX keratopathy – develops by characteristic gradual alterations of the posterior cornea (Fig. 6.3.19). Such a damaged and dysfunctional corneal endothelium increases the risk of early corneal endothelial decompensation after moderate rises in intraocular pressure, e.g., after mydriasis, or after minor intraoperative trauma (Fig. 6.3.20), and can even result in irreversible corneal endothelial decompensation requiring penetrating keratoplasty. The distinction between Fuchs' and PEX keratopathy is of clinical relevance, particularly if a simultaneous perforating keratoplasty (PKP) and extracapsular cataract extraction (ECCE) with lens implantation (triple procedure) is planned: the zonular instability and other anterior segment

Table 6.3.6. Clinical differential diagnosis of Fuchs' endothelial corneal dystrophy and pseudoexfoliation (PEX) keratopathy

	Fuchs' corneal dystrophy	PEX keratopathy
Secondary glaucoma	–	++
Cornea guttata	+++	+ atypical
Iris atrophy	–	+ → +++
Melanin dispersion	–	++
Location	Central	Diffuse
Endothelial loss	+++	++
Nuclear cataract	++	++

+ = mild, ++ = moderate, +++ = marked, – = absent

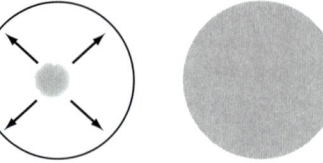

Fuchs' dystrophy (central)   PEX keratopathy (diffuse)   Pseudophakic keratopathy (peripheral)

Fig. 6.3.20. Schematic representation of the differential clinical diagnosis of corneal endothelial decompensation patterns in Fuchs' endothelial dystrophy, pseudophakic bullous keratopathy, and pseudoexfoliation (PEX) keratopathy

changes are not relevant in Fuchs' dystrophy (Table 6.3.6). However, the corneal manifestations of PEX signal a vulnerability for decompensation also in all other types of intraocular anterior segment microsurgery.

6.3.5
Microsurgical Considerations

The final results of cataract surgery and glaucoma filtering surgery in eyes with PEX in the very *early* stages are usually comparable to those in eyes without PEX. However, intraoperative and postoperative surgical complications are more common and more serious and are related to the pathological tissue alterations of the anterior segment (Table 6.3.1). As complications occur more frequently with *advanced* disease, as a general principle we prefer to recommend cataract extraction in relatively early stages of the disease to avoid late stage increased zonular instability and harder nuclei. Because long-term effects of medical therapy and laser treatment are often unsatisfactory in patients with PEX-associated open-angle glaucoma, surgical intervention may be more early and more frequently necessary than in other forms of glaucoma. However, patients need to be given realistic expectations through adequate preoperative counselling regarding the more complicated nature of the surgery, increased risk of complications, and more prolonged recovery time (Conway et al. 2004).

6.3.5.1
Intraoperative Complications

In a prospective study of 1,000 extracapsular cataract extractions the only significant risk factors for vitreous loss were the presence of *PEX* and *small pupil size*, which underscores the importance of adequate surgical access (Guzek et al. 1987). As PEX often responds poorly to mydriatics due to the iris dilator muscle atrophy and sphincter muscle fibrosis, mechanical dilatation is frequently required intraoperatively. Strategies might include removal of posterior synechiae as well as *mechanical enlargement of the pupil* including stretching, iris hooks or sphincterotomy. The presence of abnormal friable iris vessels can lead to intraoperative hemorrhage during iris manipulation, postoperative hyphema and a marked fibrin reaction as evidence of the blood-aqueous barrier breakdown in PEX irides.

Although the posterior capsule is of normal thickness, posterior capsular rupture during cataract surgery is reported to be increased 5- to 13-fold in eyes with PEX compared to eyes without PEX (Guzek et al. 1987), which may be predisposed by poor surgical access because of inadequate mydriasis and an instable zonular apparatus. The mechanical behavior of the anterior capsule is reported to be normal.

Perhaps the most serious complication associated with surgery on eyes with PEX can be attributed to zonular weakness. Zonular fragility has been associated with a three- to tenfold increased risk of zonular dialysis and lens dislocation and an approximately fivefold increased risk of vitreous loss (Naumann et al. 1988). Another study has found that anterior chamber depth asymmetry – in comparison to the fellow eye – and absolute anterior chamber depth less than 2.5 mm (presumably related to weak zonules allowing anterior lens movement) were associated with increased risk of zonular dialysis and/or vitreous loss (Küchle et al. 2000). Strategies to reduce stress on the zonules may include avoidance of excessive fluctuations in anterior chamber pressure, e.g., through the use of small incision surgery and adequate viscoelastics, as well as avoidance of quick maneuvers on the lens (Naumann et al. 1998; Conway et al. 2004). In cases with frank zonular weakness as indicated by phacodonesis and/or shallow anterior chamber, the use of a capsular tension ring that is supposed to distribute forces circumferentially is recommended to improve capsule fixation and to avoid focal stress on the zonules as well as to reduce postoperative lens decentration (Moreno-Montanes et al. 2002). This, however, may not prevent late postoperative decentration and dislocation of the lens implant.

Patients with PEX may have reduced corneal endothelial reserve due to both the reduced cell count and the direct involvement of the remaining endothelial cells in the PEX process. Awareness of this may help reduce critical intraoperative endothelial cell loss and avoid postoperative corneal endothelial failure.

6.3.5.2
Postoperative Complications

Although the outcome of glaucoma filtering surgery in PEX eyes is usually comparable to that in eyes with POAG, peri- and postoperative surgical complications, such as inflammatory responses, fibrin reactions, formation of synechiae, and intraocular pressure fluctuations, are much more common in PEX eyes. These postoperative complications can be directly attributed to the characteristic chronic defects in blood-aqueous barrier (Küchle et al. 1995), which are exaggerated by the paracentesis effect (see Chapters 2, 4) in the early postoperative phase with a more prolonged return to basal levels compared to controls (Nguyen et al. 1999; Schumacher et al. 1999). Therefore, frequent and thorough follow-up examinations are important for detection and treatment of complications in the early period. Preoperative treatment with corticosteroids and non-steroidal anti-inflammatory agents may be beneficial along with more intensive and prolonged topical postoperative corticosteroid therapy and prostaglandin inhibitors.

Late postoperative complications in PEX patients include a higher incidence of secondary cataract and late decentration or even subluxation of the lens implant including the capsular bag (Auffahrt et al. 1996). Probably because of the persistent breakdown of the blood-aqueous barrier, posterior and anterior capsular opacification/contraction due to lens epithelial proliferation and pseudofibrotic metaplasia are significantly more common in eyes with PEX [45% within 24 months in one series using polymethyl methacrylate (PMMA) lenses] (Küchle et al. 1997).

6.3.6
Conclusions

PEX syndrome is a common age-related generalized disorder of the extracellular matrix affecting a considerable proportion of our cataract and glaucoma patients. It may not only cause severe chronic open-angle glaucoma, but also a spectrum of other ocular complications including phacodonesis, lens subluxation, melanin dispersion, blood-aqueous barrier impairment, posterior synechiae, corneal endothelial decompensation, and serious intra- and postoperative complications in cataract surgery. In addition, it appears to be associated with an increased risk for cardiovascular disease. A thorough awareness of the pathology of PEX syndrome and its effects on ocular tissues is critical to understand the multifactorial causes of "spontaneous" and operative complications and thereby find ways to avoid or minimize them. Regarding the clinical management of these patients, the importance of early recognition of the pathological features, expectations of a higher complication rate, close attention to postoperative follow-up and well-informed patients before surgery have to be emphasized.

References

Asano N, Schlötzer-Schrehardt U, Naumann GOH: A histopathologic study of iris changes in pseudoexfoliation syndrome. Ophthalmology 1995, 102, 1279–1290

Auffahrt GU, Tsao K, Wesendahl TA, Sugita A, Apple DJ. Centration and fixation of posterior chamber intraocular lenses in eyes with pseudoexfoliation syndrome. Acta Ophthalmol Scand 1996, 74, 463–467

Bartholomew RS. Lens displacement associated with pseudocapsular exfoliation. A report on 19 cases in the Southern Bantu. Br J Ophthalmol 1970, 54, 744–750

Bleich S, Roedl J, von Ahsen N, Schlötzer-Schrehardt U, Reulbach U, Beck G, Kruse FE, Naumann GOH, Kornhuber J, Jünemann AGM. Elevated homocysteine levels in aqueous humor of patients with pseudoexfoliation glaucoma. Am J Ophthalmol 2004, 138, 162–164

Brooks AMV, Gillies WE. Fluorescein angiography and fluorophotometry of the iris in pseudoexfoliation of the lens capsule. Br J Ophthalmol 1983, 67, 249–254

Carpel EF. Pupillary dilation in eyes with pseudoexfoliation syndrome. Am J Ophthalmol 1988, 105, 692–694

Conway RM, Schlötzer-Schrehardt U, Küchle M, Naumann GOH. Pseudoexfoliation syndrome: pathologic manifestations of relevance to intraocular surgery. Clin Exp Ophthalmol. 2004, 32, 199–210

Cursiefen C, Händel A, Schönherr U, Naumann GOH. Pseudoexfoliation syndrome in patients with branch and central retinal vein thrombosis. Klin Monatsbl Augenheilkd 1997;211:17–21

Damji KF, Bains HS, Stefansson E, Loftsdottir M, Sverrisson T, Thorgeirsson E, Jonasson F, Gottfredsdottir M, Allingham RR. Is pseudoexfoliation syndrome inherited? A review of genetic and nongenetic factors and a new observation. Ophthalmic Genetics 1998, 19, 175–185

Dark AJ, Streeten BW. Precapsular film on the aging human lens: Precursor of pseudoexfoliation? Br J Ophthalmol 1990, 74, 717–722

Freissler K, Küchle M, Naumann GOH. Spontaneous dislocation of the lens in pseudoexfoliation syndrome. Arch Ophthalmol 1995, 113, 1095–1096

Gillies WE, Brooks AMV. Central retinal vein occlusion in pseudoexfoliation of the lens capsule. Clin Exp Ophthalmol 2002, 30, 176–178

Gottanka J, Flügel-Koch C, Martus P. Correlation of pseudoexfoliative material and optic nerve damage in pseudoexfoliation syndrome. Invest Ophthalmol Vis Sci 1997, 38, 2435–2446

Gross FJ, Tingey D, Epstein DL. Increased prevalence of occludable angles and angle-closure glaucoma in patients with pseudoexfoliation. Am J Ophthalmol 1994, 117, 333–336

Guzek JP, Holm M, Cotter JB, Cameron JA, Rademaker WJ, Wissinger DH et al. Risk factors for intraoperative complications in 1000 extracapsular cataract cases. Ophthalmology 1987, 94, 461–466

Hammer Th, Schlötzer-Schrehardt U, Naumann GOH. Unilateral or asymmetric pseudoexfoliation syndrome? An ultrastructural study. Arch Ophthalmol 2001, 119, 1023–1031

Helbig H, Schlötzer-Schrehardt U, Noske W, Kellner U, Foerster MH, Naumann GOH: Anterior chamber hypoxia and iris vasculopathy in pseudoexfoliation syndrome. German J Ophthalmol 1994, 3, 148–153

Hietanen J, Kivelä T, Vesti E, Tarkkanen A. Exfoliation syndrome in patients scheduled for cataract surgery. Acta Ophthalmol 1992, 70, 440–446

Inazumi K, Takahashi D, Taniguchi T, Yamamoto T. Ultrasound biomicroscopic classification of zonules in exfoliation syndrome. Jpn J Ophthalmol 2002, 46, 502–509

Kivelä T, Hietanen J, Uusitalo M. Autopsy analysis of clinically unilateral exfoliation syndrome. Invest Ophthalmol Vis Sci 1997, 38, 2008–2015

Knorr HLJ, Jünemann A, Händel A, Naumann GOH. Morphometrische und qualitative Veränderungen des Hornhautendothels bei Pseudoexfoliationssyndrom. Fortschr Ophthalmol 1991, 88, 786–789

Koliakos GG, Konstas AGP, Schlötzer-Schrehardt U, Hollo G, Katsimbris IE, Georgiadis N, Ritch R. 8-isoprostaglandin F2A and ascorbic acid concentration in the aqueous humour of patients with exfoliation syndrome. Br J Ophthalmol 2003; 87: 353–356

Konstas AGP, Stewart WC, Stromann GA. Clinical presentation and initial treatment patterns in patients with exfoliation glaucoma versus primary open-angle glaucoma. Ophth Surg Lasers 1997, 28, 111–117

Krause U, Helve J, Forsius H. Pseudoexfoliation of the lens capsule and liberation of iris pigment. Acta Ophthalmol 1973, 51, 39–46

Küchle M, Nguyen N, Hannappel E. The blood-aqueous barrier in eyes with pseudoexfoliation syndrome. Ophthalmic Res 1995, 27(Suppl 1), 136–142

Küchle M, Amberg A, Martus P, Nguyen NX, Naumann GOH. Pseudoexfoliation syndrome and secondary cataract. Br J Ophthalmol 1997, 81, 862–866

Küchle M, Viestenz A, Martus P, Händel A, Jünemann A, Naumann GOH. Anterior chamber depth and complications during cataract surgery in eyes with pseudoexfoliation syndrome. Am J Ophthalmol 2000, 129, 281–285

Lanzl IM, Merte RL, Graham AD. Does head positioning influence anterior chamber depth in pseudoexfoliation syndrome? J Glaucoma 2000, 9, 214–218

Lim MC, Doe EA, Vroman DT, Rosa RH, Parrish RK. Late onset lens particle glaucoma as a consequence of spontaneous dislocation of an intraocular lens in pseudoexfoliation syndrome. Am J Ophthalmol 2001, 132, 261–263

Lindberg JG. Clinical investigations on depigmentation of the pupillary border and translucency of the iris. Acta Ophthalmol 1989, 67 (Suppl 190), 1–96

Mardin CY, Schlötzer-Schrehardt U, Naumann GOH. "Masked" pseudoexfoliation syndrome in unoperated eyes with circular posterior synechiae. Arch Ophthalmol 2001, 119, 1500–1504

Mitchell P, Wang JJ, Smith W. Association of pseudoexfoliation syndrome with increased vascular risk. Am J Ophthalmol 1997, 124, 685–687

Moreno-Montanes J, Rodriguez-Conde R. Capsular tension ring in eyes with pseudoexfoliation. J Cat Refract Surg 2002;28:2241–2242

Naumann GOH, Schlötzer-Schrehardt U. Keratopathy in pseudoexfoliation syndrome as a cause of corneal endothelial decompensation. A clinicopathologic study. Ophthalmology 2000, 107, 1111–1124

Naumann GOH, "Erlanger Augenblätter-Group". Exfoliation syndrome as a risk factor for vitreous loss in extracapsular cataract surgery (preliminary report). Acta Ophthalmol 1988, 66 (Suppl 184), 129–131

Naumann GOH, Schlötzer-Schrehardt U, Küchle M. Pseudoexfoliation syndrome for the comprehensive ophthalmologist. Intraocular and systemic manifestations. Ophthalmology 1998, 105, 951–968

Nguyen NX, Küchle M, Martus P, Naumann GOH. Quantification of blood-aqueous barrier breakdown after trabeculectomy: pseudoexfoliation versus primary open-angle glaucoma. J Glaucoma 1999, 8, 18–23

Orr AC, Robitaille JM, Price PA, Hamilton JR, Falvey DM, De Saint-Sardos AG, Pasternak S, Guernsey DL. Exfoliation syndrome: clinical and genetic features. Ophthalmic Genetics 2001, 22, 171–185

Parodi MB, Bondel E, Saviano S, Ravalico G. Iris indocyanine green angiography in pseudoexfoliation syndrome and capsular glaucoma. Acta Ophthalmol Scand 2000, 78, 437–442

Prince AM, Streeten BW, Ritch R. Preclinical diagnosis of pseudoexfoliation syndrome. Arch Ophthalmol 1987, 105, 1076–1082

Ritch R. Exfoliation syndrome: the most common identifiable cause of open-angle glaucoma. J Glaucoma 1994a, 3, 176–178

Ritch R. Exfoliation syndrome and occludable angles. Trans Am Ophthalm Soc 1994b, 92, 845–944

Ritch R, Schlötzer-Schrehardt U. Exfoliation syndrome. Surv Ophthalmol 2001, 45, 265–315

Ritch R, Schlötzer-Schrehardt U, Konstas AGP. Why is glaucoma associated with exfoliation syndrome? Progr Ret Eye Res. 2003, 22, 253–275

Sampaolesi R, Zarate J, Croxato O. The chamber angle in exfoliation syndrome: Clinical and pathological findings. Acta Ophthalmol 1988, 66 (Suppl 184), 48–53

Schlötzer-Schrehardt U, Naumann GOH: A histopathologic study of zonular instability in pseudoexfoliation syndrome. Am J Ophthalmol 1994, 118, 730–743

Schlötzer-Schrehardt U, Naumann GOH: Trabecular meshwork in pseudoexfoliation syndrome with and without open-angle glaucoma. A morphometric, ultrastructural study. Invest Ophthalmol Vis Sci 1995, 36, 1750–1764

Schlötzer-Schrehardt U, Naumann GOH. Perspective – Ocular and systemic pseudoexfoliation syndrome. Am J Ophthalmol 2006, 141, 921–937

Schlötzer-Schrehardt U, Koca M, Naumann GOH, Volkholz H: Pseudoexfoliation syndrome: ocular manifestation of a systemic disorder? Arch Ophthalmol 1992, 110, 1752–1756

Schlötzer-Schrehardt U, Dörfler S, Naumann GOH: Corneal endothelial involvement in pseudoexfoliation syndrome. Arch Ophthalmol 1993, 111, 666–674

Schlötzer-Schrehardt U, Küchle M, Naumann GOH. Mechanisms of Glaucoma Development in Pseudoexfoliation Syndrome. In: Gramer E, Grehn F (eds). Pathogenesis and Risk Factors of Glaucoma. Heidelberg, Springer. Chapter 5, 1999, pp 34–49

Schlötzer-Schrehardt U, Zenkel M, Küchle M, Sakai LY, Naumann GOH. Role of transforming growth factor-β1 and its latent form binding protein in pseudoexfoliation syndrome. Exp Eye Res 2001, 73, 765–780

Schumacher S, Nguyen NX, Küchle M, Naumann GOH. Quantification of aqueous flare after phacoemulsification with intraocular lens implantation in eyes with pseudoexfoliation syndrome. Arch Ophthalmol 1999, 117, 733–735

Schumacher S, Schlötzer-Schrehardt U, Martus P, Lang W, Naumann GOH. Pseudoexfoliation syndrome and aneurysms of the abdominal aorta. Lancet 2001, 357, 359–360

Seitz B, Müller EE, Langenbucher A, Kus MM, Naumann GOH. Endotheliale Keratopathie bei Pseudoexfoliationssyndrom: quantitative und qualitative Morphometrie mittels automatisierter Videobildanalyse. Klin Monatsbl Augenheilkd 1995, 207, 167–175

Shrum KR, Hattenhauer MG, Hodge D. Cardiovascular and cerebrovascular mortality associated with ocular pseudoexfoliation. Am J Ophthalmol 2000, 129, 83–86

Streeten BW. Aberrant synthesis and aggregation of elastic tissue components in pseudoexfoliative fibrillopathy: a unifying concept. New Trends in Ophthalmology 1993, 8, 187–196

Streeten BW, Li Z-Y, Wallace RN, Eagle RC, Keshgegian AA. Pseudoexfoliative fibrillopathy in visceral organs of a patient with pseudoexfoliation syndrome. Arch Ophthalmol 1992, 110, 1757–1762

Tetsumoto K, Schlötzer-Schrehardt U, Küchle M, Dörfler S, Naumann GOH: Precapsular layer of the anterior lens capsule in early pseudoexfoliation syndrome. Graefe's Arch Clin Exp Ophthalmol 1992, 230, 252–257

Teus MA, Castejon MA, Calvo MA. Intraocular pressure as a risk factor for visual field loss in pseudoexfoliative and in primary open-angle glaucoma. Ophthalmology 1998, 105, 2225–2229

Thorleifsson G, Magnusson KP, Sulem P, et al. Common sequence variants in the LOXL1 gene confer susceptibility to exfoliation glaucoma. Science 2007, 317: 1397–1400

Vessani RM, Ritch R, Liebmann J, Jofe M. Plasma homocysteine is elevated in patients with exfoliation syndrome. Am J Ophthalmol 2003, 136, 41–46

Vogt A. Ein neues Spaltlampenbild des Pupillengebiets: Hellblauer Pupillensaumfilz mit Häutchenbildung auf der Linsenvorderkapsel. Klin Monatsbl Augenheilkd 1925, 75, 1–12

von der Lippe I, Küchle M, Naumann GOH. Pseudoexfoliation syndrome as a risk factor for acute ciliary block angle closure glaucoma. Acta Ophthalmol 1993, 71, 277–279

Wishart PK, Spaeth GL, Poryzees EM. Anterior chamber angle in the exfoliation syndrome. Br J Ophthalmol 1985, 69, 103–107

Zagórski Z, Gossler B, Naumann GOH. Effect of low oxygen tension on the growth of bovine corneal endothelial cells in vitro. Ophthalmic Res 1989, 21, 440–442

Zenkel M, Pöschl E, von der Mark K, Hofmann-Rummelt C, Naumann GOH, Kruse FE, Schlötzer-Schrehardt U. Differential gene expression in pseudoexfoliation syndrome. Invest Ophthalmol Vis Sci 2005, 46, 3742–3752

6.4 Other Generalized Diseases

G.O.H. Naumann

6.4.1
Infectious Disorders (AIDS, Sepsis)

Intraocular infections usually derive from bacteria or fungi of the lid margins from the patients themselves. Another possibility is the rare infection of infusion fluid, lens implants or instruments. Corneal grafts require the exclusion of viral infections such as hepatitis B and C or AIDS.

Generalized and epibulbar and adnexal bacterial infections are a relative contraindication for intraocular surgery. This is particularly true for patients suffering from diabetes mellitus, insufficiency of hepatic function or acquired immune deficiency syndrome (HIV, AIDS). Postoperative endophthalmitis is discussed in chapter 2, 4 and 5.5.

Chronic viral infections of the patients themselves (hepatitis B and C, HIV) are not a contraindication for intraocular microsurgery. However, it is in the surgeon's interest that these entities are excluded by history and testing as additional precautions to prevent infection of the surgical team.

6.4.2
Hematologic Disorders

Intra- and Postoperative Hemorrhage

Diseases of the vessel wall, e.g., arteriosclerosis with diabetes mellitus or arterial hypertension, alert to the risk of hemorrhage. More common are deficiency of coagulation factors in the blood – rarely congenital or acquired – most frequently with anticoagulation therapy in cardiovascular disease.

6.4.3
Neurologic and Muscular Diseases

Myotonic dystrophy – easily diagnosed by the ophthalmologist from the pathognomonic cataract – and Parkinson's disease require close cooperation with the anesthesiologist.

Visual deprivation by congenital cataract may be interpreted as "mental retardation." Older patients suffer visual deprivation with acquired cataracts, may seem confused and develop pseudodementia.

Vitreous inflammatory infiltrates originating from peripheral retinal perivasculitis (Rucker) may be useful to confirm or raise suspicion of multiple sclerosis and should alert one to performing close postoperative care to prevent posterior or anterior synechiae.

Finally *Munchausen syndrome*-autoaggressive behavior can cause severe diagnostic irritation for the ophthalmologist. This entity should only be considered if other causes of infectious or traumatic conditions are excluded (see Naumann, 1995).

References (see also page 379)

Naumann GOH. The Bowman Lecture Nr. 56, Part II: Corneal Transplantation in Anterior Segment Diseases. Eye 1995; 9: 398–421

General References

Albert DM, Jakobiec FA (eds.) Principles and Practice of Ophthalmology, Philadelphia New York; Saunders: 1994 (7 Vols)

Apple DJ, Rabb MF: Ocular Pathology – Clinical Applications and Self-Assessment, ed. 3. (Formerly Clinicopathologico Correction of Ocular Disease: A Text and Stereoscopic Atlas), Mosby, St. Louis, 1985

Apple DJ, Kincaid MC, Mamalis N, Olson RJ. Intraocular lenses. Evolution designs, complications, and pathology, Williams & Wilkins, Baltimore, 1989

Berlinger NT. Robotic Surgery – Squeezing into Tight Places. NEJ Med 2006; 354: 2099

Bornfeld N, Gragoudas ES, Höpping W et al. Tumors of the Eye, Kugler, New York, 1991

Brennen T and many coauthors. Medical Professionalism in the New Millenium: A Physician Charter, 2002; 136: 243 simultaneously published in Lancet

DeLaey JJ, Hanssens M. Vascular Tumors and Malformations of the Ocular Fundus, London Boston; Kluwer, 1990

Duke-Elder (ed): System of Ophthalmology, 15 Volumes, Vol. 1 (1958) – XV (1976), London, Henry Kimpton, London

Forrester JV, Dick Aderhaut, McMenamin PG and Lee WR. The Eye (Basic Science in Practice), Saunders, London 2002

Garner A, Klintworth GK (eds.): Pathobiology of Ocular Disease: A Dynamic Process (2 Vols), Marcel Dekker, Inc., New York, 1994

Hogan MJ, Zimmerman LE: Ophthalmic Pathology – An Atlas and Textbook, 2nd edition. W.B. Saunders Co, London Philadelphia, 1962

Jensen OA. Human Ophthalmic Pathology, Copenhagen; Munksgaard, 1986

Johnson GJ, Miniassian DC, Weale R et al. The Epidemiology of Eye Disease, Chapman & Hall Medical, London, 1998 and Arnold, London 2003

Kelman CD. Phacoemulsification and aspiration: A new technique of cataract removal. Am J Ophthalmol 1967; 64: 23 – 25

Kelman CD. The history and development of phacoemulsification. Int Ophthalmol Clinics 1994; 34: 1 – 12

Lee WR. Ophthalmic Histopathology, Heidelberg London Berlin; Springer, 1993

Lommatzsch PK. Intraokulare Tumoren, Stuttgart; Enke, 1989

Lommatzsch, PK (editor) Ophthalmologische Onkologie, Enke, Stuttgart, 1999

Lommatzsch PK and Blodi FC. Intraocular tumors, Akademie Publ. Berlin, 1983

Naumann GOH and Gloor B. Wound Healing of the Eye and its Complications. Bergmann, Munich, 1980

Naumann GOH together with Apple DJ, von Domarus D, Hinzpeter EN, Ruprecht KW, Völcker HE, and Naumann LR. Pathologie des Auges, 1043 pp., 1603 Figs. 115 schemes, drawings, 188 diff. diagnostic tables. In: Doerr-Seifert-Uehlinger (eds) Vol 12: Speziellen Anatomischen Pathologie. Heidelberg Berlin New York, Springer-Verlag, 1980

Naumann GOH and Apple DJ with contributions by von Domarus D, Hinzpeter EN, Manthey RM, Naumann LR, Ruprecht KW, Völcker HE. Pathology of the Eye (translated by Apple DJ). 998 pp, 544 Figs in 1002 parts. New York, Springer-Verlag, 1986

Naumann GOH and Apple DJ, with contributions by Domarus D, Hinzpeter EN, Mantey RM, Naumann LR, Ruprecht KW, Völcker HE. Pathology of the Eye. Japanese Edition translated by Nishi O. 1066 pp, 544 Figs in 1002 parts. Tokyo, Springer-Verlag, 1987

Naumann GOH and coauthors: Apple DJ, Deuble-Bente K, von Domarus D, Funk RHW, Hinzpeter EN†, Holbach L, Kirchhoff B, Kruse FE, Küchle M, Lang GE, Laqua H, Lüllwitz W†, Messmer E, Ruggli GH, Ruprecht KW, Rummelt V, Schlötzer-Schrehardt U, Thiel HJ, Völcker HE, Weindler J, Wenkel H. Pathologie des Auges. 2nd extended and revised edition in 2 vols. (1500 pp, 818 figs in 1638 parts, partly incolor, including 175 schematic drawings, 284 differential diagnostic tables). In: Doerr-Seifert-Uehlinger (ed). Vol 12: Speziellen Anatomischen Pathologie. Heidelberg Berlin New York, Springer-Verlag, 1997

Naumann GOH and Apple DJ, with contributions by Domarus D, Hinzpeter EN, Mantey RM, Naumann LR, Ruprecht KW, Völcker HE. Pathology of the Eye. 2nd Japanese edition translated by Nishi O. Tokyo, Springer-Verlag, 2003

Machemer R (1972) Vitrectomy. A pars plana approach. Grune & Stratton, New York, pp 1 – 136

Offret G, Dhermy P, Brini A, Bec P. Anatomie pathologique de l'oeil et de ses annexes. Paris; Masson et Cie, 1974

Okisaka S. A Textbook and Atlas of Ocular Histopathology, Tokyo, 1991

Podos SM, Yanoff M (eds.) Textbook of Ophthalmology. Vols. 1 – 10; New York London; Gower, 1993

Reese A. Tumors of the Eye (3rd ed.) Hargerstown: Harper & Row, 1976

Ridley NHL. Intraocular acrylic lenses. Trans Ophthalmol Soc UK LXXI-617-621, 1951

Ridley NHL. Intraocular acrylic lenses – 10 years development. Br J Ophthalmol 1960; 44: 705 – 712

Schieck F, Brückner A (eds.) Kurzes Handbuch der Ophthalmologie. Vols. 1 – 7, Berlin; Springer, 1932

Spencer WH, Albert DM. The Armed Forces Institute of Pathology. An Appreciation, Arch Ophthal, 2006; 124: 1332 – 34

Spencer WH (ed.), Font RL, Green WR, Howes EL Jr, Jakobiec FA, Zimmerman LE: Ophthalmic Pathology – An Atlas and Textbook (3 Vols), 4th edition. W.B. Saunders Co, Philadelphia, 1996

Spiessl B et al. (eds.). T.N.M. Atlas of Ophthalmic Tumors, International Union Against Cancer (p. 272 – 295), Heidelberg Berlin New York; Springer, 1990

T.N.M. Classification of Ophthalmic Tumors. International Union Against Cancer, Geneva, 1985

Wessely K (eds.). Spezielle Pathologie des Auges, contributions by G. Abelsdorff, A. Elschnig, S. Ginsberg, R. Greef, E. Hertel, E. v. Hippel, R. Kümmel, W. Löhlein, A. Peters, F. Schieck, E. Seidel, A.v. Szily and K. Wessely. In: Henke F, Lubarsch O. (eds.) Handbuch der Speziellen pathologischen Anatomie und Histologie, XI. volume in 3 parts, Part I 1928, part II 1931, part III 1937, Berlin; Springer

World Health Organization: International Histological Classification of Tumours, Geneva, 1969–1980

Yanoff M and Fine B: Ocular Pathology, 5th Edition, 721 pages Mosby-Wolfe 2002

Yanoff M and Duker JS (eds). Ophthalmology, 2nd Edition, Mosby, St. Louis, 2004

Zimmerman LE, Sobin L: International Histological Classification of Tumors, Nr. 24: Histological Typing of Tumours of the Eye and its Adnexa, WHO, Geneva, 1980. In addition the volumes of the International Histological Classification of Tumors, World Health Organization, Geneva:

No. 3, Histological typing of soft tissue tumors, 1969
No. 7, Histological typing of salivary gland tumors, 1972
No. 12, Histological typing of skin tumors, 1974
No. 14, Histological and cytological typing of neoplastic diseases of haematopoietic and lymphoid tissues, 1976, Geneva, WHO publications

List of Figures

Chapter 1: Introduction

Fig. 1.1. Gerd Meyer-Schwickerath, 1920–1992, Hamburg, Bonn, Essen, Germany
Fig. 1.2. Operating microscope
Fig. 1.3. Lorenz E. Zimmerman (1920–), Washington DC, USA

Chapter 2: General Opthalmic Pathology: Principal Indications and Complications, Comparing Intra- and Extraocular Surgery

Fig. 2.1. Intraocular neovascularization
Fig. 2.2. Choroidal and retinal changes with ocular hypotony due to anterior segment trauma with wound leakage
Fig. 2.3. Choroidal detachment and differential diagnosis of choroidal edema
Fig. 2.4. Progression of choroidal detachment and hemorrhage in prolonged ocular hypotony syndrome following anterior segment trauma and aqueous leakage
Fig. 2.5. Lens-iris diaphragm moving forward by uveal hyperemia and effusion ("vis a tergo")
Fig. 2.6. Blood-ocular barrier breakdown ("paracentesis effect")
Fig. 2.7. Expulsive choroidal hemorrhage
Fig. 2.8. Pupillary and ciliary block leading to angle closure glaucoma (schematic)
Fig. 2.9. Purulent panophthalmitis
Fig. 2.10. Intraocular foreign body granuloma due to intraocular wooden foreign body
Fig. 2.11. Epithelial downgrowth or ingrowth (sketch)
Fig. 2.12. Cystic epithelial ingrowth in the deep corneal stroma anterior to Descemet's membrane
Fig. 2.13. Cystic epithelial ingrowth at iris root and ciliary body following perforating trauma
Fig. 2.14. Retinopathia proliferans – vitreoretinopathy
Fig. 2.15. Hemorrhage into the vitreous
Fig. 2.16. Region of minor persistence in the biomechanics of the eye wall at limbus, insertion of straight muscles and in the optic disc region
Fig. 2.17. Deformation of globe with blunt trauma; rupture of the globe at the limbus from contusion
Fig. 2.18. Proximity of osseous orbital wall and globe: narrowest distance at 12 and 6 o'clock

Chapter 3.1: Eyelids

Fig. 3.1.1. Cross section of the upper and lower eyelid
Fig. 3.1.2. Schematic illustration of the posterior eyelid lamellae
Fig. 3.1.3. Lymphatic drainage of the eyelids into the preauricular and submandibular nodes
Fig. 3.1.4. Degree of horizontal eyelid laxity estimated clinically by gently pulling the lid away from the eye
Fig. 3.1.5. Clinical signs of involutional ectropion of the upper eyelid in floppy eyelid syndrome
Fig. 3.1.6. Involutional ectropion of the upper eyelid in floppy eyelid syndrome
Fig. 3.1.7. Light microscopy of lid sections stained by van Gieson's method for elastic fibers in floppy eyelid syndrome and control specimens
Fig. 3.1.8. Matrix metalloproteinases in the tarsal conjunctiva and tarsal plate of floppy eyelid syndrome
Fig. 3.1.9. Lateral tarsal strip procedure
Fig. 3.1.10. Involutional ectropion of the left lower eyelid medially
Fig. 3.1.11. Cicatricial ectropion of the left lower eyelid
Fig. 3.1.12. Paralytic ectropion of the left lower eyelid
Fig. 3.1.13. Involutional entropion of the right lower eyelid
Fig. 3.1.14. Recurrent involutional entropion of the left lower eyelid with horizontal laxity
Fig. 3.1.15. Cicatricial entropion of the left lower eyelid
Fig. 3.1.16. Cicatricial upper lid entropion
Fig. 3.1.17. Acquired aponeurotic blepharoptosis of the right eye
Fig. 3.1.18. Acquired dermatochalasis involving the upper and lower eyelids
Fig. 3.1.19. Acquired myogenic blepharoptosis due to chronic progressive external ophthalmoplegia
Fig. 3.1.20. Basal cell carcinoma
Fig. 3.1.21. Sebaceous gland carcinoma
Fig. 3.1.22. Squamous cell carcinoma
Fig. 3.1.23. Malignant melanoma
Fig. 3.1.24. Merkel cell carcinoma
Fig. 3.1.25. Nodular pigmented basal cell carcinoma
Fig. 3.1.26. Large nodular basal cell carcinoma of the left lower eyelid
Fig. 3.1.27. Full-thickness defect
Fig. 3.1.28. Full-thickness defect of the right lower eyelid

Chapter 3.2: Lacrimal Drainage System

Fig. 3.2.1. Schematic illustration of the lacrimal drainage system with approximate measurements
Fig. 3.2.2. Oncocytoma of the lacrimal sac

Chapter 3.3: Orbit

Fig. 3.3.1. Anatomy of the bony orbit
Fig. 3.3.2. Orbital dermoid cysts located in different parts of the orbit and periorbita
Fig. 3.3.3. Histopathology of orbital dermoid cysts
Fig. 3.3.4. Orbital rhabdomyosarcoma
Fig. 3.3.5. Nodular fasciitis
Fig. 3.3.6. Langerhans-cell histiocytosis of the orbit
Fig. 3.3.7. Orbital lymphangioma
Fig. 3.3.8. Orbital cavernous hemangioma
Fig. 3.3.9. Primary intraosseous cavernous hemangioma of the orbit
Fig. 3.3.10. Orbital hemangiopericytoma
Fig. 3.3.11. Solitary fibrous tumor of the orbit
Fig. 3.3.12. Orbital neurilemmoma (schwannoma)
Fig. 3.3.13. Orbital marginal-zone B-cell lymphoma
Fig. 3.3.14. Orbital involvement in multiple myeloma
Fig. 3.3.15. Reactive polyclonal lymphofollicular hyperplasia of the orbit and periocular xanthogranulomas
Fig. 3.3.16. Bilateral orbital metastases as the first presentation of breast adenocarcinoma
Fig. 3.3.17. Adenoid cystic carcinoma of the lacrimal gland
Fig. 3.3.18. Thyroid eye disease
Fig. 3.3.19. Thyroid eye disease

Chapter 3.4: Conjunctiva and Limbus Cornae

Fig. 3.4.1. Conjunctival lymphangioma which clinically manifested as chronic chemosis
Fig. 3.4.2. Distended, normally invisible conjunctival lymphatics which become visible through iatrogenic trauma and secondary filling with erythrocytes
Fig. 3.4.3. Follicular form and papillary form of conjunctivitis
Fig. 3.4.4. Malignant melanoma of the conjunctiva extending onto the cornea, but respecting Bowman's layer as barrier
Fig. 3.4.5. Massive lymphatic drainage to regional lymphatics with malignant melanoma of the conjunctiva
Fig. 3.4.6. Clinical and histologic appearance of conjunctival nevus with pseudocysts
Fig. 3.4.7. Extraocular extension of uveal melanoma presenting as brown epibulbar tumor
Fig. 3.4.8. Theodore's superior limbal keratitis with typical rose bengal staining

Chapter 4: General Pathology for Intraocular Microsurgery: Direct Wounds and Indirect Distant Effects

Fig. 4.1. "Erlangen sketch" for documentation of anterior segment and intraocular pathology
Fig. 4.2. Access into the eye: corneal through Bowman's layer; and limbal corneoscleral beyond Bowman's layer
Fig. 4.3. Bowman's layer is crucial for fixation of single and running sutures
Fig. 4.4. Landmarks for the anterior segment surgeon
Fig. 4.5. Seclusio pupillae: posterior synechiae; occlusio pupillae: posterior synechiae and fibrovascular membrane covering the pupil back of the cornea
Fig. 4.6. Consequences of perforating injuries
Fig. 4.7. Obvious and potential compartments of the intraocular space
Fig. 4.8. "Vagaries" of the retinal pigment epithelium in distinct pattern (schematic)
Fig. 4.9. Terminology of variation of the corneal diameter and the length of the optical axis in various congenital anomalies
Fig. 4.10. Extreme nanophthalmus with microcornea and imminent angle closure glaucoma
Fig. 4.11. Clear corneal wound: avascular wound healing (schematic)
Fig. 4.12. Limbal wound: *vascularized* wound healing; scar after perforating peripheral corneal wound with vascularization; interruption of Bowman's layer; defect in Descemet's membrane bridged by newly formed basement membrane produced by proliferating corneal endothelium
Fig. 4.13. Corneal scar, partially vascularized after penetrating injury and traumatic aphakia with incarceration of formed vitreous
Fig. 4.14. Wound rupture after cataract extraction and recent perforating keratoplasty with mycotic keratitis and epithelial invasion
Fig. 4.15. Perforating corneal wound closed with two sutures with wound leakage; vascularized corneal scar with interrupted Descemet's membrane; after elliptical corneal transplantation, cataract extraction and lens implantation
Fig. 4.16. Vascularized scars after severe perforating injury of the anterior segment
Fig. 4.17. Surgically induced necrotizing scleritis leading to limbal furrow and corneoscleral leakage

Chapter 5.1: Cornea and Limbus

Fig. 5.1.1. In vivo confocal microscopy of subbasal corneal nerves
Fig. 5.1.2. Bullous keratopathy in Fuchs' dystrophy with corneal guttae
Fig. 5.1.3. Corneal Langerhans cells interdigitating in between corneal epithelium in vivo confocal microscopy

Fig. 5.1.4. Palisades of Vogt: localization of limbal stem cells
Fig. 5.1.5. Anti-inflammatory and antiangiogenic effects of corneal epithelium
Fig. 5.1.6. Macular corneal dystrophy
Fig. 5.1.7. Acute keratoconus
Fig. 5.1.8. Transition of avascular cornea into conjunctiva
Fig. 5.1.9. After an inflammatory stimulus such as herpetic keratitis parallel ingrowths of both clinically visible blood and clinically invisible lymphatic vessels into the cornea
Fig. 5.1.10. Pathologic lymphangiogenesis in vascularized human corneas obtained after keratoplasty
Fig. 5.1.11. Time course of hem- and lymphangiogenesis after an inflammatory stimulus
Fig. 5.1.12. Immune reflex arc leading to immune rejections after penetrating keratoplasty
Fig. 5.1.13. Corneal angiogenic privilege is already in place during fetal development
Fig. 5.1.14. Limbal transition zone in fetal human eyes
Fig. 5.1.15. Retrieval of healthy limbal stem cell tissue for ex-vivo amplification
Fig. 5.1.16. Map-dot-fingerprint dystrophy (Cogan's dystrophy) with typical "fingerprint" lines; cysts and basement membrane duplications
Fig. 5.1.17. Granular corneal dystrophy with "granular" deposits in the central corneal stroma
Fig. 5.1.18. Lattice dystrophy with fine tubes extending through central stroma
Fig. 5.1.19. Corneal iron lines
Fig. 5.1.20. Corneal neovascularization causes reduction in visual acuity primarily due to secondary opacifying changes in the corneal stroma
Fig. 5.1.21. Postkeratoplasty neovascularization is a common phenomenon after low-risk keratoplasty and predisposes to subsequent immune rejections
Fig. 5.1.22. Neurotrophic keratitis after refractive surgery (LASIK)
Fig. 5.1.23. Necrotizing keratitis after bacterial superinfection of herpetic stromal keratitis; granulomatous reaction against Descemet's membrane
Fig. 5.1.24. Avascular wound healing after keratoplasty for keratokonus with both of the double-running sutures in place
Fig. 5.1.25. Different types of immune rejection can be classified from the slit-lamp appearance
Fig. 5.1.26. Pathologic new blood vessels in the human cornea are quickly covered by pericytes and no longer depend on angiogenic growth factors
Fig. 5.1.27. Antiangiogenic therapy with bevacizumab eye drops
Fig. 5.1.28. Non-mechanical excimer laser keratoplasty yields lower postoperative astigmatism and better visual acuity
Fig. 5.1.29. A loose suture after keratoplasty attracts blood vessels, lymphatic vessels and antigen-presenting cells and induces immune rejections
Fig. 5.1.30. In DSAEK (Descemet stripping automated lamellar endothelial keratoplasty), a posterior lamella of about 100 μm is cut with the microkeratome
Fig. 5.1.31. Amniotic membrane consists of a single layer of epithelium with basement membrane and avascular stroma beneath

Chapter 5.2: Glaucoma Surgery

Fig. 5.2.1. Structures of anterior segment for aqueous circulation
Fig. 5.2.2. Variation of chamber angle in unremarkable anterior segment
Fig. 5.2.3. Fundamental glaucoma patterns
Fig. 5.2.4. Chamber angle pattern by gonioscopy
Fig. 5.2.5. Angle closure glaucomas
Fig. 5.2.6. Open angle glaucomas
Fig. 5.2.7. Pattern of macrophagocytic glaucomas
Fig. 5.2.8. Secondary open angle glaucoma
Fig. 5.2.9. Anterior chamber cleavage syndromes
Fig. 5.2.10. Peters' anomaly
Fig. 5.2.11. Histology of congenital glaucomas
Fig. 5.2.12. Principles of glaucoma surgery
Fig. 5.2.13. Histopathology after goniotomy
Fig. 5.2.14. Microanatomy beneath scleral flap
Fig. 5.2.15. Scarred filtering bleb after Elliot trephination
Fig. 5.2.16. Luxuriant filtering bleb extending on the surface of the cornea anterior to Bowman's layer
Fig. 5.2.17. Experimental erbium YAG-laser trabeculotomy in donor eye

Chapter 5.3: Iris

Fig. 5.3.1. Iris microanatomy: iris root and pupillary zone are significantly thinner than the rest of the iris
Fig. 5.3.2. Open, but very narrow chamber angle
Fig. 5.3.3. Congenital anomalies and acquired deformation of the pupil
Fig. 5.3.4. Congenital anomalies of anterior uvea and cornea as a spectrum of the anterior chamber cleavage syndrome
Fig. 5.3.5. Biocytology of uveal melanocytes
Fig. 5.3.6. Melanin dispersion syndromes: diaphanoscopy pattern (schematic)
Fig. 5.3.7. Diabetic iridopathy
Fig. 5.3.8. Iridopathy of pseudoexfoliation syndrome
Fig. 5.3.9. Sectorial ischemic necrosis of iris following acute pupillary block angle closure glaucoma
Fig. 5.3.10. Microsurgical procedures to iris
Fig. 5.3.11. Iridodialysis from 7–9 o'clock, contusion cataract and lens subluxation with bulging of iris from vitreous prolapse
Fig. 5.3.12. Optical sector coloboma for central congenital cataract performed in 1939

Fig. 5.3.13. Localized iris tumors not involving iris root sparing the chamber angle without signs of tumor cells shedding in the aqueous: suitable for curative iridectomy

Fig. 5.3.14. Early melanomas of the iris (rare!) with *documented growth* sparing the chamber angle and sphincter pupillae

Fig. 5.3.15. Wound healing of the iris in the rabbit 3 weeks after iridotomy with several interrupted sutures adapting the wound margins illustrating stromal and iris-pigment epithelial wound healing

Fig. 5.3.16. Primary rhabdomyosarcoma of iris involving the iris root *and* chamber angle

Fig. 5.3.17. Malignant melanomas of the iris root with diffuse shedding of the malignant melanocytes into the aqueous

Fig. 5.3.18. Localized epithelial implantation cyst *not* involving the angle

Fig. 5.3.19. Iris prolapse with early diffuse epithelial ingrowth

Fig. 5.3.20. Diffuse epithelial ingrowth of iris root, face of ciliary body and retrocorneal surface showing epithelial tract connecting with the surface epithelium

Fig. 5.3.21. Attempted YAG-laser iridotomy for angle closure glaucoma: Descemets membrane in iris

Fig. 5.3.22. Diffuse malignant melanoma of iris; recurrence

Fig. 5.3.23. Persisting anterior synechiae of iris to cornea after perforating injury

Chapter 5.4: Ciliary Body

Fig. 5.4.1. Normal ciliary body

Fig. 5.4.2. Aging changes of ciliary epithelium

Fig. 5.4.3. Aging of the ciliary muscle (3 months – 95 years)

Fig. 5.4.4. Blood supply of the pars plicata of the ciliary body by anastomosing branches from the long posterior ciliary artery and the anterior ciliary arteria via the four straight extraocular muscles

Fig. 5.4.5. Traumatic cyclodialysis showing separation of ciliary body from sclera with focal anterior synechiae of iris root, untreated

Fig. 5.4.6. Surgically intended cyclodialysis

Fig. 5.4.7. Direct cyclopexy for cyclodialysis with persisting ocular hypotony

Fig. 5.4.8. Direct cyclopexy closing traumatic cyclodialysis with persisting ocular hypotony in steps: pre-, intra- and postoperatively

Fig. 5.4.9. Malignant melanoma of the ciliary body and iris root: invasion of sclera, Schlemm's canal and outflow channels

Fig. 5.4.10. Diffuse shedding of malignant melanocytes into aqueous and adjacent structures in different patients showed unilateral ocular hypertension or glaucoma

Fig. 5.4.11. Diffuse non-pigmented malignant melanoma of the iris (ring melanoma) masquerading as "glaucoma"

Fig. 5.4.12. Recurrence and subconjunctival extension of malignant melanoma of the anterior uvea 14 years after sector iridectomy via corneal scleral incision

Fig. 5.4.13. Primary malignant rhabdomyosarcoma of the "iris root" in 5-year-old girl treated by sector iridectomy, recurrence

Fig. 5.4.14. Block excision of tumors of the anterior uvea (schematic)

Fig. 5.4.15. Highly vascularized malignant melanoma of the iris extending into the ciliary body in a 47-year-old male, block-excision

Fig. 5.4.16. Large malignant melanoma of the anterior uvea extending to the level of the inferior temporal retinal vessel arcade located inferiorly, block excision

Fig. 5.4.17. Malignant melanoma of the anterior uvea with extension into the iris root

Fig. 5.4.18. Teratoid medulloepithelioma in 4-year-old boy with adjacent cataract treated by block excision

Fig. 5.4.19. Melanocytic nevus of iris root and anterior ciliary body with spontaneous hemorrhage into the anterior chamber, block excision

Fig. 5.4.20. Episcleral extension of melanocytoma of the ciliary body, block excision

Fig. 5.4.21. Adenoma of the non-pigmented ciliary epithelium extending into the anterior chamber in 62-year-old female patient, block excision

Fig. 5.4.22. Adenoma of the ciliary pigment epithelium in 34-year-old female patient, block excision

Fig. 5.4.23. Leiomyoma of ciliary body and choroid with collateral and distant retinal detachment in 17-year-old boy treated by enucleation

Fig. 5.4.24. Mesectodermal leiomyoma of the ciliary body treated by 10-mm block excision in 43-year-old man

Fig. 5.4.25. Some common features of epithelial ingrowth involving the chamber angle relevant for ophthalmic microsurgers

Fig. 5.4.26. Congenital large cystic epithelial ingrowth ("iris cyst") filling two-thirds of the anterior chamber after amniocentesis

Fig. 5.4.27. Surgical steps of block excision of epithelial ingrowth in sketches

Fig. 5.4.28. Rapidly growing cystic epithelial ingrowth after thorn injury 2 years previously requiring 10-mm block excision

Fig. 5.4.29. Cystic epithelial ingrowth with impression cataract extending to posterior pole of lens, block excision

Fig. 5.4.30. Cystic epithelial ingrowth with nuclear cataract in 55-year-old male, block excision

Fig. 5.4.31. Cystic epithelial ingrowth 20 years after perforating keratoplasty for herpetic scars progressing into the pupillary area, block excision

Fig. 5.4.32. Cyclodestructive procedures

Chapter 5.5: Lens and Zonular Fibers

Fig. 5.5.1. Anatomy of the lens
Fig. 5.5.2. Stages in the embryonic development of the lens
Fig. 5.5.3. Relationship between the lens and the anterior vitreous face
Fig. 5.5.4. Ultrastructure of the lens epithelium and the lens capsule
Fig. 5.5.5. Schematic view of the lens capsule showing the relative thickness of various portions
Fig. 5.5.6. Surface view of lens epithelium
Fig. 5.5.7. Schematic view of the (pre)equatorial lens epithelium differentiating into lens fibers
Fig. 5.5.8. Ultrastructure of lens fibers
Fig. 5.5.9. Schematic representation of the adult lens showing the nuclear and cortical zones and the attachment of zonular fibers at the lens capsule
Fig. 5.5.10. Schematic representation of the vitreous body and its relationship to neighboring tissues
Fig. 5.5.11. Aging changes of the lens capsule
Fig. 5.5.12. Aging changes of the lens fibers
Fig. 5.5.13. Long anterior zonules
Fig. 5.5.14. Lens coloboma
Fig. 5.5.15. Lenticonus anterior and posterior
Fig. 5.5.16. Schematic representation of persistent hyperplastic primary vitreous (PHPV)
Fig. 5.5.17. Spontaneous course of persistent hyperplastic primary vitreous
Fig. 5.5.18. Ectopia lentis
Fig. 5.5.19. Congenital cataracts
Fig. 5.5.20. Cataracts associated with systemic disorders: diabetes, generalized skin disease, myotonic dystrophy and rheumatoid arthritis
Fig. 5.5.21. Contusion cataract
Fig. 5.5.22. Degenerative alterations of cortical lens fibers by transmission electron microscopy
Fig. 5.5.23. Degenerative alterations of cortical lens fibers by transmission electron microscopy
Fig. 5.5.24. Schematic representation of abnormal proliferation of the lens epithelium
Fig. 5.5.25. Anterior subcapsular cataract
Fig. 5.5.26. Posterior subcapsular cataract
Fig. 5.5.27. Types of cortical and nuclear lens degeneration and cataract formation
Fig. 5.5.28. Age-related cortical cataract
Fig. 5.5.29. Cataracta matura, cataracta hypermatura, and cataracta Morgagni
Fig. 5.5.30. Spheroliths
Fig. 5.5.31. True exfoliation and pseudoexfoliation of the lens capsule
Fig. 5.5.32. Phacogenic uveitis; beginning of "endophthalmitis phacoanaphylactica" with foreign body giant cells
Fig. 5.5.33. Schematic representation of main loci of fixation of artificial lenses
Fig. 5.5.34. Fibrosis of the posterior and anterior capsule following extracapsular cataract surgery
Fig. 5.5.35. Pearl-type posterior capsule opacification
Fig. 5.5.36. Soemmerring's ring cataract
Fig. 5.5.37. Potential complications of cataract surgery

Chapter 5.6: Retina and Vitreous

Fig. 5.6.1. Extremely simplified structural elements of the extraordinarily complex retina
Fig. 5.6.2. Horizontal barriers (*Leitstrukturen*) and the preformed spaces
Fig. 5.6.3. Vertical barriers (*Leitstrukturen*); horizontal *Leitstrukturen*; cystoid degeneration limited by middle limiting membrane and outer limiting membrane and Müller cells; hemorrhage in the inner and outer retinal layers beyond middle limiting membrane; shrinking preretinal membrane leads to foldings of the internal limiting membrane
Fig. 5.6.4. Vitreous detachment
Fig. 5.6.5. Peripheral retinal defects
Fig. 5.6.6. Seven types of retinal processes with treatment recommendation
Fig. 5.6.7. Lattice degeneration
Fig. 5.6.8. Retinal detachment and retinoschisis
Fig. 5.6.9. Manifestations of vitreomacular traction
Fig. 5.6.10. Cross sections through macular regions close to the foveola (OCT)
Fig. 5.6.11. Normal Foveola: Sketch histology
Fig. 5.6.12. Cystoid maculopathy with macular folds
Fig. 5.6.13. Cystoid maculopathy
Fig. 5.6.14. Stages of macular holes (modified after Gass)
Fig. 5.6.15. Cystoid space; incomplete hole; full thickness hole; pseudo hole; macular hole after severe contusion
Fig. 5.6.16. Optical coherence tomography demonstrating vitreomacular traction (upper) leading to an impending hole characterized by foveal cyst formation
Fig. 5.6.17. Fixed macular folds after reversible hypotony syndrome
Fig. 5.6.18. Posterior vitreous detachment versus vitreoschisis
Fig. 5.6.19. Arteria ophthalmica splits into the central retinal artery (retinal circulation) and the short posterior ciliary arteries (choroidal circulation)
Fig. 5.6.20. Ischemic retinal microinfarct ("cotton-wool spot"); similar damage from excessive light/laser damage originating from the "oven" of the RPE leading to interruption of axons
Fig. 5.6.21. Diabetic retinopathy
Fig. 5.6.22. Preretinal neovascularization
Fig. 5.6.23. Marked thickening of retinal vessel wall by excessive collagen formation
Fig. 5.6.24. Sarcoidosis: granulomatous vasculitis of retina

Fig. 5.6.25. Familial exudative vitreoretinopathy with central retinal fold and macular dragging; lymphocytic infiltrates surrounding vessels with thickened wall
Fig. 5.6.26. Retinopathy of prematurity: schematic drawing of the stages
Fig. 5.6.27. International Classification for Retinopathy of prematurity emphasizing location and extent
Fig. 5.6.28. Topographic relation of basal laminar deposits, soft drusen, and hard drusen
Fig. 5.6.29. Histology of various types of drusen
Fig. 5.6.30. Macular "edema"
Fig. 5.6.31. Choroidal neovascularization; chorioretinal anastomosis
Fig. 5.6.32. Fibrous hemorrhagic disciform macular degeneration
Fig. 5.6.33. Retinoblastoma: exophytic and endophytic tumor growth
Fig. 5.6.34. Growth pattern of malignant melanoma of the uvea
Fig. 5.6.35. Processes involving the retinal pigment epithelium
Fig. 5.6.36. Oculocerebral non-Hodgkin lymphoma
Fig. 5.6.37. Variants of posterior vitreous detachment
Fig. 5.6.38. The "Cologne" classification of proliferating vitreoretinopathy
Fig. 5.6.39. Appearance of retinal pigment epithelium in PVR
Fig. 5.6.40. Comparison of wound-healing reactions

Chapter 5.7: Optic Nerve and Elschnig's Scleral Ring

Fig. 5.7.1. Optic atrophy: ascending (after 2 weeks), descending (after 4–6 weeks)
Fig. 5.7.2. Schematic drawing of the vascular supply of the anterior optic nerve
Fig. 5.7.3. Course of the retinal nerve fibers in the optic disc according to the position of their ganglion cells
Fig. 5.7.4. Cross section through the optic disc with its prelaminar, laminar and retrolaminar parts
Fig. 5.7.5. Variants of sickle-shaped coni at the edge of the optic disc
Fig. 5.7.6. Typical and heterotypical congenital disc coni (right eye)
Fig. 5.7.7. Physiologic defect of the blood-retina barrier at the level of the optic disc
Fig. 5.7.8. Classification of prelaminar optic atrophy at the level of the optic disc
Fig. 5.7.9. Features of optic disc atrophy at the level of the retinal nerve fiber layer, pigment epithelium, choriocapillaris, cup and rim
Fig. 5.7.10. Healthy optic disc vs progressed, glaucomatous optic disc
Fig. 5.7.11. Cavernous optic atrophy
Fig. 5.7.12. Fluorescence angiography of a patient's fundus with Kranenburg's syndrome
Fig. 5.7.13. Melanocytoma of the optic disc within the optic nerve head
Fig. 5.7.14. Radiation arteriopathy

Chapter 6.3: Pseudoexfoliation Syndrome: Pathological Manifestations of Relevance to Intraocular Surgery

Fig. 6.3.1. Light and electron micrographs showing structure and origin of PEX material
Fig. 6.3.2. Schematic representation of anterior segment tissues involved in active production and subsequent deposition of PEX material
Fig. 6.3.3. Schematic representation of clinical classification of PEX syndrome based on morphologic alterations of the anterior lens surface
Fig. 6.3.4. Various clinical appearances of PEX material deposition in PEX syndrome
Fig. 6.3.5. Classification of PEX syndrome based on ultrastructural alterations of the anterior lens capsule surface
Fig. 6.3.6. Clinical involvement of the zonular apparatus in PEX syndrome
Fig. 6.3.7. Histopathologic involvement of the lens in PEX syndrome
Fig. 6.3.8. Schematic representation of the presumed origin of lenticular PEX material
Fig. 6.3.9. Histopathologic involvement of the zonular apparatus in PEX syndrome
Fig. 6.3.10. Schematic representation of the typical localizations of zonular alterations in PEX syndrome
Fig. 6.3.11. Schematic drawing of iris involvement in PEX syndrome
Fig. 6.3.12. Histopathologic involvement of the iris in PEX syndrome
Fig. 6.3.13. Clinical appearance of the iris affected by PEX
Fig. 6.3.14. Schematic representation of the trabecular meshwork in PEX syndrome showing the localization of PEX deposits of presumed endotrabecular (local production) and exotrabecular (passive inflow) origin
Fig. 6.3.15. Light microscopic semithin sections showing involvement of the trabecular meshwork and Schlemm's canal in PEX syndrome
Fig. 6.3.16. Electron micrographs showing involvement of the trabecular meshwork in PEX syndrome
Fig. 6.3.17. Clinical appearance of corneal involvement in PEX syndrome (PEX keratopathy)
Fig. 6.3.18. Histopathologic features of PEX keratopathy
Fig. 6.3.19. Schematic representation of the posterior cornea and scanning electron micrographs of the corneal endothelium displaying the differential histopathologic diagnosis of PEX keratopathy and Fuchs' endothelial dystrophy compared with the normal structure of the posterior cornea
Fig. 6.3.20. Schematic representation of the differential clinical diagnosis of corneal endothelial decompensation patterns in Fuchs' endothelial dystrophy, pseudophakic bullous keratopathy, and pseudoexfoliation keratopathy

List of Tables

Chapter 1: Introduction

Table 1.1. Historical overview of ophthalmic surgery from antiquity to 1800
Table 1.2. Selected overview of ophthalmic surgery after 1800
Table 1.3. Milestones and personalities in ophthalmic pathology and anatomy from antiquity to the present

Chapter 2: General Opthalmic Pathology: Principal Indications and Complications, Comparing Intra- and Extraocular Surgery

Table 2.1. Special features of the eye's normal function
Table 2.2. Special risks of "open eye" microsurgery
Table 2.3. Advantages and disadvantages of local and general anesthesia
Table 2.4. Potential indications for general anesthesia

Chapter 3.1: Eyelids

Table 3.1.1. Differential diagnosis of disorders in eyelid position and movement
Table 3.1.2. Frequency of eyelid tumors

Chapter 3.2: Lacrimal Drainage System

Table 3.2.1. Differential diagnosis of lacrimal drainage system disorders causing epiphora
Table 3.2.2. Lacrimal sac tumors

Chapter 3.3: Orbit

Table 3.3.1. Frequency of orbital tumors in children
Table 3.3.2. Frequency of orbital tumors in adults
Table 3.3.3. Differential diagnosis of proptosis
Table 3.3.4. Assessment of thyroid eye disease severity
Table 3.3.5. Clinical activity score of thyroid endocrine orbitopathy

Chapter 3.4: Conjunctiva and Limbus Cornae

Table 3.4.1. Differential diagnosis: follicular hypertrophy of the conjunctiva
Table 3.4.2. Differential diagnosis of oculoglandular Parinaud conjunctivitis
Table 3.4.3. Etiology of symblepharon
Table 3.4.4. Differential diagnosis of xerosis conjunctivae
Table 3.4.5. Differential diagnosis cystic/cystoid changes of the conjunctiva
Table 3.4.6. Differential diagnosis: leukoplakia of conjunctiva
Table 3.4.7. Pigmented findings of conjunctiva and episclera
Table 3.4.8. Classification of primary acquired melanosis
Table 3.4.9. Malignant melanoma of the conjunctiva: histologic classification
Table 3.4.10. Reasons for "enlargement" of pigmented conjunctival nevus
Table 3.4.11. Localized non-pigmented processes of the conjunctiva

Chapter 4: General Pathology for Intraocular Microsurgery: Direct Wounds and Indirect Distant Effects

Table 4.1. Access into eye – principal options
Table 4.2. Mechanical "loci minores resistentiae" of the eye wall-sclera
Table 4.3. Obvious and potential compartments of intraocular space
Table 4.4. Principal options of intraocular surgery
Table 4.5. Morphologic essential requirements for sustainable functioning "minimal eye"

Chapter 5.1: Cornea and Limbus

Table 5.1.1. Differential diagnosis of Descemet's folds
Table 5.1.2. Important corneal dimensions
Table 5.1.3. Differential diagnosis of the main stromal corneal dystrophies
Table 5.1.4. Differential diagnosis of corneal band degeneration

Chapter 5.2: Glaucoma Surgery

Table 5.2.1. Principal terminology of glaucomas

Table 5.2.2. Classification of primary and secondary angle closure glaucoma
Table 5.2.3. Differential diagnosis of angle closure glaucomas
Table 5.2.4. Classification of primary and secondary open angle glaucoma
Table 5.2.5. Differential diagnosis: open but "narrow anterior chamber angle"
Table 5.2.6. Congenital/infantile glaucoma
Table 5.2.7. Critical cell populations in open angle glaucomas
Table 5.2.8. Critical cell population with aging and open angle glaucoma
Table 5.2.9. Indications for glaucoma surgery
Table 5.2.10. Terminology of mechanical glaucoma surgery
Table 5.2.11. Glaucoma surgery – selection of implant types
Table 5.2.12. Terminology of non-mechanical glaucoma surgery
Table 5.2.13. Growth factors ("scar wars")

Chapter 5.3: Iris

Table 5.3.1. Iris-pigment epithelium defects on transillumination
Table 5.3.2. Iris-stroma necrosis: differential diagnosis
Table 5.3.3. "Biocytology" of anterior uvea and anterior lens capsule
Table 5.3.4. Spontaneous hyphema: causes
Table 5.3.5. Heterochromia iridium – differential diagnosis
Table 5.3.6. Iris cysts: differential diagnosis
Table 5.3.7. Differential diagnosis: "multiple iris nodules"
Table 5.3.8. Spectrum of laser effects on eye
Table 5.3.9. Melanocytic processes of the iris
Table 5.3.10. Non-pigmented tumors of iris
Table 5.3.11. Ocular pigments

Chapter 5.4: Ciliary Body

Table 5.4.1. Concerns with direct surgery of the ciliary body
Table 5.4.2. Indications for direct cyclopexy
Table 5.4.3. Tumors of the ciliary body: differential diagnosis
Table 5.4.4. Block excision of processes of the anterior uvea in 210 patients
Table 5.4.5. Block excisions of tumors of the anterior uvea: rationale
Table 5.4.6. Block excisions of epithelial ingrowth: reasons
Table 5.4.7. Block excision of expanding ciliary body tumors involving chamber angle
Table 5.4.8. Block excision of epithelial ingrowth

Chapter 5.5: Lens and Zonular Fibers

Table 5.5.1. Phakogenic intraocular disease
Table 5.5.2. Lens measurements throughout life
Table 5.5.3. Lens capsule thickness throughout life
Table 5.5.4. Major causes of ectopia lentis
Table 5.5.5. Cataract types
Table 5.5.7. Advantages and disadvantages of intra- and extracapsular cataract extraction
Table 5.5.8. Cataract surgery: risks and complications

Chapter 5.6: Retina and Vitreous

Table 5.6.1. Common findings in the retinal periphery
Table 5.6.2. Recommendations for prophylactic laser coagulation in patients with lattice degeneration with and without retinal holes
Table 5.6.3. Peripheral microcystoid degeneration in degenerative retinoschisis
Table 5.6.4. Recommendations for a prophylactic laser photocoagulation in patients with fresh horseshoe tears
Table 5.6.5. Differential diagnosis of peripheral retinal defects
Table 5.6.6. Causes of exudative retinal detachments
Table 5.6.7. Differential diagnosis of macula hole and its early stages
Table 5.6.8. Electron microscopic criteria of periretinal membranes
Table 5.6.9. Neovascularizations originating from relative retinal hypoxia
Table 5.6.10. Retinopathy: classification of sickle cell hemoglobinopathy
Table 5.6.11. Intraocular lymphomas
Table 5.6.12. Physical properties of PFD, F6H8, their mixture and silicone oil 1,000
Table 5.6.13. SPR study comparing primary vitrectomy versus scleral buckling
Table 5.6.14. Indications for pars plana vitrectomy in uveitis patients
Table 5.6.15. Therapeutic options in malignant melanomas of choroid
Table 5.6.16. Risk factors for age-related macular degeneration

Chapter 5.7: Optic Nerve and Elschnig Scleral Ring

Table 5.7.1. Pathogenetic classification of optic atrophies
Table 5.7.2. Optic nerve head: tissue components
Table 5.7.3. Course of nerve fiber bundles in the lamina cribrosa of the human optic nerve
Table 5.7.4. Micro and macro discs
Table 5.7.5. Biomorphometric data in eyes with disc anomalies, correlating with disc area and size
Table 5.7.6. Critical details of glaucomatous disc atrophy in chronic glaucomas

Table 5.7.7. Clinical manifestations of giant cell arteritis in the eye and visual system
Table 5.7.8. Central retinal venous occlusion, variants
Table 5.7.9. Tumors of the optic nerve
Table 5.7.10. Clinical signs of the disc for optic nerve head involvement
Table 5.7.11. Differential diagnosis of papilledema (*Stauungspapille*)

Chapter 6.3: Pseudoexfoliation Syndrome: Pathological Manifestations of Relevance to Intraocular Surgery

Table 6.3.1. Diagnosis of early stages, and clinical and surgical complications of pseudoexfoliation syndrome
Table 6.3.2. Clinical stages of pseudoexfoliation syndrome
Table 6.3.3. Aqueous flare values (photon counts/ms) in normal controls, pseudoexfoliation with or without secondary open-angle glaucoma and primary open-angle glaucoma
Table 6.3.4. Differential diagnosis of pseudoexfoliation syndrome
Table 6.3.5. Pathogenetic factors of ocular hypertension and glaucoma development in PEX syndrome
Table 6.3.6. Clinical differential diagnosis of Fuchs' endothelial corneal dystrophy and pseudoexfoliation keratopathy

Subject Index

ACAID, see anterior-chamber-associated immune deviation
Acanthamoeba 116
ACG, see angle closure glaucoma
acquired anterior chamber immune deviation (ACAID) 77, 107
actin 223
Actinomyces canaliculitis 46
acute ocular hypotony 76
adenoid cystic carcinoma of the lacrimal gland 61
adenoma
– of the ciliary pigment epithelium 202
– of the non-pigmented ciliary epithelium 200
age-related macular degeneration (AMD) 9, 90, 247, 315
Alport syndrome 229, 230
Alzheimer's disease 236
amblyopia 231
AMD, see age-related macular degeneration
aminoglycoside 302
amniotic membrane transplantation 75, 125
– conjunctiva 73, 74
angioblast 318
angle closure glaucoma (ACG) 136, 137, 158, 340, 371
– after vitreoretinal surgery 319
angular
– artery 32
– vein 32
aniridia 154, 234
annulus of Zinn 50
anophthalmic socket surgery 65
anterior
– chamber
– – cleavage syndrome 154
– – hypoxia 367
– extraperiostal orbitotomy 65
– transconjunctival orbitotomy 64
– transseptal orbitotomy 64
– uvea
– – malignant melanoma 190, 196
– – tumors 177
anterior-chamber-associated immune deviation (ACAID) 105
antigen-presenting cell (APC) 97
antiglaucomatous iridotomy 3
antithrombin III defect 343
APC, see antigen-presenting cell

aphakia 23, 229, 251
apolipoprotein C 343
aponeurotic blepharoptosis 39
apoptosis photoreceptor death 302
argon-laser 92
– iridoplasty 169
– – non-penetrating coagulation 169
arterial hypertension 353, 378
arteriitis, giant cell 342
arteriosclerosis 378
artificial retinal detachment 82
asteroid hyalosis 308
astigmatism 72, 110
astrocytes 278, 280, 318, 335, 339
atypical cyclodialysis 150, 151
avascular woundhealing, cornea
Avellino dystrophy 111
Axenfeld syndrome 140, 154
axial hyperopia 337
axon 385

bacterial endophthalmitis 19
balloon cells 297
basal cell carcinoma of the eyelid 41
basal lamina 307
basal linear deposits 291
basement membrane deposit 291
Bell's phenomenon 33
Berger's space 95, 221, 226, 255
Bergmeister disc 256
bevacizumab 121
Bick procedure 36
bilateral orbital metastases 60
biocytology 7
biphakia 229
black ball hyphema 145
blepharoplasty 32, 34, 40
blepharoptosis 33, 34, 59, 61
– aponeuritic 39
– mechanical 39
– myogenic 39, 40
– neurogenic 39
blepharotomy 63, 65
Blessig-Ivanoff cyst 272
blindness, bilateral 289
block-excision
– tumors, iris-root and ciliary body see ch. 5.3; 5.4
– epithelial ingrowth in chamber angle see ch. 5.3; 5.4
blood-aqueous barrier 14–17
– ciliary body 16
– iris 15

– retinal barrier: see ch. 2; 4; 5.2; 5.4; 5.5; 5.6; 6.3
blood-ocular barrier breakdown 14–17
bony orbital wall 49
Bowman's layer 69, 76–78, 86, 98, 99, 109, 113, 120, 123, 135
– interruption 85
brachytherapy 312
brow ptosis 34
Bruch's membrane 257, 291, 302, 311
brunescence of the lens 228, 239
buckling 305
bulbar conjunctiva 67
bullous keratopathy 97, 98
– and keratoplasty 113
buphthalmus 24, 140, 337, 339
bursa macularis 256
bypass tube insertion 48

CALT, see conjunctiva-associated lymphatic tissue
canaliculo-dacryocystorhinostomy 47
canthal tendon 37
capsule contraction syndrome 249
capsulectomy, anterior 251
capsulopalpebral fascia 32
capsulorrhexis 93, 219, 226, 228, 251
cataract 234, 244
– age-related 235
– congenital 235
– – visual deprivation 378
– diabetic 351
– etiology 235
– extraction 8, 217
– – extracapsular 170, 245, 351, 373
– – intracapsular 91, 246
– – wound rupture 87
– formation 236, 319
– iatrogenic traumatic 93
– intumescent 79
– nuclear 211
– after vitrectomy 318
– optical coherence tomography 244
– surgery 3, 182, 225
– – complications 246
– – wound healing 246
– ultrasound biomicroscopy 244
cataracta
– calcarea 241
– matura 241
cavernous hemangioma of the orbit 55
cavernous optic nerve atrophy 131

central
- retinal artery obstruction 286
- retinal vein occlusion (CRVO) 136, 284, 287
- serous retinopathy 268
CHED, see congenital hereditary endothelial dystrophy
chemotaxis 4
cholesterol crystals 290
choriocapillaris 268, 311, 340
chorioretinal
- anastomosis 344
- biopsy 311
choristoma 8
choroid/choroidal
- detachment 82, 90, 193
- edema 12
- fibroblasts 269
- hemangioma 313
- hemorrhage 8, 11, 13, 94
- leiomyoma 203
- malignant melanoma 296
- neovascularization 290, 291, 311
- osteoma 298
- stroma 168
- tumors 294, 298, 312
chromorrhexis 299
chronic progressive external ophthalmoplegia (CPEO) 39, 40
cicatricial
- ectropion 36, 37
- entropion 37
ciliary body 176
- block-excision 17, 18
- blood supply 178
- blood-aqueous barrier 16, 178
- - involvement in epithelial ingrowth see ch. 5.3; 5.4
- - involvement in iris-root tumors
- leiomyoma 203, 204
- malignant melanoma 186, 187, 191
- melanocytoma 200
- muscle 12
- neurotrophic factor (CNTF) 316
- surgical anatomy 178
- tumors 186, see block-excisions (5.3; 5.4)
- wound healing 215
cilioschisis 90, 215
CIN, see conjunctival intraepithelial neoplasia
clear lens dislocation 8
cleft
- foveolar
- ora
Cloquet's canal 226, 255
CNTF, see ciliary neurotrophic factor
Coats' disease 268, 285, 290
Cogan's map-dot-fingerprint dystrophy 97, 111
COL2A1 gene 269
collagen 280, 305, 307
collateral retinal detachment 82
congenital
- bilateral blindness 289
- episcleral melanocytosis 72
- hereditary endothelial dystrophy (CHED) 113

conjunctiva/conjunctival
- amniotic membrane transplantation 73
- biopsy 71
- bleb wound dehiscence 150
- bulbar 67
- cystic/cystoid changes 70, 72
- follicular hypertrophy 68
- intraepithelial neoplasia (CIN) 125
- leukoplakia 70
- lymphangenesis 67
- lymphatic endothelial markers 67, 68
- lymphangioma 70
- lymphatics 67
- malignant melanoma 71
- malignant melanosis 73
- melanocytic nevus 72
- peritomy 108
- pigmented findings 72
- pterygium 72
- sarcoidosis 71
- squamous cell carcinoma 125
- stem cells 67
- superior limbal keratitis 74
- tumors 69, 72
conjunctiva-associated lymphatic tissue (CALT) 68
conjunctivitis 68
- iatrogenic 147
- ligneous (lignosa) 74
conjunctivochalasis 74
contusion deformity 183
contusion-cataract 237
conus, scleral 338
corectopia 154
cornea/corneal
- abrasion 125
- acquired pathologies 114
- angiogenesis 120
- angiogenic privilege 106, 99, 102
- antiangiogenic privilege 101, 105
- antigen-presenting cells (APCs) 108
- avascularity 114
- blood vessel 115
- cysts 21
- defects 7
- dendritic cells 108
- dimensions 110
- dystrophies 110-113, 127
- - COGAN 111
- - Macular 112
- - Granular 112
- - Lattice 112, 113
- ectasia 113
- endothelium 76
- - cell loss 247
- - dystrophies 113
- epithelium 67, 92, 97, 107, 108, 127
- - abrasion 114
- - ingrowth 19, 20
- erosions 351
- excision, en bloc
- - tumors iris-root and ciliary body see ch. 5.3; 5.4
- - epithelial ingrowth-chamber angle see ch. 5.3; 5.4

- grafting 3, 115
- guttata 359
- immune privilege 107
- inflammatory process 107
- innervation 108
- iron lines 113, 114
- landmarks 109
- Langerhans cells 98, 108
- LASIK, dry eye 102
- limbus 86, 108
- lymphangiogenesis 102, 103, 120
- neovascularization 114, 115
- - postkeratoplasty 116
- nerves 108
- non-vascularized 90
- opacities 8
- perforating injuries 80, 89
- pseudoexfoliation (PEX) syndrome 371 and from ch. 5.1
- scar 86
- self-sealing wound architecture 14
- stem cells 107
- stroma 67, 100, 108
- surgical anatomy 97
- suturing technique 123
- tear film 102
- transparency 105
- transplantation 108, 120, 126
- - immune reactions 119
- trauma 97, 118
- trephination, non-mechanical with Excimer Laser see ch. 5.1
- vascularized scar 89, 91
- wound healing 118, 125
corneoscleral
- defect 91
- graft after block-excisions 194, 195, 202
- limbus 107
corpora amylacea 339
corticosteroids 375
cotton-wool spot 282, 336
CPEO, see chronic progressive external ophthalmoplegia
CRVO, see central retinal vein occlusion
cryocoagulation 25, 76
cryotherapy 3, 263, 302
cyclitic membrane 81
cyclocoagulation 148
cyclodestruction 213
cyclodialysis 17, 171; see also cyclopexy
- atypical 150, 151
- iatrogenic 193
- traumatic 177, 182, 183, 193
cyclopexy 177, 183; see also cyclodialysis
- direct 184, 185, 193, 215
cystathionine-β-synthetase 233
cystic
- blebs 150, 151
- retinal tuft 261
cystoid
- macular edema 276
- maculopathy 90, 95, 151, 247
- retinal degeneration 272
cytokeratin 125
cytologic smear 74

dacryocystorhinostomy external 46, 47
– endonasal 48
dacryolithiasis 46
DALK, see deep anterior lamellar keratoplasty
daunomycin 302
daunorubicin 315
deep anterior lamellar keratoplasty (DALK) 100, 123
degenerative
– fibrillopathy 355
– retinoschisis 262
dentritic melanocytes 153
dermatochalasis 39, 40
dermoid cyst of the orbit 51, 52, 64
Descemet's
– membrane 100, 113, 123, 174, 371
– – defects 85
– stripping automated lamellar endothelial keratoplasty (DSAEK) 124
dexamethasone 315
diabetes mellitus 237, 351, 378
diabetic
– cataract 351
– cystoid maculopathy 307
– iridopathy 157, 159, 351
– retinopathy 281, 287, 305, 351
diaphanoscopy 178
diathermy 25, 213
– transscleral 76
diffuse large B-cell lymphoma (DLBCL) 298
diffuse malignant melanoma
– iris see ch. 5.3; 5.4; 5.6
– uvea see ch. 5.3; 5.4
– block excision-contraindication see ch. 5.3; 5.4; 5.6
dilatator pupillae 153
diplopia 303
disc, optic – at risk 337
– drusen 337
disciforme keratitis 116
dislocation of the clear lens 8
distichiasis 31, 39
DLBCL, see diffuse large B-cell lymphoma
dot hemorrhage 283
drusen retinal 291
drusen of the optic disc 338
drusinosis retinal 343
dry eye 68, 74, 75, 102, 116
DSAEK, see Descemet's stripping automated lamellar endothelial keratoplasty
dystrophy of corneal endothelium 113

Eales disease 281, 285, 289
ectopia lentis 232
ectropion 34, 46
– cicatricial 36, 37
– involutional 36
– paralytical 36, 37
effusion, aveal see ch. 2; 4; 5.1; 5.5
Egger's line 226
elastic microfibrils 355

electroretinography (ERG) 300
Elliot's principle 145
ELM, see external limiting membrane
Elschnig's
– pearls 248, 249
– scleral ring 35, 335, 338, 340
– spur 26, 346
embryotoxon 140
EMZL, see extranodal marginal zone B-cell lymphoma
endonasal dacryocystorhinostomy 48
endophthalmitis 14, 19, 149, 247
– hemogranulomatosa 24, 315
– phacoanaphylactica 5, 244, 245
– postoperative 76, 252
– purulent 18
endoresection 312
endothelial cells 101
enucleation 66
entropion 34, 37
– cicatricial, of the lower lid 37
– involutional, of the lower lid 37
– of the upper lid 38
epiphora 46
epiretinal membrane 279
episclera/episcleral
– melanocytosis 72
– pigmented findings 72
epithelial
– hemidesmosomes 125
– ingrowth: see block-excision
– melanosis 72
epitheloid cells 297
equatorial sclera 86
ERG, see electroretinography
Erlangen sketch 77
ethmoidal
– nerve 50
– vessel 50
evisceration 66
excavation 131
excimer laser trephination cornea 126
exenteration of the orbit 66
exfoliation syndrome: see pseudo-exfoliation syndrome (PEX)
exophthalmometry 33
expulsive choroidal hemorrhage 17, 18
exsiccosis 145
exsudative retinal detachment 82
external limiting membrane (ELM) 278
extracapsular cataract extraction 351, 373
extranodal marginal zone B-cell lymphoma (EMZL) 298
extraocular, see also intraocular surgery
– muscle 50
– – surgery 65
– solid tumor
– – choroidal metastases 297
exudative retinal detachment 266, 268
eye
– blunt trauma 183
– high myopic 94

– normal function 7
– size 94
– transcorneal access 76
eyelid
– basal cell carcinoma 41
– cicatricial entropion 37
– disorders of position and movement 33
– extraocular surgery 11
– fat pads 32
– full-thickness defect 44
– involutional entropion 37
– laxity 33, 34
– lower retractor 32
– Merkel cell carcinoma 43
– nodular tumefaction 60
– sebaceous gland carcinoma 40, 42
– skin 30
– squamous cell carcinoma 42
– surgery 65
– surgical anatomy 30
– tumors 39, 40
– upper retractor 31
– veins 32
eye-wall sclera, mechanical loci minores resistentiae 86

facial nerve 32
factor V Leyden defect 343
familial exudative vitreoretinopathy (FEVR) 268, 269, 290
FasL 259
Fenestration of the oveal sheath 342
FGF, see fibroblast growth factor
fibrillin 225
– fibrillin-1 gene 232
fibrillogenesis, fibrillopathy 355
fibrin 74, 109
fibroblast 285
– growth factor (FGF) 316
fibrocytes 317
fibronectin 306
fibrosis 248
fibrous
– astrocytes 278
– pseudo-metaplasia 239
fish-hook technique 91
fistula 17
FLA, see fluorescein angiography
flame hemorrhage 283
flap tear 262
Fleischer ring 113
Flexner-Wintersteiner rosettes 299, 313
floppy eyelid syndrome 34. 35
fluorescein angiography (FLA) 343
5-fluorouracil 147, 150, 302
follicular hypertrophy of the conjunctiva 68
foveola
– cleft 256
– slit 8
Fuchs'
– adenoma 186
– corneal dystrophy 113
– dystrophy 92, 97, 98, 374, 101, 372
– heterochromia 178
– roll 92, 93, 134, 143, 153, 169

ganglioglioma   346
gas tamponade   345
gentamicin sulfate   302
GFAP, see glial fibrillary acidic protein
giant
– cell arteritis   342
– retinal tears   268
glaucoma   131
– angle closure glaucoma (ACG)   136
– – after vitreoretinal surgery   319
– filtrating surgery   146
– hemolytic   146
– juxtapapillary damage   340
– laser application   143
– malignant   371
– melanolytic   145
– neovascular   289, 299, 371
– open angle glaucoma (OAG)   138
– phacolytic   138, 244
– primary open angle glaucoma (POAG)   138
– secondary open angle glaucoma (SOAG)   138
– siliconophagic   145, 146
– wound healing   149
glaucomatous optic disc   339, 340
glial
– cell   285
– fibrillary acidic protein (GFAP)   278, 318
glioma   4, 346
gliosis   267
– cellophane-type   279
– pucker-type   279
goblet cells   68, 74
gonioscopy   359
– landmarks   131
goniotomy   140, 145
– failure   150
– mechanical   144
graft-host-cornea wound   87
granulocytes   282
granulomatous cell reactions along Descemet's membrane   117–118
Graves' orbitopathy   62, 64
– surgical treatment   65
gulp phenomenon   14

halo glaucomatosus   340
hamartoma   8
Handmann's anomaly   337
hard drusen, retina   291
Hassal-Henle warts   101
Healon   204
heliostat   91
hemangioblast   317
hemangiogenesis   104
hemangioma, cavernous, of the orbit   55
hemangioma, intraosseous, of the orbit   56–57
hemangiopericytoma of the orbit   51, 57
hematocornea   114
hemiphakia   234
hemoglobinopathy   287, 305
hemorrhage   21
– choroidal   94

– intraocular   92
– intraoperative   215
– iris vessel   173
– spontaneous intrastromal   367
– subarachnoidal   346
– subhyaloidal   308
– vitreal   23
– vitreous   308, 309
hemosiderin   294
Henle
– fibers   257
– layer   258
heparin   302
hereditary
– progressive arthro-ophthalmopathy   269
– X-linked retinoschisis   269
herpetic keratitis   116–118
– herpetic non-necrotizing disciform keratitis with endotheliitis   116–118
– herpetic necrotizing stromal keratitis   116–118
– herpetic epithelial keratitis (dendritic and/or geographic)   116–118
herpetic keratouveitis   92
heterochromia iridium   162
high myopia   24, 269, 339
Hodgkin's disease   57
Holbach's rule   117
Homer-Wright rosettes   299
homocystinuria   193, 232
Horner's muscle   31
horseshoe tear   8, 263, 267
Horton's disease   342, 343
Hruby-Irvine-Gass syndrome   95
hyalocapsular ligament, see also Wieger's ligament   219, 226
hyalocytes   317
hydrops   113
hyperhomocysteinemia   355
hyperlysinemia   229
hypoxia, ischemia   281
hypoxia-inducible factor (HF-1a)   282

iatrogenic
– conjunctivitis   147, 150
– mydriasis   220
– traumatic cataract   93
ICG, see indocyanine green
IFIS, see intrafloppy iris syndrome
IGF-I, see insulin-like growth factor-I
ILM, see inner limiting membrane
immune reflex arc   115
impression cataract   210
indocyanine green (ICG)   278, 299
inferior
– oblique muscle   50
– orbital fissure   50
infraorbital nerve   33
infrared femtolaser   148
infusion fluid   302
inner limiting membrane (ILM)   257
– PAS-positive   305
– peeling   279
– removal   306
insulin-like growth factor-I (IGF-I)   316

interleukin-1 (IL-1)   126
intracranial hypertension   346
intraoperative floppy iris syndrome (IFIS)   22, 153, 171, 247
intraocular
– hemorrhage   92
– infection   378
– – hepatitis B/C   378
– – HIV   378
– lens implant (IOL)   225
– lymphoma   300
– microsurgery   11
– – variants   90
– neovascularization   9
– pressure (IOP)   126, 131, 147, 369
– surgery
– – wound healing   76
– trauma
– – wound healing   76
intraoperative hemorrhage   215
intraosseous cavernous hemangioma of the orbit   57
intravitreal dye   299
intumescent cataract   79
involutional
– ectropion   36
– entropion   37
IOL, see intraocular lens implant
IOP, see intraocular pressure
iridectomy   3, 161
– laser
– mechanical   170
– – peripheral   143
iridodoalysis   160
– closure   171
iridopathy
– diabetic   157, 159, 351
– of PEX syndrome   158
iridotomy   3, 152
– mechanical   170
– – peripheral   143
iris   152
– anterior border layer   153
– blood-aqueous barrier   15, 154
– blunt trauma   159
– collarette   91
– cysts   163, 206
– hook   374
– intraoperative floppy iris syndrome (IFIS)   154
– malignant melanoma   163, 166, 18, 191
– melanocytic
– – lesions   161
– – nevus   199
– microanatomy   93, 152
– microsurgical procedures   160
– multiple nodules   163
– necrosis   159
– neovascularization   289
– nevus   153
– pigment epithelium   156, 359
– plateau syndrome   136, 158, 169
– primary rhabdomyosarcoma   165, 192
– prolaps   168
– pseudoexfoliation syndrome   364, see also PEX

- root 169, 171, 172, 187
- – involvement in epithelial ingrowth   see 5.3; 5.4
- – rhabdomyosarcoma 192
- – tumors and block-excision   see 5.3; 5.4
- sectorial ischemic necrosis 159
- sphincterotomy 374
- stroma 154, 171
- – circumscribed defects 172
- – crypts 367
- surgical anatomy 153
- suture 172
- synechia 14
- tumors 161, 162, 171
- vessel 173
- – hemorrhage 173
- wound healing 164
iris-lens diaphragm 13, 94, 360
ischemia 281, 310
- damage to endothelial cells 282

jaw winking phenomenon 33
Jünemann line 114
juvenile
- retinoschisis 258
- rheumatoid arthritis 246
- uveitis 246

keratectomy 3, 108
- photorefractive (PRK) 98
keratin 107, 111, 125
keratitis 115, 116
- herpetic 116–118
- immune reaction 119–121
- mycotic 87
- necrotizing 87, 117
- – stromal 116
- neurotrophic 117
- superior limbal 74
keratoconjunctivitis, vernal 116
keratoconus 101, 113
- acute 113
keratocyte 126
keratoepithelin gene 110
keratoglobus 113
keratokonus, avascular wound healing 119
keratopathy 63
- bullous 92, 97, 98
- lipid 115
- neurotrophic 116
- pseudoexfoliation syndrome (PEX) 92
keratoplasty 38, 79, 100, 126
- DSAEK 123–124
- Excimer laser 121–123
- lamellar 121, 123–125
- low risk 115, 126
- penetrating 90, 105, 110, 113, 121, 125
- – reinnervation 126
- perforating 117, 174, 87
keratotorus 113
keratouveitis, herpetic 92
Kranenburg's syndrome 337, 344
krypton laser 92

lacrimal
- artery 32
- drainage system 45
- – surgical anatomy 45
- gland 50
- – adenoid cystic carcinoma 61
- – biopsy 65
- – pleomorphic adenoma 62
- nerve 33
- sac 45
- – oncocytoma 47
- – tumors 46
- surgery 47
lamellar keratoplasty 121, 123
lamina
- cribrosa 86
- elastica interna 342
- papyracea 49
laminin 306, 307
landmarks
- for gonioscopy 131
- for surgical corneal limbus 135
Langerhans-cell histiocytosis of the orbit 54
laser
- in situ keratomileusis (LASIK) 102, 116, 123, 126
- iridotomy 92, 93, 143, 159, 173, 174
- photocoagulation 302
- trabeculoplasty 3, 144
- trephination in PKP   see ch. 5.1
- tyndallometry 119, 166, 244, 347
LASIK, see laser in situ keratomileusis
- complications 127
- Reinervation cornea after surgery 127
lateral
- orbitotomy 65
- tarsal strip procedure 36
lattice
- degeneration 260, 261
- dystrophy 111
- – type II (Meretoja form) 112
lax eyelid syndrome 34
Leber's hemorrhagic lymphangiectasia 70
Lee syndrome 92
leiomyoma
- of the choroid 203
- of the ciliary body 203, 204
leitstructuren
- horizontal
- vertical
lens 217
- aging changes 226
- anatomy 217
- brunescence 228
- capsule 93, 219, 221, 227, 243, 354
- – aging changes 227
- – posterior 94
- – true exfoliation 243
- coloboma-like defect 229, 232
- dislocations 232
- – isolated 232
- duplication 229
- epithelium 220, 222, 223, 239
- – aging changes 227
- equator 92

- fibers 223, 224, 241
- – aging changes 227
- intraocular implant (IOL) 225
- metabolism 300
- microsurgery 219
- opacities 8, 360
- proteins 241
- pseudophacic implants 220
- subluxation 151, 360
- surgical anatomy 220
- suspensory ligament 225
- traumatic luxation 234
- zonules
- – aging changes 227
lens-induced uveitis 232
lens-iris diaphragm 219, 371
lentectomy 309
lenticonus 230
lenticular opacification 234
lentiglobus 230
leukokoria 299
leukoplakia of the conjunctiva 70
levator aponeurosis 31, 49, 65
lid, see eyelid
ligneous conjunctivitis 74
limbus/limbal 107, 135
- corneae 86
- corneoscleral 107
- definition 109
- lymphatic vessel 101
- macrophage 101
- perforation 81
- stem cells (SCs) 107
- – transplantation 109, 116, 125
- surgical anatomy 97
- vascular arcade 101
- wound 84
LIPCOF sign 74
lipid keratopathy 114
lipofuscin 314, 340   see also ch. 4; 5.1
- and other ocular pigments
- cornea 114–115
Lisch's dystrophy 110, 111
Lockwood's suspensory ligament 32
long anterior zonule syndrome 228
lymphangiogenesis 67, 103, 104, 114
lymphangioma
- of the conjunctiva 67, 70
- of the orbit 55
lymphatic endothelial marker 67, 68
lymphatic vessel 115
lymphoma 309

macrophthalmus 337
macular
- corneal dystrophy (MCD) 112
- edema 280, 309, 319
- hole 273, 276, 278
- – impending 280
- – traumatic 279
- pucker 276, 281
- retinoschisis 344
- star 193
- translocation 311
maculopathy
- cystoid 90, 95, 151, 247
- – diabetic 307

malignant
- melanocytes 188
- melanoma of the uvea 82
- melanosis of the conjunctiva 73
Marchesani's syndrome 233
Marcus-Gunn pupillary sign 343
Marfan's syndrome 225, 232
marginal-zone B-cell lymphoma of the orbit 59
Martegiani's ring 93, 255
masquerade syndrome 298
matrix metalloproteinase (MMP) 35, 357
McCannel technique 159
MCD, see macular corneal dystrophy
mechanical
- goniotomy 144
- iridectomy 170
- iridotomy 170
- mydriasis 171
- peripheral iridotomy/iridectomy 143
medial canthal swelling 46
Meesmann's dystrophy 111
Meibomian gland 31, 67
melanin 134, 155, see also ocular pigments
- dispersion syndrome 155, 16
- granule 316
- - dispersion 366
- phagocytosis 351
melanocytes 191, 294
- dentritic 153
- malignant 188
- uveal 156
melanocytic
- freckles 161
- nevus 161
- - conjunctiva 72
melanocytoma of the optic disc 345
melanophages 156
melanosis
- epithelial 72
- primary, acquired 73
melanosomes 316
mental retardation 378
Merkel cell carcinoma of the eyelid 43
metamorphopsia 307
Meyer-Schwickerath, G 4
microaneurysm 284
microcornea 84, 229
microfibrillopathy 355
microfibrils 225
microphthalmos 94, 229, 230
microspherophakia 229
microsurgery, intraocular 11, 90
middle limiting membrane (MLM) 257
mini-disc 337
minimal eye 95
mini-PEX 359
mitomycin C 147, 150
Mittendorf dot/spot 221, 256
MLM, see middle limiting membrane
Moh's surgery 43
morbus Wilson 244
Morgagnian cataract 241
morning glory syndrome 337

mouches volantes 266
mucopolysaccharide, acid 74, 341
Mucosa-transplantation 75; see ch. 3.4; 5.1
- autologons see ch. 3.4; 5.1
- nasal see ch. 3.4; 5.1
Müller cells 93, 263, 272, 278, 307
- gliosis 317
- insufficiency 317
Müller's muscle 32, 34, 65
multicoria 154
multiple myeloma, orbital involvement 58
multiple sclerosis 289
Munchhausen syndrome 378
myasthenia gravis 33
mycotic
- endophthalmitis 19
- keratitis 87
mydriasis 373
- iatrogenic 220
- mechanical 171
myofibroblasts 280
myogenic blepharoptosis 39, 40
myopia 337
myotonic dystrophy 237, 378

nanomedicine 7
nanophthalmus 84, 94
nasal mucosa transplantation 75
nasociliary nerve 33
nasolacrimal duct 50
- obstruction 46
Nd:YAG laser capsulotomy 222
necrotizing keratitis 8, 82, 87, 116, 117
neovascular glaucoma 289
neovascularization
- intraocular 9
- subretinal 9
nerve fiber course 336
nerve fiber polarimetry 339
nerve growth factor (NGF) 116
neurilemmoma of the orbit 58
neurofibromatosis 338
neurotrophic
- keratitis 117
- keratopathy 116
NGF, see nerve growth factor
nidogen 307
nodular
- fasciitis 54
- tumefaction of the eyelids 60
non-arteriitic apoplexy of the disc 337
non-Hodgkin's
- B-cell lymphoma of the orbit 59
- lymphoma, oculocerebral 295
non-proliferative diabetic retinopathy 319
Norrie's disease 285, 289, 290
- gene mutations 290
nuclear cataract 211
- after vitrectomy 318
nystagmus 229

OAG, see open angle glaucoma
occlusio pupillae 79

OCT, see optical coherence tomography
ocular
- histoplasmosis choroiditis syndrome 314
- hypertension 215
- hypotony 7, 12, 13, 17, 90, 91, 149, 151, 183, 193, 204, 215, 268
- - acute 76
- pemphigoid 37
oculocerebral syndrome of Lowe 230
oculoglandular Parinaud conjunctivitis 69
oligodendrocytes 335, 340
OLM, see outer limiting membrane
oncocytoma of the lacrimal sac 47
open angle glaucoma (OAG) 72, 138, 354
- congenital 140
- PEX-associated 374
- phacolytic 243
open trephine 208
operculum 278
ophthalmic
- artery 32
- microsurgery
- - historical overview 2
- - wound healing, vascular and avascular 1
- pathology 1
ophthalmoscopy 3, 335
optic
- atrophy 335, 336
- chiasm 347
- disc
- - swelling 346
- glioma 346
- nerve 335
- - anatomy 335
- - congenital pits 344
- - fenestration of the dural sheath 347
- - lamina cribrosa 337
- - tumor 345
- neuropathy, pseudocavernous 347
- pit (PIT) 344
optical coherence tomography (OCT) 91, 148, 269
opticotomy 343
ora
- serrata 256
- slit 8
orbicularis muscle 30
orbit/orbital
- bilateral metastases 60
- bony walls 49
- capillary hemangioma 51
- cavernous hemangioma 55
- decompression 65
- dermoid cysts 50, 52, 64
- exenteration 66
- fat prolaps 39
- hemangiopericytoma 57
- implants 65
- - enucleation 65
- inferior fissure 50
- intraosseous cavernous hemangioma 57
- Langerhans-cell histiocytosis 54

- lymphangioma 55
- marginal-zone B-cell lymphoma 59
- neurilemmoma (schwannoma) 58
- periocular xanthogranuloma 60
- rhabdomyosarcoma 51, 53
- solitary fibrous tumor 57
- superior fissure 50
- surgical anatomy 49
- tumors 50
- – excisional biopsy 62
- – incisional biopsy 62
- – surgery 64
orbitopathy, thyroid-associated 62
orbitotomy 57
- anterior
- – extraperiostal 65
- – transconjunctival 64
- – transseptal 64
- lateral 65
outer limiting membrane (OLM) 257

painful blind eye 65
palisades of Vogt 97, 99, 107, 110
panretinal photocoagulation 308, 309
papilledema 11, 193
papillophlebitis 343
paracentesis effect 14, 91; also ch. 5.2; 5.5; 5.6; see blood-ocular barriers: aqueous and retinal
paralytic ectropion 36, 37
pars
- plana 225
- – cyst 83, 90, 178, 256
- – transscleral approach 90
- – vitrectomy 3, 91, 95, 193, 247, 301, 305, 308, 309, 343
- plicata 92, 164, 176
PAS-positive
- inner limiting membrane 305
- rhabdomyoblast 165
paternoster phenomenon 153
PCNSL, see primary central nervous system lymphoma
PCO, see posterior capsule opacification
PDFG, see platelet-derived growth factor
penetrating keratoplasty 26, 90, 105, 110, 113, 121, 125
- reinnervation 126
perfluorocarbon liquid 301
perforating keratoplasty 87, 117, 174
pericytes dropout 284
periocular xanthogranuloma of the orbit 60
periorbita 50
peripheral
- microcystoid degeneration 262
- retinal hole 263
peripupillary iris pigment epithelium 359
peritomy, conjunctival 108
perlecan 307
persistent hyperplastic primary vitreous (PHPV) 230, 231
Peters' anomaly 140, 141, 154, 171
Petit's canal 255
PEX, see pseudoexfoliation
PEX syndrome 219

phacodonesis 8, 92, 360, 374
phacoemulsification 3, 18, 91, 147, 217, 245, 251
phacogenic uveitis 244, 245
phacolytic glaucoma 244
phakomatosis 5, 338
photocoagulation 313
- panretinal 309
photoreceptor
- outer segment (POS) 316
- pigment epithelial interface 258, 266
photorefractive keratectomy (PRK) 3, 98
phototoxic damage 93
PHPV, see persistent hyperplastic primary vitreous
phthisis bulbi 305
physiological pupillary resistance 92
pigmented ciliary cyst 83
pilocarpine 154
pilocytic astrocytoma 346
PIOL, see primary intraocular lymphoma
platelet-derived growth factor (PDFG) 316, 318
pleomorphic adenoma of the lacrimal gland 62
PMMA, see polymethylmethacrylate
POAG, see primary open angle glaucoma
polygeny 110
polymethylmethacrylate (PMMA) 3, 216
polyneuropathy 112
polyphenotypia 110
POS, see photoreceptor outer segment
post-detachment pucker 280
posterior
- capsule opacification (PCO) 247
- – fibrosis-type 248
- – pearl-type 249
- – prevention 251
- – treatment 251
- ciliary artery occlusion 286
- synechiae 171
- vitreous detachment (PVD) 278
postkeratoplasty neovascularization 116, 121, 123, 126
postoperative endophthalmitis 76; also ch. 2; 4; 5.1; 5.2; 5.5; 5.6
preretinal vascularization 9
presbyopia 182, 227, 245
primary
- acquired melanosis 73
- central nervous system lymphoma (PCNSL) 298
- intraocular lymphoma (PIOL) 298
- open angle glaucoma (POAG) 138, 144, 368
PRK, see photorefractive keratectomy, -Haze after 100
progressive endophthalmitis 150
proliferative vitreoretinopathy (PVR) 94, 314, 305
proptosis 58, 59
- differential diagnosis 62
pseudo-accommodation 182, 252

pseudoadenomatous hyperplasia 186
pseudocavernous optic neuropathy 347
pseudoexfoliation (PEX)
- endotrabecular material 368
- fiber formation 357
- fibrils 362
- glaucoma 368
- hydropathy 360
- iridopathy 159, 178
- – aqueous flare 359
- – laser-tyndallometry 359
- keratopathy 92, 113, 371, 372, 373
- syndrome 8, 92, 94, 101, 138, 156, 171, 193, 220, 225, 233, 237, 243, 246, 351, 354
- – asymmetry of involvement 359
- – corneal involvement 371
- – genetic: LoxL1 357
- – glaucome 371
- – iris involvement 364, 365
- – masked 359
- – pathobiology 355
- – pathogenetic concept 355
- – surgical pathology 360
- – trabecular meshwork 368
pseudoglaucomatous
- macroexcavation 337
- optic atrophy 342
pseudoglioma 267, 289
pseudohypopyon 299
pseudometaplastic epithelial cells 240
pseudonormal mini-cups 337
pseudo-operculum 278
pseudophakia 247, 251, 304
pseudophakic accomodation 182, 252 ff.
pseudophakos 216, 217, 252
pseudo-rosettes 299
pseudotumor cerebri (PTC) 347
pseudouveitis 367
PTC, see pseudotumor cerebri
pterygium of the conjunctiva 72
pupillary block 17, 18
purulent
- endophthalmitis 18
- panophthalmitis 19
PVR, see proliferative vitreoretinopathy

Quickert procedure 37

radial optic neurotomy (RONT) 343
radiation
- opticoneuropathy (RONP) 347
- retinopathy 289
Radius-Maumenee syndrome 138, 139, 146
ragged red fiber 34
RAM, see relative anterior microphthalmus
reactive polyclonal lymphofollicular hyperplasia of the orbit 60
Reis-Bückler's dystrophy 111
relative anterior microphthalmus (RAM) 94, 139
relaxing retinotomy 315
reticular retinoschisis 272

retina/retinal
- damage 301
- defect 8
- detachment 266, 267
- dialysis 268
- dystrophy 338
- ganglion cells (RGC) 272
- granulomatous vasculitis 295
- horizontal barriers (Leitstrukturen) 257
- hypoxia 310
- inner vasculature 318
- internal tamponade 300
- neovascular disease 281
- neovascularization 281
- nerve fibers (RNF) 335, 336
- occlusive disease 310
- oxygen response (ROR) 310
- periphlebitis 10
- perivasculitis 378
- photocoagulation 310
- photoreceptor layer 302
- pigment epithelium (RPE) 8, 83, 92, 93, 256
- - cells 257, 280, 316
- - scar 314
- sarcoidosis 295
- tumors 294, 312
- vasculitis 295, 309
retinoblastoma 5, 296, 298, 299, 312, 313
- systemic chemotherapy 313
- trilateral 313
retinopathia diabetica
- proliferans 9, 21–23
- simplex 351
retinopathy 276
- central serous 268
- diabetic 281, 287, 305, 351
- of prematurity (ROP) 285, 287, 288, 305, 310
- vasoproliferative 305
retinopexy 215
retinoschisis protein 272
retinoschisis 270, 345
- degenerative 262
- juvenile 258
- reticular 272
- typical 272
- X-linked 269, 272
retrocorneal membrane 91, 123
retrolental fibroplasia 287
reversible hypotony syndrome 277
RGC, see retinal ganglion cells
rhabdomyosarcoma of the orbit 51, 53
rhegmatogenous retinal detachment 260, 261, 266
rheumatoid arthritis, juvenile 246
rhinostomy 48
Rho-kinase pathway 317
Rieger's anomaly 140, 154
rim neuroretinal 339
ring melanoma 188, 189
RNF, see retinal nerve fibers
robotic surgery 7
RONP, see radiation opticoneuropathy
RONT, see radial optic neuropathy

ROP, see retinopathy of prematurity
ROR, see retinal oxygen response
RPE, see retinal pigment epithelium
rubeosis iridis 9, 21, 156, 213, 289, 306, 310, 371

Sampaolesi's line 370
sarcoidosis of the conjunctiva 71
scar war 150
schisis detachment 270
Schlemm's canal 86, 92, 131, 132, 134, 135, 148, 150, 368, 370
Schlichting's dystrophy 113
Schnabel's cavernous optic neuropathy and disc atrophy 301, 341, 342, 347
Schnyder's crystalline dystrophy 111, 113
Schwalbe's line 86, 92, 109, 131, 134–136, 370
schwannoma of the orbit 58
sclera/scleral
- buckling 303, 318
- conus 338
- ectasia 312
- equatorial 86
- indentation 303
- juxtapapillary 86
- spur 86, 135
- staphyloma 24
- wall defects 7
scleritis 24
sclerotomy overlying the pars plana 91
scotoma in the white-white perimetry 336, 337
seclusio pupillae 79
secondary
- melanin granule dispersion syndrome 351
- open angle glaucoma (SOAG) 138, 183
sector iridectomy 171
sectorial teleangiectasia 290
severe ocular trauma 315
sickle cell disease 281, 287
silicone
- oil 300, 301, 319, 347
- tubing 47
sinosotomy 139, 146
SINS, see surgically induced necrotizing scleritis
SOAG, see secondary open angle glaucoma
Soemmerring's ring 249, 250
soft drusen 291
sorbitol pathway 239
spherolith 241
sphincter pupillae muscle 153
spindle cells 297
spiral of Tillaux 50
spontaneous intrastromal hemorrhage 367
squamous cell carcinoma
- of the conjunctiva 125
- of the eyelid 42
staphyloma 337
stem cell transplantation, limbus 125
Stickler syndrome 269
strabism 346

stromal
- dystrophy 111
- edema 114
- keratocytes 125
subarachnoidal hemorrhage 346
subconjunctival scarring 75
subhyaloidal hemorrhage 308
subretinal neovascularization 9
sulfur hexafluoride 300, 301
superficial temporal artery 32
superior
- limbal keratitis 74
- orbital fissure 50
supraorbital neurovascular bundle 50
supratrochlear nerve 33
surgical corneal limbus landmarks 135
surgically induced necrotizing scleritis (SINS) 95, 247
symblepharon 70, 75
sympathetic uveitis system 32
synchisis
- nivea 308
- scintillans 308

TAC, see transit amplifying cell
tamsulosin 153
tarsal plate 31
TASS, see toxic anterior segment syndrome
tear
- film 67, 75, 102
- meniscus 46
tectonic corneoscleral graft 164, 215
teletherapy 313
temporal artery 32
- biopsy 342
Tenon's fascia 135
teratoid medulloepithelioma 198
Terson's syndrome 346
TGF-β, see transforming growth factor-β
thermic
- argon laser 92
- trabeculoplasty 150
Thiel-Behnke dystrophy 110
thrombospondin 105, 107
thymidine 107
thyroid
- endocrine orbitopathy 64
- eye disease 62, 63
- - surgical treatment 65
thyroid-associated orbitopathy 62
TIMP, see tissue inhibitor of matrix metalloprotease
tissue inhibitor of matrix metalloprotease (TIMP) 316
tobacco dust 268
toxic
- anterior segment syndrome (TASS) 22, 91, 247
- lens syndrome 252
Toxocara canis 5
toxoplasmosis retinochoroiditis 5, 314
trabeculectomy 145, 146
trabeculoplasty, thermic 150
trabeculotomy 135, 145
- ab externo 140

- mechanical 144
traction detachment 266, 269
transforming growth factor-β (TGF-β) 316
transit amplifying cell (TAC) 107
transpupillary thermotherapy (TTT) 313
transscleral
- coagulation 148
- diathermy 76
- thermic diode laser 144
traumatic ectopia 232
trephination, cornea mechanic- and laser- 121; see ch. 5.1
trichiasis 31, 37
trigeminal nerve 32, 116
trisomy 13 229
trochlea 50
true operculum 278
true pseudophakic accommodation 252
trypan blue 300
trypsin 284
- digest preparation 287
TTT, see transpupillary thermotherapy
tuberculosis 289
tuberous sclerosis 338
tubulin 223
TUNEL staining 302
tunica vaculosa lentis 307

ultrasound biomicroscopy 148
uvea/uveal
- effusion 17, 18, 268
- malignant melanoma 82, 190, 196, 294
- melanocytes 156
- melanoma, transscleral local excision 312
- reactive lymphoid hyperplasia 312
- tumors 177

uveitis 19, 309
- juvenile 246
- lens-induced 232
- phacogenic 244, 245

valve of Rosenmüller 45
vascular
- endothelial growth factor (VEGF) 105, 281, 316, 318
- - expression 310
- pannus 109
VEGF, see vascular endothelial growth factor
venous stasis retinopathy 343
Verhoeff's membrane 14, 16, 316
vernal keratoconjunctivitis 116
verteporphin 311
vimentin 223
vis a tergo 13, 353
vitreal hemorrhage 23
vitrectomy procedure 215, 266, 303, 305, 310, 319
- iatrogenic breaks 303
- loss of accommodation 304
vitreomacular traction syndrome 273, 278
vitreoretinal microsurgery 345
vitreoretinopathy 22, 269, 305
- erosive 269
- familial exudative 269
- proliferative 94, 305
vitreoschisis 256, 279, 280
vitreous
- body, surgical anatomy 255
- cavity 76, 93
- detachment 260
- hemorrhage 308, 309
- hyaloid membrane 306
- opacities, removal 308
- substitutes 300
- tamponade 279

vitritis 295
Vogt lines 113
von Szily's ring 161

Wagner disease 269
Wedl bladder cells 222, 239, 249
Weill-Marchesani syndrome 229
Whitnall's
- ligament 31
- tubercle 31
Wieger's ligament, see also hyalocapsular ligament 93, 94, 219, 221, 226, 255
wound healing
- after intraocular surgery/trauma 76
- avascular 94
- in ophthalmic microsurgery 1
- vascular 94

xenon light 91
xerosis conjunctivae 70
X-linked retinoschisis (XLRS) 272
XLRS, see X-linked retnioschisis

YAG laser, see also Nd:YAG laser 3, 92, 222
- capsulotomy 8
- iridotomy 143, 169
Yanoff syndrome 163

Zimmermann, Lorenz E 4
Zinn-Haller's circle 343
zonular fiber 217, 225
zonules 374
- of Zinn 225
zygomaticofacial
- artery 49
- nerve 49
zygomatico-frontal suture 50